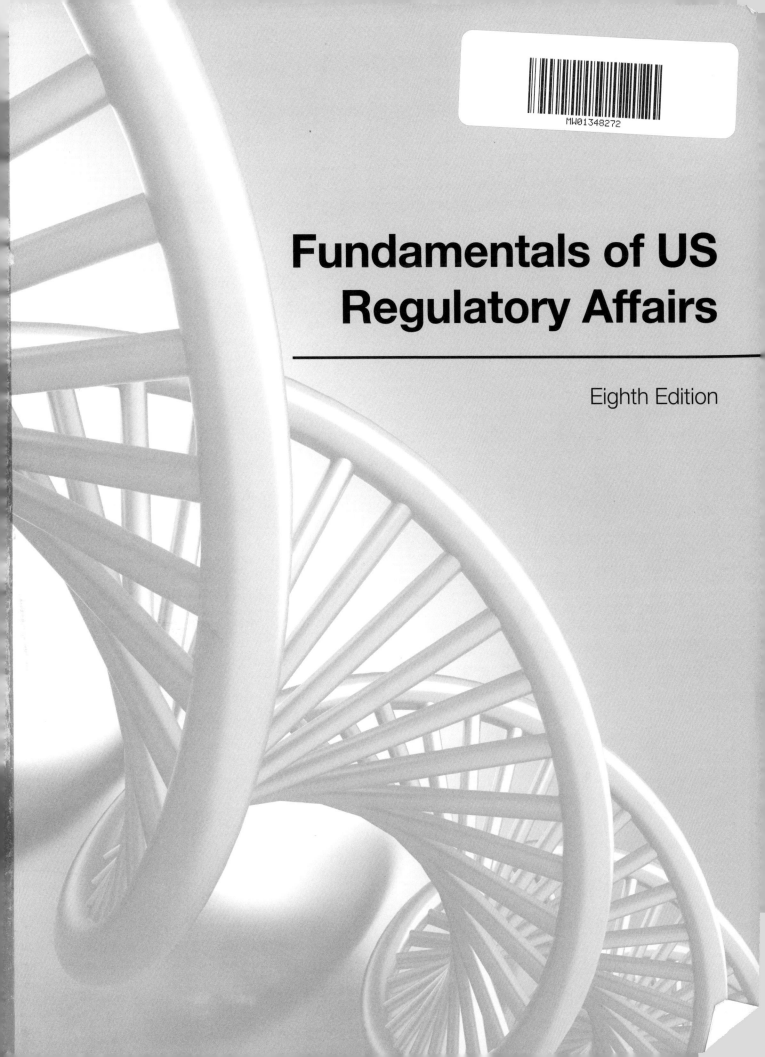

Fundamentals of US Regulatory Affairs

Eighth Edition

This book is dedicated to the memory of Clawson (Cal) Bowman, Jr., longtime RAPS member, former RAPS Board Member and a contributing author to this publication.

Copyright © 2013 by the Regulatory Affairs Professionals Society.
All rights reserved.

ISBN: 978-0-9829320-6-3

Every precaution is taken to ensure accuracy of content; however, the publisher cannot accept responsibility for the correctness of the information supplied. At the time of publication, all Internet references (URLs) in this book were valid. These references are subject to change without notice.

RAPS Global Headquarters
5635 Fishers Lane
Suite 550
Rockville, MD 20852
USA

RAPS.org

Foreword

The last two years have seen significant changes to healthcare product regulation in the US, largely stemming from the *Food and Drug Administration Safety and Innovation Act* of 2012 (*FDASIA*). There also are implications for the industry in the implementation of the *Patient Protection and Affordable Care Act*.

FDASIA expanded the powers of the US Food and Drug Administration (FDA), and new regulations from other state and federal agencies have also come into play in the two years since the seventh edition of this book was published.

Fundamentals of US Regulatory Affairs, Eighth Edition, reflects those changes and their impact on regulatory professionals. New chapters have been added that cover: crisis management, health technology assessment, pharmacovigilance, companion diagnostics and medical foods. All information is current through early 2013.

This edition of *US Fundamentals* has been organized into seven sections:
- **Section I:** General Information—topics relating to multiple products types, such as the history of US regulations and regulatory agencies, the role of FDA and other agencies, FDA meetings and communications, crisis management and GxPs
- **Section II:** Drugs—information on prescription, generic and over-the-counter drug product regulations and compliance, patents and pharmacovigilance
- **Section III:** Medical Devices—information on medical device and in vitro regulations and compliance
- **Section IV:** Biologics—biologics submissions, compliance and promotion
- **Section V:** Other Product Classifications—combination products, orphan products, blood and blood products, cell and tissue products, pediatric regulations and more
- **Section VI:** Inspection and Enforcement—FDA inspection and enforcement actions and healthcare fraud and abuse compliance
- **Section VII:** Resources—regulatory information resources

The text is accompanied by a matrix of applicable laws and regulations, a glossary and an index. *Fundamentals of US Regulatory Affairs, Eighth Edition*, is an outstanding reference text for regulatory professionals at all levels—from those new to the field to senior level executives looking for information on an unfamiliar topic. It also is an excellent study tool for those planning to take the US RAC exam.

Pamela A. Jones
Senior Editor

Acknowledgements

The Regulatory Affairs Professionals Society (RAPS) thanks the following individuals, who have shared their knowledge and expertise to advance the regulatory profession by contributing to this publication.

Alix E. Alderman,
Director, Global Product Strategy and Global Regulatory Lead
AbbVie

Patricia Anderson, RAC
VP, Strategic Regulatory Affairs
Optum

Alay Bhayani, MS, RAC
Specialist, Regulatory Affairs
Medtronic

Clawson (Cal) Bowman, JD, CQA, CQM, RAC
President
Bowman FDA Regulatory Consulting Group, LLC

Evelyn D. Cadman
Owner & Principal Consultant
Bioscience Translation & Application

Rafael Cassata, MS, RAC (US, EU)
Deputy Directory, Cellular Therapies
AABB

Melissa Cavuto, MS, MBA, RAC
Associate Director and Group Manager, Regulatory Project Management
AstraZeneca

Ojas Chandorkar
Associate Tech Lead
Stryker Global Technology Center

Min Chen, PhD, RAC
Manager, Regulatory Affairs
Ultragenyx Pharmaceutical Inc.

Joseph C. Fratantoni, MD
Senior Clinical Consultant
Biologics Consulting Group

Klaus Gottlieb, MD, MS, MBA, RAC
Medical Officer
US Food and Drug Administration, Center for Drug Evaluation and Research

Michael R. Hamrell, PhD, RQAP-GCP, RAC, FRAPS
President
MORIAH Consultants

Donna Helms, MBA, RAC
Senior Director, Special Projects
Optum Life Sciences, Strategic Regulatory and Safety

Nigel Andre Sean Hernandez, PhD, MSc, MS, MBA, GCMD, GCIRA, RAC
Chief Regulatory Science Officer
GloboScience Inc.

Hutch Humphreys, MS, RAC
Associate Director, Regulatory Affairs
Therapeutics Inc.

Treena Jackson, MS, CQA, CSSGB, RAC
President
Quality Resource Consulting Inc.

Karen Jaffe, MS, MBA, MRSc, RAC
Manager of Clinical Research and Regulatory Affairs

Jocelyn Jennings, MS, RAC
Senior Manager, Regulatory Affairs
bioMèrieux Inc.

Allison Kennedy, MSc, RAC
Manager, Regulatory Affairs
Cangene Corporation

William H. Kitchens, JD
Partner
Arnall Golden Gregory LLP

Tatiana Leshchinsky, PhD
Mamager, Regulatory Associate
InBios International Inc.

Alan Minsk, JD
Partner & Leader, Food & Drug Practice Team
Arnall Golden Gregory LLP

Brian Miyazaki, RAC
Associate Director, Global Safety
Bristol-Myers Squibb

Linda Pollitz, RAC
Director, Regulatory Affairs, Advertising & Promotion
Alkermes

Maruthi Prasad Palthur, PhD, RAC
Senior Director, Technical Operations & Regulatory Affairs
Indigene Pharmaceuticals Inc.

Giuseppe Randazzo, MS
Regulatory Scientist
US Food and Drug Administration, Center for Drug Evaluation and Research

Matthew Rycyk, MS, RAC
Principal Consultant
DS Regulatory consulting LLC

Srikonda V. Sastry, PhD, RAC
Senior Director, Pharmaceutical Product Development
InterMune

Anthony P. Schiavone, RAC
In-house Counsel

Jessica W. Smith, RAC
Regulatory/Biomedical Consultant
Kali Corporation

Michelle Sotak, MPH, MBA
Associate Director, Product Value Strategy
Optum Life Sciences

Usha Srinivasan, MS, RAC
Principal
TLUS LLC

Michael A. Swit, Esq.
Special Counsel, FDA Law Practice
Duane Morris LLP

Mya Thomae, RAC
Founder and CEO
Myraqa Inc.

Anne Tomalin
Managing Director, Pharmacovigilance and Special Projects
Optum

Laurence M. Wallman, RAC (US, EU, CAN)
Quality Systems & Regulatory Compliance Consultant

Maria Walsh, RN, MS
Associate Director for Regulatory Affairs
US Food and Drug Administration, Center for Drug Evaluation and Research, Office of Drug Evaluation III

Diane R. Whitworth, MLS
Principal Research Consultant
DRW Research & Information Services LLC

Sherry Yanez Gregor, JD, MSc
Vice President
Gregor Library

Linda Yang, PhD, MBA, RAC
President/Regulatory Consultant
KleaGen LLC

Andrew P. Zeltwanger
Director of Regulatory and Quality
Rinovum Women's Health

Jeffrey Zinza, RAC
Regulatory Specialist
Hologic Inc.

Table of Contents

Section I: General Information
Chapter 1   FDA and Related Regulatory Agencies 1
Chapter 2   History of Food, Drug and Cosmetic Laws 11
Chapter 3   Overview of Drug, Biologic and Device Regulatory Pathways 19
Chapter 4   FDA Communications and Meetings 47
Chapter 5   Preparing for Key FDA Meetings and Advisory Committee Meetings 55
Chapter 6   Crisis Management 65
Chapter 7   Health Technology Assessment 71
Chapter 8   Good Laboratory Practice Regulations 79
Chapter 9   Clinical Trials: GCPs, Regulations and Compliance 91
Chapter 10   Current Good Manufacturing Practice and Quality System Design 105

Section II: Drugs
Chapter 11   Prescription Drug Product Submissions 121
Chapter 12   Postapproval Prescription Drug Submissions and Compliance 139
Chapter 13   Generic Drug Submissions 155
Chapter 14   Patents and Exclusivity 179
Chapter 15   Over-the-Counter Drug Products 191
Chapter 16   Prescription Drug Labeling, Advertising and Promotion 199
Chapter 17   Pharmacovigilance and Risk Management 211

Section III: Medical Devices
Chapter 18   Medical Device Submissions 221
Chapter 19   Medical Device Compliance and Postmarketing Activities 237
Chapter 20   Advertising, Promotion and Labeling for Medical Devices and In Vitro Diagnostics 259
Chapter 21   In Vitro Diagnostics Submissions and Compliance 267

Section IV: Biologics
Chapter 22   Biologics Submissions 273
Chapter 23   Biologics Compliance 289
Chapter 24   Biologics Labeling, Advertising and Promotion 299

Section V: Other Product Classifications
Chapter 25   Combination Products 311
Chapter 26   Products for Small Patient Populations 319
Chapter 27   Blood and Blood Products 327
Chapter 28   Human Cell and Tissue Products 335
Chapter 29   Regulations Pertaining to Pediatrics 353
Chapter 30   Dietary Supplements and Homeopathic Products 363
Chapter 31   Cosmetics 383

Chapter 32	Veterinary Products	391
Chapter 33	Food Products	401
Chapter 34	Companion Diagnostics	421
Chapter 35	Medical Foods	427

Section VI: Inspection and Enforcement

| Chapter 36 | FDA Inspection and Enforcement | 435 |
| Chapter 37 | Healthcare Fraud and Abuse Compliance | 445 |

Section VII: Resources

| Chapter 38 | Regulatory Information Resources in Review | 455 |

Appendices

Comparative Matrix of Regulations Across Product Lines	473
Glossary	505
Index	527

Figures

Figure 1-1.	FDA Organizational Chart	3
Figure 3-1.	Decision Tree for Drug and Device Development and Approval for Situations that Require FDA Premarket Review	24
Figure 3-2.	CTD Organization	32
Figure 4-1.	NDA and BLA Submissions	49
Figure 4-2.	PMA Submissions	50
Figure 5-1.	Major Milestone Timeline	58
Figure 5-2.	Sample Project Management Chart	61
Figure 7-1.	An HTA Model	73
Figure 7-2.	Importance of the Relevant Technology for the Patient's Everyday Life (Børlum 2007)	74
Figure 10-1.	Quality System Elements	110
Figure 10-2.	ICH Q10 Pharmaceutical Quality System Model	113
Figure 10-3.	Process Model for Meeting GMP Requirements	120
Figure 11-1.	The Common Technical Document	130
Figure 11-2.	Major Steps in the NDA or BLA Review for Applications Not Under the PDUFA V "Program"	134
Figure 11-3.	New Timeline for NMEs and Original BLAs Under PDUFA V	137
Figure 13-1.	ANDA Backlog	158
Figure 13-2.	Median ANDA Approval Times	159
Figure 13-3.	FDA's ANDA Approval Process	160
Figure 15-1.	Example of an OTC Drug Facts Label	197
Figure 19-1.	Quality System Elements	245
Figure 19-2.	Relationship of Medical Device Records	246
Figure 19-3.	Total Product Lifecycle	253
Figure 28-1.	Form FDA 3356	338
Figure 28-2.	Form FDA 3486	342
Figure 30-1.	Sample Supplement Facts Boxes	368
Figure 37-1.	Fraud Detection Technology	452

Tables

Table 1-1.	CDER versus CBER Product Oversight Responsibilities	6
Table 1-2.	Selected Primary FDA Centers/Offices Involved in Sponsor Interface During the Development and Approval of Drugs, Biologics and Devices	8
Table 2-1	Other Laws, Regulations and Guidelines	16
Table 3-1.	21 CFR Parts Most Relevant to Drug and Device Development	23
Table 3-2.	Key Questions to be Addressed in a Drug Development Program	28
Table 3-3.	IND Safety Reporting Timeframes	34
Table 3-4.	Summary of Device Classification System	41
Table 4-1.	Description of FDA Product Application Meetings and Timing	52
Table 7-1.	Comparison of Health Technology Regulation and Health Technology Assessment Characteristics Health Technology Regulation	72
Table 7-2.	Choice of Type of Economic Analysis (Børlum 2007)	76
Table 7-3.	Cost-effectiveness Decision Matrix	77
Table 8-1.	21 CFR 5	83
Table 9-1.	FDA Regulations and Guidelines for Clinical Studies	95
Table 11-1.	Expedited Drug Development	124
Table 11-2.	Benefits of Breakthrough Designation	129
Table 12-1.	Postapproval CMC Supplements	144
Table 14-1.	180-Day Exclusivity Forfeiture Snapshot	185
Table 14-2.	Differences Between Applications Submitted and Approved Under FD&C Act Section 505	186
Table 15-1.	NDA vs. OTC Drug Monograph	193
Table 15-2.	OTC Monograph Therapeutic Category Subtopics Evaluated as Part of the OTC Review Process	194
Table 16-1.	PLR Format, Associated Regulations and Guidance Documents	204
Table 18-1.	Abbreviated IDE Requirements, per 21 CFR 812.2(b)	225
Table 19-1.	Domestic Establishment Registration and Listing Requirements	241
Table 19-2.	Foreign Establishment Registration and Listing Requirements	242
Table 19-3.	Registration and Listing Timelines	243
Table 22-1.	History of Biologics Regulation	275
Table 22-2.	Key CMC Guidance for Development of Biological Products	282
Table 22-3.	Timetable for BLA Review	285
Table 25-1.	Unique Proposed Postmarket Safety Reporting Provisions for Combination Products	317
Table 28-1.	21 CFR 1271 at a Glance	336
Table 28-2.	Examples of Cell and Tissue-Based Products	337
Table 28-3.	Overview of the Core CGTP Requirements (21 CFR 1271, Subpart D)	340
Table 28-4.	FDA Regulation of Minimally Manipulated Cord Blood Products	350
Table 29-1.	Definition of Pediatric Subpopulations	359
Table 38-1.	Publisher Resources	460
Table 38-2.	Commercial & Government Databases	466
Table 38-3.	Agencies Associated with Healthcare Product Regulation	468

Chapter 1

FDA and Related Regulatory Agencies

Updated by Michael R. Hamrell, PhD, RQAP-GCP, RAC, FRAPS

OBJECTIVES

❑ Introduce the US Food and Drug Administration (FDA) and provide a history of the agency's evolution over more than a century and significant laws that guided FDA's growth

❑ Discuss the structure of FDA and its relationship with other US regulatory agencies

LAWS AND REGULATIONS COVERED IN THIS CHAPTER

❑ Food and Drug Act of 1906

❑ Federal Food, Drug and Cosmetic Act of 1938

❑ Family Smoking Prevention and Tobacco Control Act of 2009

❑ Vaccine Act of 1813

❑ Federal Advisory Committee Act of 1972

❑ Federal Trade Commission Act of 1914

❑ Health Insurance Portability and Accountability Act of 1996

❑ Consumer Product Safety Act of 1972

❑ Occupational Safety and Health Act of 1970

❑ Federal Alcohol Administration Act of 1935

❑ Poultry Products Inspection Act of 1957

❑ Safe Drinking Water Act of 1974

Introduction

The US Food and Drug Administration (FDA) is part of the executive branch of government and falls under the jurisdiction of the US Department of Health and Human Services (DHHS). From its humble beginnings in 1862 as a laboratory that analyzed samples of food, fertilizers and agricultural substances, FDA has evolved over a century and a half, expanding its regulatory responsibility to include drugs, cosmetics and devices. FDA now regulates more than $1 trillion worth of consumer goods, about 25% of US consumer expenditures. This amount includes $466 billion in food sales, $275 billion in drugs, $60 billion in cosmetics and $18 billion in vitamin supplements.[1] Consistent with FDA's evolution, the agency's influence is likely to grow in the future.

FDA's Mission

FDA's current mission statement reads:
   "FDA is responsible for:
- Protecting the public health by assuring that foods are safe, wholesome, sanitary and properly labeled; human and veterinary drugs, and vaccines and other biological products and medical devices intended for human use are safe and effective
- Protecting the public from electronic product radiation
- Assuring cosmetics and dietary supplements are safe and properly labeled
- Regulating tobacco products

- Advancing the public health by helping to speed product innovations
- Helping the public get the accurate science-based information they need to use medicines, devices, and foods to improve their health

FDA's responsibilities extend to the 50 states, the District of Columbia, Puerto Rico, Guam, the Virgin Islands, American Samoa and other US territories and possessions."

FDA's History

During the 19th century, states exercised principal control over domestically produced and distributed foods and drugs, while federal authority was restricted to imported foods and drugs. The *Vaccine Act* of 1813 was one of the first federal laws dealing with consumer protection and therapeutic substances. The Division of Chemistry, which became the Bureau of Chemistry in July 1901, began investigating the adulteration of agricultural commodities as early as 1867. Dr. Harvey W. Wiley, credited as the father of US food and drug law, and who eventually became chief chemist of the US Department of Agriculture, expanded the division's research in this area. He demonstrated his concern about chemical preservatives as adulterants in the highly publicized "poison squad" experiments, in which able-bodied volunteers consumed varying amounts of questionable food additives to determine their impact on health. Wiley also unified a variety of groups behind a federal law to prohibit the adulteration and misbranding of food and drugs, which was rampant (e.g., arsenic in vinegar, sulfuric acid in pickles, woodchips in bread, alum and clay in wheat flour). Foods also were marketed with bold and unsubstantiated claims (e.g., as cures for cancer and the prevention of baldness). Upton Sinclair's description of the meatpacking industry in *The Jungle* was a precipitating force behind both a meat inspection law and a comprehensive food and drug law. On 30 June 1906, President Theodore Roosevelt signed the *Food and Drugs Act*, known simply as the *Wiley Act*.

An incident in 1937 with an untested product containing sulfanilamide, an anti-infective, mixed with a toxic solvent led to the 1938 *Food, Drug, and Cosmetic Act (FD&C Act)*, which gave FDA the authority to oversee food, drugs and cosmetics. The *FD&C Act* has been amended many times since 1938. For details on the more significant amendments, see Chapter 2.

Role of FDA

FDA is part of the Department of Health and Human Services (DHHS) of the US government. DHHS is the US government's principal agency for protecting the health of all Americans and providing essential human services, especially for those who are least able to help themselves. FDA's primary goal is to ensure the safety and effectiveness of human and veterinary drugs, biologics and medical devices, the nation's food supply (in conjunction with the US Department of Agriculture), cosmetics, dietary supplements and products that emit radiation.

Other key DHHS agencies that play an integral part in health and medical research services and interact regularly with FDA include the National Institutes of Health (NIH) and the Centers for Disease Control and Prevention (CDC) and the Center for Medicare and Medicaid Services (CMS).

Structure of FDA

FDA is an agency within DHHS and consists of multiple centers/offices:
- Office of the Commissioner (OC)
- Office of Foods and Veterinary Medicine
- Office of Medical Products and Tobacco
- Office of Operations
- Office of Global Regulatory Operations and Policy

FDA has undergone a tremendous amount of reorganization and realignment in recent years to better align personnel and resources to address the complex issues over which the agency has jurisdiction. More information on FDA's organizational structure may be found at www.fda.gov/AboutFDA/CentersOffices/default.htm and www.fda.gov/AboutFDA/CentersOffices/OrganizationCharts/default.htm.

Office of the Commissioner (OC)

The Office of the Commissioner provides centralized agency-wide direction and management to support effective administration of all programs. It is responsible for the efficient and effective implementation of FDA's mission.

Among the offices reporting directly to OC are the Office of the Chief Counsel, the Office of the Chief Scientist, the Office of Global Regulatory Operations and Policy, the Office of Women's Health, the Office of Minority Health, the Office of the Counselor to the Commissioner, the Office for Legislation, Policy and Planning and External Affairs and the Office of Operations. The current (May 2013) organizational structure of the Office of the Commissioner is depicted in **Figure 1-1**.

For more information on the Office of the Commissioner, visit www.fda.gov/AboutFDA/CentersOffices/OC/default.htm.

Office of the Chief Counsel (OCC)

The Office of the Chief Counsel represents FDA in court proceedings, handling both civil and criminal enforcement cases and defending challenges to the *FD&C Act*. It also provides legal advice and policy guidance for FDA programs. The office drafts or reviews all proposed and final FDA regulations, performs legal research and gives legal opinions on regulatory issues, actions and petitions. OCC also acts as a liaison to the Department of Justice (DOJ) and other federal agencies for programs administered by

Figure 1-1. FDA Organizational Chart

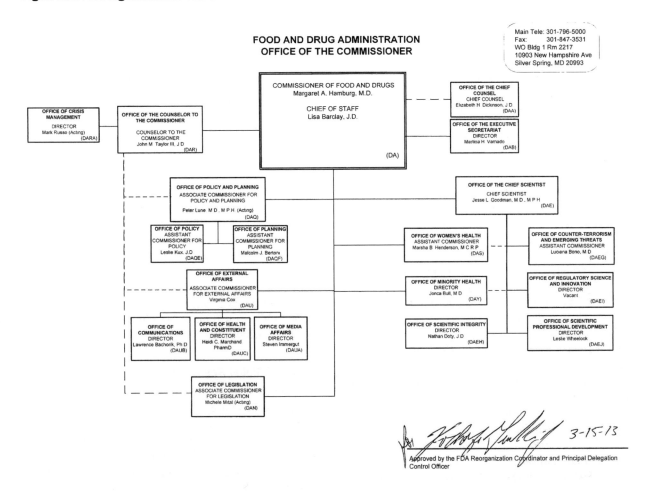

FDA. In addition, FDA attorneys are involved in explaining agency programs to Congress, regulated industry and the public. For more information about the Office of the Chief Counsel, visit www.fda.gov/AboutFDA/CentersOffices/OC/OfficeoftheChiefCounsel/default.htm.

Office of the Chief Scientist
The Office of the Chief Scientist provides strategic leadership, coordination and expertise to support scientific excellence, innovation and capacity. It fosters the development and use of innovative technologies, provides cross-agency scientific coordination and supports the professional development of FDA scientists in all areas through the Commissioner's Fellowship Program, continuing education and scientific interaction with academia. In today's environment, the office supports science and public health activities to effectively anticipate and respond to counterterrorism and emerging deliberate and natural threats (e.g., chemical, biological, radiological and nuclear) to US and global health and security. Offices under the auspices of the Office of the Chief Scientist include:

- Office of Counterterrorism and Emerging Threats
- Office of Regulatory Science and Innovation
- Office of Scientific Integrity
- Office of Scientific Professional Development
- FDA's National Center for Toxicological Research

Office of Counterterrorism and Emerging Threats
The Office of Counterterrorism and Emerging Threats' (OCET) mission is to facilitate the development and availability of safe and effective public health emergency medical countermeasures, establish policies to safeguard medical products from adulteration and prevent disruption of supplies as a result of terrorist activities.

Office of Regulatory Science and Innovation
The Office of Regulatory Science and Innovation provides strategic leadership, coordination, infrastructure and support for excellence and innovation in FDA science that will advance the agency's ability to protect and promote the public health. In addition, this office seeks input from FDA programs, stakeholders and outside advisors, including the

FDA Science Board, to help define, review and meet FDA scientific needs and priorities to support FDA's public health mission.

Office of Critical Path Programs
Included under the Office of Regulatory Science, the Critical Path Initiative (CPI) is FDA's national strategy for transforming the way FDA-regulated products are developed, evaluated and manufactured. The Division of Science Innovation and Critical Path supports CPI efforts across the agency.

Office of Scientific Integrity
Formed in 2009, the Office of Scientific Integrity (OSI) reports to the Chief Scientist and works with the Office of the Commissioner and FDA's other centers to:
- ensure that FDA's policies and procedures concerning scientific integrity at FDA are current and applied across the agency
- review and work to resolve both informal and formal scientific disputes

OSI evaluates scientific differences that are not resolved at center levels and advises the Chief Scientist and other senior FDA leaders on appropriate responses. OSI coordinates FDA's response to and evaluation of allegations of improper deviation from established procedures governing FDA's regulatory mandate.

The FDA Ombudsman
Located within OSI, the FDA Office of the Ombudsman is the agency's focal point for addressing complaints and assisting in resolving disputes between companies or individuals and FDA offices concerning fair and even-handed application of FDA policy and procedures. It serves as a neutral and independent resource for members of FDA-regulated industries when they experience problems with the regulatory process that have not been resolved at the center or district level. It works to resolve externally and internally generated problems for which there are no legal or established means of redress by finding approaches that are acceptable to both the affected party and the agency. In addition, each center has an ombudsman to handle issues within that center.

Office of Scientific Professional Development
The Office of Scientific Professional Development leads and supports FDA efforts to recruit and foster top talent by providing innovative skills development programs to prepare the staff to successfully address the regulatory challenges presented by new areas of science and medicine. FDA has designed a range of dynamic and innovative programs and activities, such as the Commissioner's Fellowship Program, collaborations with scientific institutions and academia, and scientific achievement awards.

National Center for Toxicological Research (NCTR)
In partnership with other FDA entities, government agencies, industry and academia, NCTR conducts research and provides advice and training necessary for science-based decision making and sound regulatory policy development. For example, in the areas of counterterrorism and food defense, NCTR scientists collaborate with scientists from other FDA centers and several federal and state agencies to evaluate the disease-causing potential of food-borne pathogens and to develop methods for rapid detection of bacterial pathogens. NCTR researchers, in collaboration with the National Institute of Child Health and Human Development (NICHD), initiated an animal study of a drug used to treat Attention Deficit Disorder in children to assess whether this drug causes genetic alterations in children. The only FDA center not located in the Washington, DC metropolitan area, NCTR is in Jefferson, AR. More information about NCTR is available at www.fda.gov/AboutFDA/CentersOffices/OC/OfficeofScientificandMedicalPrograms/NCTR/ucm2006206.htm.

Office of Global Regulatory Operations and Policy
The Office of Global Regulatory Operations and Policy comprises the Office of Regulatory Affairs and the Office of International Programs. The office provides executive oversight, strategic leadership and policy direction to FDA's domestic and international product quality and safety efforts, including global collaboration, global data-sharing, development and harmonization of standards, field operations, compliance and enforcement activities.

Office of Regulatory Affairs (ORA)
ORA advises and assists the FDA commissioner and other key officials on regulations and compliance matters. ORA evaluates and coordinates all proposed FDA legal actions to ascertain compliance with regulatory policy and enforcement objectives. It is the lead office for all FDA field activities and executes direct line authority over all agency field operations. It provides direction and counsel to FDA field offices in implementing FDA policies and operational guidelines. The Quality System Inspection Technique (QSIT) guide, which provides guidance to agency field staff on the inspectional process used to assess a manufacturer's compliance with the Quality System Regulation, was developed by ORA and CDRH staff. ORA also directs and coordinates the agency's emergency preparedness and civil defense programs. More information on ORA is available at www.fda.gov/AboutFDA/CentersOffices/OfficeofGlobalRegulatoryOperationsandPolicy/ORA/default.htm.

Office of International Programs

The Office of International Programs (OIP) is the focal point for all international FDA matters. It works in collaboration with international health and regulatory partners through ongoing communications, cooperation on health and regulatory issues, exchanges of information and documents, technical cooperation and training, personnel exchanges and certification of certain products exported to and from the US. As a global public health agency, FDA strives to meet its domestic mission through its essential engagement with counterpart agencies around the world.

OIP activities include bilateral arrangements such as memoranda of understanding; formal arrangements with regulatory counterparts in other countries; participation in regional programs such as the Trilateral Cooperation (US/Canada/Mexico); multilateral organizations such as the World Health Organization and Pan American Health Organization; and taking part in harmonization and multilateral activities such as the Codex Alimentarius Commission and International Conference on Harmonization.

In addition, FDA has established a permanent presence in China, India, Europe and Latin America, and there are recent efforts establishing a presence in the Middle East, Asia Pacific, sub-Saharan Africa and North Africa.

For more information about the Office of International Programs, see www.fda.gov/AboutFDA/CentersOffices/OfficeofGlobalRegulatoryOperationsandPolicy/OfficeofInternationalPrograms/default.htm.

Office of Medical Products and Tobacco

One of the recent major FDA reorganizations was to consolidate the centers related to product review into a single office. This includes the following offices:
- Office of Special Medical Programs
- Center for Drug Evaluation and Research (CDER) Center for Biologics Evaluation and Research (CBER)
- Center for Devices and Radiological Health CDRH)
- Center for Tobacco Products (CTP)

Office of Special Medical Programs

The Office of Special Medical Programs serves as the agency focal point for special programs and initiatives that are cross-cutting and clinical, scientific and/or regulatory in nature.

The Office of Special Medical Programs:
- coordinates internal and external review of pediatric science, safety, ethical and international issues as mandated by law and agency activities
- oversees the implementation of the orphan products provisions of the *FD&C Act*
- provides executive leadership to the Office of Good Clinical Practice
- oversees the functions of the Office of Combination Products as provided in the *FD&C Act*
- oversees advisory committees and management staff, working in close collaboration with all FDA centers to provide consistent operations and seek continuous improvements in the agency advisory committee program
- acts as liaison with the Office of the Secretary, the DHHS Committee Management Office, all of FDA's center advisory committee support staff and other organizations/offices within FDA
- ensures that all FDA committee management activities are consistent with the provisions of *Federal Advisory Committee Act*, departmental policies and related regulations and statutes

The Office of Special Medical Programs includes the following offices:
- Office of Combination Products
- Office of Good Clinical Practice
- Office of Orphan Product Development
- Office of Pediatric Therapeutics

More information on the Office of Special Medical Programs can be found at http://www.fda.gov/AboutFDA/CentersOffices/OfficeofMedicalProductsandTobacco/OfficeofScienceandHealthCoordination/default.htm.

Center for Drug Evaluation and Research (CDER)

CDER regulates prescription and over-the-counter drugs, including therapeutic biologics and generic drugs, throughout the product lifecycle to ensure they are safe and effective. The center routinely monitors television, radio and print drug ads to ensure they are truthful and balanced. CDER also plays a critical role in providing healthcare professionals and consumers with information on how to use drugs appropriately and safely. More information on CDER is available at www.fda.gov/AboutFDA/CentersOffices/OfficeofMedicalProductsandTobacco/CDER/default.htm.

Center for Biologics Evaluation and Research (CBER)

CBER regulates biological products for disease prevention and treatment, including vaccines, protein-based products such as monoclonal antibodies and cytokines, and blood and blood products such as plasma, blood-derived proteins, tests used to screen blood donors and devices used to make blood products. More information on CBER, including the center's organizational structure, may be found at www.fda.gov/AboutFDA/CentersOffices/OfficeofMedicalProductsandTobacco/CBER/default.htm.

Table 1-1 delineates the jurisdictions of CDER and CBER.

Table 1-1. CDER versus CBER Product Oversight Responsibilities

CDER Oversight	CBER Oversight
• Small Molecule Drugs • Therapeutic Biologics • Monoclonal antibodies • Cytokines • Growth factors • Enzymes and Interferons (including recombinant versions) • Proteins intended for therapeutic use derived from animals or microorganisms • Therapeutic immunotherapies	• Vaccines • Blood products • Plasma expanders • Gene therapy • Products composed of human or animal cells or cell parts • Allergen patch tests and allergenic extracts • Antitoxins • Antivenins • Venoms • In vitro diagnostics • Toxoids/toxins intended for immunization

Center for Devices and Radiological Health (CDRH)

CDRH is tasked with ensuring that new medical devices are safe and effective before they are marketed. CDRH regulates medical devices and radiation-emitting products such as microwaves, television sets, cell phones and lasers to ensure they meet radiation safety standards. Many of these devices are the first of a kind. The center also monitors devices throughout the product lifecycle, including a nationwide postmarket surveillance system. More information on CDRH, including the center's organizational structure, may be found at www.fda.gov/AboutFDA/CentersOffices/OfficeofMedicalProductsandTobacco/CDRH/default.htm.

Table 1-2 shows selected FDA centers and offices involved in sponsor interface for the approval of drugs, biologics and devices.

Center for Tobacco Products (CTP)

CTP is responsible for overseeing the implementation of the *Family Smoking Prevention and Tobacco Control Act*, which became law on 22 June 2009. FDA responsibilities under the law include establishing performance standards, performing premarket review for new and modified risk tobacco products, reviewing labeling and establishing and enforcing advertising and promotion restrictions. More information about CTP may be found at http://www.fda.gov/AboutFDA/CentersOffices/OfficeofMedicalProductsandTobacco/AboutheCenterforTobaccoProducts/default.htm.

Office of Foods and Veterinary Medicine

The Office of Foods and Veterinary Medicine was created in 2009 to lead a functionally unified Foods Program and enhance the agency's ability to meet the current challenges and opportunities in food and feed safety, nutrition and other critical areas. The FDA Foods Program includes the Center for Food Safety and Applied Nutrition (CFSAN) and the Center for Veterinary Medicine (CVM). It is supported by ORA and draws on the resources and expertise of NCTR and key OC staff offices.

The Office of Foods is responsible for providing all elements of FDA's Foods Program with the leadership, guidance and support to achieve the agency's public health goals. The office is also the focal point for planning implementation of the recommendations of the President's Food Safety Working Group and the new food safety authorities contained in the 2011 *FDA Food Safety Modernization Act*.

CVM

CVM helps ensure that animal food products are safe. CVM regulates the manufacture and distribution of food additives and drugs that will be given to animals. It also evaluates the safety and effectiveness of drugs used to treat companion (pet) animals. More information on CVM is available at www.fda.gov/AboutFDA/CentersOffices/OfficeofFoods/CVM/default.htm.

CFSAN

CFSAN is responsible for the safety of almost all food consumed in the US, with the exception of meat, poultry and some egg products, which are regulated by the US Department of Agriculture (USDA). CFSAN pioneered widespread use of the Hazard Analysis and Critical Control Point (HACCP) system, which places preventive controls at the most contamination-prone points in the production process. More information on CFSAN may be found at www.fda.gov/AboutFDA/CentersOffices/OfficeofFoods/CFSAN/default.htm.

Agencies With Related Responsibilities

Federal Trade Commission (FTC)

FTC enforces the *Federal Trade Commission Act*, which prohibits unfair or deceptive acts or practices in or affecting commerce. The act prohibits the dissemination of any false advertisement for the purpose of inducing the purchase of food, drugs, devices, services or cosmetics. FTC also is empowered to seek monetary redress and other relief for conduct injurious to customers.

Per a 1971 Memorandum of Understanding (MOU), FDA has primary jurisdiction over advertising of prescription drugs and restricted devices and over labeling of all products it regulates. FTC has primary jurisdiction over advertising of OTC drugs and products other than restricted devices. The two agencies cooperate in law enforcement efforts. For example, FTC and FDA both sent Warning Letters to website operators who were marketing coral calcium products claiming that coral calcium was an effective treatment or cure for cancer and/or other diseases.[2] While the FTC letter stated that such unsupported claims were false and deceptive and were unlawful under the *FTC Act*, FDA warned website operators that their products were in violation of the *FD&C Act* because of disease claims and unsubstantiated structure/function claims. FDA compliance and law enforcement personnel have access to FTC's secure, online complaint database, Consumer Sentinel, which receives thousands of complaints each year. More information on FTC is available at http://www.ftc.gov/.

Center for Medicare and Medicaid Services (CMS)

CMS is a federal agency within DHHS. Formerly the Health Care Financing Administration (HCFA), CMS is responsible for Medicare, Medicaid and other programs. While FDA's focus is on safety and effectiveness, CMS evaluates whether new technologies are necessary and reasonable. CMS is not bound by FDA decisions and expects the clinical utility of new technologies to be proven in order to assign coding and reimbursement. Currently the two agencies review products serially. Per a DHHS announcement on 14 January 2005, FDA and CMS have agreed to work together in specific areas. At the request of the applicant and with the concurrence of both agencies, parallel review may be conducted to minimize delays between marketing approval and reimbursement. With respect to postmarket surveillance, FDA may make greater use of existing CMS mechanisms for collection of new data through the Medicare drug benefit. More information on CMS may be found at www.cms.gov/.

CMS has jurisdiction over the *Health Insurance Portability and Accountability Act* (*HIPAA*), which was enacted by Congress in 1996 to create a national standard for protecting the privacy of patients' personal health information. The regulation requires safeguards to protect the security and confidentiality of an individual's protected health information (PHI). The general rule is that healthcare entities may not use or disclose PHI without an individual's written authorization, with some exceptions as permitted or required by law. *HIPAA* allows for civil and criminal penalties for privacy and security violations. *HIPAA* also standardized the electronic exchange of health-related administrative information, such as claims forms. Where a healthcare entity conducts clinical research involving PHI, physician-investigators need to understand the Privacy Rule's restrictions on its use and disclosure for research purposes. More information on the impact of *HIPAA* as it relates to clinical research may be found at http://privacyruleandresearch.nih.gov/clin_research.asp.

CMS also regulates all laboratory testing (except research) performed on humans in the US through the *Clinical Laboratory Improvement Amendments* (*CLIA*). In total, *CLIA* covers approximately 225,000 laboratory entities. The Division of Laboratory Services, within the Survey and Certification Group, under the Office of Clinical Standards and Quality (OCSQ) is responsible for implementing the *CLIA* program. FDA, through CDRH, reviews and approves laboratory tests licensed for use (as in vitro diagnostics), but *CLIA* regulates the laboratories that use these tests on humans. As a result, coordination and interaction between CMS and CDRH on laboratory tests occurs frequently. The objective of the *CLIA* program is to ensure quality laboratory testing. Although all clinical laboratories must be properly certified to receive Medicare or Medicaid payments, *CLIA* has no direct Medicare or Medicaid program responsibilities. More information can be found at: www.cms.gov/Regulations-and-Guidance/Legislation/CLIA/index.html.

Consumer Product Safety Commission (CPSC)

CPSC is responsible for ensuring the safety of consumer goods, such as household appliances (excluding those that emit radiation), paint, child-resistant packages and baby toys. Tobacco, pesticides, motor vehicles and products subject to FDA jurisdiction are expressly exempt from regulation under the *Consumer Product Safety Act* (*CPSA*). FDA and CPSC work cooperatively for consumer protection. For example, articles employed in the preparation or holding of food that may malfunction and cause contamination or spoilage (e.g., home canning equipment, pressure cookers, refrigerators, freezers and can openers) are subject to regulation as "consumer products" by CPSC under the *CPSA*. Under the *FD&C Act*, FDA may take action against manufacturers of food that has been contaminated or spoiled by such articles and shipped in interstate commerce. More information on CPSC may be found at www.cpsc.gov/.

Securities and Exchange Commission (SEC)

SEC's primary mission is to protect the investing public and maintain the integrity of the securities market. FDA assists in SEC investigations of possible violations of federal securities laws. FDA also supports SEC staff in assessing the accuracy of statements by FDA-regulated firms in SEC filings, especially where such statements can have a powerful effect on stock prices. Under measures adopted in February 2004 to improve the sharing of information between the two agencies, a reporting process was established to allow

Chapter 1

Table 1-2. Selected Primary FDA Centers/Offices Involved in Sponsor Interface During the Development and Approval of Drugs, Biologics and Devices

FDA Center/Office	Primary Responsibility
Office of the Commissioner • Office of Orphan Products Development (OOPD) • Office of Combination Products (OCP)	Review requests for orphan drug designation and review and award orphan drug grants. Review and adjudicate review assignments for combination products.
Center for Biologics Evaluation and Research (CBER) • Office of Biostatistics and Epidemiology • Office of Blood Research and Review • Office of Vaccines Research and Review • Office of Compliance and Biologics Quality • Office of Cellular, Tissue, and Gene Therapies	Evaluate and monitor the safety and effectiveness of biological products for disease prevention and treatment, including blood and blood products, vaccines, human gene therapy, xenotransplants, human tissues and cellular product and allergenics.

Center for Drug Evaluation and Research (CDER)
• Office of Compliance
  o Office of Scientific Investigations
  o Office of Manufacturing and Product Quality
• Office of Surveillance and Epidemiology
  o Office of Medication Error and Prevention and Risk Management
  o Office of Pharmacovigilance and Epidemiology
• Office of Clinical Pharmacology and Biopharmaceutics (Clin Pharm reviewers)
• Office of Medical Policy
  o Office of Prescription Drug Promotion
  o Office of Medical Policy Initiatives
• Office of Translational Sciences
  o Office of Biostatistics
  o Office of Clinical Pharmacology
• Office of New Drugs (includes OTC products)
• Office of Pharmaceutical Science
  o Office of Generic Drugs (OGD)
  o Office of New Drug Quality Assessment (CMC Reviewers and CMC Project Managers)
  o Office of Biotechnology Products
	Evaluate and monitor the safety and effectiveness of all prescription and over-the-counter drugs (including peptides and well-characterized proteins used for therapeutic purposes).

Center for Devices and Radiological Health (CDRH) • Office of Compliance • Office of Device Evaluation • Office of Surveillance and Biometrics • Office of In Vitro Diagnostic Device Evaluation and Safety	Evaluate and monitor the safety and effectiveness of new medical devices for human use and assure that radiation-emitting products (e.g., microwave ovens, cell phones, x-ray machines) meet radiation safety standards.
Center for Veterinary Medicine (CVM) • Office of New Animal Drug Evaluation • Office of Surveillance and Compliance • Office of Research • Office of Minor Use and Minor Species	Evaluate and monitor the safety and effectiveness of new drugs for animals and the safety of animal food products.

any FDA employees who suspect erroneous or exaggerated public statements by a company to bring them to the attention of SEC staff as quickly and efficiently as possible. More information on SEC is available www.sec.gov/.

Occupational Safety and Health Administration (OSHA)

The *Occupational Safety and Health Act* (*OSH*) created OSHA at the federal level within the Department of Labor. OSHA's mission is to prevent work-related injuries, illnesses and deaths by issuing and enforcing rules (called standards) for workplace safety and health. FDA's statutory authority does not extend to the occupational safety and health responsibilities of OSHA. FDA has no workplace inspection program. However, the agencies coordinate their efforts in cases of overlapping regulatory responsibility (e.g., unshielded syringes and natural rubber latex). More information on OSHA may be found at www.osha.gov/.

Tax and Trade Bureau (TTB)

The *Federal Alcohol Administration Act* (*FAAA*) provides for federal regulation of beer, wine and distilled spirits. It establishes requirements for packaging used to hold alcohol over and above those imposed by FDA for foods under the *FD&C Act*. The *FAAA* is administered by the Treasury

Department's Alcohol and Tobacco Tax and Trade Bureau (TTB). TTB consults with FDA regarding the approval of ingredients in alcoholic beverages and the requirements of label disclosure. Under a 1987 MOU, FDA is directed to contact TTB when it learns or is advised that an alcoholic beverage is or may be adulterated. More information on TTB may be found at http://www.ttb.gov/.

US Department of Agriculture (USDA)

USDA's Food Safety and Inspection Service (FSIS) has oversight over dairy, poultry, fruit and meat products, except for shell eggs, for which FDA and USDA share jurisdiction. Egg processing plants (egg washing, sorting, egg breaking and pasteurizing operations) are under USDA jurisdiction. However, FDA is responsible for egg-containing products and other egg processing not covered by USDA, e.g., restaurants, bakeries, cake mix plants, etc. The *Poultry Products Inspection Act* (*PPIA*) defines the term "poultry" as any domesticated bird. USDA has interpreted the term "poultry" to include domestic ducks, domestic geese, chickens and turkeys. FDA is responsible for all non-specified birds, including wild turkeys, wild ducks and wild geese. FDA also regulates game meats, such as venison and ostrich. FDA and USDA together published guidance on quality and environmental concerns for companies producing human and animal drugs from genetically modified plants. FDA has jurisdiction over labeling of genetically modified foods and food from cloned animals. More information on USDA may be found at www.usda.gov/wps/portal/usdahome.

Department of Commerce (DOC)

FDA operates a mandatory safety program for all fish and fishery products under the provisions of the *FD&C Act*. Seafood is one of the few FDA-regulated food groups further regulated under a system of risk prevention controls known as Hazard Analysis and Critical Control Points (HACCP). Under HACCP, domestic and foreign processors are required to prepare site- and product-specific plans that analyze potential safety hazards, determine where they are likely to occur during processing, identify control points and how they will be monitored and study how hazards are being controlled.

The National Oceanic and Atmospheric Administration (NOAA) within DOC oversees fisheries management in the US. It has its own authority for the promulgation of grade standards and for inspection and certification of fish and shellfish. NOAA Fisheries administers a voluntary, fee-for-service seafood inspection program that exceeds FDA HACCP-based requirements by providing grading, certification, label review, laboratory testing, training and consultative services. Participants may use official marks on compliant products, indicating that they are federally inspected. More information may be found at www.nmfs.noaa.gov/.

Environmental Protection Agency (EPA)

The mission of EPA is to protect human health and the environment, which includes jurisdiction over the public water supply. In the past, FDA considered drinking water to be a food. However, both agencies have determined that the passage of the *Safe Drinking Water Act* (*SDWA*) in 1974 implicitly repealed FDA's authority under the *FD&C Act* over drinking water. EPA and FDA have a 1979 Memorandum of Agreement specifying that EPA regulates and develops national standards for the safety of drinking water from municipal water supplies while FDA regulates the labeling and safety of bottled water as a consumer beverage.

Antimicrobial surface solutions applied to counter tops, table tops, food processing equipment, cutlery, dishware or cookware, to sanitize such objects after they have been washed, meet the definition of "pesticide chemical" and therefore are subject to regulation by EPA. However, any antimicrobial surface solutions used to sanitize food packaging materials are excluded from "pesticide chemical" classification and are considered food additives subject to regulation by FDA. Materials preservatives are sometimes incorporated into food-contact articles to protect the finished product from discoloration, degradation or decomposition due to microbiological activity, rather than to prevent microbial activity. These materials are regulated as food additives by FDA. Antimicrobials impregnated into food packaging to protect either the package or to extend the shelf life of the food are also regulated as food additives by FDA. More information on EPA may be found at www.epa.gov/.

FDA, USDA and EPA share responsibility for regulating pesticides. EPA determines the safety and effectiveness of the chemicals and establishes tolerance levels for residues on feed crops, as well as on raw and processed foods. FDA and USDA are responsible for monitoring the food supply to ensure that pesticide residues do not exceed the allowable levels in the products under their jurisdictions.

Drug Enforcement Administration (DEA)

Illegal drugs with no approved medical use, such as heroin and cocaine, are under the jurisdiction of DEA. FDA assists DEA in deciding how stringent DEA controls should be on drugs that are medically accepted but have a strong potential for abuse. DEA establishes limits on the amount of these prescription drugs that is permitted to be manufactured each year. More information on DEA may be found at www.usdoj.gov/dea/index.htm.

Tips for Obtaining Information

Information for consumers and industry can be obtained directly from FDA. Each agency division has its own website, containing a wide variety of information, including laws and regulations, administrative information regarding FDA's organizational structure and staff contact information, news and events, problem reporting, guidance documents, forms and links to other national and international regulatory agencies. There also are databases of products cleared or approved for marketing, adverse event reporting and recalls. The websites and databases are fully searchable.

A network of FDA offices exists to help small businesses. The Commissioner's Office of the Ombudsman liaises with the Small Business National Ombudsman to resolve complaints and answer questions. Product-specific centers each have their own ombudsmen. Also, each of the five regional offices has a small business representative available to answer questions and provide training. The Division of Small Manufacturers, International, and Consumer Assistance (DSMICA) provides assistance to medical device manufacturers and consumers. A detailed directory identifies staff by area of expertise, and a toll-free number will connect you directly to staff members during normal business hours. Similarly, CDER and the other product-specific centers have staff members available to answer inquiries from small business owners and help explain the agency's structure and rules.

Information pertaining to the rulemaking process can be found at www.regulations.gov/#!home. This website facilitates public participation in the federal rulemaking process by enabling the public to view and comment on federal regulatory actions.

Summary

FDA's regulatory responsibility has evolved over 150 years from being tasked with regulating foods to include drug, cosmetics, devices, biologics and tobacco products.

FDA is responsible for protecting the public health by assuring the safety, efficacy and security of human and veterinary drugs, biological products, medical devices, cosmetics, products that emit radiation and the food supply.

During the 19th century, states exercised principal control over domestically produced and distributed foods and drugs, while federal authority was restricted to imported foods and drugs. Dr. Harvey Wiley, the father of the food and drug laws, was concerned about the use of preservative chemicals as "adulterants" in food products. He organized various groups to support a federal law to prohibit the adulteration and misbranding of foods and drugs.

FDA is an agency within DHHS and consists of nine main centers/offices.

The Office of the Commissioner is responsible for the efficient and effective implementation of FDA's mission.

CDER evaluates all new prescription and over-the-counter drugs, as well as protein-based products, such as monoclonal antibodies and cytokines, before they are sold to ensure they are safe and effective.

CBER regulates biological products for disease prevention and treatment, including vaccines, and blood and blood products, such as plasma, blood-derived proteins, tests used to screen blood donors and devices used to make blood products.

CDRH is tasked with ensuring that new medical devices are safe and effective before they are marketed.

CVM helps ensure that animal food additives and drug products are safe.

CFSAN is responsible for the safety of most food consumed in the US, with the exception of meat, poultry and some egg products, which are regulated by the USDA.

NCTR conducts research and provides advice and training necessary for science-based decision making and developing sound regulatory policy.

CTP is responsible for overseeing the implementation of the *Family Smoking Prevention and Tobacco Control Act*, which became law on 22 June 2009.

ORA advises and assists the FDA commissioner and other key officials on regulations and compliance matters and oversees all agency field operations.

Other agencies play a role or work with FDA in the regulation of food, drugs, cosmetics and devices. These agencies include: FTC, CMS, CPSC, SEC, OSHA, TTB, USDA, DOC, EPA and DEA.

References
1. Harris G. "The Safety Gap" 2 November 2008. *The New York Times* website. www.nytimes.com/2008/11/02/magazine/02fda-t.html. Accessed 6 May 2013.
2. FTC and FDA Take New Actions in Fight Against Deceptive Marketing. FTC website. www.ftc.gov/opa/2003/06/trudeau.shtm. Accessed 6 May 2013.

Recommended Reading
- Grossman LA. "Food, Drugs and Droods: A Historical Consideration of Definitions and Categories in American Food and Drug Law." *Cornell Law Review*. Volume 93, pp. 1091–1148 (2008).
- Burditt GM. "The History of Food Law." *Food and Drug Law Journal*, 50th Anniversary Special Edition, pp 197–201 (2009).

Chapter 2

History of Food, Drug and Cosmetic Laws

Updated by Treena Jackson, MS, CQA, CSSGB, RAC

OBJECTVES

- Review the differences between laws, regulations and guidance documents
- Provide an overview of the laws, regulations, and regulatory agencies governing foods, drugs and medical products marketed in the US
- Discuss the historical context in which those laws were enacted
- Provide an overview of the rulemaking process

LAWS, REGULATIONS AND GUIDELINES COVERED IN THIS CHAPTER

- *Pure Food and Drug Act* of 1906
- *Federal Food, Drug, and Cosmetic Act* of 1938
- *Nutrition Labeling and Education Act* of 1990
- *Bioterrorism Act* of 2002
- *Food Allergen Labeling and Consumer Protection Act* of 2004
- *Color Additive Amendment* of 1960
- *Kefauver-Harris Amendments* of 1962
- *Controlled Substances Act* of 1970
- *Drug Price Competition and Patent Term Restoration Act of 1984 (Hatch-Waxman Act)*
- *Fair Packaging and Labeling Act* of 1967
- *Prescription Drug User Fee Act* of 1992
- *Food and Drug Administration Modernization Act* of 1997
- *Food and Drug Administration Amendments Act* of 2007
- *Food Safety Modernization Act* of 2011
- *Medical Device Amendments* of 1976
- *Safe Medical Devices Act* of 1990
- *Medical Devices Amendments* of 1992
- *Safe Medical Devices Act* of 1990
- *Medical Device User Fee and Modernization Act* of 2002
- *Durham-Humphrey Amendment* of 1951
- *Orphan Drug Act* of 1983
- *Prescription Drug Amendments* of 1992
- *Food and Drug Administration Safety and Innovation Act* of 2012

Chapter 2

❑ *FDA Export Reform and Enhancement Act* of 1996

❑ *Pediatric Research Equity Act* of 2003

Introduction

To understand the history of food, drug and cosmetic laws, it is important to know the history that led to such laws, the process involved to create laws and the authority and enforceability of the law. This chapter discusses these topics as well as an overall introduction to key laws and regulations related to food, drugs and cosmetics.

Laws, Regulations and Guidance

Laws begin as legislation enacted by the US Congress. A bill is introduced by one house of Congress and is considered in committee where public hearings may be held. The bill is then amended as necessary and reintroduced into committee for debate and vote. Once approved by the majority of both the House and the Senate, the bill is then submitted to the president. If the president signs the bill, it becomes a law. However, if the president disapproves the bill, he can veto the bill by refusing to sign it. If both the Senate and the House pass the bill in turn by a two-thirds majority vote, the president's veto is overruled and the bill becomes law. Laws establish general principles and clarify congressional intent; they can only be changed by Congress. The United States Code (U.S.C.) is the official compilation of codified laws by subject, and the US Statutes-at-Large is the official chronologic compilation of all laws.

Federal executive departments and administrative agencies (such as the US Food and Drug Administration (FDA)) write regulations to implement the authority of laws. Laws are therefore enforced by regulations through an agency of the executive branch. Although regulations are subordinate to laws, both laws and regulations are enforceable.

Regulations establish standards or requirements of conduct and provide details of how the law is to be followed. Regulations are both interpretive (they explain the meaning of the language of a section of the act) and substantive (they provide a specific scientific or technical basis). They are promulgated through the "rulemaking process" and have the force of law. The Code of Federal Regulations (CFR) is the official compilation of regulations. FDA follows the procedures required by the *Administrative Procedure Act*, a federal law enacted in 1946, to propose and establish FDA regulations. This typically involves a process known as "notice and comment rulemaking" that allows public input and comment on a proposed regulation before FDA issues a final regulation.

Guidance documents and guidelines establish principles or practices that represent an agency's thinking. However, they do not go through the formal rulemaking process, and therefore do not have the force of law and are not legally binding. FDA follows the procedures required by its "Good Guidance Practice" regulation (Title 21 CFR 10.115) to issue FDA guidance. FDA guidance describes the agency's current thinking on a regulatory issue.

History

The history of modern food and drug law began in the 20th century. During the 1800s, commerce in food and drugs was largely unregulated due to concerns about government interference with free trade and the inability of the individual states to control sales of products that were manufactured in other states. This led to conditions such as those described in *The Jungle* by Upton Sinclair, published in 1906. Although it was presented as a work of fiction, the book's description of the unsanitary conditions in Chicago's meat-packing plants led to widespread public outrage and a demand for legislation. In response to the demand, Congress passed the *Pure Food and Drug Act* in 1906.

Pure Food and Drug Act of 1906

The 1906 *Pure Food and Drug Act*, which the Department of Agriculture's Bureau of Chemistry was charged to enforce, prohibited the interstate commerce and transport of adulterated and misbranded food and drugs under penalty of seizure of questionable products and/or prosecution of responsible parties. Harvey Washington Wiley, chief chemist of the Bureau of Chemistry, was the driving force behind the *Pure Food and Drug Act*, which took approximately 25 years to establish. The statute stated: "The term 'food,' as used herein, shall include all articles used for food, drink, confectionary, or condiment by man or other animals, whether simple, mixed or compound." It defined "drug" as including "all medicines and preparations recognized in the *United States Pharmacopoeia* (*USP*) or *National Formulary* (*NF*) for internal or external use, and any substance or mixture of substances intended to be used for the cure, mitigation, or prevention of disease of either man or other animals." This "intended use" language, which later also was incorporated into the definition of "device," survives largely intact in the *Food, Drug, and Cosmetics Act* (*FD&C Act*) today.

The basis of the law rested on the regulation of product labeling rather than premarket approval. The food or drug label could not be false or misleading in any particular, and the presence and amount of 11 dangerous ingredients—including alcohol, heroin and cocaine—had to be listed. Specific variations from the applicable *USP* and *NF* standards for drugs were to be plainly stated on the label. Labels were not even required to state the weight or measure; only that any contents statement, if used, be truthful. If the manufacturer opted to list a food's weight or measure, the information had to be accurate. The law prohibited the addition of any ingredients that would substitute for the food, conceal damage, pose a health hazard or constitute a filthy or decomposed substance.

The law assumed that average consumers could avoid risks if they were made aware of same via product labeling; therefore, it relied on consumer vigilance to assess labeling for deception or harm. Food manufacturers were not required to submit labeling for regulatory review. The Bureau of Chemistry was tasked with actively identifying violations and bringing legal action. The law enabled the government to prosecute manufacturers of illegal products but lacked affirmative requirements to guide compliance.

The *Pure Food and Drug Act*, as revised in 1912, stated that a drug was misbranded if its label contained a "false and fraudulent" statement regarding "curative or therapeutic effect." The requirement of demonstrating fraud made this a difficult standard for the Bureau of Chemistry to satisfy. The Bureau of Chemistry's name was changed to the Food, Drug, and Insecticide Administration in July 1927, and shortened to the Food and Drug Administration in July 1930.

The Federal Food, Drug, and Cosmetics Act (FD&C Act) of 1938

The *FD&C Act* is a federal law enacted by Congress. It and other federal laws establish the statuatory framework within which FDA operates today. The *FD&C Act* and its subsequent amendments can be found in the U.S.C.

The 1938 *FD&C Act* replaced the *Pure Food and Drug Act* and revised the misbranding standard for therapeutic claims in a way that helped further differentiate food labeling from drug labeling. The 1938 act tightened the standard from "false and fraudulent" to "false or misleading in any particular," a change that greatly eased FDA's burden in proving misbranding. The 1938 act also introduced premarket drug review, requiring the manufacturer of a "new drug" (defined as a drug not generally recognized as safe) to submit a New Drug Application (NDA) to FDA, setting forth the company's evidence of the drug's safety. It prohibited false therapeutic claims for drugs, while a separate law granted the Federal Trade Commission (FTC) jurisdiction over drug advertising. The *FD&C Act* also brought cosmetics and medical devices under FDA's control and mandated legally enforceable food standards. In addition, tolerances for certain poisonous substances were addressed. The law formally authorized factory inspections and added injunctions to the enforcement tools at the agency's disposal. Below is a bulleted summary of the new provisions as a result of the act:
- extended control to cosmetics and therapeutic devices
- required new drugs to be shown safe before marketing, beginning a new system of drug regulation
- eliminated the *Sherley Amendment* requirement to prove intent to defraud in drug misbranding cases
- provided safe tolerances to be set for unavoidable poisonous substances
- authorized standards of identity, quality and fill-of-container for foods
- authorized factory inspections
- added the remedy of court injunctions to the previous penalties of seizures and prosecutions

The *Durham-Humphrey Amendment* of 1951 clarified what constituted a prescription versus an over-the-counter drug. The *Kefauver-Harris Amendments* of 1962 mandated the establishment of efficacy as well as safety before a drug could be marketed, required FDA to assess the efficacy of all drugs introduced since 1938, instituted stricter agency control over drug trials (including a requirement that patients involved must give their informed consent), transferred regulation of prescription drug advertising from FTC to FDA, established Good Manufacturing Practice (GMP) requirements for the drug industry and granted FDA greater powers to access company production and control records to verify those practices.

Regulating Devices After the 1938 FD&C Act

In 1938, when the *FD&C Act* was approved, medical devices were simple instruments such as scalpels and stethoscopes. While premarket approval in the 1938 *FD&C Act* did not apply to devices for regulatory purposes, the law equated them to drugs in every other sense.

In the post-World War II years, however, a technology boom resulted in an increase in the complexity and number of medical devices, including products such as heart-lung machines and dialysis equipment. The Cooper Commission in 1970 determined that more than 700 deaths and 10,000 injuries were associated with medical devices. Among those, 512 deaths and injuries were attributed to heart valves, 89 deaths and 186 injuries were tied to heart pacemakers and 10 deaths and 8,000 injuries were attributed to intrauterine devices (i.e., Dalkon Shield intrauterine device therapeutic disaster).

As a result of the Cooper report, Congress passed the 1976 *Medical Device Amendments* to the *FD&C Act*. This legislation established three classes of medical devices, each requiring a different level of regulatory scrutiny, up to premarket approval. The three classes were based on the degree of control necessary to assure that the devices were safe and effective. The amendments also made provisions for device listing, establishment registration and adherence to GMPs. The *Safe Medical Devices Act* of 1990 (*SMDA*) and the *Medical Devices Amendments* of 1992 revised and expanded the 1976 *Medical Device Amendments* to the *FD&C Act*.

SMDA of 1990

Under the *SMDA*, device user facilities must report device-related deaths to FDA and the manufacturer, if known. Device user facilities also must report device-related serious injuries to the manufacturer, or to FDA, if the manufacturer is not known. In addition, the *SMDA* required that device user facilities submit to FDA, on a semiannual basis, a summary of all reports submitted during that time period. The device user facility reporting section of the *SMDA* became effective on 28 November 1991.

The *SMDA* defined a "medical device" as "any instrument, apparatus, or other article that is used to prevent, diagnose, mitigate, or treat a disease or to affect the structure or function of the body, with the exception of drugs." It instituted device tracking and postmarket surveillance requirements and allowed FDA to temporarily suspend or withdraw approval of an application for premarket approval. The rule provided civil penalties for violation of a requirement of the *FD&C Act* relating to devices. The act amended the *FD&C Act* to create an incentive for the development of orphan or humanitarian use devices (HUDs), defined as devices for use in the treatment or diagnosis of diseases or conditions affecting fewer than 4,000 patients in the US each year.

The primary impact of the 1992 *Medical Device Amendments* was to clarify certain terms and to establish a single reporting standard for device user facilities, manufacturers, importers and distributors.

The Medical Device User Fee and Modernization Act of 2002 (MDUFMA)

Medical device user fees were first established by Congress in 2002. Medical device companies pay fees to FDA when they register their establishments and list their devices with the agency, whenever they submit an application or a notification to market a new medical device in the US and for certain other types of submissions. *MDUFMA* established fees for Premarket Approval applications (PMAs), supplements and 510(k) submissions. In return, FDA committed to strict performance goals for medical technology reviews.

The *Medical Device User Fee Amendments* of 2012 (*MDUFA III*) took effect in October of 2012. *MDUFA III* represented a commitment between the US medical device industry and FDA to increase the efficiency of regulatory processes in order to reduce the time it takes to bring safe and effective medical devices to the US market.

Regulating Foods After the 1938 Act

The *FD&C Act* required colors to be listed (approved) before they could be used in foods, drugs and cosmetics, and, in addition, required those made from coal tar sources to be batch certified. The Color Certification Program, supported by user fees, continues today, with nearly 18,000,000 compounds certified for composition and purity in FDA's laboratories in Fiscal 2005. The *FD&C Act* also required the label of a food to "bear its common or usual name." The food would be illegal or misbranded if it represented itself as a "standardized food" unless it conformed to that standard. Some food products were deemed "standardized foods" because there were established FDA standards for them. The act authorized three kinds of food standards—identity, quality and fill of container. In 1939, the first food standards were issued for canned tomatoes, tomato purée and tomato paste. The next standards were for jams and jellies. By 1957, additional food standards had been established for foods such as chocolate, flour, cereals, bakery products, milk, cheese, juices and eggs.

In 1950, the Delaney Committee started a congressional investigation of the safety of additives that laid the foundation for the *Food Additives Amendment* and the *Color Additive Amendments*. Rep. James Delaney (D-NY), later submitted a change to the bill proposing the *Food Additives Amendment* by inserting the "Delaney Clause," which prohibited the approval of any food additive shown to induce cancer in humans or animals in studies with a relevant route of exposure. Enacted in 1958, the *Food Additives Amendment* required manufacturers of new food additives to establish their safety to FDA's satisfaction before marketing. Also in 1958, FDA published the first list of generally recognized as safe (GRAS) substances, which contained nearly 200 substances, including ascorbic acid, papain and propylene glycol.

In 1966, the *Fair Packaging and Labeling Act (FPLA)* required products marketed on a retail basis to consumers in interstate commerce to be honestly and informatively labeled, with FDA enforcing provisions on foods, drugs, cosmetics and medical devices.

Significant amendments to the *FD&C Act* regarding the regulation of food include the *Nutrition Labeling and Education Act* of 1990, which requires manufacturers to provide standardized food labels and consistency in health claims and serving sizes. The *Dietary Supplement Health and Education Act* of 1994 was another significant amendment, classifying dietary supplements as foods and establishing a framework and requirements for labeling and GMPs, among other regulatory provisions.

The events of September 11, 2001 prompted a closer look at the food industry, leading to the *Bioterrorism Act* of 2002. This law and its implementing regulations were designed to improve the ability to trace the movement of foods through international and interstate commerce, to restrict the availability of certain biological agents and toxins and to improve the security of the drinking water supply.

The *FDA Food Safety Modernization Act (FSMA)* was signed into law by President Obama on 4 January 2011. It aimed to ensure the US food supply was safe by shifting the focus of federal regulators from responding to contamination to preventing it. This 2011 reform was noted by FDA as the most sweeping reform to US food safety law in 70 years. The law provided FDA with new enforcement authorities designed to achieve higher rates of compliance with prevention- and risk-based food safety standards and new tools to respond to and contain problems when they occur. For the first time, FDA had a legislative mandate to require comprehensive, science-based preventive controls across the food supply. The law also gave FDA new tools to hold imported foods to the same standards as domestic foods and directs the agency to build an integrated national food safety system in partnership with state and local authorities.

Regulating Cosmetics After the 1938 Act

The *Color Additive Amendments* of 1960 require manufacturers to establish the safety of color additives in foods, drugs and cosmetics and was the source of the designation of colors as FD&C (safe for foods, drugs and cosmetics), D&C (safe for drugs and cosmetics) or Ext. D&C (for externally applied products only).

Cosmetic products generally are not subject to premarket approval by FDA unless they make structure or function claims or are also intended to treat or prevent disease. Such products also are considered to be drugs and must comply with both the drug and cosmetic provisions of the law. For instance, cosmetics containing sunscreens are considered drugs because they are intended to affect the body's physiological response to solar radiation.

Current Trends in Drugs and Devices—Amending the FD&C Act

The Orphan Drug Act of 1983

The 1983 *Orphan Drug Act* originally defined the term "orphan drug" as "a drug for a disease or condition which is rare." In October 1984, the term "rare" was defined in an amendment as "any rare disease or condition which (a) affects less than 200,000 persons in the U.S. or (b) affects more than 200,000 persons in the U.S. but for which there is no reasonable expectation that the cost of developing and making available in the U.S. a drug for such disease or condition will be recovered from sales in the U.S. of such drug." The act guarantees the developer of an orphan product seven years of market exclusivity following FDA's approval of the product. Incentives also include tax credits for clinical research undertaken by a sponsor to generate data required for marketing approval.

The Drug Price Competition and Patent Term Restoration Act of 1984

Because the approval process for each new product required the submission of full safety and efficacy data, the economic pressures resulting from the lengthy review process led to the *Drug Price Competition and Patent Restoration Act* of 1984, also known as the *Hatch-Waxman Act*. This law established a process for the approval of drugs based on comparison to an already approved product and provided for exclusive marketing status for a period of time based on the length of the approval process for new drugs or the patent status of the branded drug for generics.

This act included provisions for patent term extension, which gave certain patent holders the opportunity to extend patent terms by five years for human drug products, including antibiotics and biologics, medical devices, food additives and color additives. By giving inventors a portion of the patent term lost during federal regulatory review, Congress sought to restore some of the incentive for innovation to US domestic drug companies that was weakened as federal premarket approval requirements became more expensive and time-consuming. The *Hatch Waxman Act* authorized Abbreviated New Drug Applications (ANDAs) for generic drugs and specifically provided that FDA could require only bioavailability studies for ANDAs.

The Prescription Drug User Fee Act (PDUFA)

PDUFA was first enacted in 1992 and authorized FDA to collect user fees from companies that produced certain human drug and biological products and submit applications for FDA review. In addition, companies were required to pay annual fees for each manufacturing establishment and for each prescription drug product marketed. Previously, taxpayers paid for product reviews through budgets provided by Congress. In this program, industry provides the funding in exchange for FDA's agreement to meet drug review performance goals, which emphasize timeliness.

The *Food and Drug Administration Safety and Innovation Act (FDASIA)*, was signed into law on 9 July 2012. *FDASIA* gives FDA the authority to collect user fees from industry to fund reviews of innovator drugs, medical devices, generic drugs and biosimilar biologics. It also reauthorizes two programs that encourage pediatric drug development. This is the fifth authorization of *PDUFA* (also known as '*PDUFA V*') and the third authorization of *MDUFA*. *FDASIA* helps to ensure FDA has consistent funding for Fiscal 2013–2017 to help maintain a predictable and efficient review process.

The Food and Drug Administration Modernization Act (FDAMA) of 1997

FDAMA provided additional authority for monitoring the progress of drug and biologic postmarketing studies. The provisions in this act required FDA to issue regulations that allowed clinical study sponsors to modify any investigational device or study protocol by submitting to FDA a "Notice of Change" five days after instituting such a change, where such changes did not significantly affect the study design or patient safety. The law codified the expedited review policy for certain medical devices, amended and clarified the humanitarian device provisions of *SMDA* and allowed FDA to recognize international or other national standards. *FDAMA* also directed FDA to consider the least-burdensome

Chapter 2

Table 2-1 Other Laws, Regulations and Guidelines

• Federal Meat Inspection Act of 1906
• Poultry Products Inspection Act of 1957
• Egg Products Inspection Act of 1970
• Dietary Supplement Health and Education Act of 1994
• Public Health Service Act of 1944
• GMPs for the 21st Century (2004)
• Wheeler-Lea Act of 1938
• Food Additives Amendment of 1958
• Fair Packaging and Labeling Act of 1967
• Animal Drug Amendments of 1968
• Poison Prevention Packaging Act of 1970
• Infant Formula Act of 1980
• Generic Animal Drug and Patent Term Restoration Act of 1988
• Animal Medicinal Drug Use Clarification Act of 1994
• Food Quality Protection Act of 1996
• Animal Drug Availability Act of 1996
• Best Pharmaceuticals for Children Act of 2002
• Animal Drug User Fee Act of 2003
• Minor Use and Minor Species Animal Health Act of 2001
• Dietary Supplement and Nonprescription Drug Consumer Protection Act of 2006

means of establishing substantial equivalence for certain device marketing applications. The act repealed the mandatory tracking requirements for some high-risk devices imposed by *SMDA*, and instead established requirements and a process under which FDA may order device tracking.

The Pediatric Research Equity Act (PREA) of 2003

PREA gave FDA clear authority to require pediatric studies of drugs when other approaches are insufficient to ensure drugs are safe and effective for children. If the course of a disease and the effects of the drug treatment for that disease are "sufficiently similar in adults and pediatric patients," FDA may waive the requirement if it can be concluded that "pediatric effectiveness can be extrapolated from adequate and well-controlled studies in adults."

The Food and Drug Administration Amendments Act (FDAAA) of 2007

FDAAA reauthorized a number of key programs, including *PDUFA*, *MDUFMA* and *PREA*. *FDAAA* requires all clinical trials of drugs, biologics and devices—except Phase 1 clinical trials—to be registered in a clinical trial registry databank. ClinicalTrials.gov, established by the National Institutes of Health (NIH)/National Library of Medicine (NLM) in collaboration with FDA, meets *FDAAA* mandates. The results of clinical trials that serve as the basis for an efficacy claim or postmarketing studies also are required to be posted. *FDAAA* provides civil monetary penalties of as much as $10,000 for failure to comply with the registration requirements. If violations are not corrected within 30 days, additional penalties of up to $10,000 per day of violation may accrue. *FDAAA* permits FDA to require sponsors to submit direct-to-consumer (DTC) television advertisements for agency review no later than 45 days before dissemination of the advertisement and permits FDA to impose penalties of as much as $500,000 for false and misleading DTC advertisements. In addition, civil penalties of as much as $10 million may be imposed for violations of postmarket studies, clinical trials or labeling changes required under *FDAAA*.

More information about the laws enforced by FDA can be obtained at www.fda.gov/RegulatoryInformation/Legislation/default.htm.

Other Food- and Drug-related Laws

While the discussion above covers many of the laws that form the basis of current regulations, there are many others that affect foods, drugs and medical devices. **Table 2-1** lists some of these other laws.

Rulemaking Process

Government agencies create regulations that are derived from statutes created through the legislative branch. Regulations define how FDA regulates products and are developed through the rulemaking process. Rulemaking is a transparent process that involves the public. By law, anyone can participate in this process. Public comments are gathered through proposed rules or petitions. FDA carefully considers the public's comments when drafting final rules. Final rules become federal regulations upon codification in the CFR. The *Administrative Procedure Act* of 1946 gave the public the right to participate in the rulemaking process by commenting on proposed rules. The public's rights were further extended through procedural rules that established a 60-day minimum public comment period for significant regulations. The enactment of the *Government in the Sunshine Act* of 1976 required advanced notice of rulemaking meetings, and required those meetings to be open to the public. A regulatory agenda known as the Unified Agenda is published semi-annually and summarizes each agency's planned rulemaking activities for the following six months.

Proposed Rules

New regulations or revisions to existing regulations are announced in the *Federal Register*. A Notice of Proposed Rulemaking describes the rule and provides background information. A comment period is established that defines how long the agency will accept comments. The *Federal Register* announcement marks the beginning of the comment period.

Comment Period/FDA Action

Public comments may be submitted electronically through the regulations.gov website. Comments are logged, numbered and placed in a file upon receipt by FDA. The comments become part of the public record and are available for anyone to read on the regulations.gov website or in the FDA Dockets Management Reading Room (Room 1061, 5630 Fishers Lane, Rockville, MD). Comment periods are generally at least 60 days including weekends and holidays, and can be as long as one year. Some comment periods may be shorter than 60 days. During the comment period, FDA carefully analyzes the public's comments. Upon the expiration of the comment period, FDA may perform one of three actions:
- promulgate interim or final rules
- extend the comment period
- abandon its intention to promulgate a rule

Rule Publication and Codification

Final rules are published in the *Federal Register*. Rules in the *Federal Register* are cited by volume and page number and are codified annually in the CFR. Title 21 consists of nine volumes divided into two chapters. FDA regulations are provided in Chapter 1, which are contained in the first eight volumes. DEA regulations are provided in Chapter 2 in the ninth volume.

Petitions

Agency processes may be influenced through the petition process. Requests can be made to FDA to issue, change or cancel a regulation. Petitions must contain specific information:
- action requested
- statement of grounds
- environmental impact
- official certification statement
- petitioner identifying information

FDA may request economic impact information after reviewing the petition. FDA management will decide whether to grant or deny the petition after a review period.

Summary

Food and drug law, which provides the framework for regulatory practices, is closely linked to the larger historical context of the times in which the laws were enacted. Many laws, such as the *FD&C Act*, the *Kefauver-Harris Amendments* and the *Bioterrorism Act*, were enacted in response to specific events that called attention to the need for additional authorities or controls. Based on this history, it is likely that future such events will continue to shape food and drug law and regulation.

Chapter 2

Chapter 3

Overview of Drug, Biologic and Device Regulatory Pathways

Updated by Alix Alderman

OBJECTIVES

- To provide an overview of US federal regulations and processes related to the development of drugs, biologics, devices and combination products and filing of a marketing application

- To provide an overview of the scientific questions and approaches that underpin the development process

- To provide a roadmap of the facts and related decisions that define how a drug, biologic, device or combination product needs to be developed to meet US federal regulations

LAWS, REGULATIONS AND GUIDELINES COVERED IN THIS CHAPTER

- *Food and Drug Administration Safety and Innovation Act (January 2012)*

- 21 CFR 314.92 Drug products for which abbreviated applications may be submitted

- 21 CFR 314.93 Petition to request a change from a listed drug

- 21 CFR 314.54 Procedure for submission of an application requiring investigations for approval of a new indication for, or other change from, a listed drug

- 21 CFR 310.3 Definitions and interpretations (new drugs)

- 21 CFR 316 Orphan Drugs

- 21 CFR 312 Subpart E Drugs intended to treat life-threatening and severely debilitating illnesses

- 21 CFR 314 Subpart H Accelerated approval of new drugs for serious or life-threatening illnesses

- 21 CFR 312 Investigational New Drug Application

- 21 CFR 312.50 General responsibilities of sponsors

- 21 CFR 312.60 General responsibilities of investigators

- 21 CFR 312.33 Annual reports (IND)

- 21 CFR 312.32 IND safety reports

- 21 CFR 312.23 IND content and format

- 21 CFR 312.38 Withdrawal of an IND

- 21 CFR 312.45 Inactive status (IND)

- 21 CFR 314 Applications for FDA Approval to Market a New Drug

Chapter 3

- 21 CFR 207 Registration of Producers of Drugs and Listing of Drugs in Commercial Distribution
- 21 CFR 190.6 Requirement for premarket notification (dietary supplements)
- 21 CFR 3.2(e) Assignment of agency component for review of premarket applications—Definitions
- 21 CFR 328–358 OTC Monographs
- 21 CFR 330.11 NDA deviations from applicable monograph (OTC drugs)
- 21 CFR 10.30 Citizen petition
- 21 CFR 862–892 Device Classifications
- 21 CFR 807 Subpart E Premarket notification procedures
- 21 CFR 812 Investigational Device Exemptions
- 21 CFR 814 Subpart H Humanitarian use devices
- 21 CFR 56 Institutional Review Boards
- 21 CFR 50 Protection of Human Subjects
- 21 CFR 54 Financial Disclosure by Clinical Investigators
- 21 CFR 814 Premarket Approval of Medical Devices
- 21 CFR 807 Establishment Registration and Device Listing for Manufacturers and Initial Importers of Devices
- *Guidance for Industry: Bioavailability and Bioequivalence Studies for Orally Administered Drug Products—General Considerations* (March 2003)
- *Guidance for Industry: Food-Effect Bioavailability and Fed Bioequivalence Studies* (December 2002)
- *Guidance for Industry: Bioanalytical Method Validation* (May 2001)
- *Guidance for Industry: Statistical Approaches to Establishing Bioequivalence* (January 2001)
- *Guidance for Industry: 180-Day Exclusivity When Multiple ANDAs are Submitted on the Same Day* (July 2003)
- *Guidance for Industry: Bioequivalence Recommendations for Specific Products* (June 2012)
- *Guidance for Industry: Contents of a Complete Submission for the Evaluation of Proprietary Names* (February 2010)
- *Guidance for Industry: Formal Meetings Between the FDA and Sponsors or Applicants* (May 2009)
- *Guidance for Industry: End-of-Phase 2A Meetings* (September 2009)
- *Guidance for Industry: Special Protocol Assessment* (May 2002)
- *Guidance for Industry: Fast Track Drug Development Programs—Designation, Development, and Application Review* (January 2006)
- *Guidance for Industry M4: Organization of the CTD* (August 2001)
- *Guidance for Industry M4Q: The CTD—Quality* (August 2001)
- *Guidance for Industry M4S: The CTD—Safety* (August 2001)
- *Guidance for Industry M4S: The CTD—Safety Appendices* (August 2001)
- *Guidance for Industry M4E: The CTD—Efficacy* (August 2001)
- *Guidance for Industry M2 eCTD: Electronic Common Technical Document Specification* (April 2003)
- *Draft Guidance for Industry: Animal Models— Essential Elements to Address Efficacy Under the Animal Rule* (January 2009)
- *Guidance for Industry: Estimating the Maximum Safe Starting Dose in Initial Clinical Trials for Therapeutics in Adult Healthy Volunteers* (July 2005)

- *Guidance for Industry: M3(R2) Nonclinical Safety Studies for the Conduct of Human Clinical Trials and Marketing Authorization for Pharmaceuticals (January 2010)*

- *Guidance for Industry: M3(R2) Nonclinical Safety Studies for the Conduct of Human Clinical Trials and Marketing Authorization for Pharmaceuticals – Questions and Answers(R2) (February 2013)*

- *Guidance for Industry: Immunotoxicology Evaluation of Investigational New Drugs (October 2002)*

- *Guidance for Industry: Nonclinical Evaluation of Pediatric Drug Products (February 2006)*

- *Guidance for Industry: Single Dose Acute Toxicity Testing for Pharmaceuticals (August 1996)*

- *Guidance for Industry: Dissolution Testing of Immediate Release Solid Oral Dosage Forms (August 1997)*

- *Guidance for Industry: cGMP for Phase 1 Investigational Drugs (July 2008)*

- *Draft Guidance for Industry: Analytical Procedures and Methods Validation Chemistry, Manufacturing, and Controls Documentation (August 2000)*

- *Guidance for Industry: Collection of Race and Ethnicity Data in Clinical Trials (September 2005)*

- *Guidance for Industry: Exposure-Response Relationships—Study Design, Data Analysis, and Regulatory Applications (April 2003)*

- *Guidance for Industry: Drug-Induced Liver Injury: Premarketing Clinical Evaluation (July 2009)*

- *Guidance for Industry: S1C(R2) Dose Selection for Carcinogenicity Studies (September 2008)*

- *Draft Guidance for Industry: Drug Interaction Studies—Study Design, Data Analysis, Implications for Dosing and Labeling Recommendations (February 2012)*

- *Guidance for Industry: Pharmacokinetics in Patients with Impaired Hepatic Function: Study Design, Data Analysis, and Impact on Dosing and Labeling (May 2003)*

- *Guidance for Industry: Pharmacokinetics in Patients with Impaired Renal Function: Study Design, Data Analysis, and Impact on Dosing and Labeling (May 1998)*

- *Guidance for Industry: E7 Studies in Support of Special Populations: Geriatrics (August 1994)*

- *Guidance for Industry: E7 Studies in Support of Special Populations: Geriatrics – Questions and Answers (February 2012)*

- *Draft Guidance for Industry: How to Comply with the Pediatric Research Equity Act (September 2005)*

- *Guidance for Industry and Investigators – Safety Reporting Requirements for INDs and BA/BE Studies (December 2012)*

- *Guidance for Industry: E2F Development Safety Update Report (August 2011)*

- *Draft Guidance for Industry and Review Staff: Target Product Profile—A Strategic Development Process Tool (March 2007)*

- *Guidance for Industry: Guideline for the Format and Content of the Nonclinical Pharmacology/Toxicology Section of an Application (February 1987)*

- *Guidance for Industry: Reproductive and Developmental Toxicities —Integrating Study Results to Assess Concerns (September 2011)*

- *Draft Reviewer Guidance: Integration of Study Results to Assess Concerns about Human Reproductive and Developmental Toxicities (November 2001)*

- *Guidance for Industry and Review Staff: Recommended Approaches to Integration of Genetic Toxicology Study Results (January 2006)*

- *Draft Guidance for Industry: Statistical Aspects of the Design, Analysis, and Interpretation of Chronic Rodent Carcinogenicity Studies of Pharmaceuticals (May 2001)*

- *Guideline for the Format and Content of the Clinical and Statistical Sections of an Application* (July 1988)

- *Draft Guidance for Industry: Integrated Summary of Effectiveness* (August 2008)

- *Guidance for Industry: Premarketing Risk Assessment* (March 2005)

- *Guidance for Industry: Development and Use of Risk Minimization Action Plans* (March 2005)

- *Guidance for Industry: Good Pharmacovigilance Practices and Pharmacoepidemiologic Assessment* (March 2005)

- *Guidance for Industry: Submitting Separate Marketing Applications and Clinical Data for Purposes of Assessing User Fees* (December 2004)

- *Guidance for Industry: Standards for Securing the Drug Supply Chain—Standardized Numerical Identification for Prescription Drug Packages* (March 2010)

- *Draft Guidance for Industry: Forms for Registration of Producers of Drugs and Listing of Drugs in Commercial Distribution* (April 2001)

- *Draft Guidance for Industry: Applications Covered by Section 505(b)(2)* (October 1999)

- *Guidance for Industry: Structure/Function Claims Small Entity Compliance Guide* (January 2002)

- *The New 510(k) Paradigm—Alternate Approaches to Demonstrating Substantial Equivalence in Premarket Notifications—Final Guidance* (March 1998)

- *MAPP 6020.5: Good Review Practice: OND Review Management of INDs and NDAs for Nonprescription Drug Products* (July 2007)

- *Guidance for Industry: How to Write a Request for Designation (RFD)* (April 2011)

- *Draft Guidance for Industry and FDA Staff: Classification of Products as Drugs and Devices & Additional Product Classification Issues* (June 2011)

- *Guidance for Industry: Nonclinical Safety Evaluation of Drug or Biologic Combinations* (March 2006)

Introduction

The development of drugs, biologics and devices in the modern era is a scientific process (hypothesis testing and the recognition and control of dependent and independent variables) in the context of objective and subjective interpretations of a product's potential or actual risks and benefits. The scope, interpretation and application of US federal regulations that must be met to market a drug, biologic or device have evolved over the past century (generally in a reactive fashion, see Chapter 2 History of Food, Drug and Cosmetic Laws) and are documented in the Code of Federal Regulations (CFR). In practice, this translates into agency use of scientific review, standards, manufacturing and other inspections, advertising controls, conditional approvals, laboratory product testing and postmarketing pharmacovigilance activities. In the last quarter century, a plethora of US Food and Drug Administration (FDA) and International Conference on Harmonisation (ICH) guidelines have been issued to assist the regulatory professional in interpreting and defining the processes needed to successfully develop drugs and devices for marketing in a regulated industry. Although not enforceable as regulations, FDA guidelines (usually draft versions are available for public comment before finalization) provide an understanding of the agency's current thinking on any given topic.

This chapter provides an overview of the development and approval process for prescription drug, biologic, device and combination products in an environment regulated by the US government. Other chapters in this book provide details regarding many of the development and approval aspects touched on in this chapter. The purpose of this chapter is to tie the various topics together to provide a development context and roadmap.

Regulatory professionals must understand where regulations originate and how they are organized and updated. The difference between a law and a regulation is sometimes misunderstood. Only Congress can enact laws ("acts" of Congress). Federal executive departments and agencies such as FDA write the regulations to implement the authority of laws. The US Code (USC, which contains 19 "titles") is the official compilation of codified laws by subject, while the CFR is the official compilation of regulations. The CFR is updated annually (in April for food and drugs—Title 21) while the *Federal Register* is the daily supplement to the CFR. Thus, these two publications should be used together to find the latest version of a regulation. The original *Federal Food, Drug, and Cosmetic Act* of 1938 (*FD&C Act*) and its many subsequent amendments constitute the basic food and drug law of the US. A current version of this act can be found at www.fda.gov/RegulatoryInformation/Legislation/FederalFoodDrugandCosmeticActFDCAct/default.htm.

The CFR is divided into 50 titles that represent broad subject areas. Each title is divided into chapters, which usually bear the name of the issuing agency. Each chapter is further subdivided into parts that cover specific regulatory areas. Large parts may be subdivided into subparts. Finally, parts are divided into sections. Thus, the order for citations is: Title, CFR, Part, Section. For drugs and devices, Title 21 (Food and Drugs), and Chapter 1 (Food and Drug Administration) are the most relevant. There are 1,499 parts in Title 21 with the most applicable summarized in **Table 3-1**.

The CFR is accessible online, and the following FDA website is a convenient CFR research point for drugs and devices www.accessdata.fda.gov/scripts/cdrh/cfdocs/cfcfr/CFRSearch.cfm. The full CFR can be found and searched at www.ecfr.gov.

Although this book and the current chapter describe drug, biologic and device development and approval processes in the US, modern drug development is becoming more and more globalized. Hence, in any development program, consideration should be given to the impact of regulations in other world regions (for example, the usual requirement for a positive control in safety and efficacy trials of drugs in the EU).

Finally, this chapter touches on aspects of drug, biologic and device development to explain the relationships between different technical areas. Because chemistry, manufacturing and controls (CMC) relative to drugs and biologics involves a number of unique issues that are covered in detail in other chapters (including Good Manufacturing Practices (GMPs) and Quality Systems), this aspect of drug development is not emphasized in this chapter.

Drug, Device or Combination?

FDA regulates more than 150,000 marketed drugs and medical devices. At any time, nearly 3,000 investigational new drugs are being developed. Organizationally, FDA is part of the Public Health Service (PHS) within the Department of Health and Human Services (DHHS). PHS also oversees the Centers for Disease Control and Prevention (CDC), the National Institutes of Health (NIH) and other agencies.

The workload described above is primarily distributed across three centers and the numerous regional field offices within FDA's Office of Medical Products and Tobacco. Chapter 1 describes the primary centers and offices involved in drug and device development pathways. Since 1977, FDA centers have issued numerous guidances to increase the transparency of the development process and help move products through the process more rapidly. More recently, the Center for Drug Evaluation and Research (CDER) has developed a system of manuals of policies and procedures (MAPPs), which are written statements issued by CDER

Table 3-1. 21 CFR Parts Most Relevant to Drug and Device Development

21 CFR Parts	General Topics
1–100	Administrative Issues and Protection of Human Subjects
100s	Foods (not covered in this chapter except for dietary supplements)
200s	Labeling, CGMPs, Controlled Substances
300s	Drugs for Human Use
500s	Drugs for Animal Use
600s	Biologics
700s	Cosmetics (not covered in this chapter)
800s	Medical Devices
1000s–1400s	Contain many miscellaneous topics, but 1270 Human Tissues Intended for Transplantation and 1271 Human Cells, Tissues and Tissue-Based Products are relevant

management to prescribe policies, responsibilities or procedures for the conduct of the center's work or daily operations. "MAPP 4000.1—Developing and Issuing Manuals of Policies and Procedures" (updated most recently in 2011) describes the guidance development process. All MAPPs can be accessed at www.fda.gov/AboutFDA/CentersOffices/CDER/ManualofPoliciesProcedures/default.htm. Several MAPPs regarding agency review processes are useful in understanding how FDA staff will use information from sponsors to make regulatory decisions and can help sponsors prepare more reviewer-friendly documents. The Center for Biologics Evaluation and Research (CBER) has a similar system, termed manuals of standard operating procedures and policies (SOPPs).

Figure 3-1 shows the decision tree regarding which regulations and FDA center or office will primarily govern development and approval of any given drug, device or combination product. Because the purpose of this flow diagram is to provide a simple overview for situations that require FDA premarket review, some complexities, such as the distinction between drugs and biologics and the development of combination products, OTC drugs and dietary supplements, are not highlighted but are addressed in the text of this chapter.

Drugs

Generic Drugs for Human Use and the Abbreviated New Drug Application (ANDA)

Overview

In part as a result of the thalidomide tragedy, the *Kefauver-Harris Amendments* (*Drug Amendments*) to the *FD&C Act* were passed by Congress in 1962. These amendments required drug manufacturers to prove to FDA that their

Chapter 3

Figure 3-1. Decision Tree for Drug and Device Development and Approval for Situations that Require FDA Premarket Review

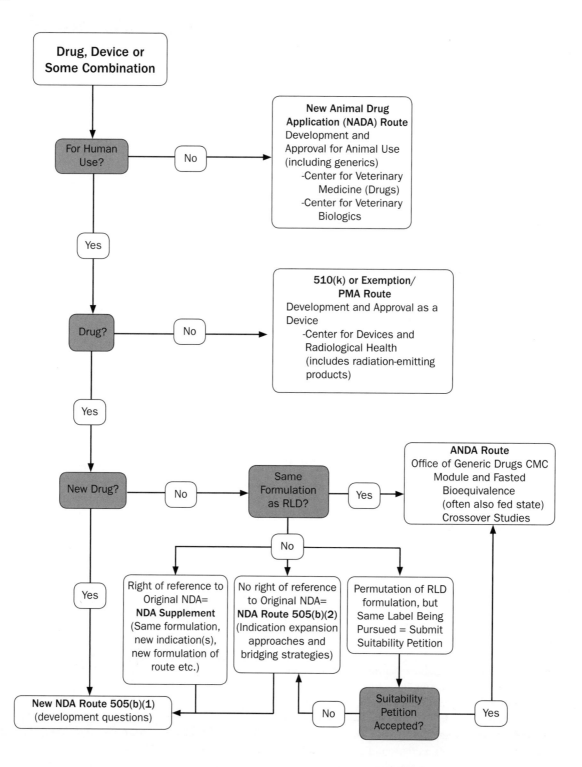

(ANDA, Abbreviated New Drug Application; CMC, Chemistry, Manufacturing, and Controls; NDA, New Drug Application; PMA, Premarket Approval; RLD, Reference Listed Drug (per *Orange Book*))

products were both safe and effective prior to marketing (only safety was required to be demonstrated in the original *FD&C Act*). The *Drug Amendments* also gave FDA control over prescription drug advertising and established GMPs and the requirement for informed consent of subjects in clinical trials. To comply, FDA contracted in 1966 with the National Academy of Sciences' National Research Council to study drugs that had been approved for safety only between 1938 and 1962 relative to the new requirement for demonstration of efficacy. The Drug Efficacy Study Implementation (DESI) program evaluated more than 3,000 separate products and 16,000 therapeutic claims. One of the early effects of the DESI program was the development of the ANDA. ANDAs were accepted for reviewed products that required changes in existing labeling to be in compliance.[1]

The modern era of generic drugs was born in 1984 with passage of the *Drug Price Competition and Patent Term Restoration Act* (the *Hatch-Waxman Act*), which represented a compromise between the innovator pharmaceutical industry and the generic pharmaceutical industry. This act expedited the availability of less-costly generic drugs by permitting FDA to approve abbreviated applications after the patent of the innovator drug had expired. They are termed "abbreviated" applications because they are not required to include animal safety and clinical data to establish safety and effectiveness, but for oral dosage forms must scientifically demonstrate that the product is bioequivalent to the innovator drug (Reference Listed Drug (RLD)). In the case of products that have a high solubility-high permeability rating (A/A rated), a waiver for *in vivo* bioequivalence testing can be obtained from FDA. To be bioequivalent, the generic drug product must deliver the same amount (within a range specified by FDA) of active ingredient into a subject's bloodstream over the same amount of time as the RLD. Specifically, a generic drug product is comparable to the innovator drug product in dosage form, strength, route of administration, quality, performance characteristics and intended use. All approved products, both innovator and generic, are listed in FDA's Approved Drug Products with Therapeutic Equivalence Evaluations (the *Orange Book*), which is accessible on FDA's website (www.accessdata.fda.gov/scripts/cder/ob/default.cfm). The *Orange Book* identifies the RLD and provides information on applicable patents and their expiration dates. A product approved under the ANDA process will have the same labeling as the RLD. Nearly 80% of total drug prescriptions dispensed in the US are generic.

The ANDA is comprised of three primary components:
- chemistry, manufacturing and controls (CMC) information
- bioequivalence data
- administrative information (including labeling and patent certification information)

ANDA requirements for CMC information and manufacture under CGMPs are not significantly different from NDA requirements. A relatively recent initiative in FDA's Office of Generic Drugs (OGD) to streamline the review process for the CMC section is submission of the ANDA Quality Overall Summary in question-based review (QbR) format (versus a more traditional non-question based summary format). The QbR questions and answers are placed in Module 2 of the Common Technical Document (CTD); therefore, QbR assumes the ANDA is submitted in CTD format, which is not mandatory but strongly suggested. OGD also has developed a standard group of summary tables (termed Model Bioequivalence Data Summary Tables) consistent with the CTD format to ensure consistent and concise data are submitted in the applicable sections of the ANDA.

The design, conduct and analysis of clinical bioequivalence studies are covered in *Guidance for Industry: Bioavailability and Bioequivalence Studies for Orally Administered Drug Products: General Considerations* (March 2003) and *Guidance for Industry: Food-Effect Bioavailability and Fed Bioequivalence Studies* (December 2002). A third guideline, *Guidance for Industry: Bioanalytical Method Validation* (May 2001), covers the requirements for validation of bioanalytical methods used to evaluate blood concentrations of the active ingredient, which also applies to drugs developed through the NDA route. OGD issued *Guidance for Industry: Bioequivalence Recommendations for Specific Products* in June 2012, indicating how and where OGD will release bioequivalence recommendations for specific products in the future.

Generally, two-way crossover bioequivalence studies (sometimes preceded by pilot studies to determine variability and group sizes) of the generic drug product versus the RLD in the fasted state are performed. If the label of the RLD indicates a food effect, a second study in the fed state (using a standardized high-fat meal) typically is required. Additional studies may be needed to demonstrate bioequivalence of different strengths if the ratio of excipients to the active pharmaceutical ingredient in each dosage strength of the generic drug is not the same. As defined by FDA, the generic is deemed bioequivalent to the RLD in any of the above studies if the 90% confidence interval for the ratio of population geometric means between the two treatments, based on log-transformed data, is contained within the equivalence limits of 80%–125% for the area under the curve (AUC) and peak serum concentration (C_{max}). A common misinterpretation of this is that levels of the active ingredient in generic drugs may vary from minus 20% to plus 25% compared to the innovator. In fact, those numbers relate to a derived statistical calculation and do not represent the actual difference in the amount of active ingredient in a patient's bloodstream, which is generally similar to the variation between different batches of the same innovator drug. For those who are statistically minded, *Guidance for Industry—Statistical Approaches to Establishing Bioequivalence* (January 2001), describes how to conduct the above analysis. If the bioequivalance studies are being conducted to support an ANDA, they do not have to be conducted under an IND, but do need to be reviewed and approved (including an informed consent form) by a duly constituted Institutional Review Board (IRB).

An ANDA must contain a statement by the applicant that one of the following patent certifications applies for the RLD:
- The patent information has not been filed (Paragraph I).
- The patent has expired (Paragraph II).
- The patent will expire on a specific date (Paragraph III), and the sponsor submitting the ANDA does not intend to market its product before that date.
- The patent is invalid or will not be infringed by the proposed drug product (Paragraph IV).

If the ANDA applicant certifies that the patent is invalid or will not be infringed (a Paragraph IV certification), the applicant is required to notify the NDA holder and patent owner. If the NDA holder brings an action for patent infringement within 45 days of this notification, FDA will not approve the ANDA for 30 months, or such shorter or longer period as a court may order, or until the date of a court decision (known as the 30-month stay). Originally, the 180-day exclusivity for generic drugs applied only to the first company to submit an ANDA with a Paragraph IV certification. However, the current approach to 180-day exclusivity (described in *Guidance to Industry: 180-Day Exclusivity When Multiple ANDAs are Submitted on the Same Day* (July 2003)) is applicable to all cases in which multiple ANDA applicants submit Paragraph IV certifications challenging the same listed patent or patents on the same first day. This provides a shared incentive for multiple companies willing to challenge a listed patent and possibly defend a patent infringement suit.

Although the development time for a generic is relatively short, ANDA review (several hundred applications each year) and approval times average approximately two years, and clearly impact the timeframe for moving generic products to the market. This suggests a proactive strategy of submitting ANDA applications well in advance of patent expiration date. A company with an approved ANDA is subject to the same postapproval reporting requirements as an NDA holder (21 CFR 314.80: Postmarketing reporting of adverse drug experiences and 21 CFR 314.81: Field alert reports and annual reports). Many of the topics above are covered in more detail in Chapter 13 Generic Drug Submissions. The OGD website is also a good resource (www.fda.gov/AboutFDA/CentersOffices/OfficeofMedicalProductsandTobacco/CDER/ucm119100.htm).

Suitability Petitions

The regulations regarding ANDAs are contained in 21 CFR 314.92 and Section 505(j) of the *FD&C Act*. In addition, 21 CFR 314.92 cross-references the limits set forth in 21 CFR 314.93 for what characteristics a generic drug not identical to the RLD can possess and still potentially be submitted as an ANDA, subject to acceptance by FDA of a suitability petition. A suitability petition by the sponsor seeks permission to file an ANDA for the drug product and contains comparisons and contrasts between the generic drug and the RLD, forming the basis for approval. FDA is required to respond to the petition within 90 days. If a suitability petition is not accepted, an NDA under Section 505(b)(2) of the *FD&C Act* may be an option. Another route is a citizen petition. Details of this latter approach are beyond the scope of this chapter.

Branded and Authorized Generics

Recently, "branded" generics have become more prevalent. Branded generics are approved in the same manner as all generics, but the ANDA applicant also applies for and receives a brand (i.e., proprietary) name under the same process used for NDAs (*Guidance for Industry: Contents of a Complete Submission for the Evaluation of Proprietary Names* (February 2010)). A brand name will allow the company to distinguish its generic from others if marketing activities are contemplated.

An "authorized generic" is a drug product for which there is a licensing agreement between the innovator company and a generic drug manufacturer. It allows the innovator company to obtain revenue through the generic process by licensing a manufacturer to market the RLD as a generic using a different "trade dress" while continuing to market the innovator drug under the original proprietary name. A list (updated quarterly) of authorized generics, including the original NDA applicant name, is available on the CDER OGD website (www.fda.gov/AboutFDA/CentersOffices/OfficeofMedicalProductsandTobacco/CDER/ucm119100.htm). The appeal of this approach is avoiding the ANDA review and approval process; instead, the generic can be added to the original NDA as a supplement or described in the NDA annual report and allows the company to continue to profit from the generic product.

In March 2010, the *Patient Protection and Affordable Care Act* was signed into law. This act contains a subtitle called the *Biologics Price Competition and Innovation Act of 2009* (*BPCI Act*) that amends Section 351 of *Public Health Service Act* and other statutes to create an abbreviated approval pathway for biological products shown to be highly similar (biosimilar) to, or interchangeable with, an FDA-licensed reference biological product. FDA is currently soliciting input regarding the agency's implementation of the statute and considering how to deal with biosimilars that are regulated under Section 505 of the

FD&C Act (well-characterized proteins and peptides). The approval process for biosimilars is more mature in the EU, and further details of the biosimilar development approach, issues and examples can be reviewed on the relevant EU websites.

Chapter 13 provides a more detailed discussion of the generic drug approval process.

New Chemical Entities and the New Drug Application for a Marketing Application for Human Use (Section 505(b)(1) of the FD&C Act)

Overview of the Approach to Drug Development and Approval

A "drug" is defined as a product used in diagnosing, curing, mitigating, treating or preventing a disease or affecting a structure or function of the body (21 CFR 310.3). Under the same regulation, a drug is considered a new drug if:
- There is a new drug use of any substance (e.g., active ingredient, excipient, carrier, coating etc.) which composes the drug.
- There is a new drug use of a combination of approved drugs.
- The proportion of the ingredients in combination is changed.
- There is a new intended use for the drug.
- The dosage, method or duration of administration or application is changed.

Thus, the following are subject to FDA approval:
1. a drug containing a novel chemical compound as its active ingredient (new chemical entity (NCE))
2. a drug containing an existing active ingredient that has never been approved for use as a medicine in the US (also an NCE)
3. a drug previously approved by FDA but now proposed for a new use or indication
4. a drug previously approved by FDA but in a dosage form, route of administration or other key condition of use different from what was originally approved

The distinction between the regulation of a drug and a biologic is primarily based on historic issues. As a result of the St. Louis tetanus contamination due to infected serum and smaller occurrences of contaminated smallpox vaccine and diphtheria antitoxin, Congress passed the *Virus Serum and Toxin Act* (also known as the *Biologics Control Act*) in 1902. The act authorized the Hygienic Laboratory of the Public Health and Marine Hospital Service (which eventually became PHS) to issue regulations governing all aspects of commercial production of vaccines, serums, toxins, antitoxin and similar products with the objective of ensuring their safety, purity and potency. In 1934, the Hygienic Laboratory (renamed NIH in 1930 by the *Ransdell Act*) issued a regulation stating that licenses to manufacture new biologics would not be granted without evidence that the products were effective. The *Public Health Service Act* of 1944 (*PHS Act*) saw the reorganization of PHS, with authority given to NIH to license, research and develop new biological products. Hence, one of the primary historical differences between biologics and drugs has been the inherent government research component of biologics as opposed to the testing and regulation emphasis for drugs.[2] In addition, because biologics are derived from living organisms, immunogenicity issues and how they are addressed in nonclinical and clinical studies often distinguish them from small-molecule drugs.

In 1972, the Division of Biological Standards (part of NIH and in turn part of PHS) was transferred to FDA and eventually became CBER. Although the *PHS Act* established the regulation of biologics licensure, biologics are classified as drugs under the *FD&C Act*, and new biologic products require approval based on safety and efficacy prior to marketing (through a Biologics License Application (BLA) as opposed to an NDA). Biologics are defined as substances derived from or made with the aid of living organisms. Review and approval of most of these products is conducted by CBER. To allow CBER to focus its expertise on vaccines, blood products and other, more-complex products such as gene therapy, FDA shifted the review and approval of biological therapeutics (primarily oncology products, peptides or well-characterized proteins) from CBER to CDER in 2003. Chapter 1 summarizes the types of products now regulated by the two centers.

The intake of any exogenous substance that has pharmacological actions on the body presents some level of risk. Drug development consists of characterizing the safety profile (risk) and the efficacy profile (benefit) as it relates to the body's exposure to the drug (pharmacokinetic profile). The most successful drugs are those with minimal risk and maximum benefit. To align development with continuous evaluation of risk and benefit, it is often productive to consider questions and answers that affect decisions on whether to continue a drug's development to the point of submitting a marketing application. The order and importance of these questions are different for each drug based on aspects such as the product (formulation) chemical and physical characteristics, the route of administration, the target patient population, the medical need, the ability to monitor safety, the ability to predict potential benefits from pharmacodynamic measures (surrogate endpoints) and the duration of treatment needed to demonstrate efficacy.

Table 3-2 lists some of the key questions FDA expects to be addressed as a drug is developed. Generally, due to risk, cost and time, evaluations are performed in the following order:
- *in vitro*
- live animals (juvenile if applicable)

Table 3-2. Key Questions to be Addressed in a Drug Development Program

In Vitro—Animals—Adults—Children		
Safety (Risk)	**Pharmacokinetics** (What the body does to the drug)	**Pharmacodynamics/Efficacy** (Benefit)
How do you maximize the intellectual property aspect of the product?		
What is the known safety profile of other drugs like yours or the class of drugs in general? For a new class of drugs or mechanism of action this will not necessarily be known and hence associated with more risk.	Are there competitor drugs that have a less than ideal route of administration or pharmacokinetic profile (e.g., substrates, inhibitors or inducers of more commonly used cytochrome P [CYP] 450 isoenzyme pathways)?	What endpoints have been accepted by FDA for other drugs developed to treat the target disease, or is this a first-in-class drug?
What safety profile would provide a competitive advantage?	What pharmacokinetic (including route of administration) profile would provide a competitive advantage?	What is the potential breadth of the target indication(s)?
What do you want to say in your label? (this will drive the development of your product)		
What are the target organs/systems for toxicity?	What exposure profiles produce target organ/system effects?	What are the target organs/systems for pharmacological effects?
What toxicity is observed acutely versus chronically?	How is the time course of the effects related to the time-concentration curves of the parent drug and its metabolites?	What is the time course and duration of pharmacological/ therapeutic effects?
Can the toxicities be monitored?	Are there potential or actual interactions with other drugs (especially those most commonly used by the target patient population)?	How do you measure the benefits?
Are the toxicities reversible?	What are the single-dose versus steady-state pharmacokinetics of the drug and its metabolites?	What happens to the therapeutic effects when you stop dosing?
What is the maximum tolerated dose and what are risks of overdose?	Is the pharmacokinetic profile linear?	What is the minimal effective dose and duration of treatment?
What are the frequency and severity of safety findings?	How variable (intra- and inter-subject) are drug concentrations (may be impacted by drug bioavailability or greater involvement of the more commonly used CYP isoenzyme systems)?	How reproducible and clinically relevant are the pharmacodynamic and/or efficacy endpoints (speaks to the validity of the endpoints)?

- adult humans (often in healthy subjects before patients)
- children (if applicable)

However, as information is gained, new hypotheses may need to be tested. Therefore, drug development often is an iterative, dynamic process that involves ongoing effective communication between all the disciplines involved.

Table 3-2 identifies key questions to be addressed in a drug development program, i.e., how a company can maximize the market share of its product and realize the maximum return on investment with the least amount of risk. The sections below describe key aspects of the drug development process and regulatory tools and approaches to help reach these goals.

FDA Interface and Development Leverage Options

The relationship between FDA and an investigational drug product sponsor can begin very early in the process (before the sponsor submits an IND to test the product in humans) and extends through the typical IND development process (often defined as Phases 1, 2 and 3) to a marketing application and postapproval commitments, safety surveillance and product lifecycle management. It is important to structure the presentation to meet FDA expectations. To succeed, it is important to learn—through experience or interaction—the relevant review division's approach to issues under its purview. The most effective interfaces between sponsors and FDA are typically formal meetings and Special Protocol Assessment (SPA) requests.

FDA–Sponsor Meetings

Sponsor meetings with FDA prior to 1997 took whatever form the reviewing divison chose to follow. It was not until the reauthorization of the 1992 *Prescription Drug User Fee Act* in 1997 (*PDUFA II*) that a formal process for meetings (with expectations and commitments from both parties) was established. Processes for the request and classification of meetings are covered in *Guidance for Industry: Formal Meetings Between the FDA and Sponsors or Applicants* (May 2009). Different kinds of meetings are categorized as Type A, B or C, with different associated timelines (see aforementioned guidance). Meetings can be requested at any time for any valid reason, but FDA will decide whether there is sufficient justification for a meeting (usually dictated by the product background and draft questions submitted in a written meeting request) or if a written response to questions and/or a teleconference would suffice. Most commonly, meetings are classified as either Pre-IND, End-of-Phase 2 (see also, *Guidance for Industry: End-of Phase 2A Meetings* (September 2009)) or Pre-NDA. For products that have been granted accelerated approval or fast track, an End-of-Phase 1 meeting generally will be granted.

For any meeting with FDA, it is important to submit clear and meaningful draft questions and a supporting pre-meeting package that is not merely a summary of what is known about a given drug (e.g., submission of only an Investigator's Brochure). Chapter 4 FDA Communications and Meetings provides a more detailed discussion of this topic.

SPA

The SPA process is described in *Guidance for Industry: Special Protocol Assessment* (May 2002). Although prior to 1997, FDA reviewed draft protocols on a case-by-case basis, the process often took several months and did not always address all the issues. As a result of *PDUFA II*, the SPA process was established. When appropriate, FDA will evaluate certain protocols and related issues within 45 days of receipt to determine whether they meet scientific and regulatory requirements identified by the sponsor (in the form of specific questions). Three types of protocols are eligible for an SPA under the *PDUFA* goals:

1. animal carcinogenicity protocols
2. final product stability protocols
3. clinical protocols for Phase 3 trials, the data from which will form the basis for an efficacy claim (i.e., a pivotal trial) if the trials were discussed at an End-of-Phase 2/Pre-Phase 3 meeting with the review division, or in some cases, if the division is aware of the developmental context in which the protocol is being reviewed and the questions are being posed

The clinical protocols for Phase 3 trials can relate to efficacy claims that will be part of an original NDA/BLA or an efficacy supplement to an approved NDA/BLA. Although the initial 45-day period is generally adhered to, depending upon FDA's responses to the questions, there could be several review/response cycles (that are no longer part of the timeframe) to reach a final understanding with the sponsor. If documentation of the final agreement is not provided by the FDA review division, the sponsor should request written communication from FDA acknowledging the final agreement.

In addition, sponsors have several available avenues to help focus FDA attention on the drug development program and expedite marketing application approval. These include orphan drug designation (when eligible) and, for drugs indicated for serious or life-threatening conditions, fast track development designation with opportunities for a "rolling NDA or BLA" and priority review. Sponsors also may seek accelerated NDA review based on a surrogate endpoint or an effect on a clinical endpoint other than survival or irreversible morbidity. Details are described in 21 CFR 314.510, Subpart H Accelerated Approval of New Drugs for Serious or Life-threatening Illnesses. Confirmatory studies are likely to be required if FDA approves an NDA under Subpart H.

Orphan Drug Designation

The *Orphan Drug Act* was signed into law in 1983 and, for the first time, provided incentives for development of drugs necessary, and often lifesaving, for patients with rare diseases but with minimal prospects for commercial return on investment. The *Orphan Drug Act* is codified in 21 CFR 316.

Since 1983, Congress has amended the act several times.

- The 1984 amendment redefined "rare disease or condition" as affecting fewer than 200,000 persons in the US at a given point or for which there is no reasonable expectation of recovering development costs through US sales.
- The 1985 amendment extended the marketing exclusivity to patentable as well as unpatentable drugs and allowed federal grants for the clinical evaluation of orphan-designated drugs.
- The 1988 amendment required industry sponsors to apply for orphan designation prior to submission of a marketing application.
- The *Food and Drug Administration Modernization Act* of 1997 (*FDAMA*) included a provision that exempted designated orphan drug products from paying new drug application fees (user fees). It also allowed sponsors to seek waivers of annual postapproval establishment and product fees on a case-by-case, year-by-year basis.
- The *Food and Drug Administration Safety and Innovation Act (FDASIA),* signed in July 2012, expanded the accelerated approval pathway, defined a new "breakthrough therapy" designation and increased FDA's communication with rare disease medical experts.

The *Orphan Drug Act* provides a number of specific incentives for sponsors:
- seven years of exclusive marketing rights for the designated indication once the drug receives FDA marketing approval
- a tax credit for up to 50% of qualified clinical research expenses incurred in developing a designated orphan product (This tax credit has a provision that allows the sponsor to carry the excess credit back one tax year if unable to use part or all of the credit because of tax liability limits, and then to carry forward any additional unused credit for up to 20 years after the year of the credit. The latter is important to start-up companies that may not make any profits until the drug is on the market. The US Internal Revenue Service administers the tax credit provisions of the *Orphan Drug Act*.)
- eligibility to apply for orphan drug grants

There is no formal application for orphan drug designation in the US; however, the European Medicines Agency (EMA) and FDA's Office of Orphan Products Development (OOPD) have developed a common application, benefitting sponsors seeking orphan drug designation in both regions. For US-only applications, the OOPD/EMA common application may be used, or sponsors can produce a request consistent with the provisions of 21 CFR 316.20, which identifies the information to be included in a complete, signed and dated document. Essentially, it is a text document with appropriate literature references appended. References are provided to support the incidence statements and can increase the total size of the submission to approximately one to three volumes of paper (a volume is generally defined as between 250 and 350 pages).

An application for orphan drug designation generally includes:
- specific rare disease or condition for which designation is being requested
- sponsor contact, drug names and sources
- description of the rare disease or condition with a medically plausible rationale for any patient subset type of approach
- description of the drug and the scientific rationale for its use for the rare disease or condition
- summary of the drug's regulatory status and marketing history
- for a treatment indication, documentation that the disease or condition affects fewer than 200,000 people in the US (prevalence)
- for a prevention indication, documentation that the disease or condition affects fewer than 200,000 people in the US per year (incidence)
- alternatively, a rationale for why there is no reasonable expectation that costs of research and development for the indication can be recovered by US sales

Specifics on the submission format and other details are available on FDA's website (www.fda.gov/ForIndustry/DevelopingProductsforRareDiseasesConditions/default.htm). Once the request for designation has been received, OOPD will send a receipt letter, and a formal response will take one to three months. Upon notification of orphan drug designation, the sponsor's name and the proposed rare disease or condition will be published in the *Federal Register*.

Once an orphan drug designation has been granted by FDA, it can only be revoked if the application is found to contain false data or there is insufficient drug product to supply market needs. Notably, the designation cannot be revoked even if post-designation prevalence exceeds the original estimates. Finally, the sponsor must provide annual updates that contain a brief summary of any ongoing or completed nonclinical or clinical studies; a description of the investigational plan for the coming year; as well as any anticipated difficulties in development, testing and marketing; and a brief discussion of any changes that may affect the product's orphan drug status. Further details are covered in Chapter 26 Regulation of Products for Small Patient Populations.

Fast Track Designation

The Fast Track Drug Development Program designation process is described in *Guidance for Industry: Fast Track Drug Development Programs—Designation, Development, and Application Review* (January 2006). FDA better defined the program (see 21 CFR 312 Subpart E) as a result of *FDAMA* in 1997. The fast track program is designed to facilitate the development and expedite the review of new drugs intended to treat serious or life-threatening conditions and that demonstrate the potential to address unmet medical needs. A disease is considered serious based on the likelihood that if left untreated, it will progress from a less-severe to a more-severe condition (e.g., AIDS, Alzheimer's disease, heart failure and cancer, but also epilepsy, depression and diabetes). FDA defines "meeting an unmet medical need" as providing a therapy where none exists or that may be superior to existing therapy by either:
- showing superior effectiveness
- avoiding serious side effects of an available treatment
- improving the diagnosis of a serious disease where early diagnosis results in an improved outcome
- decreasing a clinically significant toxicity of an accepted treatment

Depending upon the stage of drug development, data that become available should support the drug's potential to address unmet medical needs, and the development plan should be designed to assess this potential. The agency will rely on summaries of available data to determine whether the potential to address unmet medical needs has been demonstrated and will provide a designation response within 60 days of receipt of the request. When fast track designation is no longer supported by emerging data or the designated drug development program is no longer being pursued, FDA may choose to send a letter notifying the sponsor that the product is no longer classified as fast track.

A sponsor may request fast track designation at any point in the development process. A product that is in a fast track development program is eligible for heightened interest by FDA in sponsor meetings, a greater probability of priority review of the marketing application (six months versus the standard 10 months) and piecemeal submission of portions (complete CTD modules—constituting a "reviewable unit") of a marketing application (referred to as a "rolling NDA or BLA"). Note that this latter provision is unique to fast track programs, but needs to be specifically requested. Moreover, the FDA review clock for the rolling NDA does not start until the marketing application submission is complete.

Breakthrough Therapy Designation

The goal of the breakthrough therapy initiative is to expedite the development and review of a potential new medicine if it is "intended, alone or in combination with one or more other drugs, to treat a serious or life-threatening disease or condition, and preliminary clinical evidence indicates that the drug may demonstrate substantial improvement over existing therapies on one or more clinically significant endpoints, such as substantial treatment effects observed early in clinical development." The designation of a drug as a breakthrough therapy was enacted as part of *FDASIA*.

Section 902 of *FDASIA* includes a provision that allows sponsors to request that their drug be designated as a breakthrough therapy. FDA is in the process of developing guidance related to this designation. Until guidance is developed, a request for breakthrough therapy designation should be submitted concurrently with, or as an amendment to an IND with a cover letter, a completed Form FDA 1571, and identification in the cover letter of the submission as a REQUEST FOR BREAKTHROUGH THERAPY DESIGNATION. No later than 60 days after receipt of the submission, a determination will be made to either grant or deny the request for breakthrough therapy designation in the form of a designation letter (for requests granted) and a non-designation letter (for requests denied). FDA has posted "Fact Sheet: Breakthrough Therapies" to guide sponsors who may be seeking this designation on their website (www.fda.gov/RegulatoryInformation/Legislation/FederalFoodDrugandCosmeticActFDCAct/SignificantAmendmentstotheFDCAct/FDASIA/ucm329491.htm). Frequently asked questions about breakthrough therapies can also be found on the FDA website (www.fda.gov/RegulatoryInformation/Legislation/FederalFoodDrugandCosmeticActFDCAct/SignificantAmendmentstotheFDCAct/FDASIA/ucm341027.htm).

ICH and FDA Guidelines and Their Relationship to the Development Process

ICH and the CTD Format

ICH was formed in 1990. It is a unique project that brings together the regulatory authorities of EU, Japan and the US and experts from the pharmaceutical industry in the three regions to discuss scientific and technical aspects of product registration. ICH recommends ways to achieve greater harmonization in the interpretation and application of technical guidelines and requirements for product registration to reduce or avoid duplicating testing during the research and development of new drugs. The objectives are conservation of human, animal and material resources and elimination of unnecessary delays in global development and availability of new medicines, while safeguarding quality, safety and efficacy and protecting public health.

The ICH process has resulted in numerous guidelines in four major categories:

1. Quality—topics relating to chemical and pharmaceutical quality assurance, including stability testing and impurity testing
2. Safety—topics relating to *in vitro* and *in vivo* nonclinical studies, including carcinogenicity testing and genotoxicity testing
3. Efficacy—topics relating to clinical studies in human subjects, including dose-response studies and GCPs
4. Multidisciplinary—topics covering cross-disciplinary issues or not uniquely fitting into one of the other categories, including *Medical Dictionary for Regulatory Activities* (*MedDRA*) terminology, the CTD and electronic CTD (eCTD) submissions

Copies of these guidelines and information on their history and status in the four-step review and consensus process are available at www.ich.org/products/guidelines.html. The majority of these guidelines have been accepted by FDA as reflecting current agency thinking (as documented in *Federal Register* announcements).

Two important aspects of the ICH endeavor are the CTD concept and *MedDRA*. The CTD is divided into five modules as shown in **Figure 3-2,** with a hierarchical structure with the most detail at the base leading to higher and higher level summaries and integration. *Guidance for Industry M4: Organization of the CTD* (2001) provides further details.

Module 1 is region-specific (US, EU, Japan). Modules 2, 3, 4 and 5 are intended to be common for all regions. For US submissions, Module 1 will contain various FDA forms, draft labeling, Risk Evaluation and Mitigation Strategies (REMS) plans, key FDA correspondence (e.g., FDA meeting minutes), patent information and the Investigator's

Figure 3-2. CTD Organization

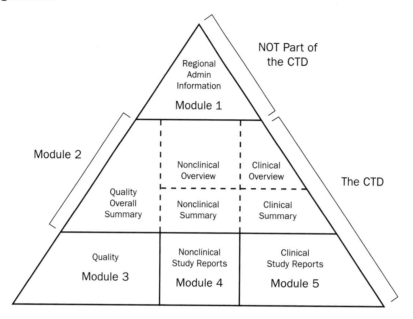

Brochure (IB) (important if the CTD format is used at the IND stage). Module 2 contains CTD summaries of the three technical areas:

- Module 3 Quality (see *Guidance for Industry M4Q: The CTD—Quality* (August 2001)) and corresponding summary in Module 2.3
- Module 4 Nonclinical/Safety (see *Guidance for Industry M4S: The CTD—Safety* (August 2001) and *Guidance for Industry M4S: The CTD—Safety Appendices* (August 2001)) and corresponding summaries in Module 2.4 Nonclinical Overview and 2.6 Nonclinical Written and Tabulated Summaries
- Module 5 Clinical (see *Guidance for Industry M4E: The CTD—Efficacy* (August 2001)) and corresponding summaries in Module 2.5 Clinical Overview and 2.7 Clinical Summary

Module 2 also has several sections, the goal of which is to provide a concise context for the reviewer and integrate key risk/benefit data. The above-cited guidelines contain not only information on their respective modules, but also what should be included in the related portions of Module 2. If submitting electronically, *Guidance for Industry M2 eCTD: Electronic Common Technical Document Specification* (April 2003) is a key starting point.

MedDRA, the currently accepted international medical terminology dictionary developed by ICH, is designed to support the classification, retrieval, presentation and communication of medical information throughout the regulatory cycle for drugs and medical devices. It is particularly important in the electronic transmission of adverse event reporting and the coding of clinical trial data. Further details are available at www.meddramsso.com/public_subscribe_meddra.asp and in associated ICH *MedDRA* specific guidelines. *MedDRA* replaces the older *Coding Symbols for a Thesaurus of Adverse Reaction Terms* (COSTART) dictionary.

Guidance Documents

Collectively, CDER and CBER have issued more than 800 guidelines since 1977. These range from general topics addressing a number of the issues. They are not regulations, but do represent FDA's current thinking on a given topic. However, some guidelines are relatively old, so the definition of "current thinking" often needs to be validated by recent experience with the agency in the area covered by the guidance. Because they are guidance documents, they should not be blindly followed, but consideration should be given to their intent and applicability to a given development issue.

The Initial IND and the IND Amendment Process

Before initiating a clinical trial in the US (other than bioequivalence studies to support an ANDA), the drug product sponsor must submit nonclinical, CMC and previous human experience data (if applicable) to FDA in a notice of claimed investigational exemption for a new drug in the form of an IND. The IND application requests permission to initiate clinical trials. IND regulations are detailed in 21 CFR 312.

The IND application is not a request for approval; rather, it is a request for exemption from federal law. Federal law requires that prior to transporting or distributing a drug in interstate commerce, an NDA or BLA must be approved by FDA. Because in most cases the drug product must be shipped to investigative sites across state lines to be used in clinical trials, the sponsor must receive an exemption from this legal requirement.

After receipt of the initial IND application, FDA will send the sponsor a letter with the assigned IND number (note that an IND number with a "P" preface can be obtained at a pre-IND meeting, and the final IND number is the same minus this preface). The letter will indicate that the proposed clinical trial cannot begin until 30 calendar days after receipt of the IND. This 30-day safety review period gives FDA an opportunity to determine whether the data in the IND application support the safety of subjects in the proposed clinical trial. Following review, rather than providing formal approval, the agency will take action on the application as follows. If the proposed study is judged not to be reasonably safe for human subjects, FDA is required to inform the sponsor within 30 calendar days of receipt of the IND application that it may not begin the clinical trial (clinical hold). If the sponsor is not contacted by FDA within 30 days, approval to initiate clinical trials is implicit. In the latter case, it is advisable for the sponsor to contact the FDA project manager assigned to the IND to develop a relationship and to confirm the results of the review.

For the initial IND (the same is true for NDAs), FDA assigns a review team led by a regulatory project manager (RPM) that includes a medical reviewer and pharmacology/toxicology reviewer from the review division. Generally, a CMC reviewer from the Office of New Drug Quality Assessment (ONDQA) is assigned. Depending upon the proposed study, a clinical pharmacologist from the Office of Clinical Pharmacology and a statistician from the Office of Biostatistics may be assigned as well. The team generally will meet the week that the 30-day review period ends and, with the division director, decide whether the proposed study may proceed. In some cases, the RPM may contact the sponsor to request additional information or to propose that the study may be initiated if certain amendments are made to the study protocol. In the latter case, or in the case of clinical hold, FDA eventually will issue a letter containing the details of any requested modifications to the protocol or supporting data.

If a Pre-IND meeting was held with FDA, the assigned P-IND number becomes the IND number (the "P" is removed), and the initial submission is given a serial number (SN) 0000. Form FDA 1571 must accompany any submission (except a Pre-IND meeting request) to the IND (termed an IND amendment), and each submission is given the next consecutive SN by the sponsor. This form is completed and signed by the sponsor or its authorized representative to acknowledge sponsor responsibilities as codified in 21 CFR 312.50. Form FDA 1571 contains sponsor and drug product information and an indication of what the submission contains. Any initial IND submission must contain a clinical study protocol and at least one (if a multicenter study) completed Form FDA 1572. This form contains study site details and IRB name and address, as well as a signoff by the investigator acknowledging legal responsibilities as indicated on the form and in 21 CFR 312.60. The investigator's curriculum vitae, documenting qualifications to conduct the proposed study, is submitted with the Form FDA 1572. There is no 30-day review period for IND amendments.

Where previous clinical studies have not been conducted for an NCE, the initial IND is a major milestone because it summarizes the data that support moving a drug from *in vitro* and animal testing into evaluation in humans. There are a number of guidances (some in draft stage) on the content and issues relating to either first-in-human or IND clinical trials, including:

- *Draft Guidance for Industry: Animal Models—Essential Elements to Address Efficacy Under the Animal Rule* (January 2009)
- *Guidance for Industry: Estimating the Maximum Safe Starting Dose in Initial Clinical Trials for Therapeutics in Adult Healthy Volunteers* (July 2005)
- *ICH Guideline for Industry M3(R2): Guidance on Nonclinical Safety Studies for the Conduct of Human Clinical Trials and Marketing Authorization for Pharmaceuticals* (June 2009)
- *Guidance for Industry: M3(R2) Nonclinical Safety Studies for the Conduct of Human Clinical Trials and Marketing Authorization for Pharmaceuticals – Questions and Answers(R2)* (February 2013)
- *Guidance for Industry: Immunotoxicology Evaluation of Investigational New Drugs* (October 2002)
- *Guidance for Industry: Nonclinical Evaluation of Pediatric Drug Products* (February 2006)
- *Guidance for Industry: Single Dose Acute Toxicity Testing for Pharmaceuticals* (August 1996)
- *Guidance for Industry: Dissolution Testing of Immediate Release Solid Oral Dosage Forms* (August 1997)
- *Guidance for Industry: cGMP for Phase 1 Investigational Drugs* (July 2008)
- *Draft Guidance for Industry: Analytical Procedures and Methods Validation Chemistry, Manufacturing, and Controls Documentation* (August 2000)
- *Guidance for Industry: Collection of Race and Ethnicity Data in Clinical Trials* (September 2005)
- *Guidance for Industry: Exposure-Response Relationships—Study Design, Data Analysis, and Regulatory Applications* (April 2003)
- *Guidance for Industry: Drug-Induced Liver Injury: Premarketing Clinical Evaluation* (July 2009)
- *Guidance for Industry: S1C(R2) Dose Selection for Carcinogenicity Studies* (September 2008)

Table 3-3. IND Safety Reporting Timeframes

SAE Outcome	Deadline for Reporting
Fatal or life-threatening	7 calendar days, by phone or facsimile, followed by a written report within 8 additional calendar days
All other outcomes	15 calendar days, in writing

- *Draft Guidance for Industry: Drug Interaction Studies—Study Design, Data Analysis, Implications for Dosing and Labeling Recommendations* (February 2012)
- *Guidance for Industry: Pharmacokinetics in Patients with Impaired Hepatic Function: Study Design, Data Analysis, and Impact on Dosing and Labeling* (May 2003)
- *Guidance for Industry: Pharmacokinetics in Patients with Impaired Renal Function: Study Design, Data Analysis, and Impact on Dosing and Labeling* (May 1998)
- *Guideline for Industry: Studies in Support of Special Populations: Geriatrics* (August 1994)
- *Draft Guidance for Industry: How to Comply with the Pediatric Research Equity Act* (September 2005)

In addition, a number of other FDA guidelines specific to certain therapeutic indications should be consulted when relevant.

The content and format of an initial IND are described in 21 CFR 312.23. Traditionally, the content follows the items listed in Section 12 of Form FDA 1571 and includes an IB, clinical protocol, CMC information, nonclinical pharmacology and toxicology information and previous human experience information (the latter only if relevant). Although an initial IND can still be submitted in paper format (three copies of the submission are required), using the CTD format for the initial IND submission is becoming more common and is accepted by FDA. The advantage of this approach, especially when done electronically, is that it begins building a CTD for an eventual marketing application that is progressively updated during the course of drug development under the IND. The disadvantages are that the CTD structure in some areas (especially Module 1 and 2) does not easily fit the information available at an initial IND stage, and Section 12 of FDA Form 1571 (application contents) does not currently directly correlate with the CTD structure. If submitted electronically, the initial IND must be in eCTD format (with the same considerations as for an electronically submitted NDA). However, once an IND is submitted electronically, all future IND submissions also must be submitted electronically.

For active INDs (an IND can be withdrawn (21 CFR 312.38) or considered inactive (21CFR 312.45)), sponsors are required to submit expedited safety reports for serious, unexpected adverse reactions to the IND (IND Safety Reports) as per the definitions provided in 21 CFR 312.32. A serious adverse event (SAE) is any untoward medical occurrence that results in death, is life-threatening, requires subject hospitalization or prolongation of existing hospitalization, results in persistent or significant disability/incapacity or is a congenital anomaly/birth defect. Submission of IND safety reports to FDA is time sensitive. The date that the sponsor is notified of the SAE by the study site is considered Day 1, and all reporting timeframes are tied to this notification. **Table 3-3** summarizes these requirements. *Guidance for Industry and Investigators—Safety Reporting Requirements for INDs and BA/BE Studies* (December 2012) provides further details and covers SAE reporting requirements for bioavailability (BA) and bioequivalence (BE) studies.

IND sponsors are required to submit annual reports to the IND within 60 days of the anniversary of the date the IND went into effect (21 CFR 312.33). The annual report focuses on safety signals (deaths or other SAEs, dropouts due to adverse events and new nonclinical safety findings) and includes an outline of the development plan for the coming year. *Guidance for Industry: E2F Development Safety Update Report* (August 2011) describes a new approach for annual safety reporting and is intended to replace the IND annual report with a comprehensive, harmonized safety summary that represents a common standard for the ICH regions.

Finally, FDA requires clinical trials to be registered with the Clinical Trials Data Bank (maintained by NIH's National Library of Medicine). This initiative began in 2001 with the posting of clinical studies for serious or life-threatening diseases and, under the *Food and Drug Administration Amendments Act* of 2007 (*FDAAA*), was expanded to include all controlled clinical trials in patients (i.e., other than Phase 1 studies). The Clinical Trials Data Bank can be accessed at www.clinicaltrials.gov/. To date, the database has registered hundreds of thousands of trials in virtually every country in the world and can be a good resource for clinical study design information.

NDA and Risk/Benefit
General Considerations

The culmination of a drug or biologic development program is the preparation and submission of a marketing application (NDA or BLA). This is accomplished either through studies conducted by (or with a right of reference from the sponsor (505(b)(1) approach) or by reference to FDA's finding of safety and effectiveness for a previously approved product (Section 505(b)(2) approach). Through frequent interactions with FDA during the development program, including a pre-NDA meeting (usually held no later than three months prior to the target filing date), sponsor and agency expectations should be reasonably well aligned. One tool suggested by FDA for late-stage discussions is the

Target Product Profile (see *Draft Guidance for Industry and Review Staff: Target Product Profile—A Strategic Development Process Tool* (March 2007)). The marketing application should contain sufficient data for FDA to decide whether the drug's benefits outweigh its risks in the context of the sponsor's proposed label.

There are a number of key FDA guidances (some in draft stage) regarding the content and approaches to data organization in marketing applications, including:

- *Guidance for Industry: Guideline for the Format and Content of the Nonclinical Pharmacology/Toxicology Section of an Application* (February 1987)
- *Draft Reviewer Guidance on the Integration of Study Results to Assess Concerns about Human Reproductive and Developmental Toxicities* (November 2001)
- *Guidance for Industry and Review Staff: Recommended Approaches to Integration of Genetic Toxicology Study Results* (January 2006)
- *Draft Guidance for Industry: Statistical Aspects of the Design, Analysis, and Interpretation of Chronic Rodent Carcinogenicity Studies of Pharmaceuticals* (May 2001)
- *Guideline for the Format and Content of the Clinical and Statistical Sections of an Application* (July 1988)
- *Draft Guidance for Industry: Integrated Summary of Effectiveness* (August 2008)
- *Guidance for Industry: Premarketing Risk Assessment* (March 2005)

An NDA number for an application in paper format can be requested by contacting the Central Document Room at CDER by telephone. A number may be assigned directly over the phone upon provision of the review division name, sponsor's name, drug name, indication and the contact person's name and phone number. For electronic applications, specific instructions are available on FDA's website for requesting a pre-assigned eCTD application number via secure email (www.fda.gov/Drugs/DevelopmentApprovalProcess/FormsSubmissionRequirements/ElectronicSubmissions/UCM085361).

Package Insert

Federal regulations pertaining to marketing applications are contained in 21 CFR 314. In addition to the study reports supporting the drug's safety and efficacy and the associated summaries, the core of the NDA is the draft package insert (or prescribing information, also referred to as simply the "label") which, since 2005, is required to be in structured product label (SPL) format in an XML (Extended Machine Language) backbone to meet FDA filing requirements. SPL is a model-derived standard adopted for exchange of FDA-regulated product information in the content of the labeling, coded information from the content of the labeling (data elements) and a "wrapper" for electronic listing elements. In addition, most review divisions will request a copy of the label in Microsoft Word to be able to communicate in the label negotiation process using the track changes function. This should be confirmed either in the pre-NDA meeting or with the FDA project manager assigned to the NDA prior to filing. When a final label is agreed to, the sponsor will submit a revised copy of the label to the NDA in SPL format. Moreover, since 2006, new NDAs must follow the format required by the Physician Labeling Rule (PLR), which is made up of three parts: highlights (one page), contents and full prescribing information. The PLR format identifies and dates recent major changes to the prescribing information and includes the date of initial US approval for the active ingredient. Further information (including links to specific FDA guidelines on the content of different sections of the label) is available at www.fda.gov/Drugs/GuidanceComplianceRegulatoryInformation/LawsActsandRules/ucm084159.htm.

Electronic Submission

Since January 2008, sponsors submitting NDAs electronically have been required to use the eCTD format. Waivers are available for those who would like to submit electronically but are unable to do so in eCTD format. For further information, FDA maintains a useful Electronic Regulatory Submissions and Review website at www.fda.gov/Drugs/DevelopmentApprovalProcess/FormsSubmissionRequirements/ElectronicSubmissions/UCM085361. For an NDA, the content and format are dictated by the CTD format described above.

REMS

Evaluation of a product's risk potential has always been a difficult aspect of FDA drug approval. Generally, it is difficult to extrapolate from data derived from a few thousand patients exposed to the drug under relatively well-controlled conditions to millions of patients with much less oversight. FDA's mandate to mitigate potential risks of drugs throughout their development and marketing lifecycle led to the issuance of three guidances in 2005 (*Guidance for Industry: Premarketing Risk Assessment*, *Guidance for Industry: Development and Use of Risk Minimization Action Plans* and *Guidance for Industry: Good Pharmacovigilance Practices and Pharmacoepidemiologic Assessment*). For drugs in development, FDA wanted to know how a sponsor planned to mitigate actual and potential risks (Risk MAP) if a marketing application was approved and how risk would be monitored post-approval. However, the agency did not have the statutory authority to require these assessments. This was rectified as part of *FDAAA*, which gave FDA the authority to require sponsors to submit a Risk Evaluation and Mitigation Strategy (REMS) plan prior to approval. A REMS may be as simple as inclusion of a medication guide with the package insert or as complex as a patient and pharmacist training program (additional elements to assure safe use). The REMS includes, at a minimum, a postapproval evaluation by the sponsor at 18 months, three years and seven years. However, given the newness of this requirement, only recently has more granularity on FDA expectations for these evaluations become available.

Proprietary Name

If not previously submitted, a request for review of the sponsor's proposed proprietary name(s) should be made to the review division under the IND (*Draft Guidance for Industry: Contents of a Complete Submission for the Evaluation of Proprietary Names* (February 2010)) or as a separate supplemental submission following submission of the initial NDA. Although the guidance states that this request may be submitted as early as at the end of Phase 2, FDA has begun to delay designating a proprietary name until close to the approval date. The review division will forward the proprietary name request to the Office of Postmarketing Drug Risk Assessment, Division of Drug Risk Evaluation, which will perform the primary review in consultation with the Office of Prescription Drug Promotion (OPDP).

User Fees

Under the original *PDUFA* of 1992 (and subsequent amendments), user fees were levied on each "human drug application," including applications for:
- approval of a new drug submitted under section 505(b)(1) after 1 September 1992
- approval of a new drug submitted pursuant to section 505(b)(2) after 30 September 1992 for certain molecular entities or indications for use
- licensure of certain biological products under section 351 of the *PHS Act* submitted after 1 September 1992

PDUFA specifies different user fees for original applications depending upon whether they are accompanied by clinical data on safety and/or efficacy (other than BA or BE studies). The act also levies fees on supplements to human drug applications that require clinical data. Under the fee schedules provided in the act, original applications without clinical data and supplements that require clinical data are assessed approximately one-half the fee of original applications. Further details are provided in *Guidance for Industry: Submitting Separate Marketing Applications and Clinical Data for Purposes of Assessing User Fees* (December 2004). The user fee for a full submission has increased every year since it was implemented and is currently well over $1 million. FDA also levies annual establishment and product fees. Further information on these fees can be found at www.fda.gov/Drugs/DevelopmentApprovalProcess/SmallBusinessAssistance/ucm069943.htm. The Office of Regulatory Policy within CDER is responsible for all the above fees.

PAI

One of FDA's objectives in the NDA review process is to determine whether the methods used in manufacturing the drug and the controls used to maintain its quality are adequate to preserve the drug's identity, strength, quality and purity. In conjunction with this evaluation, FDA field inspectors conduct a CGMP preapproval inspection (PAI) of the drug product manufacturing site if it has not recently been inspected by FDA with a favorable outcome. A PAI can occur as early as 90 days after an NDA submission. An adequate PAI generally is required for NDA approval.

Periapproval Activities

There are a number of periapproval activities that should be part of the overall submission and approval plan. A safety update is required to be submitted as an amendment to the NDA within 120 days. In addition, approximately one month prior to the FDA action date, the FDA RPM will contact the sponsor and begin label negotiations. At this time (if not previously done), the sponsor should submit a request for a National Drug Code (NDC) assignment (*Guidance for Industry: Standards for Securing the Drug Supply Chain—Standardized Numerical Identification for Prescription Drug Packages* (March 2010)). Historically, FDA has provided these NDC numbers months before approval of the application, but recently has limited this to the periapproval timeframe due to drug piracy concerns. Thus, the drug label, packaging artwork and labels and promotional material cannot be finalized until very close to the approval date.

In 1972, Congress passed the *Federal Advisory Committee Act*, which prescribed the formal use of Advisory Committees throughout the federal government. With the increasing complexity of benefit:risk decisions, FDA has increasingly used Advisory Committees to provide independent advice that will contribute to the quality of the agency's regulatory decision making and lend credibility to the product review process in cases where additional input is desired by FDA. Chapter 5 provides a detailed description of FDA Advisory Committees and the timing of these in the periapproval process when FDA requests such a meeting.

Establishment Listing

Under 21 CFR 207, FDA requires establishments (e.g., manufacturers, repackers and relabelers) upon first engaging in the manufacture, preparation, propagation, compounding or processing of human drugs, veterinary drugs and biological products, with certain exceptions, to register their establishments and submit listing information for all drugs and biological products in commercial distribution. Registrants also are required to submit, on or before 31 December each year, updates in registration information for their establishments. Form FDA 2656 is used for registration of the drug establishment (and also the labeler code assignment) and Form FDA 2657 is used for drug product listing purposes. In 2008, FDA began a pilot program to allow submission of the above information in an electronic format and, since 1 June 2009, all submissions are required to be completely electronic and in XML format, unless a waiver is granted. Further information is available in *Draft Guidance for Industry: Forms for Registration of Producers of Drugs and Listing of Drugs in Commercial Distribution* (April 2001) and at www.fda.gov/Drugs/GuidanceComplianceRegulatoryInformation/DrugRegistrationandListing/ucm084014.htm.

Patent Restoration
The passage of the *Drug Price Competition and Patent Term Restoration Act* (the *Hatch-Waxman Act*) in 1984 represented a compromise between the innovator pharmaceutical industry and the generic pharmaceutical industry. It allowed the innovator pharmaceutical companies to apply for up to five years of additional patent protection for new drugs to make up for time lost while their products were going through the development and regulatory review process. The drug (animal or human), medical device, biologic or food or color additive must be the first commercial marketing or use of the product under the provision of the law for which regulatory review occurred. FDA assists the Patent and Trademark Office (PTO) in determining a product's eligibility for patent extension, but PTO ultimately is responsible for determining the period of patent extension. Similarly, up to three years of exclusivity are granted for a change in an approved drug product where approval requires new clinical investigations other than BA studies (e.g., new indication, strength, dosage form or route of administration). The following website provides further details on the patent term restoration program www.fda.gov/Drugs/DevelopmentApprovalProcess/SmallBusinessAssistance/ucm069959.htm. Six months of pediatric exclusivity (FDA's incentive to conduct more studies of the use of the drug in pediatric populations) also can be requested; see www.fda.gov/Drugs/DevelopmentApprovalProcess/DevelopmentResources/UCM049867.htm for additional details.

NDA Amendments
Finally, an NDA amendment is submitted to change or add information to an unapproved NDA or NDA supplement. With the exception of the required 120-day safety update, sponsors should try to avoid initiating NDA amendments because they will potentially reset the review clock (especially if submitted in the final three months of the review period).

The 505(b)(2) NDA
Overview
The "paper" NDA approach was created after the 1962 passage of the *Drug Amendments* to the *FD&C Act*. It created a means by which duplicates (now known as generic drugs) of post-1962 drugs could be approved because the DESI program and the ANDA did not apply to drugs approved after 1962. The paper NDA policy allowed applicants to use published literature to satisfy the requirements for full reports of safety and effectiveness. The *Hatch-Waxman Act* eliminated the paper NDA policy because it provided a mechanism to approve duplicates of post-1962 drugs, including situations where the applicant did not have the right of reference to the original NDA submitted and approved under Section 505(b)(1) of the *FD&C Act*.

The 505(b)(2) NDA is a submission type that shares characteristics of both traditional NDAs and ANDAs and is named after the section of the *FD&C Act* that describes it. **Figure 3-1** outlines how this type of NDA potentially fits into the overall development and approval scheme for a drug. As with an NDA, a 505(b)(2) application is submitted under Section 505(b)(1) and is considered a complete application. Like a traditional NDA, it is approved under Section 505(c) of the act. Like an ANDA, a 505(b)(2) application may refer to FDA's finding of safety and effectiveness for a previously approved product, and its approval is subject to patent exclusivity limitations. The applicant also may rely on published literature. *Draft Guidance for Industry: Applications Covered by Section 505(b)(2)* (October 1999) provides additional details. The regulations for this type of application are codified in 21 CFR 314.54.

Bridging and Expansion Issues and Approaches
The most common uses of the 505(b)(2) route are for:
- change in drug product dosage form (including route of administration), formulation, strength and/or dosing regimen, including changes that were not accepted by OGD in a Suitability Petition
- change in active ingredient (different salt, acid or base)
- new combination product in which the active ingredients have been previously approved individually
- change from a prescription indication to an over-the-counter (OTC) indication
- indication that has not been previously approved for the active moiety
- NCE that is a prodrug or active metabolite of a drug approved in the US

If the applicant is the original NDA holder or has right of reference to that NDA from the holder, the above changes become supplements to the original NDA as outlined in **Figure 3-1**.

Chapter 3

The data most commonly required in a 505(b)(2) approach provide a bridge between the data forming the basis for approval of the referenced NDA (and agreed to by FDA in the approved drug product label) and the different or additional claims in the 505(b)(2) NDA label. For active ingredient modifications, bridging centers on changes in impurity profiles and/or bioavailability and subsequent exposure. For drug product modifications, bridging centers on differences in the exposure profile. In both cases, a bridging toxicology program usually includes multiple-dose toxicology studies (between 14 and 90 days), with toxicokinetics in appropriate species, as well as mutagenicity and genotoxicity studies. The bridging program generally should not be initiated until agreement is reached with FDA in a formal meeting and the IND is in effect.

The above types of changes also will require additional bridging clinical pharmacokinetic studies. The product should be at least as bioavailable as the RLD unless it has some other advantage such as a smaller peak/trough exposure ratio. Moreover, the pattern of release of the proposed product, although different, should be at least as favorable as that of the RLD. Clinical studies conducted for a 505(b)(2) application generally should be performed under an IND. A 505(b)(2) application may itself be granted three years of exclusivity if one or more of the clinical investigations, other than BA/BE studies, was essential to approval and was conducted for or sponsored by the applicant. A 505(b)(2) application also may be granted five years of exclusivity if it is for an NCE.

Between 1996 and 2004, 126 Section 505(b)(2) applications were filed,[3] and this continues to be a productive approach for moving older drugs into new technology platforms and/or better characterized and understood therapeutic areas. Tuttle[4] provides a concise description of how the regulatory professional can research this development approach.

Dietary Supplements and Natural Health Products

A dietary supplement is a product taken by mouth that contains a "dietary ingredient" intended to supplement the diet. These dietary ingredients may be vitamins, minerals, herbs or other botanicals, amino acids or substances such as enzymes, organ tissues, glandulars and metabolites.

Until 1994, dietary supplements were subject to the same regulatory requirements as other foods. Based on the belief in a positive relationship between sound dietary practices and health, Congress passed the *Dietary Supplement Health and Education Act (DSHEA)* in 1994, which amended the *FD&C Act* to create a new regulatory framework for the safety and labeling of dietary supplements (yet still under the regulatory umbrella of foods). Provisions of *DSHEA* define dietary supplements and dietary ingredients and describe the proper use of statements of nutritional support. *DSHEA* also set forth new labeling requirements and required manufacturers of dietary supplements to notify FDA of new dietary ingredients (after 1994; 21 CFR 190.6) prior to marketing. Interestingly, it also authorized FDA to prescribe GMPs for the industry. A final rule on this latter aspect was not forthcoming until 2007. The *Final Rule on cGMPs in Manufacturing, Packaging, Labeling, or Holding Operations for Dietary Supplements* established dietary supplement CGMPs for all domestic and foreign companies that manufacture, package, label or hold these supplements, including those involved with testing, quality control, packaging and labeling and distribution in the US. The dietary supplement CGMPs bear a stronger resemblance to drug CGMPs than to the rather general food CGMPs; however, dietary supplement CGMPs do not require process validation, which is mandated for drug CGMPs.

Dietary supplements do not require premarket approval by FDA. The manufacturer is responsible for ensuring that a dietary supplement is safe before it is marketed. *DSHEA* places the burden on FDA to prove that a marketed dietary supplement is unsafe prior to any action to remove the product from the market. Because of this requirement and the fact that FDA received numerous reports of safety concerns for a number of products,[5] Congress passed the *Dietary Supplement and Nonprescription Drug Consumer Protection Act* in 2006. It mandates the same type of adverse event reporting for dietary supplements as for prescription drugs.

Dietary supplement claims allowed under *DSHEA* include:

- claims of benefits related to nutrient deficiencies (if the prevalence of the disease in the US is disclosed)
- claims describing the role of the dietary supplement's effects on structure or function in humans (e.g., "calcium builds strong bones")
- claims describing the mechanism of effects on structure or function (e.g., "fiber maintains bowel regularity")
- claims of general well being

Manufacturers cannot make an express or implied claim that a product will diagnose, mitigate, treat, cure or prevent a specific disease or class of diseases. Examples of prohibited statements include: "protects against the development of cancer" or "reduces the pain and stiffness associated with arthritis." Examples of allowable structure/function claims include: "helps promote urinary tract health," "helps maintain cardiovascular function" or "promotes relaxation." Further details can be found in *Guidance for Industry: Structure/Function Claims Small Entity Compliance Guide* (January 2002). Also see Chapter 30 Dietary Supplements and Homeopathic Products.

Over-the-Counter (OTC) Drugs

An OTC product is a drug product marketed for use by the consumer without the intervention of a healthcare professional. There are more than 80 therapeutic categories of OTC drugs, and more than 100,000 OTC drug products are marketed in the US, encompassing approximately 800 active ingredients. Oversight of OTC drugs is performed by CDER's Office of Nonprescription Drugs.

The distinction between drugs that do and do not require a physician prescription dates back to the 1951 *Durham-Humphrey Amendment* to the *FD&C Act*.[6] FDA applied the principle of retrospective review to OTC drugs starting in 1972. The OTC review by panels of experts focused on active ingredients (initially, approximately 1,000 different moieties). The agency published the results as a series of monographs in 21 CFR 328–358, specifying the active ingredient(s), restrictions on formulations and labeling by therapeutic category for those drugs deemed appropriate for OTC use.

If the standards of the relevant monograph are met, marketing preclearance of an OTC is not required. An NDA 505(b)(2) can be used to request approval of an OTC drug that deviates in any respect from a monograph that has become final (21 CFR 330.11). However, a citizen petition (see 21 CFR 10.30) is an alternate route that bypasses the requirement of *PDUFA* user fees.

"Prescription-to-OTC switch" refers to over-the-counter marketing of a former prescription drug product for the same indication, strength, dose, duration of use, dosage form, population and route of administration. An efficacy supplement to an approved NDA for a prescription product should be submitted if the sponsor plans to switch a drug product covered under an NDA to OTC status in its entirety without a change in the previously approved dosage form or route of administration. An NDA under Section 505(b)(1) should be submitted if the sponsor is proposing to convert some, but not all, of the approved prescription indications to OTC marketing status. An original NDA ((505)(b)(1) or 505(b)(2)) needs to be submitted if the sponsor plans to market a new product whose active substance, indication or dosage form has never previously been marketed OTC (refer to CDER MAPP 6020.5: "Good Review Practice: OND Review Management of INDs and NDAs for Nonprescription Drug Products" (July 2007).

FDA has approved the switch of a number of drugs from prescription to OTC status under NDAs:
- antidiarrheals (loperamide)
- topical antifungals (clotrimazole, terbinafine)
- antihistamines (clemastine fumarate)
- vaginal antifungals (clotrimazole, miconazole nitrate)
- analgesics (ketoprofen, naproxen sodium)
- acid reducers (cimetidine, famotidine)
- hair growth treatments (minoxidil)
- smoking cessation drugs (nicotine polacrilex)

In allowing these drugs to be sold OTC, FDA considered safety and effectiveness, benefit:risk ratio and whether clear and understandable labeling could be written to enable consumers to safely self-medicate. In 21 CFR 201.66, the agency established standardized content and format for OTC drug product labeling. In addition, manufacturers commonly are required to conduct studies to determine whether consumers understand the proposed OTC labeling and can use the products in a safe and effective manner.[7] OTC product labeling has always contained usage and safety information for consumers. With the introduction of the "Drug Facts" label regulation in 1999, the information became more uniform and easier to read and understand. Patterned after the Nutrition Facts food label, the Drug Facts label uses simple language and an easy-to-read format to help people compare and select OTC medicines and follow dosage instructions. The following information must appear in the indicated order:

- product's active ingredients, including the amount in each dosage unit
- purpose of the product
- product uses (indications)
- specific warnings, including when the product should not be used under any circumstances and when it is appropriate to consult with a doctor or pharmacist; this section also describes possible side effects and substances or activities to avoid
- dosage instructions—when, how and how often to take the product
- inactive ingredients, to help consumers avoid ingredients that could cause an allergic reaction

OTC guidances can be found on the FDA website at www.fda.gov/Drugs/GuidanceComplianceRegulatoryInformation/Guidances/ucm065013.htm. See Chapter 15 Over-the-Counter Drugs for more information.

Medical Devices

Overview and Medical Device Classification

A "device" is defined by FDA as an instrument, apparatus, implement, machine, contrivance, implant, in vitro reagent or other similar or related article, including a component part, or accessory which is:

- recognized in the official *National Formulary* or the *United States Pharmacopoeia* or any supplement to them
- intended for use in the diagnosis of disease or other conditions, or in the cure, mitigation, treatment or prevention of disease in man or other animals
- intended to affect the structure or any function of the body of man or other animals, and which does

not achieve any of its primary intended purposes through chemical action within or on the body of man or other animals and which is not dependent upon being metabolized for the achievement of any of its primary intended purposes

Devices first became subject to regulation under the *FD&C Act* (which also defined medical devices for the first time). As a result of the increasing hazards that could result from new, more-complicated devices that were being introduced in the 1960s and 1970s (e.g., pacemakers, kidney dialysis machines, replacement heart valves), Congress passed the *Medical Device Amendments* in 1976 and heralded the modern age of device regulation. These amendments included the following major provisions:

- redefined medical devices to make them more distinct from drugs and expanded the definition to include diagnostics for conditions other than disease
- established safety and efficacy requirements for devices
- established premarket review by FDA
- established the medical device classification system
- created two routes to market (premarket notification and premarket approval) and established Investigational Device Exemptions (IDEs)

A second milestone in device regulation was the passage of the *Safe Medical Device Act* (*SMDA*) in 1990. This act included the following major provisions:

- extended adverse device incident reporting to user facilities, including hospitals, ambulatory surgical facilities and nursing homes (This was a landmark event because FDA had never extended its jurisdiction so broadly. When a user facility receives information regarding a death caused by a device, it must report it to FDA and the manufacturer. If a user facility receives information about a serious injury or illness caused by a device, it must report it to the manufacturer. A user facility must also submit to FDA an annual summary of its reports to the agency.)
- required device tracking requirements for high-risk devices
- defined substantial equivalence
- required that submitters of 510(k)s receive clearance by FDA prior to marketing
- gave FDA the authority to regulate combination products
- defined the humanitarian device exemption
- gave FDA recall authority

These regulatory milestones gave rise to most of the modern components of the regulations used by FDA's Center for Devices and Radiological Health (CDRH) to fulfill its responsibilities for regulating firms that manufacture, repackage, relabel and/or import medical devices sold in the US.

Because medical devices vary widely in complexity and risks or benefits, they do not all require the same degree of regulation. Thus, FDA places medical devices into one of three regulatory classes based on the level of control necessary to assure safety and effectiveness. Device classification depends on intended use as well as indications for use. In addition, classification is based upon the risk the device poses to the patient and/or the user. Class I includes devices with the lowest risk and Class III includes those with the greatest risk. The class to which a device is assigned determines the type of premarketing submission/application required for marketing. **Table 3-4** summarizes this system.

General controls for all classes include:

- establishment registration of companies required to register under 21 CFR 807.20, such as manufacturers, distributors, repackagers and relabelers; foreign establishments, however, are not required to register with FDA
- medical device listing with FDA
- manufacturing devices in accordance with GMP in 21 CFR 820
- labeling devices in accordance with labeling regulations in 21 CFR 801 or 809
- submission of a premarket notification (510(k)) (unless exempt) before marketing a device

Special controls may include special labeling requirements, mandatory performance standards and postmarket surveillance.

Premarket approval is the required process of scientific review to ensure the safety and effectiveness of Class III devices, the most stringent regulatory category. Class III devices are those for which insufficient information exists to assure safety and effectiveness solely through general or special controls. They usually support or sustain human life, are of substantial importance in preventing impairment of human health or present a potential, unreasonable risk of illness or injury.

FDA has established classifications for approximately 1,700 different generic types of devices and grouped them into 16 medical specialties, referred to as "panels." Classification of a device can be obtained through the CFR or the CDRH database.

CBER reviews marketing and investigational device submissions (510(k)s, PMAs and IDEs) for medical devices associated with blood collection and processing procedures, as well as those associated with cellular therapies and vaccines. Although these products are reviewed by CBER, the medical device laws and regulations still apply.

It is important for the regulatory professional to ensure that a general product definition is available for new devices.

Table 3-4. Summary of Device Classification System

Class	Required Controls			Exemptions	Examples
	General	Special	Premarket Approval		
I	X			**Exempt** = subject to limitations on exemptions covered under 21 CFR xxx.9, where xxx refers to Parts 862–892. Class I devices are usually exempt. **Nonexempt** = 510(k) required for marketing	Elastic bandages, examination gloves, hand-held surgical instruments
II	X	X			Powered wheelchairs, infusion pumps, surgical drapes
III	X	X	X	Exempt if it is a preamendment device (i.e., on the market prior to the passage of the *Medical Device Amendments* in 1976 or substantially equivalent to such a device) and PMAs have not been called for. In that case, a 510(k) will be the route to market	Heart valves, silicone gel-filled breast implants, implanted cerebellar stimulators

Responses to the following questions will help to guide this effort:
- What will the device do? (intended use)
- For what clinical conditions or patient population will the device be used? (indications for use)
- How does the device work? (principles of operation)
- What are the features of the product? For example, is it electronic versus mechanical, controlled by software or other mechanism, invasive or noninvasive, implanted versus not, sterile versus nonsterile, disposable versus reusable? (product characteristics)
- What are the risks inherent in the use of the device? (risks)

A designation similar to that for an orphan drug provides an incentive for the development of devices for use in the treatment or diagnosis of diseases affecting small populations. A Humanitarian Use Device (HUD) is intended to benefit patients by treating or diagnosing a disease or condition that affects or is manifested in fewer than 4,000 individuals in the US per year. A request for HUD designation (21 CFR 807) needs to be submitted to FDA; if so designated, the device is eligible for a humanitarian device exemption (HDE). An HDE submission is similar in both form and content to a premarket approval (PMA) application, but is exempt from the effectiveness requirements of a PMA.

An approved HDE authorizes marketing of the HUD. However, an HUD may only be used in facilities that have established a local IRB to supervise clinical testing of devices and after the IRB has approved the use of the device to treat or diagnose the specific disease. The device labeling must state that it is a humanitarian use device and that, although authorized by federal law, its effectiveness for the specific indication has not been demonstrated.

The CDRH website has a number of useful, searchable databases, including one for device classifications, one for 510(k)s, a similar one for PMAs and one for registrations and listings. There is also Device Advice (www.fda.gov/MedicalDevices/DeviceRegulationandGuidance/default.htm), which is very helpful, and a relatively new CDRH Learn site (www.fda.gov/MedicalDevices/ResourcesforYou/Industry/ucm126230.htm) that provides both visual and audio components. Finally, Chapters 18, 19, 20 and 21 of this book are devoted to devices and provide more detailed coverage.

Premarket Notification 510(k) and Exemptions

A sponsor wishing to market a Class I, II or III device intended for human use in the US, for which a PMA is not required, must submit a 510(k) **exemption** to FDA unless the device is exempt from those requirements and does not exceed the limitations of exemptions in the CFR device classifications as detailed below.

FD&C Act Section 513(d)(2)(A) authorizes FDA to exempt certain generic types of Class I devices from the premarket notification (510(k)) requirement. FDA has exempted more than 800 generic types of Class I devices and 60 Class II devices from the requirement. It is important to confirm the exempt status and any limitations that apply with 21 CFR 862–892, the CDRH Product Code Classification Database or subsequent *Federal Register* announcements on Class I or II exemptions. The 510(k) exemption has certain limitations, which are so noted in ".9" of each chapter of the regulation.

There is no 510(k) form; however, 21 CFR 807 Subpart E describes requirements for a 510(k) submission. This premarket submission to FDA demonstrates that the device to be marketed is as safe and effective as (i.e., substantially equivalent to) a legally marketed predicate device that is not subject to PMA. A predicate device can be:

1. a preamendment device (a currently marketed device that was on the market prior to 1976)
2. a device reclassified from Class III to Class II or I

3. a device found to be substantially equivalent to a device in the one of the above two categories

A device is substantially equivalent if, in comparison to a predicate, it:
- has the same intended use and the same technological characteristics as the predicate

or
- has the same intended use as the predicate and different technological characteristics and the information submitted to FDA
  - does not raise new questions of safety and effectiveness
  - demonstrates that the device is at least as safe and effective as the legally marketed device

A claim of substantial equivalence does not mean that the new device and the predicate device must be identical. Substantial equivalence is established with respect to intended use, design, energy used or delivered, materials, performance, safety, effectiveness, biocompatibility, standards and other applicable characteristics (e.g., sterility).

FDA determines substantial equivalence, usually within 90 days. If the device is determined to be substantially equivalent, it can be marketed in the US when the submitter receives a letter from the agency (and the sponsor has complied with the general controls provisions). If FDA determines that a device is **not** substantially equivalent, the applicant may:
- resubmit another 510(k) with new data
- request a Class I or II designation through the *de novo* process
- file a reclassification petition
- submit a PMA

FDASIA included the *Medical Device User Fee Amendments of 2012* (*MDUFA III*), which introduced, in exchange for user application fees, new performance goals for FDA decision making with respect to a variety of medical device submission types (such as whether or not to clear a premarket notification or 510(k) within 90 days of active FDA review for at least 91% of submissions accepted in Fiscal 2013).

A 510(k)'s content and complexity can vary significantly depending upon the amount of information needed to establish substantial equivalence to the predicate. A typical 510(k) is between 15 and 100 pages. There are three subtypes of 510(k)s: a traditional 510(k), described in 21 CFR 807; a special 510(k); and an abbreviated 510(k) The latter two are described in *The New 510(k) Paradigm—Alternate Approaches to Demonstrating Substantial Equivalence in Premarket Notifications: Final Guidance* (March 1998).

Investigational Device Exemption (IDE) and Premarket Approval (PMA) Process

An IDE (21 CFR 812) allows the investigational device to be used in a clinical study to collect safety and effectiveness data required to support a PMA application or a Premarket Notification (510(k)) submission to FDA. Clinical studies are most often conducted to support a PMA. Only a small percentage of 510(k)s require clinical data to support the application. Investigational use also includes clinical evaluation of certain modifications or new intended uses of legally marketed devices. All clinical evaluations of investigational devices, unless exempt, must have an approved IDE before the study is initiated. The IDE is similar in content and organization to an IND. The sponsor may begin clinical trials 30 days after FDA receives the IDE, unless the agency objects.

Clinical evaluation of devices that have not been cleared for marketing requires:
- an IDE approved by an IRB; if the study involves a significant risk device, the IDE must also be approved by FDA
- informed consent from all patients
- labeling for investigational use only
- study monitoring
- records and reports

An approved IDE permits a device to be shipped lawfully for the purpose of conducting investigations without complying with other requirements of the *FD&C Act* that apply to devices in commercial distribution. Sponsors need not submit a PMA or Premarket Notification 510(k), register their establishment or list the device while it is under investigation. IDE sponsors also are exempt from the Quality System Regulation (QSR) except for the requirements for design control.

In an industry of 15,000 manufacturers, where half have fewer than 10 employees, the planning and conduct of a clinical study can take a significant proportion of resources. For significant risk devices, where trials can be relatively complex and expensive, following the types of processes used for industry-sponsored drug trials is advisable to protect the validity of the company's investment. This should include the use of clinical study protocols, informed consent forms that meet FDA regulations (21 CFR 50) and are reviewed by duly constituted IRBs (21 CFR 56), source documents at the investigational sites, clinical study reports and well-written investigator agreements that include not only financial aspects (see 21 CFR 54), but also compliance with the study protocol and IDE responsibilities.

PMA is FDA's review process to evaluate the safety and effectiveness of Class III medical devices. Due to the level of risk associated with Class III devices, FDA has determined that general and special controls alone are insufficient to assure their safety and effectiveness. Therefore, these devices require a PMA application (21 CFR 814).

A PMA is the most stringent type of device marketing application required by FDA. The applicant must receive FDA approval of its PMA application prior to marketing the device. Approval is based on a determination by FDA that the PMA contains sufficient valid scientific evidence to assure that the device is safe and effective for its intended use(s). An approved PMA is, in effect, a private license granting the applicant (or owner) permission to market the device. The PMA owner, however, can authorize use of its data by another.

The PMA application is similar in content and organization to a traditional (non-CTD format) NDA application, although with much less clinical data required. FDA has observed problems with study designs, study conduct, data analyses, presentations and conclusions. Sponsors should always consult all applicable FDA guidance documents, industry standards and recommended practices. Numerous device-specific FDA guidance documents are available. Although FDA has 180 days to review the PMA, in reality this usually takes longer, due to the frequent involvement of an Advisory Committee.

Establishment Registration and Medical Device Listing

Establishments involved in the production and distribution of medical devices intended for marketing or leasing (commercial distribution) in the US are required to register with FDA. This process is known as establishment registration. Registration provides FDA with the location of medical device manufacturing facilities and importers. An establishment is defined as any place of business under one management at one physical location at which a device is manufactured, assembled or otherwise processed for commercial distribution. The "owner/operator" is defined as the corporation, subsidiary, affiliated company, partnership or proprietor directly responsible for the activities of the registering establishment. The owner/operator is responsible for registering the establishment.

The regulations for establishment registration are provided in 21 CFR 807. As of 1 October 2007, all establishment registrations and listings must be submitted electronically using FDA's Unified Registration and Listing System (FURLS)/Device Registration and Listing Module (DRLM), unless a waiver has been granted. Congress also authorized FDA to implement a user fee for certain types of establishment registrations processed after 30 September 2007 (for 2013 this fee is $4,960). Registration of an establishment is not an approval of the establishment or its products by FDA. That is, it does not provide FDA clearance to market. Unless exempt, premarketing clearance or approval is required before a device can be placed into commercial distribution in the US.

Most medical device establishments required to register with FDA also must identify the devices they have in commercial distribution, including those produced exclusively for export. This process is known as medical device listing and is a means of keeping FDA advised of the generic category(s) of devices an establishment is manufacturing or marketing. The regulations for medical device listing also are provided in 21 CFR 807.

Quality Systems for Manufacturing

The CGMP requirements set forth in the QSR require domestic or foreign manufacturers to have a quality system for the design, manufacture, packaging, labeling, storage, installation and servicing of finished medical devices intended for commercial distribution in the US. The regulation requires:

- various specifications and controls to be established for devices
- devices to be designed under a quality system to meet their specifications
- devices to be manufactured under a quality system
- finished devices to meet their specifications
- devices to be correctly installed, checked and serviced
- quality data to be analyzed to identify and correct quality problems
- complaints to be processed

FDA monitors device problem data and inspects the operations and records of device developers and manufacturers to determine compliance with the GMP requirements in the QSR.

The QSR is contained in 21 CFR 820. It covers quality management and organization, device design, buildings, equipment, purchasing and handling of components, production and process controls, packaging and labeling control, device evaluation, distribution, installation, complaint handling, servicing and records.

Combination Drug-Device and Drug-Drug Products

Combination products (i.e., drug-device, drug-biologic and device-biologic products, formally defined in 21 CFR 3.2(e)) have been regulated for decades. Prior to 1990, FDA regulated such products on a case-by-case basis. Generally, the sponsor and FDA negotiated an ad hoc regulatory approach without explicit statutory guidance. As combination products multiplied and increased in complexity, the ad hoc approach was no longer satisfactory, and in 1990, Congress enacted the *SMDA*. This provision required the agency to designate a center (CDER, CBER or CDRH) with primary jurisdiction based on the product's primary mode of action. FDA issued intercenter agreements between

Chapter 3

the three centers in 1991; however, there were still a number of problems with this approach.[8]

As part of the *Medical Device User Fee and Modernization Act* of 2002 (*MDUFMA*), Congress established the Office of Combination Products (OCP) within FDA's Office of the Commissioner to ensure prompt assignment of combination products to FDA centers and oversee coordination of the development and approval processes.

By submitting a Request for Designation (RFD), a company may obtain a formal agency determination of a combination product's primary mode of action and assignment of the lead center for the product's premarket review and regulation. OCP will make a determination within 60 days of receipt of the RFD. *Guidance for Industry: How to Write a Request for Designation* (April 2011) and *Draft Guidance for Industry and FDA Staff: Classification of Products as Drugs and Devices & Additional Product Classification Issues* (June 2011) each provide more specifics. Chapter 25 Combination Products also gives additional details.

In recent years, in part as pharmaceutical companies strive to reduce the inherent risks of drug development, drug-drug combinations have become increasingly common. Combination drug products are convenient and can improve dosing compliance, especially in polypharmacy scenarios. Moreover, by combining drugs with different mechanisms of action, lower doses can be used, which may decrease adverse effects (e.g., diuretics combined with angiotensin-converting enzyme (ACE) inhibitors, angiotensin receptor blockers or beta-adrenergic blockers for the treatment of hypertension, or some antiretroviral agents combining up to three drugs in one dosage form).

The type of development program for drug-drug combinations will depend upon whether one, both or neither component of a two-drug (or greater) combination product has been previously approved. From a nonclinical perspective, FDA has issued *Guidance for Industry: Nonclinical Safety Evaluation of Drug or Biologic Combinations* (March 2006). Similar principles would apply to the clinical portion of the development program. However, in both cases, proposed development approaches should be discussed with FDA in the early stages.

Summary

The development of drugs and devices is a scientific process in the context of objective and subjective interpretations of a product's potential or actual risks and benefits. The scope, interpretation and application of US federal regulations that must be met to market a drug or device have evolved over the past century and are documented in the CFR. This translates into agency use of scientific review, standards, manufacturing and other inspections, advertising controls, conditional approvals, laboratory product testing and postmarketing pharmacovigilance activities. Over the last 25 years, a plethora of FDA and ICH guidelines have been issued to assist in interpreting and defining the processes needed to successfully develop drugs, biologics and devices for marketing in a regulated industry.

The modern era of generic drugs was born with passage of the *Hatch-Waxman Act*. This act expedited the availability of less-costly generic drugs by permitting FDA to approve abbreviated applications after the patent of the innovator drug had expired. These abbreviated applications generally are not required to include animal safety and clinical data to establish safety and effectiveness. Specifically, a generic drug product is comparable to the innovator drug product in dosage form, strength, route of administration, quality, performance characteristics and intended use.

A "drug" is defined as a product used in diagnosing, curing, mitigating, treating or preventing a disease or affecting a structure or function of the body. A "biologic" is defined as a substance derived from or made with the aid of living organisms. Drug development consists of characterizing the safety profile (risk) and the efficacy profile (benefit) as it relates to the body's exposure to the drug (pharmacokinetic profile). The most successful drugs are those with minimal risk and maximum benefit.

The relationship between FDA and an investigational drug product sponsor can begin very early in the process (before the sponsor submits an IND) and extends through the typical IND development process (often defined as Phases 1, 2 and 3) to a marketing application and post-approval commitments, safety surveillance and product lifecycle management. Meetings with FDA are an important component of the IND process. Meetings can be requested at any time for any valid reason, but FDA will decide whether there is sufficient justification for a meeting (usually dictated by the product background and draft questions submitted in a written meeting request) or if a written response to questions and/or a teleconference would suffice.

Sponsors can submit a request for a Special Protocol Assessment (SPA). Within 45 days of receipt, FDA will evaluate certain protocols and related issues to determine whether they meet scientific and regulatory requirements identified by the sponsor. Three types of protocols are eligible for an SPA under the *PDUFA* goals—animal carcinogenicity protocols, final product stability protocols and clinical protocols for Phase 3 trials whose data will form the basis for an efficacy claim (i.e., a pivotal trial).

The *Orphan Drug Act*, for the first time, provided incentives for development of drugs necessary, and often lifesaving, for patients with rare diseases (defined as a US prevalence of less than 200,000 patients) but with minimal prospects for commercial return on investment.

The Fast Track Drug Development Program is designed to facilitate the development and expedite the review of new drugs intended to treat serious or life-threatening conditions and demonstrate the potential to address unmet medical needs. A disease is considered serious based upon the likelihood that if left untreated, it will progress from a less-severe to a more-severe condition. FDA defines "meeting an unmet medical need" as providing a therapy where none exists or that may be superior to existing therapy by meeting a number of conditions. A sponsor may request fast track designation at any point in the development process. A product in a fast track development program is eligible for heightened interest by FDA in sponsor meetings, a greater probability of priority review of the marketing application and piecemeal submission of portions (complete CTD modules) of a marketing application ("rolling NDA/BLA").

ICH was formed in 1990. It brings together the regulatory authorities of Europe, Japan and the US and experts from the pharmaceutical industry in the three regions to discuss scientific and technical aspects of product registration. ICH recommends ways to achieve greater harmonization in the interpretation and application of technical guidelines and requirements for product registration to reduce or avoid duplicating testing during the research and development of new drugs.

The ICH process has resulted in numerous guidelines into four major categories—quality, safety, efficacy and multidisciplinary. Two important aspects of the ICH endeavor are the CTD concept and *MedDRA*.

Before initiating a clinical trial in the US (other than bioequivalence studies to support an ANDA), the sponsor must submit nonclinical, CMC and previous human experience data (if applicable) to FDA in the form of an IND. The IND application requests permission to initiate clinical trials. It is not a request for approval; rather, it is a request for exemption from federal law requiring an approved NDA or BLA prior to transporting or distributing a drug in interstate commerce. For a new chemical entity (NCE), the initial IND is a major milestone because it summarizes the data that support moving a drug from *in vitro* and animal testing into evaluation in humans. Sponsors are able to initiate their proposed clinical trial if they have not received any communication from FDA within 30 days of FDA receipt of the initial IND application.

The culmination of a drug or biologic development program is the preparation and submission of a marketing application (NDA or BLA). This is accomplished either through studies conducted by (or with a right of reference from) the sponsor (505(b)(1) approach) or by reference to FDA's finding of safety and effectiveness for a previously approved product (Section 505(b)(2) approach). Through frequent interactions with FDA during the development program, including a pre-NDA meeting, sponsor and agency expectations should be reasonably well aligned. Items to be considered when preparing a marketing application include package inserts (labeling), electronic submissions, risk evaluation and mitigation strategies (REMS), proprietary names, user fees, preapproval inspections (PAIs), establishment listings, patent restoration, other periapproval activities and NDA amendments and supplements.

A dietary supplement is a product taken by mouth that contains a "dietary ingredient" intended to supplement the diet. *DSHEA* created a new regulatory framework for the safety and labeling of dietary supplements (yet still under the regulatory umbrella of foods). Provisions of *DSHEA* define dietary supplements and dietary ingredients and describe the proper use of statements of nutritional support. *DSHEA* set forth new labeling requirements and required manufacturers of dietary supplements to notify FDA of new dietary ingredients prior to marketing. It also authorized FDA to prescribe GMPs for the industry. Dietary supplements do not require premarket approval by FDA. The manufacturer is responsible for ensuring that a dietary supplement is safe before it is marketed. *DSHEA* places the burden on FDA to prove that a marketed dietary supplement is unsafe (including noncompliance with CGMPs) prior to any action to remove the product from the market.

An OTC product is a drug product marketed for use by the consumer without the intervention of a healthcare professional. Oversight of OTC drugs is performed by CDER's Office of Nonprescription Drugs. In allowing drugs to be sold OTC, FDA considers safety and effectiveness, benefit:risk ratio and whether clear and understandable labeling can be written to enable consumers to safely self-medicate.

A "device" is defined as an instrument, apparatus, implement, machine, contrivance, implant, in vitro reagent or other similar or related article, including a component part or accessory that meets a number of conditions.

FDA places medical devices into one of three regulatory classes based on the level of control necessary to assure safety and effectiveness. Device classification depends upon intended use as well as indications for use, and the risk the device poses to the patient and/or user. Class I includes devices with the lowest risk and Class III includes those with the greatest risk. The class to which a device is assigned determines the type of premarketing submission/application required for marketing.

A sponsor wishing to market a Class I, II or III device intended for human use, for which a PMA is not required, must submit a 510(k) exemption to FDA unless the device is exempt from those requirements and does not exceed the limitations of exemptions in the CFR device classifications. A 510(k)'s content and complexity can vary significantly depending upon the amount of information needed to establish substantial equivalence to the proposed predicate.

Premarket approval is the required process of scientific review to ensure the safety and effectiveness of Class III devices. Class III devices are those for which insufficient information exists to assure safety and effectiveness solely through general or special controls. They usually support or sustain human life, are of substantial importance in preventing impairment of human health or present a potential, unreasonable risk of illness or injury. An IDE allows the investigational device to be used in a clinical study to collect safety and effectiveness data required to support a PMA application or a Premarket Notification (510(k)) submission.

Establishments involved in the production and distribution of medical devices intended for commercial distribution in the US are required to register with FDA (establishment registration). In addition, the QSR requires domestic or foreign manufacturers to have a quality system for the design, manufacture, packaging, labeling, storage, installation and servicing of finished medical devices intended for commercial distribution in the US.

Combination products are defined as drug-device, drug-biologic and device-biologic products. As part of *MDUFMA*, Congress established the Office of Combination Products to ensure prompt assignment of combination products to FDA centers and oversee coordination of the development and approval processes. By submitting a Request for Designation (RFD), a company may obtain a formal agency determination of a combination product's primary mode of action and assignment of the lead center for the product's premarket review and regulation.

References

1. FDA. Abbreviated New Drug Application (ANDA): Generics. FDA website. www.fda.gov/Drugs/DevelopmentApprovalProcess/HowDrugsareDevelopedandApproved/ApprovalApplications/AbbreviatedNewDrugApplicationANDAGenerics/. Accessed 24 April 2013.
2. Bren L. "The Road to the Biologic Revolution—Highlights of 100 Years of Biologics Regulation." FDA Consumer Magazine, January–February 2006. http://www.fda.gov/AboutFDA/WhatWeDo/History/FOrgsHistory/CBER/ucm135758.htm. Accessed 24 April 2013.
3. Tuttle ME. "Researching the 505(b)(2) Application." *Regulatory Affairs Focus*, May 2004; pp. 12–14.
4. Ibid.
5. Jiang T and Zhang S. "Stringent Laws and Regulations for Dietary Supplements." *Drug Information Journal*, Vol. 43; No. 1. pp. 75–81. (2009)
6. Op cit 1.
7. Hellbusch SJ. "Involving the End User in the Development of Label Wording." *Regulatory Affairs Focus*, May 2004, pp. 48–51.
8. Kahan JS and Shapiro JK. "FDA's Regulation of Combination Products: The Road Ahead." *Regulatory Compliance Newsletter*. November 2003, pp. 37–40.

Chapter 4

FDA Communications and Meetings

Updated by Clawson (Cal) Bowman, JD, CQA, CQM, RAC

OBJECTIVES

- To provide the reader a solid understanding of the four basic/essential types of FDA communications and meetings

    o   Regulatory communications

    o   Product application communications and meetings

    o   Administrative communications and meetings

    o   Public administrative proceedings

LAWS, REGULATIONS AND GUIDELINES COVERED IN THIS CHAPTER

- 21 CFR 10 Administrative Practices and Procedures

- 21 CRF Formal Evidentiary Public Hearing

- 21 CFR 13 Public Hearing Before a Public Advisory Committee

- 21 CFR 15 Public Hearing Before the Commissioner

- 21 CFR 16 Regulatory Hearing Before the Food and Drug Administration

- 21 CFR 312 Investigational New Drug Application

- 21 CFR 812 Investigational Device Exemptions

- *Guidance for Industry: Formal Meetings Between the FDA and Sponsors or Applicants* (May 2009)

- *Guidance for the Public, FDA Advisory Committee Members, and FDA Staff on Procedures for Determining Conflict of Interest and Eligibility for Participation in FDA Advisory Committee* (August 2008)

- *Draft Guidance for the Public, FDA Advisory Committee Members, and FDA Staff: Public Availability of Advisory Committee Members' Financial Interest Information and Waivers* (March 2010)

- *Guidance for FDA Advisory Committee Members and FDA Staff: Voting Procedures for Advisory Committee Meetings* (August 2008)

- *Guidance for Industry: Advisory Committee Meetings—Preparation and Public Availability of Information Given to Advisory Committee Members* (August 2008)

Introduction

Excellent communications between the US Food and Drug Administration (FDA) and the industries it regulates are key components in successful product development and promoting an understanding of the regulation process and regulatory compliance.

Understanding the various types of communications and meetings, their purposes, formats and timelines is critical to the success of regulatory professionals and the organizations they represent and is vital if they are to achieve their desired objectives in the most efficient and effective way.

Types of FDA Communications

There are four basic types of regulatory interactions that apply to drugs, biologics and devices. These are:
1. regulatory communications
2. product application meetings
3. administrative meetings or communications
4. public administrative proceedings

FDA has issued significant guidances to address the above interactions. They describe for sponsors when and how to request and execute the various types of administrative communications and meetings. Following the published guidances has numerous benefits, including:
- design testing and development plans that will expedite reviews and approvals
- saving sponsors time and money
- providing a more collaborative approach
- significantly reducing the possibilities of development surprises[1]

Regulatory Communications

Title 21 Part 10 of the Code of Federal Regulations (CFR) governs the practices and procedures for preparing and communicating FDA regulations, guidances and recommendations. With limited exceptions, regulations are published in the *Federal Register* and are available for public comment. Proposed regulations generally are subject to a 60-day comment period, which can be shortened or lengthened depending on FDA's opinion of what is a reasonable time for industry to review and comment. Comments from industry are evaluated by FDA and are published in the preamble to regulations.

Guidance Documents

Guidance documents describe the agency's current thinking on a topic and should be viewed only as recommendations, unless specific regulatory or statutory requirements are cited.[2] They differ from a regulation because they are non-binding (not legally enforceable) on FDA or the public. They are prepared by FDA staff, with input from sponsors or the public. Good Guidance Practices govern the preparation, dissemination and use of guidance documents.

Recommendations

Recommendations are FDA's advice on specific regulatory policy. They may be disseminated in the *Federal Register* or via emails to a specific audience. Generally, they provide specific advice that does not involve direct regulatory action under law.

Background and Types of Regulatory Communications

Citizen Petitions

A Citizen Petition is a formal written request to FDA asking the agency to take or refrain from taking an administrative action. By regulation, FDA must respond within 180 days of receipt. Citizen Petitions are filed in FDA's document management system and assigned a docket number. Subsequent submissions or comments on the petition must reference the docket number and become an official part of the docket file. Under FDA regulation, a Citizen Petition should contain the following:
- action requested
- statement of grounds
- environmental impact
- economic impact
- a certification by the submitter

Suitability Petitions

Suitability Petitions are a specific type of Citizen Petition used to file an abbreviated application for a new human or animal drug whose active ingredients, route of administration, dosage form or strength differ from that of the approved drug. According to statute, FDA will approve or deny a suitability petition within 90 days of the submission date.

Advisory Opinion

An advisory opinion is FDA's formal position on a matter. Interested parties may request an advisory opinion on a matter of general applicability. The regulations provide FDA great latitude in determining whether to grant a request for an advisory opinion. FDA statements of policy, such as the preamble to a final rule or the Compliance Policy Guides Manual, constitute advisory opinions.

Pharmaceutical or Biologics Product Application Communications and Meetings

There are three main types of product application meetings for pharmaceuticals and biologics: Type A, Type B and Type C (*Guidance for Industry: Formal Meetings Between the FDA and Sponsors or Applicants*). These communications and meetings are requested at critical product development points to establish or confirm that a company's product development plan will lead to an FDA marketing approval.

Application meetings are requested by the sponsor and are private, two-way communications (either by phone or in person) between FDA and the sponsor. These meetings

FDA Communications and Meetings

Figure 4-1. NDA and BLA Submissions

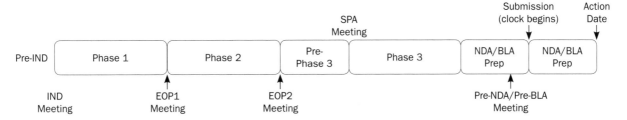

follow a systematic approach and well-established FDA procedures.

The timeline for drug and biologic submissions and meetings is shown in **Figure 4-1**.

Type A meetings are those that are immediately necessary to address and resolve issues with a product submission—one that is delaying FDA's review. Type A meetings generally are reserved for dispute resolution, discussion of clinical holds or Special Protocol Assessments.

FDA guidance advises notifying the appropriate review division of the Center for Drug Evaluation and Research (CDER) or the Center for Biologics Evaluation and Research (CBER) prior to submitting an official request for all types of meetings.[3] Official meeting requests should be submitted to the appropriate review division in writing and should include a complete listing of questions the sponsor wishes to address or resolve. The request should clearly explain the rationale for the request and the issues to be discussed. According to FDA guidance, a Type A meeting should be held within 30 days of FDA's receipt of a written request. A meeting package should be submitted to FDA at least four weeks before the meeting. A summary of meeting types and timelines is found in **Table 4-2**.

FDA reserves the right to grant or deny Type A, B or C meeting requests. If a meeting is granted or denied, FDA will notify the sponsor. In the case of a denial, FDA will include an explanation for the denial. Notification from FDA for Type A meetings usually occur within 14 days and within 21 days for Types B and C.

Type B meetings are pivotal development meetings that occur prior to progression to the next development stage. Type B meeting requests, like those for Type A and C meetings, should be discussed with the appropriate review division before submission of the formal request. According to FDA guidance, the agency will schedule Type B meetings within 60 days of receipt of a written request. FDA expects the sponsor to submit a meeting package at least four weeks before the formal meeting.

Type B meetings generally occur in the following order:
- Pre-Investigational New Drug (IND) meetings (21 CFR 312.82)
- Certain End-of-Phase 1 meetings (21 CFR 312.82)
- End of Phase 2 meetings/Pre-Phase 3 meetings (21 CFR 312.47
- Pre-NDA/Biologic License Application (BLA) meetings (21 CFR 312.47)

Each sponsor should only request one of each of these Type B meetings. For example: a pre-IND meeting, an end of Phase 2 or Pre-Phase 3 meeting and a pre-NDA or BLA meeting. The Pre-NDA meeting is intended to discuss formatting of the submission.

Type C meetings are any other product development meeting not included in Type A or B. According to FDA guidance, the agency will schedule Type C meetings within 75 days of receipt of a written request. The process for requesting a meeting is the same as for Types A and B. Type C meeting packages should be submitted to FDA at least four weeks before the formal meeting.

Meeting Requests by Sponsors or Applicants Should Include

- product name
- application number, if applicable and assigned
- chemical name and structure
- proposed indication(s) or context of product development
- type of meeting requested (Type A, B or C)
- brief statement of the meeting purpose and objectives (The statement should include a brief background of the issues underlying the agenda. It should provide enough information to facilitate understanding of the issues.)
- proposed agenda
- list of proposed questions grouped by discipline (For each question, there should be a brief explanation of the context and purpose of the question.)
- list of individuals (including titles) who will attend the meeting representing the sponsor's organization
- list of FDA staff, by title or discipline, requested by the sponsor to participate in the meeting
- suggested dates and times for the meeting
- meeting format (face-to-face, teleconference or videoconference)[4]

Figure 4-2. PMA Submissions

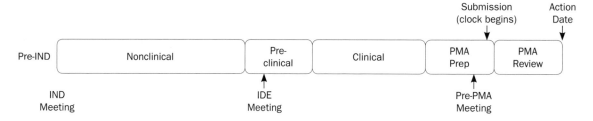

Meeting packages generally should include the following information:
- product name and application number (if applicable)
- chemical name and structure
- proposed indication
- dosage form, route of administration and dosing regimen
- an updated list of sponsor or applicant attendees, affiliations and titles
- background section that includes:
  o a brief history of the development program and the events leading up to the meeting
  o the status of the product development (e.g., the target indication for use)
- brief statement summarizing the purpose of the meeting
- proposed agenda
- list of final questions for discussion grouped by discipline with brief summary of each question to explain the need or context of the questions
- data to support discussion organized by discipline and question

Communications During and After FDA Meetings

The sponsor should assign individuals to take careful notes during the course of FDA meetings so commitments and action items are captured. The sponsor should immediately make a summary of the minutes of the meeting available to all participants for review and comment and then should publish internally the company's minutes of the meeting.

FDA will prepare official meeting minutes, summarizing meeting outcomes, agreements, unresolved issues and action items. Generally, within 30 days of the formal meeting, FDA will issue the official minutes to the sponsor.[5] In those rare situations when FDA exceeds the 30-day limit for publishing its meeting minutes, the sponsor may consider submitting to FDA its formal meeting minutes.

Medical Device Application Meetings

There are five basic types of meetings available to sponsors of medical device applications submitted to the Center for Devices and Radiological Health (CDRH):
- Agreement
- Determination
- Pre-Investigational Device Exemption (Pre-IDE)
- Pre-PMA
- PMA day 100

The timeline for medical device-related meetings is shown in **Figure 4-2**.

Agreement Meetings

The purpose of an Agreement Meeting is to reach concurrence on the key parameters of the investigational plan. A sponsor that intends to perform a clinical study of any class of device has the opportunity to present its investigational plan to FDA and obtain agreement on the plan before applying for an Investigation Device Exemption (IDE). Agreements reached in the meeting are documented in writing, shared with the sponsor and made part of the administrative record. The written agreement is binding on FDA and may be changed only with the written agreement of the sponsor or when there is a substantial scientific issue essential to determining the device's safety or effectiveness. Requests for Agreement Meetings must be submitted to the appropriate CDRH review division in writing. Generally, the request should include the information listed above for IND meetings. Additionally, the sponsor should provide the device classification and code number.

Determination Meetings

Determination Meetings are limited to PMAs or product development protocol (PDP) applications. The purpose is to determine the type of valid scientific evidence required to demonstrate that a device is safe and effective for its intended use. Discussions at these meetings will include the types of clinical studies (e.g., concurrent randomized controls, non-randomized controls and historical controls) or other types of evidence that will support effectiveness and the least burdensome way of evaluating effectiveness.

Pre-IDE Meetings

Pre-IDE Meetings are established, formal medical device collaboration meetings. The purpose of the Pre-IDE Meeting is to expedite the regulatory review process and minimize product development delays. They provide the sponsor an opportunity to present its product development plan to FDA and obtain an official acceptance.[6] Contrary to its name, a Pre-IDE meeting does not need to occur prior to filing an IDE and is available for medical devices that do not require an IDE.[7] Submissions made under the Pre-IDE process are not official IDE applications as described in 21 CFR 812.

Pre-IDE Meetings may address but are not limited to:
- analytical protocols
- clinical protocols
- proposed study designs
- statistical plan
- preclinical (animal) safety testing to support initiation of a clinical trial
- guidance on significant versus non-significant device determinations
- feasibility study protocols
- guidance on appropriate regulatory approval pathways
- Primary and Secondary Clinical endpoints

Pre-PMA Meetings

Pre-PMA meetings are intended to help guide the development of PMA submissions. They include such topics as the result of preclinical testing not included in the IDE submission, reliability testing, CMC issues and clinical results. The meeting also may include a discussion of the formatting of the application.[8] FDA guidance advises sponsors to notify the appropriate review division of their intent in requesting a Pre-PMA Meeting before making the official request. The official request should be addressed to the appropriate review division's director. The appropriate addresses are provided on CDRH's webpage.

PMA Day-100 Meetings

The PMA Day-100 Meetings are scheduled to occur 100 days after a PMA is accepted for filing. The meetings are intended to provide an opportunity to discuss the application's review status and obtain additional information, if any, required to complete the PMA review. Generally, FDA will inform the applicant in writing of any identified deficiencies and what additional information is required to correct those deficiencies or complete the review.

Administrative Meetings and Communications

Administrative meetings or communications are ad hoc, private two-way communications (phone, mail or in person) between FDA and outside parties on matters within FDA's jurisdiction.[9] These meetings generally occur between FDA, a healthcare company, a medical association, an advocacy group or a private individual. FDA or the sponsor may request a meeting. The purpose of administrative meetings or communications is to address scientific issues that warrant discussion with FDA. Following the meetings, FDA generally will issue non-binding advice.

Administrative meetings have a specific timeline for scheduling, filing of appropriate documents and the meeting, based on FDA classification of the meeting as a Type A or Type C meeting as referenced in the guidance for product application meetings.

Public Administrative Proceedings

In response to the public's demand for greater transparency of FDA policy and procedures, FDA has established four types of Public Administrative Proceedings (meetings):[10]
1. formal evidentiary hearings
2. public board of inquiry
3. hearing before the commissioner
4. Advisory Committee meetings

Public administrative meetings occur as needed except Advisory Committee meetings that generally occur prior to the *Prescription Drug User Fee Act* (*PDUFA*) action date.[11] These proceedings occur as specified by regulation, when ordered by the commissioner or when requested by a sponsor or affected public parties and approved by the commissioner.

Evidentiary Hearing

A formal evidentiary hearing is the administrative equivalent of a civil court hearing with comparable preparation and procedural controls.[12] Evidentiary hearings occur when specifically provided by law, when mandated by Congress or when ordered by the FDA commissioner in order to discuss public health concerns for a product or review proposed guidances, such as Risk Evaluation and Mitigation Strategies (REMS).

Board of Inquiry

Boards of inquiry are called when specifically authorized by regulation, at the discretion of the FDA commissioner or as an alternative to a formal evidentiary public hearing.[13] A board of inquiry is a hearing to review medical, scientific and technical issues.[14] The proceedings are conducted as a scientific inquiry and therefore are not comparable to a legal trial.[15]

Table 4-1. Description of FDA Product Application Meetings and Timing

	Type A Meeting	Type B Meeting	Type C Meeting
Meeting description	Dispute resolution Clinical holds Special Protocol Assessment (SPA)	Pre-IND EOP1 EOP2 Pre-NDA/Pre-BLA	Any other meeting not identified as Type A or B meeting
Confirmation of scheduling following sponsor request	14 days from time of request	21 days from time of request	21 days from time of request
Timing window for meeting to occur	30 days from time of request	60 days from time of request	75 days from time of request
Briefing information and relevant questions for discussion due to FDA	14 days prior to meeting	28 days prior to meeting	28 days prior to meeting

Public Hearing

A public hearing occurs when the commissioner determines that it is in the public interest to permit persons to present information and views at a public hearing on matters pending before the agency. These meetings are intended to solicit general views and information from interested parties on a particular topic. Under 21 CFR 16, public hearings are called at the discretion of the commissioner when considering regulatory action or when provided by law or regulation. Withdrawal of a PMA or disqualification of an IRB are examples of possible regulatory hearings.

Advisory Committee Meetings

Advisory Committee meetings are held by FDA to obtain recommendations and advice from subject matter experts on the safety and efficacy of foods, drugs, biologics and medical devices. Advisory Committees are composed of independent experts and public representatives. Most commonly, they provide medical expertise on product approvals, labeling conditions, scientific issues and research projects.[16] The Food and Drug Administration Amendment Act of 2007 (FDAAA) explicitly mandates that FDA must either convene an Advisory Committee panel for all new molecular entities or provide a written explanation as to why one is not required.[17]

In addition to the new regulations listed below, there has been an increased public focus on the transparency of Advisory Committees and the potential for conflict of interest of committee members.[18]

Currently, there are 50[19] Advisory Committees organized by the different centers within FDA (drugs, devices, biologics and food). Each committee is subject to a two-year renewal unless otherwise chartered. There are two types of committees: technical advisory committees that focus on product-related regulatory decisions and policy advisory committees that focus on general policy issues. Prior to an Advisory Committee meeting, FDA generally provides the committee a meeting package and specific questions to guide their discussions. A typical Advisory Committee meeting is open to the public,[20] and it is important to note that materials provided to an Advisory Committee must be made available to the public.[21] Advisory Committee meetings include a 45–90 minute presentation by the drug, biologic or device sponsor; a presentation by FDA; a public comment period; a question and answer (Q&A) session; a deliberations session; and, ultimately, a vote.

Any individual or company presenting at an Advisory Committee must understand that if any of the information declared as proprietary has been shared in a public forum, such as a scientific meeting, filed under patent, published, given to a customer, provided to financial analysts and stockholders or otherwise distributed upon request, it is not exempt from disclosure.[22]

Advisory Committee votes or recommendations are not binding on FDA, but they are given significant consideration.

In 2008, FDA issued the following final guidance documents on Advisory Panels:

- Guidance for the Public, FDA Advisory Committee Members, and FDA Staff on Procedures for Determining Conflict of Interest and Eligibility for Participation in FDA Advisory Committee
- Guidance for the Public, FDA Advisory Committee Members, and FDA Staff: Public Availability of Advisory Committee Members' Financial Interest Information and Waivers
- Guidance for FDA Advisory Committee Members and FDA Staff: Voting Procedures for Advisory Committee Meetings
- Guidance for Industry: Advisory Committee Meetings—Preparation and Public Availability of Information Given to Advisory Committee Member

Chapter 5 addresses Advisory Committee meetings in greater detail.

Summary

Collaborative communications between FDA, sponsors, Advisory Committees, and the public are generally divided into four categories or forms: regulatory communications, product applications meetings, administrative meetings or communications and public administrative proceedings. Each category or form has a specific purpose or objective. It is critical to regulatory professionals' success that they and their organization be totally familiar with each basic category or form and their proper application.[23]

FDA publishes numerous guidance documents on successfully communicating with the agency. Before any communication or meeting with FDA, regulatory professionals should ensure they and their organizations have reviewed the most recent FDA guidance documents on communication and meetings. Regulatory professionals should ensure participating parties are thoroughly trained and meetings are completely planned. They should also make sure the results of their communications are adequately recorded internally and they obtain a copy of FDA's communication record. If the sponsor's record of the communication is substantially different from FDA's record, the sponsor should request a further communication to discuss the differences.

References

1. "Understanding the Pre-IDE Program: FDA Perspective." Presentation by Captain Stephen P. Rhodes,USPHS, Director IDE and HDE Programs, Office of Device Evaluation. AdvaMed Audio Conference, 17 October 2007. Slide 3. Slide Serve website. www.slideserve.com/kordell/understanding-the-pre-ide-program-fda-perspective. Accessed 7 May 2013.
2. 21 CFR 10.115(b) Good guidance practices. FDA website. www.accessdata.fda.gov/scripts/cdrh/cfdocs/cfcfr/CFRSearch.cfm?fr=10.115. Accessed 7 May 2013.
3. FDA. *Guidance for Industry: Formal Meetings between the FDA and Sponsors or Applicants* (May 2009). Page 3. FDA website. www.fda.gov/downloads/Drugs/GuidanceComplianceRegulatoryInformation/Guidances/UCM153222.pdf. Accessed 5 May 2013.
4. Ibid pages 4–5.
5. Ibid page 10.
6. FDA. "FY 2004 Performance Report to the President and the Congress for the Medical Device User Fee and Modernization Act" which states "the more formal types of meetings (agreement meetings, determination meetings, 100-day meetings) are not used as frequently by premarket applicants." FDA website. www.fda.gov/AboutFDA/ReportsManualsForms/Reports/UserFeeReports/FinancialReports/MDUFMA/ucm135560.htm. Accessed 5 May 2013.
7. FDA. IDE Guidance #D99-1. Pre-IDE Program: Issues and Answers (March 1999). FDA website. www.fda.gov/MedicalDevices/DeviceRegulationandGuidance/GuidanceDocuments/ucm126600.htm. Accessed 5 May 2013.
8. FDA. *Early Collaboration Meetings under the FDA Modernization Act (FDAMA); Final Guidance for Industry and for CDRH Staff* (February 2001). Page 3. FDA website. www.fda.gov/MedicalDevices/DeviceRegulationandGuidance/GuidanceDocuments/ucm073604.htm. Accessed 7 May 2013.
9. 21 CFR 10.65(a) Meetings and correspondence. FDA website. www.accessdata.fda.gov/scripts/cdrh/cfdocs/cfcfr/CFRSearch.cfm?fr=10.65. Accessed 7 May 2013.
10. 21 CFR 10.203 Definitions. GPO website. www.gpo.gov/fdsys/pkg/CFR-2012-title21-vol1/pdf/CFR-2012-title21-vol1-sec10-203.pdf. Accessed 7 May 2013.
11. PDUFA action due date (or user fee goal date) is the date by which an action is due on a marketing application under the timeframes negotiated as a result of the Prescription Drug User Fee Act of 1992 (PDUFA) and subsequent legislation amending that act. SOPP 8401.3: Filing Action: Communication Options, FDA website. www.fda.gov/BiologicsBloodVaccines/GuidanceComplianceRegulatoryInformation/ProceduresSOPPs/ucm073085.htm. Accessed 7 May 2013.
12. FDA. *Guidance for Industry on Medical Device Appeals and Complaints: A Guidance on Dispute Resolution* (February 1998). Page 8. FDA website. www.fda.gov/downloads/MedicalDevices/DeviceRegulationandGuidance/GuidanceDocuments/ucm094523.htm. Accessed 5 May 2013
13. Ibid.
14. Ibid.
15. Ibid.
16. 21 CFR 14 Public Hearing Before a Public Advisory Committee. FDA website. www.accessdata.fda.gov/scripts/cdrh/cfdocs/cfcfr/CFRSearch.cfm?CFRPart=14. Accessed 7 May 2013.
17. Section 918 of the *Food and Drug Administration Amendments Act* of 2007 (P.L. 110-85, in effect March 2008).
18. Food and Drug Administration Amendments Act of 2007 (FDAAA). FDA website. www.fda.gov/RegulatoryInformation/Legislation/FederalFoodDrugandCosmeticActFDCAct/SignificantAmendmentstotheFDCAct/FoodandDrugAdministrationAmendmentsActof2007/FullTextofFDAAALaw/default.htm. Accessed 7 May 2013.
19. FDA Committees and Meeting Materials webpage. FDA website. www.fda.gov/AdvisoryCommittees/CommitteesMeetingMaterials/default.htm.. Accessed 7 May 2013.
20. Op cit 17.
21. Op cit 18.
22. 21 CFR 14.27 Determination to close portions of advisory committee meetings. GPO website. www.gpo.gov/fdsys/pkg/CFR-1999-title21-vol1/pdf/CFR-1999-title21-vol1-sec14-27.pdf. Accessed 7 May 2013.
23. *The FDA Advisory Committee Survival Manual: A Step-by-Step Guide to Preparing for a Successful Meeting*. Published by 3D Communications (2008). Available at: www.3dcommunications.us/FDAsurvivalguide.html. Accessed 5 May 2013.

Chapter 5

Preparing for Key FDA Meetings and Advisory Committee Meetings

Updated by Allison Kennedy, MSc, RAC

OBJECTIVES

- Provide general recommendations for preparing for FDA meetings
- Detail the extensive preparation process for Advisory Committee presentations

LAWS, REGULATIONS AND GUIDELINES COVERED IN THIS CHAPTER

- *Guidance for Industry: Formal Meetings Between the FDA and Sponsors or Applicants* (May 2009)

- *Guidance for the Public, FDA Advisory Committee Members, and FDA Staff on Procedures for Determining Conflict of Interest and Eligibility for Participation in FDA Advisory Committee* (August 2008)

- *Guidance for the Public, FDA Advisory Committee Members, and FDA Staff: Public Availability of Advisory Committee Members' Financial Interest Information and Waivers* (March 2012)

- *Guidance for FDA Advisory Committee Members and FDA Staff: Voting Procedures for Advisory Committee Meetings* (August 2008)

- *Guidance for Industry: Advisory Committee Meetings—Preparation and Public Availability of Information Given to Advisory Committee Members* (August 2008)

- *Guidance for the Public, FDA Advisory Committee Members, and FDA Staff: The Open Public Hearing at FDA Advisory Committee Meetings* (December 2010)

Introduction

The various types of meetings with the US Food and Drug Administration (FDA) outlined in Chapter 4 require different levels of preparation by the company, ranging from regulatory communications, which require less preparation, to highly publicized Advisory Committee meetings, requiring intensive preparation.

All meetings should begin with a goal of maximizing the opportunities provided by FDA interactions. Establishing an open and forthright relationship with the FDA division and demonstrating credibility for the company's product or issue is paramount in every interaction.

This chapter highlights the general steps that companies should consider in preparing for all FDA meetings and outlines the more detailed and comprehensive process of preparing for an Advisory Committee meeting.

General Preparation for FDA Meetings

Importantly, before requesting any meeting, make sure the company is actually ready to have a meeting, as briefing packages are generally due four weeks prior to meeting (two weeks for Type A). Regardless of the type of meeting, the product category for which a company may be requesting approval or any issues playing out in the external environment, there is one commonality for all FDA meetings—the need to tell a clear story and to set the data or issue in context. Just as FDA has a process for determining whether a drug or device should be approved, a company needs a process to keep its team on track and prepare in the most efficient and effective way. A good process will incorporate the following objectives: developing a strategy to best attain company goals; understanding the various FDA audiences; prioritizing data and other information; preparing speakers to articulate the information and effectively answer questions; and testing and measuring progress with well-organized practice and rehearsals.

Prior to all meetings with FDA, whether in person or by telephone, companies should consider the following 10 steps:

1. Know Your Audience
- Research FDA personnel who will be in attendance at the meeting. Learn about their experiences, biases and backgrounds in order to better anticipate their opinions.

2. Know the Issues
- Review recent relevant precedents and actions by the FDA division responsible for evaluating the product; understand published or implied FDA guidances and consider explicitly incorporating them into the sponsor's strategy or presentation.

3. Set a Goal for Each FDA Conversation or Meeting
- Determine the meeting's objective or purpose, whether it is to obtain FDA guidance, present the development program or obtain FDA agreement.
- Determine the issues and questions that will be addressed and who will attend on behalf of the company and the agency.
- Stay focused on the goal during each meeting. Seek specific answers and commitments from FDA to achieve that goal.
- Strive for agreement on main issues. Try to get clarity, direction and, if possible, commitment on these issues.

4. Know Your Position
- Conduct a high-level messaging session before filing a new drug or device application for consistency across all communications. In this session:
    o Analyze key data with a public forum and media in mind.
    o Brainstorm and identify potential issues among all stakeholders.
    o Develop high-level messages to provide the basis for conversations with FDA.
- Make sure the team clearly understands and is aligned with the company's position and knows how to articulate it.

5. Provide Pertinent Materials for Each Meeting in a Timely Manner to Allow FDA to Adequately Analyze the Information
- Be succinct. Do not overwhelm FDA with thousands of pages of background information; streamline the information, and focus it on the issues and goal of each meeting. Include a preliminary proposed agenda, focused questions and a background package or briefing document that includes the sponsor's position, an outline of the product data and the sponsor's development recommendation.

6. Anticipate Concerns and Interests; Be Prepared to Sufficiently Answer Likely FDA Questions
- Understand potential risks from a difference in data interpretation or recommended data requests and proactively prepare acceptable contingency scenarios that could resolve them.
- In addition to FDA concerns, proactively address resolutions to any issues regarding therapeutic area, class perception and public concern.

7. Be Organized
- Manage the meeting time carefully to ensure adequate discussion and clear understanding of answers and recommendations within the allotted meeting time.
- Define attendees' roles in advance and bring the appropriate people to the meeting to discuss the sponsor's questions and provide any necessary clarification to FDA.

8. Listen Carefully to What FDA is Actually Saying
- During in-person meetings, pay attention to body language, internal dynamics and offhand remarks. During phone meetings, listen to voice tone.
- Immediately correct any misinterpretations or misconceptions FDA may have.

9. Record Feedback
- Strive for clear agreement on critical decisions and make sure they are documented in the FDA meeting minutes.
- Keep an ongoing list of all issues raised by FDA officials during the meetings and conference calls. Record how many times specific issues are raised to gauge their importance. Remember to note which agency representative is raising them.
- Explicitly document when FDA mutes the phone. This usually indicates either an important question they want to refine or internal disagreement and

may help you determine what issues are still causing internal dissent or confusion at the agency. Consider additional data or programs that could clarify or resolve these issues.
- Save the last five minutes of the meeting to summarize the discussion and obtain agreement on action steps.

10. **Foster a Flexible, Collaborative and Non-adversarial Relationship**
    - Keep the lines of communication open—even if FDA's message is negative.
    - Do not take a divergent point of view personally. Always retain composure if FDA takes the opposite position. Do not debate policy—unless it is clearly on the agenda and has been "briefed."
    - Listen to FDA's requests and provide answers where possible. Look for opportunities to resolve issues before they become obstacles to approval.
    - Be respectful, but not meek.
    - Be prepared to calibrate the communications strategy in light of shifting issues, an evolving environment and changes within the FDA review team.
    - Anticipate potential data requirements beyond those being articulated by FDA in case the agency shifts direction or changes its mind.
    - Do not include any off-agenda items—avoid surprises.
    - Do not hide information—the last thing a sponsor wants is for FDA to find out about a negative issue that you have not introduced.
    - Do not stress commercial or corporate concerns over science.

Overview of Advisory Committee Meetings

Because the *Food and Drug Administration Amendments Act of 2007 (FDAAA)* mandates that Advisory Committees be convened for all new molecular entities, or requires FDA to provide a written explanation as to why there will not be a meeting, the sponsor of a new drug or device must plan for the likelihood that an Advisory Committee will be part of its regulatory processes. However, a sponsor often does not know whether its product will have to face a committee hearing until a few months before the actual event. Thus, strategic planning for a potential meeting must be an integral part of any product's development process.

An Advisory Committee meeting to review a new drug or device application is unlike most other FDA meetings. It is not only a scientific discussion of the data and issues surrounding a drug or device, it is also a high-profile regulatory, financial and legal event—a very public day in court for the sponsor and its product.

Advisory Committee meetings are typically attended by rival pharmaceutical or device companies, the media and key stakeholders, including patient and advocacy groups. The voting members on an Advisory Committee are not a typical scientific audience. Due to concerns regarding conflicts of interest, FDA often is prohibited from including on the panel any experts who may have collaborated on the study or may have contributed to the product's development. This means the panel's clinicians, academicians and statisticians, while experts in their respective fields, may know little more about the specific issues than what they read in the FDA and sponsor briefing books and will hear at the meeting. Sponsors need to be aware of this and be careful not to assume in-depth, product-specific knowledge on the part of the committee members.

The order of events for Advisory Committee meetings can vary considerably. Most meetings begin with a call to order by the chairperson, followed by an introduction of the panel and its members. A statement regarding the conflicts of interest of committee members is read. The chairperson will welcome attendees on behalf of FDA and focus the issues in terms of the meeting agenda. The opening events are then followed by the open public hearing (minimum of one hour), followed by presentations by the sponsor and the FDA, as listed in the meeting agenda. Committee discussion and a question and answer session ensue, followed by a committee vote, and finally, adjournment of the meeting. "Affected persons" are then informed of the agency's decision (i.e., in light of the committee recommendation) within 90 days of the advisory committee meeting.

Under the *Federal Advisory Committee Act*, a part of every Advisory Committee meeting must be open to the public. Examples of "open sessions" are those in which NDAs, supplements, postapproval safety and risk versus benefit issues are discussed. Sessions that are not open to the public, the so-called "closed sessions," include those in which trade secrets or commercial confidential information (e.g., INDs and review division updates to the committee) are discussed. Only special government employees (SGEs), FDA employees and invited sponsor representatives are allowed to attend closed sessions of Advisory Committee meetings. (See Chapter 4 for more detailed information on the purpose and format of Advisory Committee meetings.)

Preparing for an Advisory Committee Meeting

A three-step approach to preparing for an Advisory Committee comprises analysis, content development and testing of the strategy and materials.

The analysis step includes: understanding the audience (FDA division heads, medical reviewers and Advisory Committee members); evaluating the data and science; analyzing the external environment and assembling the

Chapter 5

Figure 5-1. Major Milestone Timeline

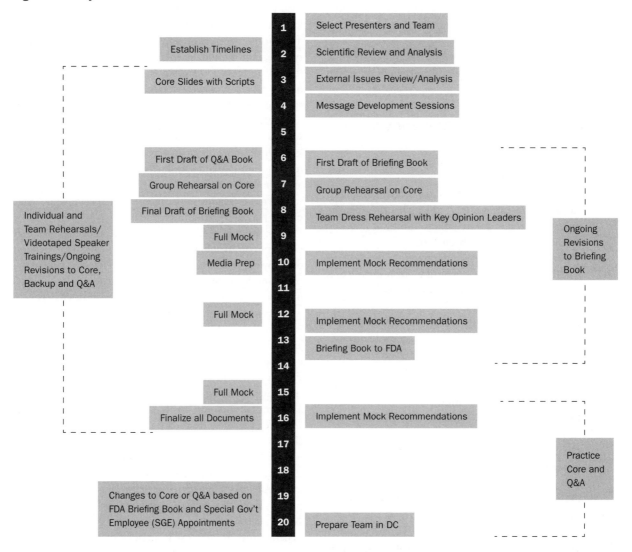

preparation team. The content development step involves creating a communications strategy and materials, including the core presentation, slides, briefing materials and advocacy outreach. The testing step comprises rehearsals, expert feedback and, ultimately, adjustment of the strategy and materials.

Selecting the Team

Most sponsors underestimate the amount of time it will take to sufficiently prepare for an FDA Advisory Committee meeting. Thus, it is critical to select the right team, assign them the proper roles and set ground rules and realistic expectations. A key starting point in team selection is identifying a senior person in research and development or regulatory to champion the project and ensure Advisory Committee preparation is the presentation team's top priority. The ideal team should include representatives from a variety of areas: regulatory, medical, clinical, toxicology, statistics, pharmacovigilance and commercial. Each brings individual expertise and a unique perspective that can help secure a positive recommendation from the committee and attain the target label. Orchestrating the team, considering and weighing its input and selecting the proper role for each team member are as much an art as a science.

The size of an Advisory Committee preparation team will vary according to the company and its resources. Frequently, an overlap of responsibilities will exist among sub-teams, with some people performing more than one role. Although there are many ways to organize a team, a typical breakdown of roles and responsibilities follows:

- Presentation team—core presenters and back-up presenters

- Data/slide triage team—people who compile and organize data and slides
- Briefing book team—main author and data triage team members
- Internal and/or external scientific advisors—content experts and responders for question and answer development
- Regulatory team—regulatory executives who manage communication and scheduling with FDA throughout the Advisory Committee process
- Communications team—presentation support team of writers, editors, presentation coaches, marketing, brand, public relations executives and media trainers
- Slide development and slide logistics team
- Logistics team—project manager, meeting organizers, schedulers and administrative support

Once the team has been selected, it is important to brief members on what to expect during the preparation process and at the hearing. Team members should be briefed on everything from how the slide process will work and what the room layout will be, to how the Advisory Committee hearing schedule will flow and anticipated media interest.

Organizational tools such as a major milestone timeline (**Figure 5-1**) and a project management chart (**Figure 5-2**) are highly effective ways to brief the team and keep it on track. These tools provide an overview of the process, the tasks, the assignments and the schedule and provide a realistic view of the required team member time commitment and how their roles are critical to achieving the goal.

Researching and Analyzing the Advisory Committee Members

Each Advisory Committee member has his or her own individual style and concerns, which can affect what questions are asked during the meeting, how they are asked and how members ultimately vote. Knowing who is on the committee, their backgrounds and how they may influence one another is critical, as it helps frame a relevant presentation, predict questions and prepare answers.

To analyze Advisory Committee members, the team may:

- Study past votes and discussions around issues similar to the sponsor's. Companies can gain a wealth of information by reviewing transcripts of previous meetings from FDA's website (www.fda.gov) or viewing videos of meetings on FDA Live (www.fdalive.com). Panel members often ask similar questions at different Advisory Committee hearings, so it is highly instructive to learn what they have asked in the past and, of equal importance, to analyze their comments.
- Analyze their interests and positions on specific issues, including scientific studies they have authored, associations with which they are affiliated, practice guideline committees on which they serve, public comments in presentations and media interviews on specific issues.
- Identify the relationships among committee members, including what associations, universities and company affiliations they may have in common.
- See the committee in action. Reviewing old Advisory Committee tapes and taking the team on a "field trip" to an Advisory Committee meeting are invaluable ways to analyze what types of questions are being asked, how they are being asked and give the team the full flavor and experience of the event.

Leveraging Advocacy

Because FDA and Advisory Committee members are influenced by the public and the political environment, sponsors must consider these external influences in the planning process. Sponsors should have a well-thought-out plan to communicate with key stakeholders—from patient advocacy groups and healthcare associations to key opinion leaders and policy groups.

Third-party advocates, key opinion leaders and medical experts can fill a variety of valuable roles in supporting the sponsor's goals. Assuming all ties with the sponsor are clearly revealed, they can publish articles on the data or the need for the product, speak at medical symposia, answer highly technical or specific questions from the Advisory Committee during the hearing, testify during the public comment period and speak to the media. Sponsors should utilize the experience offered by such experts as much as possible. Key opinion leaders also should be considered as presenters at the Advisory Committee meeting, as they can bring a great deal of credibility to a company's presentation.

It is important to note that engaging key opinion leaders and groups has never been more complicated, so any compensation must come with no strings attached. All financial relationships should be appropriately disclosed. In today's environment, transparency is extremely important.

Some key steps in creating an effective advocacy program are:

- identifying the most influential patient and consumer groups and healthcare associations and ranking them in terms of leadership and influence
- assessing opinions of medical experts in the field, as well as the position statements of medical societies
- listening to what financial analysts are saying about the product and how they are characterizing its impact on the company

Finally, it is important to prioritize the information and factor it into the communications strategy and core messages for all communications, including the Advisory Committee presentation, the briefing book, the Q&A book and media outreach. As part of this process, it is also important to brief advocacy groups and, when appropriate, enlist their support.

Preparing the Briefing Materials, Core Presentation, and Q&A Book

There is no substitute for good data. But good data alone are not always sufficient to secure a positive recommendation at an Advisory Committee meeting. A well-constructed scientific story that provides context for that data is the backbone of a sponsor's briefing book and presentation.

To ensure consistency of messages across all materials, no content should be developed until a strategic messaging session is conducted. The messaging should drive the direction of the briefing book, the presentation script, the slides and answers to key questions. This process should begin as soon as the sponsor has selected and organized its team and is analyzing the environment, the audiences and its issues.

The primary steps in creating, prioritizing and harmonizing content are:
- Conduct a brainstorming session with key people from the sponsor's team. Set a goal for the content. What is it the sponsor really wants to communicate to the audience about its product? Focus on the high-level messages that will serve as the foundation of the presentation to the Advisory Committee. These messages should be based on the medical need for the product, the strength of the data and the benefit the product provides.
- Discuss and prioritize the data, outlining all relevant studies for easy reference and outlining key metrics of each study (e.g., meaningful endpoints, results, sample size, demographics). Rank the studies to determine which to emphasize during the presentation.
- Incorporate the data into a message matrix to serve as a guide to outline and develop the presentations and the questions and answers (Q&A), and prioritize the messages by rating what is most important by considering the strengths of the product and science, the issues FDA officials have highlighted and the areas of interest from Advisory Committee members.
- Finally, assign individual "owners" to issues by topic, assigning responsibility and accountability to specific team members for gathering data, drafting the first set of answers to questions and developing supporting documentation in the form of charts, graphs or tables for slides.

Once the key messages and data for the briefing materials and presentation have been determined, it is time to construct the flow of the presentation and the briefing book.

Although the content and flow of both of these will vary depending upon the product and the issues, there are some general guidelines to follow.

For both the presentation and the briefing book, follow the rules of clear writing and logical organization. Headline main points. Be succinct, and write in short sentences. Summarize key messages at the beginning and end of the documents.

Writing the Briefing Book

Because the Advisory Committee members will get briefing books from both FDA and the sponsor, it is best to keep the book short, concise and well-organized, so it can be easily read and understood. Aim for approximately 100 to 150 pages in length, depending upon the extent of the clinical program.

For the purposes of efficiency, consistency and clarity, be sure to base the briefing book on the clinical section of the New Drug Application (NDA), Biologics License Application (BLA) or Premarket Approval Application (PMA), focusing on information directly related to the issues being considered by the committee. Edit out information and data not directly related to these issues. Consider how the product will fit into current treatment patterns in order to address treatment issues, barriers or beliefs. Never include new data in the book that have not been submitted in the NDA, BLA or PMA and have therefore not been reviewed by FDA. Finally, avoid any statements or suggestions that can be viewed as misleading or promotional or that can be misconstrued as a recommendation of off-label product use.

Structure the book in an organized way by dividing it into distinct sections, beginning with a clear executive summary that provides an overview of the main points of the book and makes the best case for the product or issue. Summarize and synthesize the data within each section. In all cases, sponsors should keep in mind that the Advisory Committee members have limited time to prepare for the meeting, so the briefing package should be a well-organized and easily readable summary of the data.

Make certain that all presenters know the contents of the briefing book and can answer questions that arise from the book as well as the presentation.

Scripting the Core Presentation

Sponsors typically have between 45 and 90 minutes to deliver the core presentation, something that can be negotiated with the agency in advance. As a result, every word counts. The core presentation is the sponsor's opportunity to make its strongest case to a "jury" deciding its fate. Because this is not a typical scientific presentation but rather a persuasive

Figure 5-2. Sample Project Management Chart

ID	Task Name	Start	Finish
1	**Strategic Definition of Key Focus**	2/7	2/21
2	Define team members (roles/responsibilities)	2/11	2/12
3	Initiate team charter	2/12	2/12
4	Identify potential Advisory Committee (AC) meeting	2/7	2/12
5	Team assembled timeline, resource, communications plan	2/13	2/19
6	Approval of timeline, resource, comms plan	2/21	2/22
7	Work initiated following plan approval	2/25	2/25
8	**Regulatory Background Review**	2/13	3/4
9	Summary of AC member background compiled	2/15	2/21
10	Summary of agency correspondence, meeting minutes, issues, etc.	2/25	2/29
11	**Identification of Relevant Advisory Commitee Meetings**	2/13	3/4
12	Obtain copies of transcripts and/or video	2/13	3/4
13	Obtain copies of briefing pkgs	2/13	3/4
14	Host AC review session with Core Team	3/6	3/6
15	**Key Messages Outlined**	2/28	3/7
16	Identify Key Messages	2/28	3/5
17	Submit Key Messages to Management for approval	3/6	3/6
18	Team finalizes Key Messages	3/6	3/7
19	**Key Issues Identified**	3/6	3/26
20	Identify Key Issues (Draft list)	3/6	3/12
21	Team review of Key Issues	3/13	3/13
22	Submit Key Issues to Management for input	3/13	3/14
23	Draft outline of responses to issues with team input	3/17	3/21
24	Team approval of outline responses to Key Issues	3/24	3/24
25	Submit outline (issues response) to Management	3/25	3/25
26	Team review of outline (issues response)	3/25	3/25
27	**Slide Production Key Presentations**	3/6	4/25
28	Develop outline of Primary Presentation	3/6	3/12
29	Team approves draft outline of core	3/13	3/13
30	Management approval of outline of core	3/14	3/17
31	Primary Presentation	3/18	4/25

argument with a singular goal, controlling the story around the data is critical. The science does not speak for itself; not everyone will interpret the same data in the same way; therefore, context and clear explanation are essential components of success. In general, all Advisory Committee members want to see and hear a clear, concise and convincing scientific story that creates confidence that the team knows its product well and has shared fully with the committee the product's positive, negative and unknown attributes.

While sponsors routinely create core presentations from pre-developed slides, outlining and scripting the presentation before developing core slides will allow the messages to drive the presentation rather than data without context. Scripting every word of the presentation is also a must, as this will ensure the precision and clarity of the message and reduce the chances of "surprises" surfacing during the presentation.

As previously mentioned, the most effective and efficient way to develop a core presentation is to start with the goal and high-level messages from the brainstorming session. From those messages, create an outline to develop a story flow for the overall presentation and then do the same for each individual presentation. Look for opportunities to weave in and reinforce the main messages of the overall presentation for consistency.

Because the core is delivered as the spoken versus the written word, it is important that the script be written for the ear and not the eye. That means using short sentences and an active voice that can easily be delivered by the presenter and understood by the audience the first time. The goal of the presentation is that everyone listening understands the data in the same way.

Writing the Q&A Book

The same rules apply when developing answers to questions. Answers should be clearly headlined so the responses and messages are clear and direct. In addition, the questions and answers should be ordered in a well-organized book, so responders learn the answers and identify the appropriate slides. The book should serve as a practice tool as well as a map for the day of the hearing. This dynamic document will change as information is incorporated from new studies, agency feedback and external sources, such as stakeholders and the media. The Q&A book should be organized by topic and identify not only the question and answer, but also the appropriate responder and what, if any, slides support the point.

Developing and Managing Slides

Once the script is written, and as answers to questions are being crafted, slides should be developed to visually reinforce the information. The purpose of a slide is to support the presenter's message—not confuse it. As a result, slides should follow the same rules of clear communication. Choose a simple, clear slide template with mid- to dark-blue backgrounds and a simple sans-serif font to reduce eye strain. For graph slides, make sure the x- and y-axes are thick and vibrant enough to be seen in the back of a large meeting room and are clearly labeled with easy-to-find legends. For text slides, the fewer words the better. The goal of any slide is to pass the "glance test," so the audience immediately understands the slide's message. It is better to have multiple slides that "build" and explain a point than to crowd too much information on one slide. Too much information on one slide can lead committee members to focus on different information and confuse the message. With slides, as with writing, less is more.

To help in both the development and management of slides, a specific process should be followed and a team assigned. This team has several important functions. One function is to compile and organize data and slides for each component of the core presentation. A second function is to gather data and prepare backup slides for the questions the Advisory Committee members may ask. A third function is to quickly and calmly locate a requested backup slide for responders during the Q&A sessions. A fourth function is to help a presenter answer a question by prompting the presenter with an appropriately chosen slide on the preview monitor.

It is common for sponsors to have several thousand backup slides for the Q&A portion of the Advisory Committee meeting. Ideally, a slide should be displayed within a few seconds of the question being asked. For this to occur, it is best for sponsors to use an automated slide recall process. This system should allow responders to preview a slide on a monitor that only they can see, and then, in real time, decide whether to show that slide or call for another.

The intricate and important process of developing and locating the right slide at the right moment starts with the data triage team. The backup slides are typically organized by topic matter (e.g., safety, efficacy, unmet need, postmarketing surveillance). Each team member is responsible for at least one of these areas and is an expert.

Conducting Perfect Practice Through Rehearsals

As the content is being developed, it also needs to be tested. Sponsor teams frequently wait too long in the process to begin testing. This is a lost opportunity because testing through practice is the best way to refine content. In addition to internal team rehearsals, sponsors should also run several realistic rehearsals with external experts role-playing the Advisory Committee members.

A mock Advisory Committee hearing is a rehearsal "on steroids," and is where the sponsor's team gets its first taste of what it is like to present to a potentially critical audience and answer questions under pressure. If done correctly, it will provide a reality check for the sponsor. The more realistic the mock panel, the better prepared the presenters and other responders will be for the actual hearing.

The key to a realistic mock panel is convening one that mirrors the actual Advisory Committee as closely as possible. This increases the opportunity for mock members to examine, interpret and challenge the data in the same way as Advisory Committee members. This is one area in which effective profiles of committee members provide benefits. The mock Advisory Committee hearing should be constructed like a dress rehearsal. The room should be set up in the same formation as it will be on the day of the hearing. Mock members should stay in role to provide presenters with a realistic run-through. The sponsor should provide briefing books to the mock Advisory Committee members prior to the rehearsal so they will go into the meeting with the same information as the actual committee. This book should be a near-complete draft of the final briefing book that will be submitted. The panel should critique the value of the book and the consistency of information provided with the presentations.

Following the rehearsal, the mock panelists should provide a tough, insightful critique and give honest feedback about the presenters as well as the presentation. This feedback should be used to adjust and enhance strategy, core messages and responses for the Q&A session.

The sponsor's internal team should schedule a debrief immediately following each mock hearing and document what worked well and what can de done differently in preparation for the next mock hearing.

Maximizing the Final Days before the Advisory Committee Meeting

In the few days leading up to the meeting, sponsor teams should set up rehearsals on or near the FDA meeting site, near Washington, DC. Forty-eight hours before the meeting, FDA will release final names of the Advisory Committee members, as well as the specific questions they will pose to the committee. This is the time to readjust strategy, if necessary, edit the final presentation and refine Q&A responses.

A logistics plan should be in place to help facilitate and control communications among team members during the meeting. Given the pressure and time constraints of Advisory Committee day, discipline in communications is critical. Only vital issues should be discussed, and that discussion should be fast, focused and confidential.

Whatever system is chosen, it must be thought through in advance and communicated to everyone involved. This includes everything from ensuring the availability of enough meeting rooms with working computers, printers, copiers and faxes, to ensuring the presence of a solid security system to guard against breaches. Whether a company hires a professional meeting planning company or security firm, or handles these tasks internally, organization and security are crucial components to ensuring that the meeting runs smoothly.

Summary

With Advisory Committee meetings becoming more like adversarial proceedings than presentations of scientific data, companies must prepare as they would for a big court case that has major implications on everything from the company's stock price to its reputation. Clear and persuasive communication is the key to success in this challenging environment.

Strategic communications planning is critical and must begin early in the product's lifecycle. Companies must honestly assess and analyze their products and be open to criticism and perceptions, right or wrong, that exist in the external environment. It is imperative to understand the concerns of the various audiences and to be proactive and persuasive in addressing their issues through an effective communication plan. By applying these principles zealously to the Advisory Committee meeting preparation process, companies can hope to achieve their goal of a positive Advisory Committee recommendation and, ultimately, FDA approval of their product.

Chapter 6
Crisis Management

By Donna Helms, MBA, RAC

OBJECTIVES

❑ Provide some perspective not only for known issues that arise in the industry but also to project that perspective to address future potential crises

❑ Learn how to apply scientific and management techniques to handle a crisis

❑ Review management activities to avert crises

❑ Learn leadership skills, effective communication skills and how to understand customers and environments

Introduction

A crisis, as defined here, is a situation that specifically involves a pharmaceutical product, medical device or activity with potentially significant adverse implications for regulatory agencies, healthcare providers, patients, media, the public or external and/or internal company stakeholders. The situation can involve a drug or device in either the investigational phase or the marketed phase.

Examples of an investigational pharmaceutical or device-related crisis include:
- investigator or employee fraud
- development program discontinuation due to safety concerns
- use of an investigational product outside IND requirements
- promotion of an investigational product
- Clinical Hold
- refusal to file an application
- Health Authority review issues affecting product approval
- pre-inspection issues

Examples of a marketed product-related crisis include:
- reports of serious adverse drug or device events or safety findings that may affect the product's benefit:risk evaluation
- reports of serious adverse drug or device events or safety findings of a similar product or similar disease
- drug/device shortages
- reports of tampering
- product recall
- litigation reports and discovery activities
- off-label promotion
- inspection issue
- Warning Letter
- regulatory or political actions
- social media events
- Application Integrity Policy
- Corporate Integrity Agreement

The regulatory discipline crosses almost all other disciplines within an organization, including nonclinical, clinical, CMC, adverse events, compliance, and marketing and promotion. To support all of these areas throughout the organization, regulatory staff should be aware of all the relevant environments—internal, health authority, patients, the healthcare industry, marketplace and political—and implications of the issues in the global environment. Regulatory staff must ensure the maintenance and appropriate management of effective relationships with the regulatory agencies. Regulatory staff are also in a position to evaluate potential compliance concerns and to provide assessments to avert any crises. A regulatory professional's leadership during times of a crisis is crucial.

Crisis Management

This chapter will not go into all of the potential areas where a crisis could occur and what the regulations are for each of those areas, but rather will address the core concepts required for managing a crisis once it occurs and discuss how to avert a crisis.

The mission of any Health Authority is to protect the public health and to ensure the safety, effectiveness and security of regulated products. These Health Authorities and other related agencies are key customers. However, the patient and healthcare practitioners are the primary customers; quality patient care is the ultimate goal. Additionally, there are many other stakeholders who also would be impacted by a crisis and its resolution.

In any crisis, the regulatory environment needs to be understood. Are there specific safety issues for which the Health Authority is watching? Have there been multiple occurrences of similar issues and the agencies are now enforcing stricter consequences? Are the authorities looking for reasons to support their own agendas? Consideration also must be given to the marketplace environment. Are there reimbursement issues? Are there competitor issues? What are the expectations of the marketplace? In addition, the political environment must be acknowledged. What are the current relevant political "hot buttons?" Will politicians feel the need to become involved in your crisis?

A priority in any crisis is to identify the stakeholders and audiences that could be impacted by the issue and might be interested in the outcome. Effective communications are key to the success of the crisis management.

The management of a crisis can have an extreme impact on the organization—positively, resulting in increased competence, or negatively, if not done correctly. With good management, a crisis well-handled can enhance the organization internally and can benefit its external image. Without good management, a crisis can worsen quickly and spread to other company activities and products. Effective crisis management not only protects the well-being of patients, but also protects the company from further adverse consequences. Effective internal communication will guide the company to resolution of the crisis and move the company forward. Effective external communication will ameliorate the potential for confusion, fear and skepticism. Above all, a crisis needs to be handled as expeditiously as possible.

Internal Management of a Crisis

Once a crisis occurs, it is essential to clearly identify the issue and its root cause. This is true for both the investigational and the marketed product phases. It normally will take a cadre of various disciplines to investigate and isolate the issue.

A Crisis Management Team (CMT) should be put into place, again with assurance that the right expertise and experience are represented. This should not be just a technical team but should also incorporate other relevant disciplines and management levels. The focus should first be on identifying the causative issue, ensuring it is specifically defined, and how and when it occurred are determined. The situation should be assessed to determine whether the issue is isolated, whether it has occurred with other products, or whether it could happen again. This should incorporate an evaluation of areas or other products that could be directly or indirectly affected.

For example, if the issue is one of investigator fraud, once the single issue is identified, the CMT should address the reason it happened, the impact on the investigator's patients, the impact on the study as a whole (remediation that may be needed, e.g., a re-analysis without that investigator's data), and the impact on other studies that included that investigator. If the product is being investigated globally, there should be an assessment of additional actions needed. The action plan would have to identify who else in the organization should be notified or brought in to assist in the resolution, in this case, legal.

Depending on the issue, it is possible that external experts will need to be involved in the assessment and potential resolutions.

The communications plan is very important. Communications must be: timely, before rumors emerge; clear and simple, especially if the issue is complex; and balanced, considering risk and benefit. The communication plan needs to identify who needs to be notified, in what timeframe, and whether the communication should be verbal, written or both.

The CMT therefore must convene strategic planning meetings to put together a plan to:
- identify the issue and understand the fundamental concerns
- determine the root cause
- ask whether it is an isolated incident, has occurred with other products or could happen again
- prepare a gap analysis and potential mitigations
- assess applicability to other operations or products
- determine frequency of event
- identify the significance of the risk and who or what it impacts
- evaluate impact for other geographic regions, as applicable
- engage other experts as necessary, to assist in problem-solving
- define activities, solutions, resources and timelines in a master document, identifying the responsible person or group
- prepare remediation plans
- document decisions, actions and resolutions

- determine level of confidentiality required
- identify internal groups that need to have special communications developed (e.g., sales force)
- develop effective internal communications strategy for the organization
- identify all external stakeholders and audiences and develop a communications plan
- oversee the corrective actions

Documentation of the issue, the situation and causes, and the actions to resolve it should be clear and factual. Decisions must be communicated clearly and effectively. The strategy and mitigation plan must be executed quickly. This is particularly critical if patient safety is a concern. However, in any case, speed is a key determinant of success.

It is imperative to inform management at all levels, as appropriate; meetings should be held with management to ensure they are engaged and supportive of the CMT recommendations for corrective actions and communications.

The CMT must have the full support of upper management. It is critical that the team and the organization not include "blame" or finger-pointing; all aspects of the issue must be reviewed and assigning blame is not productive. Defining the issue and identifying potential resolutions and a mitigation plan are paramount. Assessing blame for a situation will only serve to push reactive problem-solving, rather than constructive, competent assessment and resolution. Openness and transparency regarding the issue and how it occurred will enable better informed decisions and development of options.

The regulatory staff play a key role in management of the crisis. Regulatory staff should share not only the regulations and guidances issued by Health Authorities, but also should provide the interpretation of those documents and convey the expectations of the Health Authorities. All activities should be carried out with the goal of patient protection and compliance with all regulatory and legal requirements.

The same basic process should be followed for a marketed product issue, except that there are additional stakeholders and interested parties that would have to be included in an action plan (see External Management of a Crisis, below).

External Management of a Crisis

Informing the regulatory authorities as soon as possible regarding a new issue, or working with the authorities as soon as an issue is identified externally, is critical. As regulatory staff are the liaisons with the Health Authority, it is critical to have good management techniques and communication skills. Presentation of the issue and proposals for remediation will be important to the effective handling of the crisis. Information exchange and discussions with the Health Authorities should occur as early as possible. Depending on the issue, this may start with a notification of a potential concern and an overview of what is being done to investigate and remediate. Broader and more detailed discussions would follow. Regular updates are critical for a partnership to develop. A comprehensive plan should be reviewed with the appropriate Health Authority or agency(ies).

In today's regulatory environment, the word "negotiation" has lost a lot of its original intent. The world of negotiation is built on data, compliance actions and resolution in a timely fashion. The CMT must demonstrate credibility, commitment and trust in the regulatory discussions. Most of the communication in the early stage of crisis management probably will be verbal, so those communication skills need to be excellent. Later, written communications will need to clearly address the Health Authority's expectations. It is important that the Health Authority feel assured that the regulatory contact, representing the company, is forthright, collaborative, presents a complete response, and will monitor the resolution appropriately.

The applicability of regulatory options should be evaluated. Depending on the issue, meetings should be scheduled with the Health Authority, requests for alternative review procedures could be made, or an Advisory Committee review may be requested. Also, the impact or need to communicate with other country regulatory agencies must be discussed and plans put in place to do so in a timely fashion; regulators in different countries do not like surprises either. The obligation of regulatory is to inform them as appropriate for the issue.

Management of a crisis most often requires communication with other stakeholders. For example, patients and the healthcare community must receive communications about the issue and the resolution for a marketed product issue. New programs may need to be developed to address patient risk; this could be the establishment of a registry or development of informational or educational tools. The organization should supply support for patients and physicians for any risk assessment.

Other stakeholders could be vendors, partners, shareholders, the financial community, the legal community, the media and the public. Depending on the issue, it is important to understand the compliance and ethics requirements for the financial and legal communities, as there could be considerable consequences for staff and the company (e.g., insider trading, discovery for litigation) if not handled correctly. Stakeholder engagement and understanding of the fundamental issue are central to success.

The same work must be done for external stakeholders as under internal management of a crisis. Effective communications will need to reach multiple audiences with varying levels of understanding. The communications need to inform, explain and educate. Regulatory staff should be involved in the preparation or review of these communications.

Additional activities for management of the external stakeholders include:

- identifying all external stakeholders or other relevant audiences
- developing communications strategies and planning with internal experts
- including appropriate external experts, if needed
- training internal staff to respond to inquiries (e.g., sales force)
- preparing briefing documents, if necessary
- revising labeling, developing educational tools
- developing Q&As for external inquiries

Post-resolution Assessment

All information obtained should be used to improve knowledge and current and future practices. Analyses of systems, procedures and operations should be conducted, with recommendations for required changes. Documentation should be developed and training should be conducted, through preparation or modification of standard operating procedures (SOPs) or guidances. Lessons Learned should be shared within the organization and imbedded into the institutional memory.

Averting a Crisis

While not every crisis can be averted, it would be extremely beneficial for the organization to develop an ongoing process to obtain information and analyze operations within the company in an effort to minimize any crises derived from in-company issues. Most companies do this through SOPs, training and audits. Regulatory and quality assurance staff play key roles in assisting in these endeavors. Early involvement of regulatory in the risk evaluation process is an important part of a proactive approach.

Also useful would be a study of other crises: what was done, were the actions successful or did they fail? Why? What could have been done differently? Again, while every crisis will be different, knowledge and experience enhance the opportunity for success, should a crisis occur in the company. This knowledge could easily be extended to understand established risks versus emerging risks. The risk potential is constantly changing as new assessment tools and algorithms are developed and new focuses for issues are brought forward by regulators or the , or arise from the political environment. It is critical to share communication of the risks and the risk environment with management. Understanding the impact is important for lessening the risk before it occurs. This takes collaboration and transparency, and regulatory should play a key role.

With the above knowledge, it would be valuable to develop a crisis management guide that would lay out general steps to be addressed in most crises. Major categories could be:
- process for establishing a CMT
- team member roles
- team responsibilities
- identifying the issue and cause
- key stakeholders
- developing a task list
- timeline requirements
- Good Documentation Practices
- correction action plan
- internal and external communication plan

Such a guide would streamline the process if a crisis should occur, save time in resolving the issue and help ensure that nothing is forgotten. Teams could practice by developing major scenarios, with processes and plans to address them. It is important to build the knowledge, systems and networks of expertise before they are needed on an urgent basis. Being proactive provides the best chance for success.

Skill Sets Required

It is imperative that the regulatory professional have some specific skill sets to be successful. Of course analytical skills are needed, but as important are the negotiation and conflict-handing skills with both co-workers and Health Authority personnel. Developing trust and respect is built on integrity, personal commitment and initiative. Teamwork and excellent communication skills provide opportunities for success. Adaptability and flexibility are needed to manage the situation as the risk unfolds.

Conclusion

The complexity of the healthcare products industry and the extensive interfaces, stakeholders, multiple products and global impact make it susceptible to a major crisis at any time. Effective management of a crisis in the healthcare products sector is critical for the organizational life—its employees, its customers and partners, the regulators, and the financial and legal communities. Traditional media, social media and political oversight can amplify negative attention and have an overwhelming adverse effect on a company's reputation. As a leader in the organization, regulatory can assist in the effective management of the crisis and can help avert a crisis.

Managing a crisis should prevent fear, confusion and skepticism. It also should consider the employees and the stress they may be under; stress is not conducive to planning and assessment or resolution of issues. Effective internal and external communications—professional, sensitive, complete, not false or misleading—provide the basis for success.

The goal is to assess patient risk, identify corrective actions as soon as possible, and minimize confusion and chaos resulting from a major unexpected adverse situation. A solid strategic plan that incorporates decision making and actions is necessary. Transparency and collaboration are key elements in this plan.

Regulatory staff should champion efforts to avert a crisis, but should one occur, being proactive will lessen the time to action. Conducting a "lessons learned" session afterward can help in creating or improving upon the company's crisis management guidance.

Chapter 7

Health Technology Assessment

By Patricia Anderson, RAC and Michelle Sotak, MPH, MBA

OBJECTIVES

- Introduce regulatory professionals to the concept of health technology assessment (HTA) and its increasing importance in the development of pharmaceuticals, devices, biologics and other healthcare products

- Understand the basic terminology and methodology used for HTAs

- Understand the use and impact of HTA on the development of healthcare products and on the ability for those products to be reimbursed and/or purchased

EXAMPLE HTA GUIDELINES

- Health Technology Assessment of Medical Devices. World Health Organization 2011. http://whqlibdoc.who.int/publications/2011/9789241501361_eng.pdf

- Børlum Kristensen F, Sigmund H, eds. *Health technology assessment handbook.* Copenhagen, National Board of Health. http://www.sst.dk/publ/publ2008/mtv/metode/hta_handbook_net_final.pdf

- National Institute of Health and Care Excellence. Specification for manufacturer/sponsor submission for Single Technology Appraisal (STA). http://www.nice.org.uk/aboutnice/howwework/devnicetech/technologyappraisalprocessguides/singletechnologyappraisalsprocess/specification_for_manufacturer_sponsor_submission_for_single_technology_appraisal_sta.jsp

Introduction

The development and use of health technology (HT) are facing greater challenges due to increasing evidence requirements for new technologies. Payers, politicians, government agencies and others increasingly insist that prior to the approval, acquisition, or payment for a healthcare technology, there must be well-founded data to support its use in a specific healthcare environment. The growth and development of health technology assessment (HTA) is in response to that need. The US Food and Drug Administration (FDA) is not involved in this type of assessment, nor is it within its scope or mandate. Other regulatory agencies (European Medicines Agency (EMA), the UK's Medicines and Healthcare Products Regulatory Agency (MHRA), and Sweden's Medical Product Agency (MPA) are actively collaborating with HTA agencies and allowing joint scientific advice meetings with manufacturers or sponsors of HTs.

The definition of HTA by the International Network of Agencies for Health Technology Assessment (INHATA) is the systematic evaluation of properties, effects and/or impacts of healthcare technology. It may address the direct, intended consequences of technologies as well as their indirect, unintended consequences. Its main purpose is to inform technology-related policymaking in healthcare. HTA is conducted by interdisciplinary groups using explicit analytical frameworks drawing from a variety of methods."[1] The European network for Health Technology Assessment (EUnetHTA) provides a similar definition, stating that "HTA is a multidisciplinary process that summarizes

Chapter 7

Table 7-1. Comparison of Health Technology Regulation and Health Technology Assessment Characteristics Health Technology Regulation

Characteristics	Health Technology Regulations	Health Technology Assessment
Perspective	Safety and efficacy	Efficacy, effectiveness and appropriateness
Requirement	Mandatory	Recommendation on complex technologies
Role	Prevent harm	Maximize clinical and cost effectiveness

information about the medical, social, economic and ethical issues related to the use of a health technology in a systematic, transparent, unbiased, robust manner" with the aim "to inform the formulation of safe, effective, health policies that are patient focused and seek to achieve best value."[2]

HTA methods are evolving and their applications are varied. This chapter introduces fundamental aspects of HTA and issues related to these methods. The demand for HTA, in particular from the for-profit private sector as well as from government agencies, is pushing the field to evolve assessment processes and reports. Methods for HTA vary by organization; while several organizations such as the National Institute for Health and Care Excellence (NICE) in the UK or the Canadian Agency for Drugs and Technologies in Health (CADTH) in Canada have been utilizing HTA methods for many years, other countries are still in the process of developing or refining methods for conducting HTAs and using HTAs in decision making.

A word of caution to the contents below: The process is explained with an introductory mind-set. The processes involved can be very complex and the system requires increasingly technical expertise.

Health Technology Assessment Process

Table 7-1 indicates the different characteristics of regulatory requirements versus those of HTA as presented in the WHO document *Health Technology Assessment of Medical Devices*. This reference document provides an introduction to the concept and program of health technology assessment (HTA) around the world and highlights the contributions that HTA can make to informed policy and decision making.

The *Health Technology Assessment Handbook* by the Danish Centre for Health Technology Assessment provides an excellent overview of HTA methodologies. The following section is a distillation of the Danish HTA process.

Figure 7-1 from the Danish Handbook 2007, provides a process flow of an HTA process.

Step 1—Formulation of the Policy Question

Careful formulation of the policy question is a critical factor to ensure an appropriate, useful HTA is produced since the policy questions are the focus of the decision maker's eventual conclusion. The Danish Handbook offers this example:

If a public offer of vaccination against HPV is requested, who should receive the offer, how should it be organized and with what effects and costs?

Step 2—HTA Question

The HTA question that follows the policy question must be phrased in such a way that the assessment will offer the information needed by the decision makers or the target group to come to a decision on the policy question. To that end, HTA questions must be clearly formulated, defined and answerable. The HTA questions in the Danish HTA process usually encompass technology, patient, organization and economy as well as any ethical aspects, although other approaches also are used.

For the policy question above, the corollary derived HTA questions are:

- What are the effects and side effects of HPV vaccination?
- Are there any interactions with other vaccines in the childhood immunization program?
- Are there any ethical problems in relation to the HPV vaccination?
- What organizational consequences will different vaccination strategies have?
- What are the benefits compared with the costs for different models of the vaccination program?

Step 3 Gather the Evidence and Complete the Analysis of the HTA Question

Four Basic Areas Related to HTA

The model described above from the Danish HTA process speaks to the gathering of evidence encompassing four basic areas related to the derived HTA question:

- technology
- organization
- patient
- economy

Technology

The properties of health technology include performance characteristics and conformity with specifications for design, composition, manufacturing, tolerances, reliability, ease of use, maintenance, etc. Safety is the assessment of the acceptability of risk (a measure of the probability of an adverse outcome and its severity) associated with using a technology in a specific environment or situation, e.g., for a patient with a particular health problem, by a clinician with certain training and/or in a specified treatment setting.

Comparative efficacy and effectiveness answer how well a technology works to improve patient health, usually based on changes in one or more health outcomes or "endpoints." A technology that works under controlled conditions and with carefully selected patients (such as in Phase 3 trials) does not always work as well in "real world settings" or once in the marketplace. In HTA, effectiveness is more important than efficacy and refers to the benefit of using a technology for a particular problem under general or routine conditions in a "real world" setting. Note: When discussing efficacy vs. effectiveness, effectiveness relates to how well a treatment works in the practice of medicine and is required for marketing authorization, as opposed to efficacy, which measures how well treatment works in clinical trials or studies

The health technology will have a certain degree of maturity and diffusion and this also becomes part of the HTA:[3]

- Future—a technology at the conceptual stage or at the earliest stage of development
- Experimental—the technology is tested in laboratories, e.g., in animal models or cell cultures
- Tested—the technology is tested in clinical studies, e.g., in patients with specific diseases or applied in a few institutions or in limited parts of the healthcare system as part of a study
- Established—the technology is considered to be standard treatment or routine practice and generally applied in the healthcare system
- Obsolete—new, safer or more effective technologies have surpassed or replaced older technology

Organization

Health technologies cannot merely be implemented since technologies introduced into an organization (e.g., hospital, health system) may influence organizational structures, tasks and the organization's staff (people) and vice versa.[4] For example, a new surgical technology may change how physicians perform surgical procedures. This organizational form(s) in which the technology will be placed must be taken into consideration given the impact to that organization. This consideration is outlined in the process description below.

Process Description of the technology is presented via, for instance, preparation of work flow diagram:[5]

- Work flow
  o How is the technology applied specifically? Describe patient flow and work processes.
  o How are existing patient flow and work processes influenced?
  o How is ongoing control and evaluation ensured?
- Staff, training and resources
  o Which players participate and what resources do they need to apply to the new technology?
  o Is extra staff required?
  o Are other staff or further training required?
  o Who decides which patients are to receive the treatment? On what basis?
- Interaction and communication
  o Interaction with other parts of the structure (other treatment units and interdisciplinary functions, e.g. financial management)—state consequences for other treatments and other treatment units inside and outside the department.
  o Interaction and communication with patients and relatives—state changes and new requirements.
  o Interaction with external actors (other hospitals, general practitioners, municipalities, pharmacies, technical consultants, etc.)—state changes.
  o Are there requirements for change in financial reporting and payment structure?
  o Can potential bottlenecks be identified (staff, funding, knowledge/information) in the work process?

Patient

Figure 7-2 illustrates those areas that have been identified as being relevant in exploring patient aspects for an HTA. Often, this will focus on a patient's knowledge of and experience with a given technology, patient resources and the importance of the technology in question for the patient's

Figure 7-1. An HTA Model

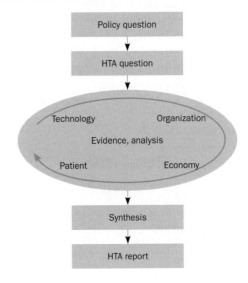

Figure 7-2. Importance of the Relevant Technology for the Patient's Everyday Life (Børlum 2007)

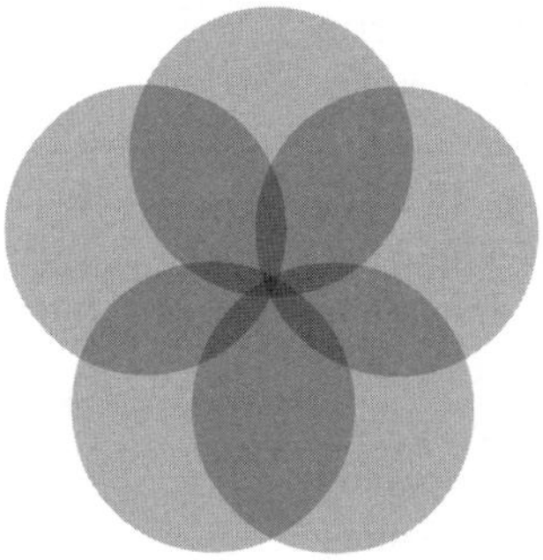

```
                    Social aspects
   Communicative aspects      Economic aspects

              [Venn diagram of four overlapping circles]

       Individual aspects         thical aspects
          Patient's experience with a given technology
```

everyday life. This demonstrates that the various focus areas cannot be considered in isolation. Some examples of what can be investigated within each area are set out below. Central research questions will therefore typically be aimed at:
- social aspects
- economic aspects
- ethical aspects
- individual aspects
- communicative aspects[6]

Social Aspects
This covers whether, from a patient perspective, the technology will have or has, for example:
- a direct and/or indirect influence on or significance for:
  o work and training
  o family life and leisure time
  o lifestyle and quality of life

Economic Aspects
This covers whether, from a patient perspective, the technology entails, for example:
- direct and/or indirect costs in relation to
  o work
  o family life
  o leisure time
  o lifestyle and quality of life

Ethical Aspects
This covers whether, from a patient perspective, the technology entails, for example:
- ethical considerations
- ethical choices
- ethical dilemmas

Individual Aspects
This covers whether, from a patient perspective, the technology entails:
- existential experiences, e.g., insecurity, worry, hope or anxiety
- patient roles and stigmatization
- courage to face life
- satisfaction
- use of one's own resources (self-care, empowerment)

Communicative Aspects
This covers whether, from a patient perspective, the technology will have or has an influence on:
- exchange of information
- patients' knowledge and understanding of the technology
- modified relations between the patient and health professionals
- involvement in decision making

As an example of an HTA from the perspective of the patient, Boothroyd et al presented issues for patients, caregivers and the healthcare system with home-based chemotherapy for the treatment of cancer.[7]

Economy
Economic analyses may help determine how resources can be used best in the healthcare sector. While economic analyses are not included in all HTAs, many agencies consider this a critical aspect of the decision-making process.

Once the policy and HTA questions are defined, the next step is to gather the available evidence on the health technology and conduct the assessment.

Assessment of Literature
Careful formulation of a literature search strategy, the literature search and the selection of studies to include in the analysis are the usual first steps in this stage of the HTA process. This step may in fact be circular in that the research offers up information that stimulates further requirements to investigate, such as when a reviewed article provides additional references that may be valuable. A systematic approach to evaluating the literature is important in order to ensure an unbiased assessment of the available evidence, and the steps in the literature review should be fully documented to enable replicable results. Information from the "gray literature" or that is not available in peer-reviewed publications is often included as well to ensure a full review.

Some useful advice and suggestions for this step include: primarily select the literature with the highest class of evidence, such as randomized controlled trials; use the focused HTA question when assessing whether the article is of relevance; use checklists in the review of the individual articles; and use internationally recognized standards for the assessment of articles.

Information obtained for an HTA is often classified in terms of the hierarchy of evidence: (most rigorous to least rigorous):
- meta-analyses and systematic reviews (among others, Cochrane reviews[8])
- randomized controlled trials (RCTs)
- non-randomized controlled trials
- cohort studies
- case control studies
- descriptive studies, limited series
- position papers, non-systematic reviews, leading articles, expert opinions

The quality of available information is often assessed using quality assessment tools such as the NICE or Grading of Recommendations Assessment, Development and Evaluation (GRADE) rating tools, as the quality of literature can vary widely. These tools evaluate the quality of evidence and strength of recommendations of individual studies and provide a systematic method of evaluating studies.

Data Generation, Analysis and Assessment
Various methods are available for the generation, analysis, assessment and use of data for an HTA. There are qualitative methods involving interviews, participant observation and fieldwork and also procedures for questionnaire-based and registry studies. This entails descriptions of methods which 1) encompass both qualitative and quantitative approaches, and 2) are related to more than one HTA element.

Conducting primary investigations for an HTA typically is considered only if the knowledge cannot be gained from a thorough review of the literature, and then only if the information is of vital importance.

Economic Analysis
As described above, while not all HTAs include economic analyses, many HTA organizations consider an economic analysis as an important component of their decision making. The four types of socioeconomic analysis are summarized in **Table 7-2**.

Quality-adjusted Life Years
An important concept in HTA is the Quality-adjusted Life Year (QALY). Health technologies have effects with more dimensions than can be measured in natural units. Cost:utility analysis should be employed if the use of a health technology is expected to lead to changes in health-related quality of life for patients or an extension of life with impaired health. In cost:utility analysis, the effects are measured and valuated in QALYs. A unit of outcome of an intervention where gains (or losses) of years of life subsequent to this intervention are adjusted on the basis of the quality of life during those years. For example, interventions that have a negative impact on quality of life would have fewer QALYs than an intervention with the same gain in years of life but a positive impact on quality of life (QoL).

Note: This parameter can provide a common unit for comparing cost-utility across different interventions and health problems. Disability-adjusted life years (DALY) and healthy-years equivalent (HYE) are QALY-analogous units.[9]

Generic Instruments as Utility Measures
Besides functioning as a profile measure for describing a patient's self-assessed health, certain health status instruments also can be used as utility measures in economic evaluations.

In this context, the instrument must be able to generate a simple preference-based index score (on a scale of 0-1) for health status, e.g., for various patient groups or treatment alternatives. Five generic instruments, have either been developed primarily as utility measures (EQ-5D, 15D, Health Utilities Index (HUI), Assessment of Quality of Life (AQoL)) or aim at this on the basis of broad use as a profile measure (e.g., Short-Form 36 (SF-36)) Whereas the 15D and AQoL are relatively new, the other instruments are widely used and perform well with respect to validity and reliability.

Cost-effectiveness Decision Matrix
To be able to determine the comparative cost-effectiveness of the health technologies and conclude which should be preferred from an economic perspective, the total costs assessed must be compared with the total effects assessed for each of the technologies. **Table 7-3** illustrates the resulting decision matrix with the nine possible responses.

Table 7-2. Choice of Type of Economic Analysis (Børlum 2007)

Type of Economic Analysis	Definition (HTA Glossary.net)	When should the individual type of analysis be chosen?
Cost minimization analysis (CMA)	An economic evaluation that compares the costs of various options presumed to produce equivalent outcomes and determines the least costly of those options.	1. When the technologies compared are equally effective—then it is only necessary to collect data about costs
Cost-effectiveness analysis (CEA)	An economic evaluation that compares various options, in which costs are measured in monetary units, then aggregated, and outcomes are expressed in natural (non-monetary) units.	1. When activities with the same purpose and measure of effectiveness are compared 2. When the effectiveness of the technologies compared is different, i.e., the difference in costs must be weighed against the difference in effectiveness
Cost-utility analysis (CUA)	An economic evaluation that compares various options, in which costs are measured in monetary units and outcomes are measured in utility units, usually in terms of utility to the patient (using quality-adjusted life years, for example). Note: This is a form of cost-effectiveness analysis in which the effectiveness of an option is adjusted on the basis of quality of life.	1. When health-related quality of life is an important outcome 2. When activities across the healthcare sector are compared
Cost-benefit analysis	An economic evaluation that compares various options, in which costs and outcomes are quantified in common monetary units.	1. When non-health effects are also important, e.g., the treatment process itself, the utility of information, etc. 2. When only one technology is assessed (net benefit) 3. When lives are to be valued in monetary units (e.g., dollars) 4. When activities across society are to be compared

Budget Impact Analysis

In addition to the analyses described above, many organizations also conduct a budget impact analysis to understand the overall financial impact of paying for a new technology on their organizations or on society as a whole.

Step 4 The Synthesis Process in HTA

The synthesis is designed to summarize and assess the findings while also providing one or more summary conclusions and, possibly, recommendations. It has been stressed that during this process great importance must be placed on transparency in terms of documents and methodology. Both advantages and disadvantages of various solutions also must be described.

Step 5 The HTA Report

General Aspects of the Utilization of HTA

It has been stressed that an HTA is not a decision, but rather it provides input or recommendations for decision-making. Decision makers are therefore the primary target user group for an HTA. The HTA may go directly to the decision makers or pass through several administrative stages where it is adapted or supplemented before the decision is made. There is a distinction between conducting HTAs and making decisions on the basis of HTAs. HTA development is based primarily in a research domain, while the outputs of HTA are used in a decision-making domain. Examples of HTAs can be found on various websites such as CADTH in Canada (http://www.cadth.ca/), NICE in the UK (http://www.nice.org.uk/) or the UK's National Health Service, which give researchers access to more than 10,000.[10]

Public and Private Agencies Using or Producing HTA Reports in the US[11]

While in most cases, the US uses HTA less formally in decision making than in other countries such as Canada, public and private healthcare organizations do produce HTA evaluations and utilize these evaluations in their decision making. The following section briefly outlines some of the major HTA-related organizations in the US.

Agency for Healthcare Research and Quality

The Agency for Healthcare Research and Quality (AHRQ) is the primary government agency in the US responsible for developing and funding HTA. AHRQ supports HTA research through three external research networks:
1. Evidence-Based Practice Centers (EPCs)
2. |Centers for Education and Research on Therapeutics (CERT)

3. Developing Evidence to Inform Decisions about Effectiveness (DEcIDE) Program

AHRQ also conducts technology assessments in-house. AHRQ assessments typically focus on a systematic review of the literature and data synthesis from multiple studies.[12] The Centers for Medicare and Medicaid Services (CMS) is the primary user of AHRQ technology assessments which are used to inform coverage policies for the national and local Medicare programs.[13]

Medicare/Medicaid

In the US, the largest government-sponsored healthcare organizations are Medicare and Medicaid. Medicare provides coverage for US citizens aged 65 and over while Medicaid serves the young, indigent and disabled. HTA assessments within these two agencies can occur at both the national and local levels. CMS is the agency responsible for oversight, financing and implementation of both the Medicare and Medicaid programs. As mentioned previously, AHRQ performs most technology assessments used by CMS staff in developing coverage decisions. The Medicare Evidence Development and Coverage Advisory Committee (MedCAC) is a group of external experts who review and weigh the evidence from HTAs such as those produced by AHRQ in open public meetings. The dossiers, public submissions of evidence submitted by the manufacturers and the final decisions for the Medicare program by CMS are placed on the CMS coverage website (http://www.cms.gov/medicare-coverage-database/indexes/technology-assessments-index.aspx).

Drug Effectiveness Review Project

The state of Oregon started the Drug Effectiveness Review Project (DERP) in 2000 to manage increasing Medicaid program costs by assessing pharmaceuticals for the state Medicaid Preferred Drug List.[14] DERP is a collaboration between the Oregon Evidence-based Practice Center (EPC) at the Oregon Health Sciences University and several states. Currently multiple state Medicaid programs and other organizations are part of DERP and utilize its assessments in their decision-making processes. Current participants includes CADTH (Canada), Oregon, Washington, Idaho, Missouri, Montana, New York, Arkansas, Colorado, Wisconsin and Wyoming.

Other Federal Programs

The Department of Veterans Affairs (VA) includes the VA Technology Assessment Program (VATAP) (http://www.va.gov/vatap/). VATAP produces technology assessments including systematic reviews and evidence-based reports targeted at informing decisions within the VA program.[15]

Private Sector Health Technology Assessment

Private health insurers and pharmacy benefits managers (PBMs) in the US use evidence evaluation techniques similar to HTA as part of their decision-making processes. Pharmaceutical and therapeutic (P&T) committees review the available evidence for a product and make recommendations for coverage and formulary placement. For example, the Blue Cross Blue Shield (BCBS) Association funds the BCBS Technology Evaluation Center (TEC), which produces technology assessment reports for the Blue Cross plans that are also available to the public (http://www.bcbs.com/blueresources/tec/press/).

Conclusions

HTA and the resulting policy decisions are a growing consideration for the development and ongoing lifecycles of healthcare technologies. An understanding of this consideration is an important tool for regulatory professionals. Tools to expedite HTA early in the development of the HT could be a consideration.

References
1. INAHTA (International Network of Agencies for Health Technology Assessment). (June 8, 2009). "HTA glossary". INAHTA. http://inahta.episerverhotell.net/Glossary/. Accessed 9 May 2013.
2. Børlum Kristensen F. Presentation on Better use of new technologies through collaboration on HTA. Learning from differences – European collaboration on health systems research conference. Montreux 16

Table 7-3. Cost-effectiveness Decision Matrix

New Technology assessed against Old Technology	Smaller effect en < eo	Same effect en = eo	Greater effect en > eo
Lower cost cn < co	1. no clear decision—no dominance	4. Introduce new technology—new dominates old	7. Introduce new technology—new dominates old
Same cost cn = co	2. keep old technology—old dominates new	5. the technologies are equally good	8. Introduce new technology—new dominates
Higher cost cn > co	3. keep old technology—old dominates new	6. keep old technology—old dominates new	9. no clear decision—no dominance

Source: (Børlum2007)

November 2010. EC website. http://ec.europa.eu/research/health/public-health/public-health-and-health-systems/pdf/finn-borlum-kristensen_en.pdf. Slide 3. Accessed 9 May 2013.
3. Børlum Kristensen F, Sigmund H, eds. *Health technology assessment handbook*. Copenhagen, National Board of Health. 2007. www.sst.dk/~/media/Planlaegning%20og%20kvalitet/MTV%20metode/HTA_Handbook_net_final.ashx. Accessed 9 May 2013.
4. Ibid.
5. Ibid.
6. Ibid.
7. Boothroyd L, Lehoux P. Home-Based Chemotherapy for Cancer: Issues for Patients, Caregivers and the Health Care System. Quebec: AETMIS. Quebec; 2004. (http://www.aetmis.gouv.qc.ca/site/home.phtml)
8. Cochrane AL. *Effectiveness and Efficiency: Random Reflections on Health Services*. London, England: Nuffield Provincial Hospitals Trust; 1972.
9. HTA Glossary.net. http://htaglossary.net/HomePage. Accessed 9 May 2013.
10. NHS. Centre for Reviews and Dissemination. University of York website. http://www.crd.york.ac.uk/crdweb/.
11. Sullivan SD, Watkins J, Sweet B, Ramsey SD. Health Technology Assessment in Health-Care Decisions in the United States, Value in Health, 2009;12, Supp 2.
12. AHRQ Technology Assessments. AHRQ website. http://www.ahrq.gov/research/findings/ta/index.html. Accessed 23 May 2013.
13. Ibid.
14 About DERP. Oregon Health & Science University website. http://www.ohsu.edu/xd/research/centers-institutes/evidence-based-policy-center/derp/about/index.cfm. Accessed 23 May 2013.
16. VA Technology Assessment Program. US Department of Veterans Affairs website. http://www.va.gov/VATAP/About_TAP.asp. Accessed 23 May 2013.

Recommended Reading
- Goodman CS. HTA 101: Introduction to Health Technology Assessment. The Lewin Group. January 2004. www.nlm.nih.gov/nichsr/hta101/ta101_c1.html.

Chapter 8

Good Laboratory Practice Regulations

Updated by Srikonda V. Sastry, PhD, RAC

OBJECTIVES

- Review the history and purpose of GLP regulations

- Learn the key GLP regulation components

- Examine the implications of noncompliance with GLP regulations

---

LAWS, REGULATIONS AND GUIDELINES COVERED IN THIS CHAPTER

- Section 701(a) of the *Federal Food, Drug, and Cosmetic Act* of 1938

- US Food and Drug Administration, 21 CFR Part 58, Good Laboratory Practice for Nonclinical Laboratory Studies, Final Rule (1987)

- Organization for Economic Cooperation and Development, *Principles of Good Laboratory Practice* (Revised 1997)

- Japanese Ministry of Health, Labour and Welfare, *Good Laboratory Practice Standards*, Ordinance No. 21 (Revised 2008)

- US Environmental Protection Agency, 40 CFR Part 792, *Toxic Substances Control Act*, Good Laboratory Practice Standards (29 December 1983)

- US Environmental Protection Agency, 40 CFR Part 160, *Federal Insecticide, Fungicide, and Rodenticide Act*, Good Laboratory Practice Standards (2 May 1984)

- US Department of Health and Human Services, Food and Drug Administration, Office of Regulatory Affairs, Comparison Chart of FDA and EPA Good Laboratory Practice (GLP) Regulations and the OECD Principles of GLP (June 2004)

- US Food and Drug Administration, Office of Regulatory Affairs, *Bioresearch Monitoring Good Laboratory Practice Compliance Program Guidance 7348.808 (Nonclinical Laboratories)* (21 February 2001)

- Food and Drug Administration Compliance Program Guidance Manual, Program 7348.808A, *Good Laboratory Practice Program (Nonclinical Laboratories) EPA Data Audit Inspections*, (25 August 2000)

Introduction

The *Federal Food, Drug, and Cosmetic Act (FD&C Act)* and the *Public Health Service Act* impose the burden on manufacturers of demonstrating that their products meet the safety and effectiveness requirements of the law and that they are not misbranded for their intended use and ensuring the highest degree of consumer protection. The US Food and Drug Administration (FDA) requires manufacturers of human drugs, biopharmaceuticals and biological products, animal drugs, medical devices, electronic products and food additives to demonstrate the safety of their products prior to use in humans or, in the case of animal drugs, prior to use in the indicated species. Hence, FDA requires that extensive animal and other types of testing be performed. Preclinical studies on drugs are of particular importance in deciding whether a new drug can be safely tested in humans to assess its potential use as a therapeutic agent. Compliance with Title 21 of the Code of Federal Regulations (CFR) Part 58, the Good Laboratory Practice (GLP) regulation, is intended to ensure the quality and integrity of the safety data used to support applications for research or marketing permits for FDA-regulated products. Compliance with GLPs allows accurate reconstruction of the conduct of a nonclinical study based on quality recordkeeping and reporting. GLP regulations are promulgated by the FDA commissioner under the general authority of the *FD&C Act* of 1938.

The US Environmental Protection Agency (EPA) requires manufacturers of chemical substances and mixtures and pesticide products to conduct studies to evaluate their health effects, environmental effects and chemical fate. Compliance with EPA's *Toxic Substances Control Act* (*TSCA*) Good Laboratory Practice Standards regulation, 40 CFR 792, and the *Federal Insecticide, Fungicide, and Rodenticide Act* (*FIFRA*) Good Laboratory Practice Standards regulation, 40 CFR 160, is intended to assure data quality for the testing of chemical substances and mixtures and pesticides, respectively.

The Organization for Economic Cooperation and Development (OECD), which includes member countries throughout North America, Europe and Asia, developed a set of principles very similar to FDA GLP regulations. Like FDA GLPs, the OECD regulations are applicable to nonclinical safety studies for pharmaceutical products, animal drugs and food additives, but also are applicable to studies to evaluate the safety of pesticides and industrial chemicals. The Japanese Ministry of Health, Labour and Welfare (MHLW) also has issued regulations similar to the FDA GLPs. Studies conducted in compliance with OECD and MHLW GLPs generally are accepted by FDA under mutual recognition agreements.

FDA, EPA and MHLW GLPs are regulations and are required by law, whereas the OECD GLP principles are voluntary procedures that must be adopted as a regulation within each member country.[1]

FDA's Office of Regulatory Affairs (ORA) issued a "Comparison Chart of FDA and EPA Good Laboratory Practice (GLP) Regulations and the OECD Principles of GLP" in June 2004. The comparison chart provides a listing of the similarities and differences among the three GLP regulations.[2]

GLPs, whether put forth by FDA, EPA or OECD, "were designed to ensure data quality and to reduce fraud by requiring that specific documentation be kept regarding several key areas that include laboratory staff, facilities and operations, equipment, test and control articles, protocol, conduct of the study, quality assurance and archiving of data, records and specimens."[3]

Most drug and biologic developers will not need to refer to the EPA GLPs, and because the focus of this book is on US regulations, the remainder of this chapter is devoted to a discussion of the FDA GLP regulation as set forth in 21 CFR 58. However, it is not uncommon for nonclinical studies to be conducted in accordance with FDA, OECD and MHLW GLP regulations, depending on the intended market for the product, so familiarity with the OECD and MHLW GLPs may be helpful.

Definition and Scope of 21 CFR 58

21 CFR 58 "prescribes good laboratory practices for conducting nonclinical laboratory studies that support or are intended to support applications for research or marketing permits for products regulated by the Food and Drug Administration, including food and color additives, animal food additives, human and animal drugs, medical devices for human use, biological products, and electronic products. Compliance with this part is intended to assure the quality and integrity of the safety data filed pursuant to sections 406, 408, 409, 502, 503, 505, 506, 510, 512-516, 518-520, 721, and 801 of the Federal Food, Drug, and Cosmetic Act and sections 351 and 354-360F of the Public Health Service Act."[4]

A "nonclinical laboratory study means *in vivo* or *in vitro* experiments in which test articles are studied prospectively in test systems under laboratory conditions to determine their safety. The term does not include studies utilizing human subjects or clinical studies or field trials in animals. The term does not include basic exploratory studies carried out to determine whether a test article has any potential utility or to determine the physical or chemical characteristics of a test article."[5]

Studies that are expected to be in compliance with GLPs include, but are not limited to:

- acute, subchronic and chronic toxicology studies, including developmental, reproductive, carcinogenic, mutagenic and degenerative toxicology studies based on appearance of these effects in laboratory animals
- biochemistry, nutrition, immunology, microbiology (both *in vitro* and *in vivo*) studies
- dermal/eye/venous/muscle irritation studies
- safety pharmacology studies (core battery)
- bioanalytical studies of samples from dose groups of study animals
- studies to validate the analytical methods to be used for samples from GLP studies (e.g., bioanalysis and test article formulation analysis)
- if the target species in animal drugs is a food-producing animal, data relating to human safety as result of use of the drug in the animal is also needed and needs to be conducted per GLP requirements

- medical device safety data obtained from *in vivo* and *in vitro* studies involving animals, as well as physical and chemical experiments
- animal testing for establishment of safety of color and food additives

Laboratories that analyze samples generated from GLP studies, such as clinical chemistry, histology and pathology, are subject to GLP regulations.

Examples of studies that are not subject to GLPs include, but are not limited to:
- basic research
- proof of concept studies
- exploratory pharmacokinetic studies (absorption, distribution, metabolism and elimination)
- dose-range finding studies
- primary pharmacodynamic studies
- analytical quality control testing for clinical and commercial products
- stability testing of clinical and commercial products
- studies using human subjects
- field trials in animals

Analytical and quality control laboratories that test raw materials and in-process samples; perform release testing for active pharmaceutical ingredients, drug products and medical devices; and perform stability testing are not subject to GLP regulations. These laboratories are subject to Good Manufacturing Practice regulations.

There are no specific FDA regulations or guidances for laboratories that perform testing of clinical samples from human clinical trials. GLPs state that nonclinical laboratory studies do not include studies utilizing human subjects or clinical studies. The *Clinical Laboratories Improvement Amendments* (*CLIA*) regulations are not applicable to research laboratories that test human specimens and do not report patient-specific results for the diagnosis, prevention or treatment of any disease or impairment of, or the assessment of the health of individual patients.[6]

GLPs and *CLIA* share similar goals in terms of assuring the quality and integrity of data produced during laboratory testing. Because there are no specific regulations or guidances for the testing of human clinical samples, many organizations—i.e., clinical trial sponsors—use the GLP and/or *CLIA* regulations as audit standards when assessing the quality of the laboratories used to test human clinical samples. The College of American Pathologists (CAP) serves as an accreditation organization under *CLIA* and has published its own guidelines for GLPs for testing of human samples.[7] The CAP guidelines have some similarity to FDA GLPs, but are focused more on laboratory process quality rather than study quality as a whole.

History of FDA GLPs

Throughout the 1960s and 1970s, the use of chemicals became more prevalent in the US. The fear of negative health effects caused by the widespread use of chemicals was shared by the public and the government. As a result, there was an increase in the number of federal laws applicable to chemical and pharmaceutical companies and an increase in the amount of product testing required. In 1969, FDA developed a plan to inspect laboratories that conducted animal research. The plan included directed inspections of facilities whose submitted studies contained inconsistencies or had questionable data integrity, where there was simultaneous performance of a large number of complex studies or where a tip had been received alleging scientific misconduct. The results of the initial investigations showed significant data quality problems and a lack of industry standards in animal toxicology testing.[8]

In 1975, FDA conducted a facility inspection of G.D. Searle and Company of Skokie, IL. Searle manufactured several pharmaceutical products and had submitted toxicology data to FDA in support of product applications. The inspection found questionable test data due to sloppy work; untrained personnel; and poor data collection, analyses, review and reporting practices.[9] In another case, numerous instances of scientific misconduct were found when FDA inspected Industrial Bio-Test Laboratories (IBT), a contract testing laboratory located in Northbrook, IL, in 1976. Some of the findings noted by FDA were fabrication of data, replacement of dead study animals with healthy ones that had not received drug treatment, changes in the interpretation of histopathology slides and changes in report conclusions to make them look more favorable.[10]

In 1976, as a result of numerous scientific integrity and data quality problems found when inspecting toxicology laboratories, FDA proposed GLP regulations. The final regulations were published in 1978 and became law in 1979. Proposed changes to the GLPs were published in 1984, and after revisions were made, the GLP regulations, final rule, were published in 1987. FDA published a request for comments on proposed revisions to the current regulations in 2010, discussed later in this chapter.

FDA GLP Subparts and Sections

To predict safety prior to use in humans or therapeutic use in animals, nonclinical studies are required for FDA-regulated products such as human and animal drugs, biopharmaceuticals, biological products, food and color additives, animal food additives, medical devices for human use and electronic products. The data obtained from the GLP nonclinical studies and submitted to FDA are used to make decisions on the product's overall toxicity profile, including the dose level at which there were no observed adverse effects, the potential adverse effects and risks associated with clinical studies involving humans or animals, the product's teratogenic and/

or carcinogenic potential, and the dose level, frequency and duration of use that can be approved.[11]

Strict adherence to scientific principles, data integrity and quality assurance provide the foundation for the GLP regulations. As mentioned above, the GLPs are codified in 21 CFR 58. The GLP regulations specify the minimum standards for the conduct and reporting of nonclinical laboratory studies that are to be used in support of a marketing application in the US. The GLPs are organized into subparts A through K with subparts H and I reserved. The subparts and their sections are noted in **Table 8-1**.

Key Elements of FDA GLPs
Key elements of the GLPs that merit discussion include:

Subpart A:
§58.3 Definitions
It is important to read and understand the definitions used in 21 CFR 58. A thorough understanding of the definitions is critical to correct interpretation of and compliance with the regulations in this section.

§58.10 Applicability to Studies Performed under Grants and Contracts
When electing to use a contract research organization (CRO) or a contractor to perform all or part of a nonclinical laboratory study intended to be submitted to FDA in support of an application or marketing permit, the sponsor is responsible for notifying the CRO or contractor that the study must be conducted in compliance with GLPs. The study protocol should include a statement about the regulatory standards under which the study will be conducted.

Though not specifically stated, there is an expectation that the sponsor will ensure the GLP capabilities of the contracted facility prior to initiation of work. The sponsor usually evaluates the facility's regulatory inspection history and/or performs a GLP prequalification audit. This is important because a facility may claim GLP compliance without a full understanding of the intricacies of 21 CFR 58. A sponsor should be wary of a facility, in the US or abroad, that claims GLP compliance but has never been inspected by FDA or contributed data to a submission reviewed by FDA.

Subpart B:
§58.29 Personnel
An adequate number of personnel, appropriately qualified by education, training, experience or a combination thereof are required by the regulations. Job qualifications are defined by laboratory management and not the regulations; however, the sponsor should ensure that appropriately qualified personnel are available to conduct the study. Maintenance of a comprehensive training file for each individual is required to document these qualifications.

§58.31, 58.33, 58.35 Testing Facility Management, Study Director, and Quality Assurance Unit (QAU), respectively
The GLP regulations are very specific regarding the responsibilities of these three functions. Testing facility management is responsible for approving all test facility standard operating procedures (SOPs). Facility management is responsible for designating a study director prior to the initiation of the study and promptly replacing the study director, if necessary, during the conduct of the study. Facility management must ensure that test and control articles and mixtures thereof have been appropriately tested for identity, purity, stability or other defining characteristics. Facility management also has the authority to provide resources and implement changes necessary to comply with GLP requirements and, if necessary, to ensure corrective actions are taken to address audit findings.

The study director is the single point of control for a nonclinical study. The study director has overall responsibility for the study's design, conduct and reporting, including compliance with the study protocol and GLP regulations. The study director must ensure that all circumstances that could affect the study's integrity are documented and assessed for impact and that corrective actions are taken as necessary. This should include evaluation of unexpected events occurring at other test sites that contribute data to the study.

The study director usually resides at the testing facility where the test article is administered to the test system. It has become common practice to conduct nonclinical studies across multiple test sites with an individual (usually called a contributing scientist or principal investigator) identified to oversee the work conducted at each facility. It is important that this individual not be referred to as a study director because he or she does not have the same responsibilities or authority for the overall study.

The Quality Assurance Unit (QAU) is responsible for ensuring that studies are conducted in accordance with the study protocol and GLPs. The QAU must remain independent from the study and must not report to the director conducting the study.

QAU personnel maintain a master schedule of GLP studies and copies of the study protocol and amendments, and ensure that no deviations from approved procedures and study protocols are made without proper authorization and documentation. QAU personnel inspect facilities on a schedule defined by an SOP to ensure GLP compliance within the facility. These inspections include equipment maintenance, training records, etc. The findings from these inspections are sent to facility management for remedial actions. QAU personnel inspect studies at intervals appropriate to assure integrity, provide inspection findings and prepare final reports, which include a statement specifying

Table 8-1. 21 CFR 5

Subpart	Section
Subpart A - General Provisions	§58.1 Scope
	§58.3 Definitions
	§58.10 Applicability to studies performed under grants and contracts
	§58.15 Inspection of a testing facility
Subpart B - Organization and Personnel	§58.29 Personnel
	§58.31 Testing facility management
	§58.33 Study director
	§58.35 Quality assurance unit
Subpart C - Facilities	§58.41 General
	§58.43 Animal care facilities
	§58.45 Animal supply facilities
	§58.47 Facilities for handling test and control articles
	§58.49 Laboratory operation areas
	§58.51 Specimen and data storage facilities
Subpart D - Equipment	§58.61 Equipment design
	§58.63 Maintenance and calibration of equipment
Subpart E - Testing Facilities Operation	§58.81 Standard operating procedures
	§58.83 Reagents and solutions
	§58.90 Animal care
Subpart F - Test and Control Articles	§58.105 Test and control article characterization
	§58.107 Test and control article handling
	§58.113 Mixtures of articles with carriers
Subpart G - Protocol for and Conduct of a Nonclinical Laboratory Study	§58.120 Protocol
	§58.130 Conduct of a nonclinical laboratory study
Subpart J - Records and Reports	§58.185 Reporting of nonclinical laboratory study results
	§58.190 Storage and retrieval of records and data
	§58.195 Retention of records
Subpart K - Disqualification of Testing Facilities	§58.200 Purpose
	§58.202 Grounds for disqualification
	§58.204 Notice of and opportunity for hearing on proposed disqualification
	§58.206 Final order on disqualification
	§58.210 Actions upon disqualification
	§58.213 Public disclosure of information regarding disqualification
	§58.215 Alternative or additional actions to disqualification
	§58.217 Suspension or termination of a testing facility by a sponsor
	§58.219 Reinstatement of a disqualified testing facility

the dates of the inspection, to the study director and facility management.

Subpart D:
§58.61 and §58.63, Equipment Design and Maintenance and Calibration of Equipment

The GLP regulations do not have a section specific to the requirements for computer systems, and they do not contain the term "computerized system," but a review of the *Bioresearch Monitoring Good Laboratory Practice Compliance Program 7348.808*, Appendix A, shows that computer systems and computer operations are included in an FDA inspection of a GLP test facility. If computerized systems are used to generate, measure, assess and store data, appropriate procedures and controls must be established and followed to ensure the quality and integrity of the study.

Chapter 8

As revised in 2002, 21 CRF 11, Electronic Records; Electronic Signatures, established FDA's "criteria under which the agency considers electronic records, electronic signatures, and handwritten signatures executed to electronic records to be trustworthy, reliable, and generally equivalent to paper records and handwritten signatures executed on paper." While Part 11 is separate from the GLPs, the two are closely linked when computerized systems are used during GLP-compliant studies. The current trend among nonclinical CROs is the use of computerized systems for all recordkeeping, and FDA expects these systems will be compliant with 21 CFR 11.

Subpart E:
§58.81. Standard Operating Procedures
Standard Operating Procedures (SOPs) are an integral part of the conduct and recreation of GLP studies. SOPs are intended to ensure that laboratory procedures and processes are consistently performed by all individuals throughout the facility. Accordingly, SOPs should be readily available to all laboratory staff, and a mandatory review of SOPs should be performed and documented. Test facility management is responsible for periodically reviewing and updating SOPs as needed.

In general, the study protocol outlines "what" is to be done during a nonclinical study, but SOPs describe "how" those procedures are to be performed. For example, the protocol would instruct you to administer an intravenous injection, but the SOP would tell you what size needle and syringe to use, the appropriate vein for the injection, the proper method of restraint for the animal, etc. A comprehensive set of SOPs should address all aspects of study conduct from pre-initiation work through archiving data and specimens after study completion. SOPs should also describe the processes in place to address each requirement outlined in 21 CFR 58.

All deviations from SOPs that occur during a study should be documented, authorized by the study director, and assessed for impact on study integrity. Specific instructions given in the study protocol supersede SOPs, and in this case, it should not be considered a deviation if SOPs are not followed.

Subpart F:
§58.105, 58.107, 58.113. Test and Control Article Characterization and Handling and Mixtures of Articles with Carriers
"Test article" means any food additive, color additive, drug, biopharmaceutical, biological product, medical device or electronic product intended for human use. "Control article" means any article other than the test article that is intended to serve as a control in the study; it typically establishes a basis for comparison with the test article.

GLPs require that characterization, stability testing, sample retention and inventory for the test and control articles be performed and documented. Characterization and stability testing may be performed by the test facility conducting the study, by the sponsor or by a laboratory contracted by the sponsor. Responsibility for the testing should be stated in the study protocol. Stability testing of the test and control articles and mixtures thereof can be performed prior to initiation or concomitantly with conduct of the study. It is important to demonstrate stability under both the conditions of storage and the conditions of use during the study. Stability of the mixture of a test article with a carrier (vehicle) must be established for a range of concentrations that bracket those used during the study.

Proper handling of the test and control articles is essential to the quality and integrity of the nonclinical study. Section 58.107 requires sponsors to establish procedures for the proper storage, distribution, identification and receipt/distribution of the articles.

Although the term "chain of custody" is not used in the GLP regulations, there is an expectation that documentation showing all movements and locations of the test and control articles from the time of sponsor shipment to final disposition will be generated and maintained.

Subpart G:
§58.120 and §58.130. Protocol for and Conduct of a Nonclinical Laboratory Study
Each GLP study is conducted according to a formal plan, i.e., study protocol. There can be only one protocol for each study. A document that describes subcontracted work conducted by a contributing scientist in support of a GLP study should not be titled as a protocol. The GLP regulations provide a list of items to be included, as applicable, in the study protocol. The order of the items presented in the study protocol may vary, provided that all relevant items are included. The study director must sign the study protocol prior to the generation of any study-specific data. The sponsor is not required to sign the protocol, but the date of the sponsor's approval must be documented within.

During the execution of the study protocol, changes to the protocol may be needed. Planned changes from the protocol, i.e., changes before they occur, are made by issuing protocol amendments, which are approved by the individuals who approved the initial study protocol. Following approval, all relevant parties should be notified of a protocol amendment.

Study deviations—those specific to the study protocol or to SOPs applicable to the conduct of the study—may occur during the course of the study. These unplanned events must be documented and assessed for study impact by the study director and reviewed by the QAU.

Quality data and the ability to accurately recreate a study are major goals of the GLPs. To this end, Section 58.130(e) is very specific about the handling of raw data. Data generated by hand are to be recorded "directly, promptly, and legibly in ink." Each entry must be accompanied by the date and the signature or initials of the recorder. Changes to data must not obscure the original entry and must be accompanied by an explanation or justification and the signature or initials of the person making the change. Prompt recording of data is important so changes made to an entry at a later date must include strong supporting documentation and justification. The same general processes apply to data generated electronically and are also related to the requirements set forth in 21 CFR 11, Electronic Records; Electronic Signatures.

Subpart J:
§58.185 Reporting of Nonclinical Study Results

The GLP regulations provide a list of required elements to be included in the final study report. A final report should be prepared for each study conducted. The date the study director signs the final report is the study completion date.

Instructions defined in Compliance Program 7348.808 specify that FDA inspectors are to verify that study reports contain all the required elements. If a subcontractor was used, the subcontractor's name and facility address and the portion of the study that the subcontractor executed must be included. There must be a description of any computer program changes. The dated signature of the study director is required and, if any changes or additions were made to the final report after it has been signed, it must include a statement and signature that the changes/additions were made in accordance with the requirements of Section 58.185.

The study director is responsible for documenting in the final study report all circumstances that may affect the study's quality and integrity. This should include, at a minimum, descriptions of deviations from the study protocol.

Although the GLP regulations do not specifically require the final report to contain a statement of GLP compliance, it is common practice for the study director to include such a statement. Sponsors generally find this preferable because they are ultimately required to make such a statement, when applicable, by 21 CFR 312.23(a)(8)(b)(iii), Investigational New Application, and 314.50 (d)(2)(v), Application for FDA Approval to Market a New Drug. Both regulations state that "for each nonclinical laboratory study subject to the good laboratory practice regulations under Part 58, a statement that the study was conducted in compliance with the good laboratory practice regulations in Part 58, or, if the study was not conducted in compliance with those regulations, a brief statement of the reason for the noncompliance" must be submitted. For studies conducted across multiple sites, each contributing scientist is expected to provide a statement to the study director that attests to the GLP compliance of the work conducted at his or her facility. This, along with QAU inspection reports, allows the study director to make an accurate statement of GLP compliance for all aspects of the study.

Full compliance with GLPs for studies subject to the regulation is always preferable, but FDA indicated in its Questions and Answers document that nonclinical laboratory safety studies with areas of noncompliance may be acceptable, provided the noncompliance did not compromise the study's quality and integrity.[12]

§58.190. Storage and Retrieval of Records and Data

The GLPs are specific with regard to the establishment of an archive for the storage of raw data, documentation, protocols, specimens and interim and final reports from completed studies. The regulations also require that an individual be assigned responsibility for the archives. At the conclusion of the study, i.e., after the study director has signed the final study report, all the raw data, protocols, amendments, analytical data and specimens are transferred to a secure storage area. The records and data are maintained under appropriate conditions in accordance with the record retention requirements specified in Section 58.195.

Guidance for Industry

FDA has issued its current thinking on all subparts of 21CFR 58, GLP, in the form of a Questions and Answers document. The document consolidated all GLP questions answered by the agency during the two-year period after 20 June 1979.[12] The review provides the current agency position on various subparts of 21 CFR 58; however, the agency is of the opinion that the answers appear somewhat cryptic and therefore cautions the reader on the limitations of the utility of correspondence. The following sections provide a brief compilation of the correspondence for each subpart of the GLP regulations. For a complete version of the guidance document, the reader is referred to FDA's website (www.fda.gov/ICECI/EnforcementActions/BioresearchMonitoring/NonclinicalLaboratoriesInspectedunderGoodLaboratoryPractices/ucm072738.htm).

GLPs apply to over dosage studies in the target species, animal safety studies, tissue residue accumulation and depletion studies and udder irritation studies. The regulations need to be followed in chemical procedures to characterize the: test article, stability determination on the test article, concentration of test article mixtures and chemical analysis of specimens (clinical chemistry, urinalysis, etc.). However, FDA clarified that validation trials to confirm analytical methods used to determine the concentrations of the test article in animal studies need not comply with GLPs. Studies conducted at a subcontractor's laboratory, including ophthalmology exams; reading of animal ECGs, EEGs and

> **Glossary**[a]
>
> **Inspection Classification Codes:**
>
> **CAN:** Canceled
>
> **NAI:** No Action Indicated. No objectionable conditions or practices were found during the inspection (or the objectionable conditions found do not justify further regulatory action).
>
> **NCC:** Non Classified
>
> **NIM:** No Inspection Made.`
>
> **OAI:** Official Action Indicated. Regulatory and administrative actions will be recommended.
>
> **PEN:** Pending review and classification.
>
> **RTC:** Refer to Center: Establishment Inspection Report had been forwarded to Center for final review and classification.
>
> **VAI:** Voluntary Action Indicated. Objectionable conditions or practices were found, but the agency is not prepared to take or recommend any administrative or regulatory action.
>
> **WO:** Washout: Firm was visited or inspected, however, not performing regulated studies at time of inspection.

a. Archive of Lab Inspection List - Nonclinical Laboratories Inspected Under FDA GLP Regulations (Title 21, Code of Federal Regulations, Part 58) SINCE FISCAL YEAR 1990. www.fda.gov/ICECI/EnforcementActions/BioresearchMonitoring/NonclinicalLaboratoriesInspectedunderGoodLaboratoryPractices/ActiveLabsInspectionList/default.htm#Codes.

EMGs; preparation of blocks and slides from tissues; statistical analysis; and hematology experiments, need to comply with GLPs. Any nonclinical studies conducted in foreign laboratories also must comply with GLPs, and it is the responsibility of the sponsor to ensure the foreign laboratory complies with US GLP regulations. On a different note, the safety studies on cosmetic products and food organoleptic evaluation studies need not comply with GLPs.

Animal cage cards usually are not considered raw data; however, if an original observation is put on the cards, then all the cards are required to be saved as raw data. Quarantine records, animal receipt, environmental monitoring, instrument calibration and photocopies of raw data that are dated and verified by signature of the copier are considered raw data. All necroscopy data recorded by the prosecutor and the signed and dated report of the pathologist also are considered raw data. However, the computer printout from the laboratory data sheets is not considered to be raw data. GLPs do not preclude the manual transcription of raw data into notebooks that are verified, signed and dated, but due to the chance of transcriptional errors occurring, such an approach should be used only when necessary. In these circumstances, GLPs require the retention of raw data. GLP animal quarantine and isolation procedures need to be followed in diagnosing, treating and certifying the animals to be "well" for use in nonclinical studies. GLPs do not specify quarantine periods for each test system. While GLPs do not prohibit the use of primates for multiple nonclinical laboratory studies, the potential impact of multiple uses on study interpretation should be assessed carefully. GLPs do not address the genetic quality of animals used in a nonclinical laboratory, and the suitability of the test system is a protocol matter that should be addressed scientifically.

GLPs require feed samples from nonclinical studies to be retained, but it is not necessary to retain reserve samples of feed that involve test article administration by routes other than feed. The stability of the test article is usually unknown during the nonclinical studies; therefore, the test article label should contain a statement such as "see protocol" or "see periodic analysis results" that allows users to know the current analytical data prior to its use. GLPs require tests on homogeneity, concentration and stability on control article mixtures. It is also necessary to analyze the test article mixtures that are used in acute studies. GLPs do not require assay analysis on each batch of test or control article mixtures, but require periodic analysis of the material. For liquid test article mixtures where the concentrations are adjusted by dilution, it is adequate to analyze the lowest dose since it would confirm the efficiency of the dilution process. While homogeneity analysis is required for suspensions of test articles, the true solutions need not be analyzed.

GLPs permit the designation of different study directors for each study under contract. Usually, it is testing center management's responsibility to approve the study director for the contracted study; GLPs do not require sponsor approval.

Sponsors do not need to reveal toxicology data already collected on a test article to a contract lab unless the test article poses a potential danger to laboratory personnel. In that case, the contract laboratory should be advised to take appropriate precautions.

FDA performs four kinds of GLP and nonclinical laboratory-related inspections: periodic/routine inspections; data audit inspection to verify the data in a final report submitted to FDA; directed inspection to evaluate questionable data in the final report; and a follow up inspection to assure that proper corrective actions have been taken.

GLP investigators do not have the authority to comment on a protocol's scientific merits; their function is only to note observations and verifications. The investigators usually select studies in accord with agency priorities, i.e., the longest-term study on the most significant product. Prior to the inspection, the investigators usually review the GLP regulations, management briefing post-conference report, GLP compliance program, protocol or final report of the ongoing study, if available, and reports from the most recent inspection. Laboratory management is notified of all routine GLP inspections; however, special compliance inspections need not be pre-announced.

In case of significant GLP deviations, FDA sends a letter and requests a response within 10 days. Even though there is no specific timetable, this is determined by FDA compliance staff based on the particular situation. The observations that are identified in the Form FDA 483 require management to initiate corrective actions as soon as possible.

Personnel and their job descriptions should be available for each individual engaged in or supervising the GLP studies. Any contracted specialists, such as pathologists, statisticians, etc., need to be identified in the final report. There is no requirement for the QAU to be composed of technical personnel. However, management is responsible for assuring the appropriate combination of education, experience and/or training. GLPs also require that the functions of the study director and those of the QAU director be separate and that the QAU not report to the study director to avoid any conflict of interest. Study records should identify the designated deputy or acting study director, and it is mandatory that the study director adheres to the GLPs.

QAU personnel are not expected to perform scientific evaluations or question scientific procedures. They are expected to ensure that the GLPs, SOPs and protocols are followed and that the data in the final report reflect the study results accurately. The QAU maintains all protocols and only those SOPs that concern the QAU's operations and procedures. Individuals involved in a nonclinical study cannot perform QAU functions; however, an individual can perform a QAU function for a study with which he or she is not involved. All final report amendments must be reviewed by the QAU, which also is responsible for maintaining the laboratory archives.

GLPs do not require clean/dirty separation for animal care areas or separate animal rooms to house the test systems and conduct different studies. However, GLPs do require separate areas adequate to assure separation of test systems, individual projects and animal quarantine.

Test and control articles need not be in locked storage units, but accurate records of accountability must be maintained. FDA has not established guidelines for the frequency of equipment calibration of balances used in nonclinical studies, but it is suggested that a suitable calibration program be instituted to assure data validity. All reagents used in the laboratory should be labeled for identity, storage and expiration date. GLPs do not require the use of product accountability procedures for reagents and chemicals used in the laboratory.

While no specific limits on details are defined by FDA for the GLP SOPs, they need to be adequate to address the systems. The adequacy of the SOPs is a key management responsibility. Management also is responsible for the approval of all SOPs, including the QAU SOPs. GLPs do not specify the content of SOPs for computerized data acquisition, but they should include the purpose, specifications, procedures, end products, language, interactions with other programs and other such details.

The nonclinical study becomes a regulated study once the protocol is signed by both the study director and management, if indicated, and the study must be entered on the Master Schedule Sheet. Each nonclinical study also requires a sponsor-approved specific protocol. Subsequently, the study is carried on the master schedule sheet until the study director submits a signed and dated final report. Therefore, the starting and completion dates of the nonclinical study are useful for the purposes of the Master Schedule Sheet and the study final report. For Master Schedule Sheet purposes, the starting date of the study is the date the protocol is approved by management, and the completion date is the date the study director signs the final report. At the completion of the study, QAU records and inspection reports should be retained in the archives.

Proposed Changes to Current FDA GLPs

In December 2010, FDA issued a public request for comments on proposed revisions to the GLPs.[13] In the time since the final regulations were published in 1978, there have been changes in the complexity and logistics of conducting nonclinical studies, most notably in the conduct of studies across multiple test sites. FDA established a working group in 2007 to evaluate the adequacy of the current GLPs relative to modern nonclinical studies, and the group concluded that changes to certain aspects of the regulations may be needed. Areas identified for potential revision include addressing multi-site studies, expanding sponsor responsibilities, monitoring QAU inspection findings, test and control article information and implementation of GLP quality systems at nonclinical laboratories. A timeline for implementing the changes has not been set.

FDA Inspection of GLP Laboratories and the Consequences of Noncompliance

All laboratories operating within the US that perform nonclinical laboratory studies are subject to inspection by FDA. The agency also conducts GLP inspections of laboratories outside the US, but only after it has requested and received consent from the laboratory.

FDA has established a Bioresearch Monitoring Program (BIMO) to address both domestic and international inspections of nonclinical testing laboratories operating under US GLPs. FDA and ORA issued *Compliance Program Guidance 7348*.808,[14] which represents FDA's current thinking on the inspection of GLP facilities and studies. The guidance provides insight into how nonclinical testing laboratory inspections are conducted and likely focal areas for the inspection.

A review of archived FDA Warning Letters from 1996 through 2010 showed the most frequently cited GLP violations involved the failure of QAUs and study directors to fulfill their responsibilities. Lack of a QAU and inadequate qualification of QAU personnel also were cited in the Warning Letters. Other selected GLP violations cited included: failure to follow the study protocol, inadequate final report, failure to establish SOPs adequate to ensure the quality and integrity of the data, failure of the test facility management to fulfill their responsibilities and failure to archive study records and data. A similar review of archived FDA inspectional observational summaries for Form FDA 483s issued from Fiscal 2006 through 2012 showed that at least 16% of 483s were for GLP-related issues. The citations included inadequate QAU systems and QAU personnel; issues related to the facility management, study director assignment, deviations from filing and archiving the study reports by study directors, inadequate qualified personnel, inadequate educational qualifications for laboratory personnel, inadequate testing of both control and test articles and others.[15]

While most of the requirements established in the GLPs are clearly described, FDA inspectors' interpretations of the regulations can evolve over time. A recent example applies to preparation of final study reports that include sub-reports from contributing scientists.[16] Per Section 58.185(a)(12), a final report shall include "the signed and dated reports of each of the individual scientists or other professionals involved in the study." It is common practice among CROs to prepare a draft final report using unsigned contributor reports and then submit it for review by the sponsor and QAU. However, FDA has recently cited at least three CROs for preparing draft final reports using unsigned contributor reports, noting that, as a result, the report "lacked accountability and confirmation that the contributing scientists' raw data was accurate."[17] In addition, allowing the sponsor to review and edit the final report before it is signed by the study director implies that "bias in data interpretation and reporting cannot be ruled out."

The consequences of noncompliance with GLP regulations can be severe. Deficiencies, such as those found during the inspections of IBT and Searle, made it impossible to either prove or disprove the safety of the products; consequently, numerous studies were declared invalid. Noncompliance with GLPs can result in research applications being placed on clinical hold and marketing permits being delayed or refused.

The measures FDA can take against a nonclinical test facility can range from the issuance of FDA inspectional observations (Form FDA 483) to Warning Letters to consent agreements to disqualification of a testing facility for conducting nonclinical laboratory studies.

If noncompliance with GLPs results in disqualification of the testing laboratory, any nonclinical laboratory study conducted by the laboratory that is submitted to FDA in an application for research or a marketing permit before or after the laboratory is disqualified may be presumed to be unacceptable, and the application may be deemed unacceptable.

Summary

GLP compliance is expected for studies that support or are intended to support FDA-regulated applications, including INDs, NDAs, IDEs, PMAs, etc. Compliance with GLPs ensures the quality, integrity, accuracy and reproducibility of data submitted for review by FDA. GLPs set minimum requirements for facility management, study personnel, study conduct, standardization of procedures, reporting, record retention and quality control systems.

References

1. Swidersky P. "Quality Assurance and Good Lab Practice, Examining the FDA's & OECD's GLPs." *Contract Pharma*. 76–83, May 2007.
2. US Department of Health and Human Services, Food and Drug Administration, Office of Regulatory Affairs, Comparison Chart of FDA and EPA Good Laboratory Practice (GLP) Regulations and the OECD Principles of GLP (Issue date: June 2004). FDA website. www.fda.gov/downloads/ICECI/EnforcementActions/BioresearchMonitoring/UCM133724.pdf. Accessed 4 April 2013.
3. Op cit 1.
4. 21 CFR Part 58, Good Laboratory Practice for Nonclinical Laboratory Studies, Final Rule, 1987. FDA website. www.accessdata.fda.gov/scripts/cdrh/cfdocs/cfcfr/cfrsearch.cfm?cfrpart=58. Accessed 4 April 2013.
5. Ibid.
6. *Clinical Laboratories Improvement Amendments (CLIA)*, 42 CFR Part 493.3. CDC website. wwwn.cdc.gov/clia/pdf/cfr493_1097.pdf. Accessed 4 April 2013.
7. Centers for Disease Control and Prevention. "Good Laboratory Practices for Waived Testing Sites." *Morbidity and Mortality Weekly Report*. 54(No. RR-13), November 2005. CDC website. www.cdc.gov/mmwr/PDF/rr/rr5413.pdf. Accessed 4 April 2013.
8. Baldeshwiler A. "History of FDA Good Laboratory Practices." *Qual Assur J*. 7: 157–161 (2003).
9. Weisskopf C. "Here's another fine mess you've gotten us into." *Washington State University, Agrichemical and Environmental News*. May 1998.

10. Marshall E. "The murky world of toxicity testing." *Science*. 220:1130–1132 (1983).
11. *Compliance Program Guidance 7348.808, Bioresearch Monitoring, Good Laboratory Practice, Compliance Program Guidance 7348.808 (Nonclinical Laboratories)* (21 February 2001). FDA website. www.fda.gov/downloads/ICECI/EnforcementActions/BioresearchMonitoring/ucm133765.pdf. Accessed 4 April 2013.
12. *Guidance for Industry, Good Laboratory Practices Questions and Answers*. June 1981, revised December 1999 and July 2007. FDA website. www.fda.gov/downloads/ICECI/EnforcementActions/BioresearchMonitoring/ucm133748.pdf. Accessed 4 April 2013.
13. "Good Laboratory Practice for Nonclinical Laboratory Studies; Advanced Notice of Proposed Rulemaking," *Federal Register* 75 (21 December 2010), pp. 80011–80013. GPO website. www.gpo.gov/fdsys/pkg/FR-2010-12-21/html/2010-31888.htm. Accessed 4 April 2013.
14. Op cit 11.
15. *Summary of the number of FDA Form 483s issued from the TURBO EIR System including the number of times an area of regulation was cited as an observation by product or program area*. FDA website. www.fda.gov/ICECI/EnforcementActions/ucm250720.htm. Accessed 25 February 2013.
16. Snyder S. "Regulatory Shockwaves: An FDA Ruling Stuns the Industry." *Contract Pharma*. October 2010. Contract Pharma website. www.contractpharma.com/issues/2010-10/view_preclinical-outsourcing/regulatory-shockwaves/. Accessed 4 April 2013.
17. Warning Letter (to SNBL USA, Ltd.). Issued 9 August 2010. FDA website. www.fda.gov/ICECI/EnforcementActions/WarningLetters/ucm222775.htm Accessed 4 April 2013.

Recommended Reading

- Cataneo R. "Good Laboratory Practice for Nonclinical Laboratory Studies: A Review." *Regulatory Focus* July 2008: 31–35.
- US Department of Health and Human Services, Food and Drug Administration, Bioresearch Monitoring Staff (HFC-30), GLP Regulations (Management Briefings) Post Conference Report, Rockville, MD. August 1979: 5–12.
- US Department of Health and Human Services, Food and Drug Administration, Bioresearch Monitoring Staff (HFC-30), *Guidance for Industry, Good Laboratory Practices Questions and Answers*. June 1981, revised December 1999 and September 2000.
- US Department of Health and Human Services, Food and Drug Administration, Office of Regulatory Affairs, *Compliance Program Guidance 7348.808, Bioresearch Monitoring, Good Laboratory Practice, Compliance Program Guidance 7348.808 (Nonclinical Laboratories)* (Issued 21 February 2001).
- US Department of Health and Human Services, Food and Drug Administration, Bioresearch Monitoring. *Good Laboratory Practices Regulation* (Issued 4 September 1987).

Chapter 9

Clinical Trials: GCPs, Regulations and Compliance

Updated by Mya Thomae, RAC, Jessica W. Smith, RAC, and Tatiana Leshchinsky, PhD

OBJECTIVES

- Provide framework of regulatory laws, regulations and guidelines covering human subjects protections during clinical studies
- Discuss the purpose of Good Clinical Practice (GCP)
- Define purpose and the obligations of the Institutional Review Board (IRB)
- Define requirements for investigational products
- Provide requirements for sponsors of research and investigators
- Provide overview of clinical studies, protocols and informed consent form requirements

LAWS, REGULATIONS, AND GUIDANCES COVERED IN THIS CHAPTER

- 21 CFR 50 Protection of Human Subjects
- 21 CFR 54 Financial Disclosure by Clinical Investigator
- 21 CFR 56 Institutional Review Board
- 21 CFR 312 Investigational New Drug Application
- 21 CFR 812 Investigational Device Exemption
- 21 CFR 46 Protection of Human Subjects
- 21 CFR 201 Labeling
- 21 CFR 320 Bioavailability and Bioequivalence Requirements
- Privacy Act, 5 U.S.C. §552a (1974)
- Health Insurance Portability and Accountability Act (1996) (HIPAA Privacy Rule: Standards for Privacy of Individually Identifiable Health Information, Final Rule, 45 CFR parts 160 and 164 (2002) and HIPAA Security Rule, 45 CFR parts 160, 162, and 164)
- *Guidance for Institutional Review Boards, Clinical Investigators, and Sponsors: Exemption from Informed Consent Requirements for Emergency Research*
- *Guidance for Industry: Financial Disclosure by Clinical Investigators*
- *Guidance for Clinical Trial Sponsors: Data Monitoring Committees, Establishment and Operation of Clinical Trial.*
- *Guidance for Industry: Investigator Responsibilities*
- *Guidance for Industry: Monitoring of Clinical Investigators*

Regulatory Affairs Professionals Society

- *Guidance for Clinical Investigators, Sponsors, and IRBs: Adverse Event Reporting to IRBs – Improving Human Subject Protection*
- *Guidance for Industry on Using a Centralized IRB Process in Multi Center Clinical Trials*
- *Guidance for IRBs, Clinical Investigators, and Sponsors: IRB Continuing Review*
- *Design Control Guidance for Medical Device Manufacturers*
- *Guidance for Industry: E6 Good Clinical Practice: Consolidated Guidance*
- *International Compilation of Human Research Standards, 2013 edition*
- *Guidance on Engagement of Institutions in Human Subjects Research*

Introduction

The main purpose of a clinical study is to advance medical knowledge. More specifically, clinical studies may be conducted to:
- evaluate one or more interventions (e.g., drugs, medical devices, approaches to surgery or radiation therapy) for treating a disease, syndrome, or condition
- find ways to prevent the initial development or recurrence of a disease or condition, which may include drug therapies, vaccines or lifestyle changes, among other approaches
- evaluate one or more interventions aimed at identifying or diagnosing a particular disease or condition
- examine methods for identifying a condition or risk factors for that condition
- explore and measure ways to improve the quality of life for people with chronic illness through supportive care[1]

Prior to the conduct of a clinical trial, it is critical to ensure protection of human subjects with proper review of the study design, monitoring and reporting procedures, as well as potential conflicts of interest by sponsors, clinical investigators and others who may be involved in the research.

Protection of Human Subjects

Protection of human subjects during clinical studies has its foundation in the Code of Medical Ethics, originally drafted in 1847 by the American Medical Association (AMA). Since then, basic ethical codes have been violated in several research studies where humans were unknowingly and/or involuntarily exposed to dangerous and often lethal procedures, experimental drugs and medical interventions. As a result of these violations of basic human rights, regulations were enacted for the primary purpose of protecting humans in biomedical research. Key legislative events that had the most profound impact on the development of human subject protection principles are summarized below.

Nuremberg Code of 1947

The *Nuremberg Code* of 1947 is a set of research ethics principles for human experimentation that was created as a result of atrocities involving medical experimentation on humans during World War II.[2] The subsequent Nuremberg Trials were held, and verdicts were delivered against several physicians who were responsible for conducting unethical research on human subjects and prisoners of war. The outcome of the trial was a set of 10 ethical principles that defined legitimate medical research, which constitute the *Nuremberg Code*.

While the *Nuremberg Code* has not been officially adopted as a legal document, it forms the basis, along with the *Declaration of Helsinki* (see below), of the Code of Federal Regulations (CFR) Title 45 Volume 46, which outlines regulations for conducting federally funded research involving human subjects in the US. The primary principles of the *Nuremberg Code* include:
- informed consent and absence of coercion
- properly formulated scientific experimentation
- beneficence of research for experiment participants

Declaration of Geneva (1948)

The *Declaration of Geneva* is a declaration made by physicians regarding the humanitarian goals of medicine that has its roots in the *Hippocratic Oath*, which is based on the beliefs and practices of the ancient Greek physician, Hippocrates (circa 400 BC). Hippocrates believed the practice of medicine should include kindness to the patient, as well as rigor, discipline and professionalism. The *Declaration of Geneva* was born from these ideas and originally was adopted by the World Medical Association (WMA) at Geneva in 1948. It was subsequently amended five times, with the most recent revision in 2006. Some of the current *Declaration of Geneva*'s main tenets include:
- giving teachers the respect and gratitude that is their due
- respecting the patient's privacy
- not permitting considerations of age, disease or disability, creed, ethnic origin or other factors to intervene in the physician's duty to his patient
- maintaining the utmost respect for human life
- not using medical knowledge to violate human rights and civil liberties

Declaration of Helsinki (1964)

The *Declaration of Helsinki*, originally developed in 1964 by the World Medical Association, is considered the cornerstone of human research ethics.[3] More specifically, the declaration combines the principles first outlined in the *Nuremberg Code* with those outlined in the *Declaration of Geneva* to form the basis for current clinical research ethics principles. The fundamental principle of the *Declaration of Helsinki* is respect for the individual. This principle guides the role of the investigator to protect the patient or volunteer, first and foremost. That is, the subject's welfare always takes precedence over the interests of the research goals. Further, the declaration specifies that the benefits of the proposed research must be based on a comprehensive understanding and knowledge of the scientific background that provides the foundation of the research, and the results must have a reasonable likelihood of benefiting the population being studied.

Since the original version, the declaration has undergone six revisions, most recently in 2008. The first revision, drafted in 1975, introduced the concept of an "independent committee" that provides oversight of clinical research with the primary purpose of ensuring protection of human subjects. This concept was adopted in the US as the Institutional Review Board (IRB) and exists in other countries as various forms of research ethics committees. The IRB remains a critical component of clinical research involving human subjects, and approval is required for all legally conducted clinical research in the US, as outlined in 21 CFR Part 56.[4]

Good Clinical Practice (GCP)

While the *Declaration of Helsinki* was a key contribution to forming basic ethical principles regarding clinical research, the US Food and Drug Administration (FDA) did not adopt it. Instead, FDA replaced the declaration with Good Clinical Practice (GCP) guidelines in October 2008. The objectives of GCPs are to define standards for conducting clinical research to test drugs, medical devices and biologics on human subjects or human samples.

The basic tenets of GCPs include an IRB-approved protocol, valid informed consent, monitoring plan, adverse effect reporting, proper documentation and valid data collection/reporting procedures. Ultimately, the responsibility of following GCPs rests on the sponsor, clinical investigators, IRBs, contract research organizations (CROs), clinical research coordinators, medical monitors, data entry personnel and any others who may be involved in conducting research. Thus, it is critical that anyone participating in the conduct of clinical research be appropriately trained and informed on GCPs to ensure appropriate steps are taken to ensure protection of human subjects.

The adequate protection of human participants involved in clinical research is recognized universally as a key component of GCPs. Internationally, GCPs are established by the International Conference on Harmonisation (ICH) (with input from the regulatory agencies of Japan, the EU and the US). FDA's GCP Program coordinates FDA policies, provides leadership and direction, contributes to ICH harmonization activities, plans and conducts training and serves as a liaison between the Office for Human Research Protections (OHRP) and other federal agencies and external organizations involved in protecting human research participants. Many countries have adopted GCP practices as law and/or regulations.

Belmont Report (1979)

The *Belmont Report*[5] was issued in 1979 and published in the *Federal Register* on 18 April 1979. Its full title is the *Belmont Report: Ethical Principles and Guidelines for the Protection of Human Subjects of Research, Report of the National Commission for the Protection of Human Subjects of Biomedical and Behavioral Research*. The *Belmont Report* summarizes the "basic ethical principles" that underlie the conduct of biomedical and behavioral research involving human subjects. It also provides guidelines that should be followed to ensure such research is conducted in accordance with those principles. The *Belmont Report* is a key reference for IRB members, to ensure the research conforms to the ethical principles described in the report, which include:

1. respect for persons
2. beneficence
3. justice

The general principles of conducting research lead to the requirements of:

1. informed consent
2. benefit:risk assessment
3. selection of subjects for research

The Department of Health and Human Services (DHHS) subsequently revised and expanded its regulations for the protection of human subjects, under 45 CFR part 46 subpart A, based on the principles outlined in the *Belmont Report*. In 1991, the *Federal Policy for the Protection of Human Subjects*, also referred to as the "Common Rule," adopted these unified guidelines.

Oversight of Human Research in the US and Internationally

Department of Health and Human Services

DHHS is the US government agency responsible for protecting the health of all Americans and providing essential human services, especially for those who are least able to help themselves. There are a total of 11 operating divisions under DHHS, which include FDA, the National Institutes of Health (NIH), Centers for Disease Control and

Prevention (CDC) and Centers for Medicare & Medicaid Services (CMS), among others.

The DHHS human subjects protection regulations, first issued in 1974, are defined under 45 CFR Part 46. The rules for protection of human subjects in research are embedded in Subparts A–D of these guidelines:
- Subpart A—Subpart A outlines the basic set of protections for all human subjects of research conducted or supported by DHHS. In 1991, the set of regulations (i.e., "Common Rule") was adopted by 14 additional US federal departments and agencies in an effort to promote uniformity, understanding and compliance with human subject protections.

Additional subparts outline protections for vulnerable subject groups:
- Subpart B—Subpart B provides additional protections for pregnant women, human fetuses and neonates involved in research.
- Subpart C—Subpart C includes additional protections for prisoners participating in biomedical and behavioral research.
- Subpart D—Subpart D provides additional protections for children involved as subjects in research.

Food and Drug Administration (FDA)

FDA is the DHHS agency that regulates clinical investigations of products such as drugs, biological products and medical devices, which fall under its jurisdiction. Every time Congress establishes a law affecting FDA-regulated products, the agency develops rules and regulations to implement such law. The federal regulations are published in the CFR. The *CFR* is divided into 50 titles that represent broad areas subject to federal regulations. CFR Title 21 covers food and drugs and is available at www.accessdata.fda.gov/scripts/cdrh/cfdocs/cfcfr/cfrsearch.cfm.

To establish an FDA rule as industry practice, the agency undertakes different approaches to solicit public opinion on legal issues to create practical guidelines and guidance for the rule. FDA does this by publishing a notice about or draft of the proposed guideline in the *Federal Register* with a request for comments and contact information for the relevant FDA office. After soliciting comments, FDA finalizes the rule as guidance to the industry. The guidance is not a law, but provides FDA's current opinion on how the law should be interpreted in practice.

FDA has created several such guidelines on clinical trials. These guidelines define terminology and establish guidance for the conduct of clinical trials, labeling requirements for investigational products, responsibilities of parties involved in conducting clinical trials, requirements for human subject consent and study reports. Some FDA guidelines pertinent to clinical studies are listed in **Table 9-1** and in the Recommended Reading section at the end of this chapter.

On 9 May 1997, FDA adopted a guideline for international clinical trials based on the latest version of the ICH guideline that covers the conduct of clinical trials in the member regions. This guideline, however, is not binding on FDA or the public and serves only as a recommendation in the US.

Office for Human Research Protections (OHRP)

OHRP is a small office within DHHS, the primary purpose of which is to provide leadership in the protection of the rights, welfare and well-being of subjects involved in research conducted or supported by DHHS. The OHRP's main duty is to implement 45 CFR Part 46, but it also develops educational programs and materials for IRBs and researchers, guidance on research ethics and advice to the Secretary's Advisory Committee on Human Protections regarding medical ethics issues. The OHRP policy and guidance can be found at www.hhs.gov/ohrp/policy/. The following list summarizes OHRP duties:
- Compliance—The Division of Compliance Oversight evaluates potential noncompliance with 45 CFR Part 46, and determines whether and what regulatory action is necessary.
- Education—The Division of Education and Development provides guidance to individuals and institutions conducting DHHS-supported human subjects research; conducts national and regional conferences and participates in professional, academic and association conferences; and develops and distributes resource materials to improve protections for human subjects.
- Policy and Assurances—The Division of Policy and Assurances interprets existing policies and creates new policies and guidance documents regarding human subjects protection and disseminates this information to the research community.
- Secretary's Advisory Committee—The Secretary's Advisory Committee on Human Research Protections advises the DHHS secretary on issues of human subjects protections.
- International Activities—OHRP provides training to institutions involved in international research to ensure ethical protections are being applied to those who participate in research outside the US.

There is some overlap between OHRP and FDA regulations. In general, if the research study is intended to evaluate an FDA-regulated product and the study is designed to satisfy FDA product clearance requirements (or to be

Clinical Trials: GCPs, Regulations and Compliance

Table 9-1. FDA Regulations and Guidelines for Clinical Studies

Regulations	Drugs	Devices
Investigational New Drug/Device Application	21 CFR 312	21 CFR 812
IND/IDE Application Process	21 CFR 312.23	21 CFR 812.20, 812.25 and 812.27
Form FDA 1571 (IND)	21 CFR 312.23(a)(1)	
Form FDA 1572 (Statement of Investigator)	21 CFR 312.53(c)	21 CFR 812.43(c) – Form FDA 1572 not required by devices
Foreign Clinical Trials not Conducted under an IND	21 CFR 312.120	
Legal Representation (Transfer of Obligations)	21 CFR 312.52	
Labeling	21 CFR 201 and 312.6	21 CFR 812.5
Responsibilities of Sponsors and Investigators	21 CFR 312 Subpart D	21 CFR 812 Subpart C and E
Record and Reports	21 CFR 312.57 21 CFR 312.58 21 CFR 312.6221 CFR 312.64 21 CFR 312.68	21 CFR 812.140 21 CFR 812.150
Safety Reporting	21 CFR 312.32	31 CFR 803
Bioavailability and Bioequivalence Requirements	21 CFR 320	
Quality System Regulations		21 CFR 820
Electronic records; Electronic Signature	21 CFR 11	Same as drugs
Protection of Human Subjects (Informed Consent)	21 CFR 50	Same as drugs
Financial Disclosure by Clinical Investigators	21 CFR 54	Same as drugs
Institutional Review Boards	21 CFR 56	Same as drugs
Form FDA 3674 (Certification)	*Food and Drug Administration Amendments Act of 2007*	Same as drugs
Data protection Rules Applicable to Clinical trials (*HIPPA*)	1. Privacy Act, 5 U.S.C. §552a (1974): 2. *Health Insurance Portability and Accountability Act* (1996) (*HIPAA* Privacy Rule: Standards for Privacy of Individually Identifiable Health Information, Final Rule, 45 CFR parts 160 and 164 (2002) and *HIPAA* Security Rule, 45 CFR parts 160, 162, and 164)	Same as drugs
Pediatric Clinical Trials	21 CFR 50, Subpart D – Additional Safeguards for Children in Clinical Investigations	Same as drugs
Orphan Drugs	21 CFR Part 316	

submitted to FDA), it must comply with FDA regulations. Some federally funded research that does not lead to FDA submission for product approval may only be covered by OHRP regulations.

Health Insurance Portability and Accountability Act (HIPAA) Regulations

The *Health Insurance Portability and Accountability Act* of 1996 (*HIPAA*), in addition to other provisions, includes requirements for protecting patients' health information in medical records and in transactions with health insurance companies. Any research study that involves health information from medical records is covered by *HIPAA* regulations. Studies that do not require review of medical records or where medical information may be obtained through interviewing patients do not require *HIPAA* compliance. Regardless of whether the study falls under *HIPAA* regulations, patient confidentiality and associated medical information are always required by OHRP and FDA regulations.

State Regulations

In addition to federal requirements, each state has its own set of clinical trial regulations. Compliance with federal regulations does not ensure compliance with state regulations. Only some states' regulations are broader than the federal requirements. Most states defer to the federal regulations for federally funded research. State regulations primarily determine whether the costs of medical procedures (including routing medical care) for patients involved in clinical trials will be covered by patients' health insurance. Some states require insurance companies to cover routine medical care for patients involved in clinical trials. As a general rule, however, the study sponsor is responsible for covering the costs of medical procedures, doctors' visits, tests and any other costs associated with the conduct of the clinical trial.

International Regulations

An ICH guideline covers the conduct of clinical trials in the member regions. FDA and ICH clinical research regulations have minor differences, and even though ICH regulations were adopted by FDA in 1997, the agency did not enact them into law.

In 1995, the World Health Organization (WHO) established "Guidelines for Good Clinical Practice (GCP) for Trials on Pharmaceutical Products," published in WHO Technical Report (TR) series No. 850, Annex 3. These guidelines are designed for pharmaceutical products and are somewhat applicable to biomedical research. They were developed in consultation with regulatory authorities of WHO Member States. The WHO guidelines were designed to ensure scientific and ethical integrity of clinical trials and are recognized by Member States as compatible with their existing national provisions, although FDA is not bound by these regulations.

Institutional Review Boards (IRBs), Review Process and Responsibilities

Definition of IRB

An IRB is a review panel that is responsible for ensuring the protection of the rights, safety and well-being of human subjects involved in a clinical study and providing oversight of compliance with the regulations.

The general standards for the composition, operation and responsibilities of an IRB are described in 21 CFR Part 56. While the vast majority of clinical trials require IRB approval prior to initiation, there are a few exceptions. Two examples of exemptions are (1) investigations commenced before 27 July 1981 and (2) emergency use of an investigational product.

An IRB is composed of a minimum of five individuals with varying backgrounds. The IRB must not consist entirely of either men or women, and must include at least one member whose primary concerns involve scientific areas and at least one member whose primary concerns are in nonscientific areas.

The primary functions of the IRB include: initial and continuing review of research, and reporting the research findings and actions to the investigator and institution; determining the frequency of review; ensuring the prompt reporting of unanticipated problems involving risks to human subjects or others; and reviewing and making recommendations of approval or rejection of proposed research. Further, the IRB has the authority to require modifications and/or disapprove proposed research activities.

To approve research, the IRB also must determine whether the following requirements are satisfied:
a. risks to subjects are minimized
b. risks to subjects are reasonable in relation to the anticipated benefits, if any.
c. selection of subjects is equitable
d. informed consent will be sought from each prospective subject or the subject's authorized representative
e. informed consent will be appropriately documented
f. where appropriate, the research plan makes adequate provision for monitoring the data collected to ensure the safety of subjects
g. where appropriate, there are adequate provisions to protect the privacy of subjects to maintain the confidentiality of data
h. when some or all of the subjects are from a vulnerable population, additional safeguards are in place to protect the rights and welfare of these subjects
i. where research is to be performed in children only, the research is in compliance with 21 CFR Part 50, Subpart D

IRB Compliance for a Multi-center Study

The clinical study may be designed in a manner that requires the participation of several organizations and transfer of data or samples collected during the study among different study site locations. The study sites may be located in different geographic areas of one state or in different states or countries. For this type of multi-center study, the regulatory requirements for each study site must be fulfilled.

Reporting to IRB

Changes to the Protocol and Consent

During the course of the study, the sponsor is required to report to the IRB all changes in the study protocol and/or informed consent, changes in staff performing the study and new financial interests of the study staff. The IRB must review and approve these changes before they are implemented.

Annual Reports
An annual study renewal form must be submitted to all appropriate IRBs to continue the study. This form documents changes relevant to the clinical study and the number of subjects consented and/or enrolled at each clinical site.

Study Closure Report
Upon study completion, a study closure report must be submitted to all appropriate IRBs.

FDA Documentation for Investigational Products
Some clinical studies require FDA approval prior to initiation. This requirement is based on level of risk, type of investigational product and purpose of the study. FDA approval for a clinical study design is obtained through an Investigational New Drug (IND) application (for new drugs) or an Investigational Device Exemption (IDE) (for medical devices).

IND
An IND application is required for all drug products not previously authorized for marketing in the US prior to being used in humans. The primary purpose of the IND submission is to ensure protection of human subjects. Guidance for contents of IND submissions can be found in 21 CFR 312.23. The key components of an IND submission include:
- information on a clinical development plan
- chemistry, manufacturing and controls information
- pharmacology and toxicology information
- previous human experience, if any, with the investigational candidate or related compounds

While current regulations allow flexibility regarding the extent of data required for an IND application, based on the goals of the investigation, the specific human testing being proposed and the expected risks, all clinical investigations performed under an IND must abide by the regulations set forth in 21 CFR regarding the conduct of clinical investigations.

Investigational Device Exemption (IDE)
The concept of an IDE is similar to that for an IND but applies to devices and allows an investigational device to be used in humans for the purposes of collecting data regarding safety and effectiveness. An approved IDE is required for all clinical evaluations of investigational devices, unless exempt, prior to study initiation. The class of medical device (Class I—low risk; Class II—medium risk; and Class III—high risk) determines the regulatory approval route. With few exceptions, Class III devices are reviewed via Premarket Applications (PMAs) and require clinical studies for approval. Class II devices typically are cleared via a 510(k) and generally do not require a clinical study for clearance. FDA does not require most Class I exempt devices to obtain FDA approval prior to marketing of the product, but the device must be registered and listed with FDA.

An IDE also is required for clinical evaluations performed for the purpose of providing evidence of safety and effectiveness for modifications to an approved use of legally marketed devices. In general, a clinical evaluation of an investigational device that has not been cleared for marketing requires the following:
- an IDE approved by an IRB (for nonsignificant risk devices) or approved by FDA for significant risk devices
- IRB approval for clinical protocol and consent
- completed informed consent from all subjects
- labeling for "investigational use only"
- study monitoring
- required records and reports

An approved IDE permits a device to be shipped lawfully within the US for the purpose of conducting investigations of the device without complying with requirements of the *Food, Drug, and Cosmetic Act (FD&C Act)* that apply to cleared or approved products in commercial distribution. IDEs also are exempt from the Quality System Regulation, with the exception of design controls. However, the clinical study must be registered with FDA at www.clinicaltrials.gov and comply with regulations and requirements for conducting a clinical study (as discussed above).

Investigational Products (Requirements & Labeling)
Requirements for Investigational Medical Devices and Pharmaceuticals
Investigational medical devices, drugs and biologics should be developed through a systematic research and development process that adheres to FDA requirements for INDs (21 CFR 312) and Design Control regulations included in the device Quality System Regulation (21 CFR 820). Prior to the initiation of a clinical trial, the study sponsor shall demonstrate through preliminary testing that the drug/device/biologic is at the final investigational prototype stage.

Usually, the clinical trial sponsor establishes the following for the investigational product before entering into a clinical study:
1. the product's regulatory classification
2. FDA submission route
3. product passes preclinical testing and demonstrates desired performance parameters
4. design transfer of the investigational product is initiated and product can be manufactured under Good Manufacturing Practice (GMP) for clinical

Chapter 9

testing (All corresponding GMP documentation for the investigational product is completed, including establishment of quality control procedures.)
5. risk analysis has been performed to evaluate the investigational product's potential risks
6. appropriate labeling has been developed for the investigational product

Labeling of Investigational Products
Drugs
Investigational new drug labeling is addressed in 21 CFR 312.6. The packaging for an investigational new drug shall be labeled with the statement "Caution: New Drug--Limited by Federal (or US) Law to Investigational Use." The labeling shall not have any statements that could be misinterpreted or could be false or misleading. It should not represent the investigational new drug as safe or effective for the purposes for which it is being investigated.

In some cases, an investigational drug may be granted an exemption from this rule as per 21 CFR 201.26 or 610.68. This provision may allow an exception or an alternative labeling of the investigational new drug for specified lots, batches, or other units that is or will be included in the Strategic National Stockpile, the national repository of medical countermeasures.

Devices
In general, FDA defines a "label" as any information that accompanies the device. This includes information on the outer packaging of a device, information on the individual components of a kit, the product insert and any information included into the shipping container. Devices that are still in research and development shall be labeled "For Research Use Only (RUO). Not for use in diagnostic procedures."

Devices that are ready for clinical testing and will be used in the studies directed to assess performance of the device shall be labeled "For Investigational Use Only. The performance characteristics of this product have not been established."

An in vitro diagnostic (IVD) product labeled for RUO should not be used for clinical investigation or clinical diagnostic use. FDA would consider such an IVD product to be misbranded under *FD&C Act* Section 502(a) of the Act, 21 U.S.C. 352(a).

Charging for Investigational Products
FDA allows sponsors to charge for investigational products, services and treatments. The regulations for drugs and biologics differ from those for medical devices. In general, any costs associated with clinical trials must be disclosed in the informed consent (21CFR 50.25(b) (3)), and reviewed and approved by IRB. The IRB ensures that any costs are reasonable and appropriate.

For medical devices, the cost of the investigational products is discussed in IDE exemption regulations (21 CFR 812.7(b)). The cost should not exceed the cost of research and development, manufacturing and handling of investigational devices. The study sponsor has to justify why charging for the investigational product does not constitute commercialization.

Accountability for Investigational Products During the Clinical Trial and Upon Study Closeout
The investigational product should be stored in a location separate from products that are intended for a similar use or have similar packaging or appearance. The investigational product inventory should be established and maintained during the study by the study site investigator or his staff. Upon study closeout, the investigational products should be either returned to the study sponsor or disposed of as required by the study sponsor and study protocol.

"Off-label" and Investigational Use of Marketed Drugs, Biologics and Medical Devices
Physicians in the US can legally use available drugs, biologics and medical devices according to their best knowledge and judgment, which include "off-label" uses of these products. If a physician makes a decision to use a product for an indication not specified in the approved product labeling, he or she is responsible for making that decision based on a scientific rationale and sound medical judgment. It becomes a physician's responsibility to maintain records of the product's "off-label" use and effects. The "off-label" use of a marketed product, with *the intent to "practice medicine,"* does not require IRB review of the submission of an IND or IDE.

In some cases, an investigational product may be classified as an "emergency use investigational product" and be exempt from IRB requirements. "Emergency use" is defined as the use of an investigational product in a human subject in a life-threatening situation for which no standard acceptable treatment is available and for which there is not sufficient time to obtain IRB approval (21 CFR 56.102(d)). This exemption usually is granted for individual situations, and FDA regulations explicitly state that any subsequent use of the investigational product should be performed under IRB-approved protocols. At the same time, FDA states that no patient in the same life-threatening situation should be denied access to the investigational product.

Responsibilities of Study Sponsor
The sponsor is the entity that has responsibility for and initiates a clinical investigation. The sponsor can be an individual, organization, manufacturer or federal agency. The sponsor is often, but not always, the entity that funds the clinical research.

In some cases of federally funded research, the funding agency is designated as the research sponsor and must comply with the requirements of 21 CFR 812.2(b). In this case, the discussion among FDA, the study sponsor, the manufacturer of the investigational product and the clinical investigator may define the regulatory responsibilities for each party as follows:

Sponsor's responsibilities to direct the clinical study include:
- Identify appropriate sites and study coordinators for clinical studies.
- Establish research protocol and prepare the consent forms (if required).
- Obtain IRB approval.
- Designate appropriately qualified medical personnel who will be readily available to advise on trial-related medical questions or problems. An outside consultant also may be used for this purpose.
- "Initiate" the site by providing training on the protocol and consent process, obtaining relevant site-specific information and arranging the shipment of test materials.
- Communicate changes in the protocol and/or consent to IRB(s).
- If the sponsor is an administrative site, then the sponsor will conduct an oversight of the research at clinical sites to monitor the study progress and ensure that consent procedure and the protocol are followed (21 CFR 812.46). An appropriately qualified individual shall be assigned to supervise the overall conduct of the trial, to handle the data, to verify the data, to conduct statistical analyses and to prepare the trial reports. The monitoring shall ensure:
  a. compliance with investigation plan
  b. record keeping—site personnel must maintain the study records in the designated storage unit throughout the study and for two years after termination of the study or when no longer needed in support of FDA submission. Examples of the records that must be maintained include:
     o protocol and any amendments
     o product labeling
     o all approved versions of informed consent forms
     o completed consent forms
     o data-collection instructions
     o IRB submissions, correspondence and approvals
     o copies of financial disclosure forms
     o subject recruitment and retention records
     o correspondence
- Review the final study report and ensure that the clinical study fulfills all the requirements and review any other issues that arise as a result of the study.
- If the study is extended, submit Continuing Review Report Form (CRRF) Work Sheet annually, or as requested by appropriate IRBs.
  a. Conduct internal discussion of the study results and file any regulatory documentation pertinent to the study with corporate records (Design History File, technical files, etc.).
  b. Recruit any additional expert advice for data interpretation and statistical analysis.
  c. If required, obtain approval of study results by the federal agency sponsoring the research.
  d. Provide study closure report to appropriate IRB(s).
- If necessary, make arrangement for a follow-up (repeat) of clinical study.

The sponsor, investigator or any person acting for or on behalf of a sponsor or investigator shall not (21 CFR 812.7):
- promote or test market an investigational device until after FDA has approved the device for commercial distribution
- commercialize an investigational device by charging the subjects or investigators for a device at a price higher than necessary to recover costs of manufacture, research, development and handling
- unduly prolong an investigation
- represent an investigational device as being safe or effective for the purposes for which it is being investigated

Financial Disclosure

Sponsors and/or investigators of human subjects research are required to disclose financial arrangements based on applicable regulations, including 21 CFR Parts 54, 312, 314, 320, 300, 601, 807, 812, 814 and 860. The reason for financial disclosure is to ensure that the financial interests and arrangements that could affect the reliability of data submitted to FDA are identified and disclosed by the applicant. Based on FDA's *Guidance for Industry: Financial Disclosure by Clinical Investigators,* the requirements for financial disclosure, which took effect 2 February 1999, apply to any clinical study submitted in a marketing application that the applicant or FDA relies on to establish the product's effectiveness and any study in which a single investigator makes a significant contribution to the demonstration of safety.

An applicant is required to submit to FDA a list of clinical investigators who conducted covered clinical studies and certify and/or disclose certain financial arrangements. These disclosures are summarized below:

- any financial arrangements to the investigator that could be affected by study outcomes
- any proprietary interest in tested product, including, but not limited to, a patent, trademark, copyright or licensing agreement
- significant equity interest in the sponsor of the covered study, which may include ownership interest, stock options or other financial interest whose value cannot be readily determined through reference to public prices
- an equity interest in a publicly held company that exceeds $50k in value (This applies to interests held during the time the clinical investigator is carrying out the study, and for one year following completion of the study.)
- the investigator has not received significant payments of other sorts, which have a cumulative monetary value of $25,000 or more, made by the sponsor of a covered study to the investigator or the investigator's institution (This applies to the time period the investigator is carrying out the clinical study and for one year following completion of the study.)

General Requirements for Study Site(s) and Study Investigators

Study sites shall be professionally recognized institutions or organizations with expertise in the required disease or condition. The clinical study investigator shall be an expert in the disease, condition and/or experimental methodology. The investigator shall:

- be able to recruit the required number of suitable subjects within the agreed recruitment period
- be able to properly conduct and complete the trial within the specified timeframe
- maintain a list of qualified persons who will be involved in conducting the clinical trial. (These persons should be trained to perform the study, and the training should be documented.)
- allow the sponsor or its designees to monitor the site
- provide timely progress reports, final report and other relevant information for the IRB(s), sponsor or study monitor
- report any changes or deviations from the protocol (The changes have to be reported as soon as possible to the research sponsor, central IRB and site-specific IRBs and appropriate regulatory authority.)
- obtain consent from subjects in an appropriate way as specified by the approved protocol
- retain essential documents pertinent to the clinical study for two years after formal closure of the study
- report serious adverse events immediately to the sponsor
- provide a written explanation to the appropriate regulatory agencies and sponsor if the study is terminated by the investigator

Clinical Study Initiation

To initiate the study, the sponsor must collect the following documents for each study site:

- IRB or Ethics Committee approval(s)
- documentation demonstrating clinical investigators' qualifications (professional license for medical professionals and Curriculum Vitae for other research personnel) and FDA number for the organization conducting clinical study (if available)
- in some cases where financial transactions are involved (e.g., grant-funded research), a finalized contractual arrangement
- assurance that the study will be performed in compliance with GCP and other applicable regulations, including site-specific regional and local regulations as well as sponsor or grant agency requirements (FDA Form 1572)
- verification of training on the study protocol

Clinical Study Reporting

The investigator shall provide prompt progress reports at specified intervals during the course of the study. Reporting requirements are determined by the sponsor and the regulatory and granting agencies. The protocol often includes a template (case report forms (CRFs)) for raw data collection. Raw data are required to be submitted independently of data analysis and are filed with the investigational product history file.

It is recommended that the following information be included in the study report:

- type of evaluation performed
- name of the investigational product
- name and contact information for site-specific study investigator
- name and contact information for the person performing the evaluation at the study site
- completed CRFs (raw data collected during the investigation)

Clinical Study Design

FDA has defined *"clinical investigation,"* also called *"clinical trial,"* to be synonymous with *"research." Clinical investigation* means any experiment that involves an experimental drug, device or biologic and one or more human subjects. It must meet the requirements for a prior submission to FDA, or the investigation's results must be intended to be submitted at a later date to, or held for inspection by, FDA as part of an application for research on or marketing of the drug, device or biologic. FDA further clarifies the definition of *"human subject" as* an individual who is a participant in research, either as a recipient of the experimental drug, device or biologic or as a control. A subject may be either a healthy individual or a patient.

It is the sponsor's responsibility to determine the appropriate study design and to prepare a protocol with specific study details. The protocol is the cornerstone for the development of the clinical study. There are two primary types of clinical trials: clinical (also referred to as interventional) studies and observational studies. For some types of medical devices, an accuracy study also may be performed. It is important to recognize that within these clinical study types, there are several different subtypes that involve randomization, placebo-control and blinding of either the investigator and subjects or both, among others. Below is a summary of the basic types of clinical studies.

Clinical (or Interventional) Trials
In clinical trials, participants receive specific interventions, which may involve a medical device, drug therapy, a medical procedure or changes to a participants' behavior, such as diet or exercise therapy, among others. These interventions, which are outlined in the research plan, may involve a comparison between a new medical procedure involving a medical device to a standard of care, a placebo that contains no active ingredients to active drug therapy, or two currently available interventions to each other. These trials may be randomized, placebo-controlled and/or blinded, which serves to increase the accuracy and reduce bias in a study.

In drug development trials, clinical trials are typically described by phases. Descriptions of each phase, as defined by FDA (www.fda.gov/drugs/resourcesforyou/consumers/ucm143534.htm), follow:
- Phase 0—exploratory study involving very limited human exposure to the drug, with no therapeutic or diagnostic goals (e.g., screening studies and microdose studies).
- Phase 1—studies that usually are conducted with healthy volunteers and that emphasize safety. The goal is to find out what the drug's most frequent and serious adverse events are and, often, how the drug is metabolized and excreted.
- Phase 2—studies that gather preliminary data on effectiveness (whether the drug works in people who have a certain disease or condition). For example, subjects receiving the drug may be compared with similar subjects receiving a different treatment, usually an inactive substance (called a placebo) or a different drug. Safety continues to be evaluated and short-term adverse events are studied.
- Phase 3—studies that gather more information about safety and effectiveness by studying different populations and different dosages and by using the drug in combination with other drugs.
- Phase 4—studies that are conducted after FDA has approved a drug for marketing (i.e., postmarketing studies). These include postmarket requirements and commitment studies that may be required or agreed to by the sponsor. These studies gather additional information about a drug's safety, efficacy or optimal use in the general population.

The gold standard of interventional studies is a randomized controlled trial (RCT). An RCT tests the efficacy of an intervention on a patient population in a way that minimizes bias. The trial is designed to compare a group of patients that received the treatment or intervention (the treatment group) with a second group of subjects who typically do not receive the treatment (the placebo group). This type of trial design is common in pharmaceutical studies and is also used for some medical device studies.

The "randomized" part of an RCT means that study subjects are randomly assigned to either the treatment group or the placebo group. Subjects are informed of how randomization is performed in the informed consent form. Randomization for clinical trials has to take many issues into account (e.g., site demographics, number of sites, etc.) but can be thought of as a process like flipping a coin: heads, the subject receives the treatment; tails, the subject is in the placebo group.

The "controlled" portion of an RCT means that both the treatment (either device or drug) is standardized for the clinical trial (e.g., formulation, dosage, model, size, etc.). The population that will be included in the trial also is controlled. The study protocol needs to clearly state specific inclusion and exclusion criteria to ensure that only the appropriate patients are enrolled. Inclusion and exclusion criteria typically include factors such as age, disease status, prior treatment status, general health status or perhaps the presence or absence of genetic markers.

Often, there are multiple treatment groups (also called "arms") in an RCT. This may occur when the study is designed to test multiple dosage levels of a drug or multiple sizes or models of a medical device. For example, a drug company may want to study the effects of two concentrations of a drug and will develop a three-arm study (e.g., 10 mg, 20 mg and placebo).

Most often, randomized trials are also "blinded." In blinded studies, information about the arm or group to which each study subject is assigned is withheld from study participants. Blinding is a method for reducing bias in evaluations and isolating the effects of the intervention from choices that might be made based on treatment information. In general, studies are either single-blind or double-blind. In a single-blind study, study subjects are unaware of the arm or group of the study to which they have been assigned;

however, the investigators and study staff are not "blinded." A double-blind study means that everyone involved in the day-to-day running of the trial (including monitors, study staff and investigators) is "blinded" as to the arm to which any individual subject has been assigned. Typically, significant procedures are put into place for single-blind studies to avoid investigators introducing bias into the trial.

There are numerous varieties of study designs that may be utilized in treatment studies. For example, some treatment studies have subjects cross-over between treatment and placebo or cluster treatment and placebo groups. Also, adaptive clinical study designs are beginning to gain acceptance. Additional information can be found on acceptable trial designs in the FDA guidance documents included at the end of this chapter.

Observational Studies
Observational studies typically are conducted to observe and report on a group of people, usually through office visits or surveys, for epidemiological purposes. When study subjects are observed over a period of time, the study is said to be "following" them. For example, investigators may choose to follow a group of people with particular characteristics (such as smokers) and follow another group of people with contrasting characteristics (non-smokers, in this case). In contrast to an interventional study, an observational study is not intended for the intervention or treatment of patients (e.g., by encouraging them to stop smoking), but rather is used to simply study both groups over time to see if any significant difference in a particular health outcome (such as lung disease) can be measured. These types of studies are not used very frequently for initial regulatory applications or for medical device trials, but may be required as postmarket studies for some products. For example, a manufacturer may be required to study patients who are given an approved drug to determine if their overall risk of suffering an adverse event or unrelated condition is higher or lower than patients who were not given the drug.

Accuracy Studies
For some types of medical devices, trials may be designed to compare the performance of the investigational device with the performance of either a predicate device (one previously cleared/approved by FDA) or a reference method that is considered to be a gold standard. The goal of such a study is not to demonstrate the superiority of the investigational method, but to show concordance (agreement) between the investigational method and the reference method or predicate device. Such studies are typically performed in support of a traditional 510(k) application, where the standard for clearance is demonstration of "substantial equivalence" to an existing cleared product (a predicate device). In general, the cost and complication of conducting an accuracy study is significantly lower than that of conducting either an interventional or an observational study.

Accuracy studies frequently are required for in vitro diagnostic products because many innovations in IVDs consist of developing new techniques for detecting or measuring known analytes. A company that develops a new method for detecting a known analyte (such as glucose) may opt to establish new performance claims for its method by conducting an intervention study and filing a PMA or may choose to take the (generally) easier path to market by demonstrating equivalence with a predicate and filing a 510(k). In cases where the developer chooses the 510(k) pathway, it generally is required to perform an accuracy study to substantiate its claim of equivalence to the predicate or reference method.

An accuracy trial must be performed with appropriate GCPs in place, including protocols, informed consent forms, IRB approval and site monitoring. Typically, these studies are much shorter than interventional or observational studies. There usually are very few adverse events to track since subject involvement is frequently limited to providing a specimen for analysis.

Accuracy trials often are considered non-significant risk trials and may be able to proceed without filing an IDE with FDA. The IRB acts as the IDE in these cases (see the previous section on FDA for more information on IDEs). However, if specimen acquisition requires any invasive measures that normally would not be a part of the course of treatment for the patient (e.g., a liver biopsy), the study may be categorized as significant risk and would require IDE approval from FDA.

Research Subjects, Study Inclusion and Exclusion Criteria and Study Protocol
The mechanisms for selecting or screening research subjects for participation in clinical trials should be defined in the study protocol. The inclusion/exclusion criteria set in the protocol must define the parameters used for selecting the clinical study participants. In addition, the IRB ensures that these criteria: do not discriminate against any subgroups of the general population and include all categories of patients who can benefit from the experimental product in the study; and adequately protect vulnerable subgroups of the population such as pregnant women, children, mentally compromised individuals and institutionalized patients.

The discussion of inclusion/exclusion criteria is key in developing a study protocol for both scientific and regulatory reasons. To conduct scientifically sound research, the investigator must select patients who are most likely to benefit from a drug even in a research setting. From the regulatory and marketing viewpoints, the inclusion/exclusion criteria must fully define the population of subjects intended to use the investigational device after FDA approval. A new drug or device may be marketed only to the patient population for which it is proven safe and effective.

Recently, FDA has expressed concern about clinical trial designs that prospectively exclude subjects based on specific genetic markers. Although there may be more predictable efficacy in a marker-positive patient population, prospective exclusion raises concern because it is common to also observe a drug's effect in the marker-negative population. FDA is becoming increasingly concerned that trials, particularly in the oncology field, define the population for the clinical trial too narrowly (via genetic markers or other criteria). This may meet short-term commercial goals but could have the long-term effect of leaving too many patients without treatment options.

Informed Consent Form (ICF)

The ICF is one of the required key documents to be included in the study protocol. The ICF is the primary means by which the investigator communicates with the person who will decide whether to participate in the study. The required elements for informed consent are contained in 45 CFR Part 46. The study sponsor must ensure that investigators obtain and document informed consent from each subject according to 21 CFR 50, Protection of Human Subjects, and local authorities (for studies outside the US), unless this documentation is waived by an IRB in accordance with 21 CFR 56.109(c).

The ICF should explain, in lay terms, the study's purpose, the nature of the testing that will be done, any potential side effects, alternative treatment options and financial aspects of participating in the clinical study. The IRB is responsible for determining whether the ICF provides sufficient information for the potential study participant to make a decision on whether to participate in the study.

ICFs may vary between study sites based on specific IRB requirements that are beyond the scope of those of FDA. All changes to the ICF must be reviewed and approved by the IRB in the same way as changes to the study protocol.

In some cases, a waiver of the consent is requested. The request is submitted to the IRB simultaneously with submission of the study protocol. Research activities involving the collection or study of existing publicly available data, documents, records, pathological specimens or diagnostic specimens may be exempt from the consent requirements. The same is true if information is recorded by investigator in a manner that prevents subjects from being identified, directly or through identifiers linked to them. In some cases, where the investigational product is of low risk and consent is the only document that connects the patient's personal information to the study data, the waiver of subject consent also may be granted.

Summary

GCPs not only ensure protection of privacy and well-being of persons participating in a clinical investigation, they also establish the guidelines for the proper conduct of the clinical investigation, based on established ethical norms, and define roles and responsibilities of study participants. GCP regulations increase the integrity of research, diminish financial bias and help to ensure unbiased study results.

Clinical trial regulatory guidance documents cover many different areas. This chapter focused on a basic representation of the major areas involved in clinical investigations for both drug therapies and medical devices. Due to the complexity of regulatory requirements, this chapter provides a broad overview of the requirements that pertain to both industries.

References
1. Clinicaltrials.gov. A service of the US National Institutes of Health, "Learn about Clinical Studies." ClinicalTrials.gov website. www.clinicaltrials.gov/ct2/about-studies/learn#WhatIs. Accessed 10 April 2013.
2. *The Nuremberg Code*. DHHS website. www.hhs.gov/ohrp/archive/nurcode.html. Accessed 10 April 2013.
3. World Medical Association. WMA Declaration of Helsinki—Ethical Principles for Medical Research Involving Human Subjects. WMA website. www.wma.net/en/30publications/10policies/b3/index.html. Accessed 10 April 2013.
4. FDA. Title 21—Food and Drug Administration, Department of Health and Human Services, Subchapter A – General, Part 56: Institutional Review Boards. FDA website. www.accessdata.fda.gov/scripts/cdrh/cfdocs/cfcfr/CFRSearch.cfm?CFRPart=56. Accessed 10 April 2013.
5. *The Belmont Report, Office of the Secretary, Ethical Principles and Guidelines for the Protection of Human Subjects of Research.* The National Commission for the Protection of Human Subjects of Biomedical and Behavioral Research. 18 April 1970. OHRP website. www.hhs.gov/ohrp/humansubjects/guidance/belmont.html. Accessed 10 April 2013.

Recommended Reading
- FDA and Clinical Drug Trials: A Short History: FDA website. www.fda.gov/AboutFDA/WhatWeDo/History/Overviews/ucm304485.htm. Accessed 10 April 2013.
- Drug Study Designs—Information Sheet: Guidance for Institutional Review Boards and Clinical Investigators. FDA website. www.fda.gov/RegulatoryInformation/Guidances/ucm126501.htm.
- Office for Human Research Protections (OHRP) Policy & Guidance Library: OHRP website. www.hhs.gov/ohrp/policy/.
- *The Belmont Report, Office of the Secretary, Ethical Principles and Guidelines for the Protection of Human Subjects of Research.* OHRP website. www.hhs.gov/ohrp/humansubjects/guidance/belmont.html.
- FDA Good Clinical Practice Guidance. FDA website. www.fda.gov/AboutFDA/CentersOffices/OfficeofMedicalProductsandTobacco/CDER/ucm090259.htm.
- 21 CFR 50.54, Process for Handling Referrals to FDA under, Guidance for Clinical Investigators, Institutional Review Boards and Sponsors. FDA website. www.accessdata.fda.gov/scripts/cdrh/cfdocs/cfcfr/CFRSearch.cfm?fr=50.54.
- *Guidance for Clinical Trials Sponsors: Establishment and Operation of Clinical Trials Data Monitoring Committees.* FDA website. www.fda.gov/downloads/Regulatoryinformation/Guidances/ucm127073.pdf.

Chapter 9

- *Guidance for Sponsors, Clinical Investigators, and IRBs: Data Retention When Subjects Withdraw from FDA-Regulated Clinical Trials*. FDA website. www.fda.gov/downloads/RegulatoryInformation/Guidances/ucm126489.pdf.
- *Structure and Content of Clinical Study Reports E3*. ICH website. www.ich.org/fileadmin/Public_Web_Site/ICH_Products/Guidelines/Efficacy/E3/E3_Guideline.pdf.
- Ethnic factors in the Acceptability of Foreign Clinical Data E5(R1). ICH website. www.ich.org/fileadmin/Public_Web_Site/ICH_Products/Guidelines/Efficacy/E5_R1/Step4/E5_R1__Guideline.pdf.
- Guideline for Good Clinical Practice E6(R1). ICH website. www.ich.org/fileadmin/Public_Web_Site/ICH_Products/Guidelines/Efficacy/E6_R1/Step4/E6_R1__Guideline.pdf.
- Institutional Review Boards Frequently Asked Questions—Information Sheet . FDA website. www.fda.gov/RegulatoryInformation/Guidances/ucm126420.htm. Accessed 10 April 2013.
- Guidance for Industry: Investigator Responsibilities—Protecting the Rights, Safety, and Welfare of Study Subjects. FDA website. www.fda.gov/downloads/Drugs/GuidanceComplianceRegulatoryInformation/Guidances/UCM187772.pdf. .
- FDA. *Statistical Guidance on Reporting Results from Studies Evaluating Diagnostic Tests* (13 March 2007). FDA website. www.fda.gov/MedicalDevices/DeviceRegulationandGuidance/GuidanceDocuments/ucm071148.htm.. NIAID Protocol Template Extramural Guidance, Version 2.0 (Extra), 16 July, 2008.
- Health and Human Services (HHS) Regulations on research with human beings (45 CFR 46 Subparts A, B, C, and D). OHRP website. www.hhs.gov/ohrp/humansubjects/guidance/45cfr46.html.
- Privacy rule (45 CFR Parts 160 and 164 of the *HIPAA*). DHHS website.

Chapter 10

Current Good Manufacturing Practice and Quality System Design

Updated by Laurence M. Wallman, RAC (US, EU, CAN)

OBJECTIVES

❑ Understand basic Current Good Manufacturing Practice (GMP) requirements and provide compliance recommendations

❑ Understand basic quality system concepts and quality system regulations

❑ Gain an overview of the most significant GMP regulations and guidance documents that affect drug and device development and manufacturing

❑ Understand the differences and similarities between pharmaceutical and medical device quality systems

❑ Describe concepts of clean design and importance of process validation

❑ Outline basic elements of sanitary equipment design for key manufacturing components

❑ Discuss aspects of effective cleaning and sanitization programs

❑ Provide required elements of an effective corrective and preventive action (CAPA) system

❑ Understand basic concepts regarding cross-contamination risk within the manufacturing environment

LAWS, REGULATIONS AND GUIDELINES COVERED IN THIS CHAPTER

❑ 21 CFR 210 Current Good Manufacturing Practice in Manufacturing, Processing, Packaging, or Holding of Drugs; General

❑ 21 CFR 211 Current Good Manufacturing Practice for Finished Pharmaceuticals

❑ 21 CFR 600 Biological Products: General

❑ 21 CFR 820 Quality System Regulation

❑ 21 CFR Part 4, Subpart A Current Good Manufacturing Practice Requirements for Combination Products

❑ *Compliance Program Guidance Manual 7356.002, Drug Manufacturing Inspections* (2002)

❑ *Compliance Program Guidance Manual 7382.845 Inspection of Medical Device Manufacturers* (2011)

❑ *Guide to Inspections of Pharmaceutical Quality Control Laboratories* (July 1993)

❑ *Guidance for Industry: Quality Systems Approach to Pharmaceutical Current Good Manufacturing Practice Regulations* (September 2006)

- Guide to Inspections of Sterile Drug Substance Manufacturers (July 1994)
- Guide to Inspections of Dosage Form Drug Manufacturers (October 1993)
- Guide to Inspections of Medical Device Manufacturers (December 1997)
- Quality System Inspection Technique – QSIT (August 1999)
- CDER 2007 Update Compliance Oversight
- Pharmaceutical cGMPs for the 21st Century – A Risk-based Approach, Final Report (September 2004)
- ONDC's New Risk-Based Pharmaceutical Quality Assessment System (July 2005)
- Guidance for Industry: Investigating Out-of-Specification Test Results for Pharmaceutical Production (October 2006)
- Draft Guidance for Industry: Manufacturing, Processing, or Holding Active Pharmaceutical Ingredients (March 1998)
- Guidance for Industry: Part 11, Electronic Records; Electronic Signatures—Scope and Application (August 2003)
- Guidance for Industry: PAT—A Framework for Innovative Pharmaceutical Development, Manufacturing, and Quality Assurance (September 2004)
- Guidance for Industry: Process Validation: General Principles and Practices (January 2011)
- Guidance for Industry: Q8(R2) Pharmaceutical Development (November 2009)
- Guidance for Industry: Q9 Quality Risk Management (June 2006)
- Guidance for Industry: Q10 Pharmaceutical Quality System (April 2009)
- Guidance for Industry: Q11 Development and Manufacture of Drug Substances (November 2012)
- Guidance for Industry: Sterile Drug Products Produced by Aseptic Processing—Current Good Manufacturing Practice (September 2004)
- Guidance for Industry: Q7A Good Manufacturing Practice Guidance for Active Pharmaceutical Ingredients (August 2001)
- Guidance for Industry: Current Good Manufacturing Practice for Phase 1 Investigational Drugs (July 2008)
- Guidance for Industry: Formal Dispute Resolution: Scientific and Technical Issues Related to Pharmaceutical CGMP (January 2006)
- Questions and Answers on Current Good Manufacturing Practice (CGMP) for Drugs (Updated 2012)
- Pharmaceutical cGMPs for the 21st Century—A Risk-Based Approach (September 2004)
- Human Factors Implications of the New GMP Rule Overall Requirements of the New Quality System Regulation (July 2008)
- Draft Guidance for Industry: Powder Blends and Finished Dosage Units—Stratified In-Process Dosage Unit Sampling and Assessment (October 2003)
- Guidance for Industry: Guideline for the Monitoring of Clinical Investigations (January 1998)
- Expiration Dating of Unit-Dose Repackaged Drugs: Compliance Policy Guide (May 2005)
- Guidance for Industry: Computerized Systems Used in Clinical Trials (May 2007)
- Draft Guidance for Industry: Analytical Procedures and Methods Validation—Chemistry, Manufacturing, and Controls Documentation (August 2000)

Introduction

The regulations set forth in Title 21 of the Code of Federal Regulations (CFR) Parts 210 and 211 contain the minimum current Good Manufacturing Practices (CGMPs) for methods to be used in, and the facilities or controls to be used for, the manufacture, processing, packing or holding of a drug to assure that such drug meets the requirements of the act as to safety, and has the identity and strength and meets the quality and purity characteristics that it purports or is represented to possess. These GMP regulations in the CFR were substantially revised in 1978 but are essentially unchanged since then.

From the US Food and Drug Administration's (FDA) perspective, the CGMP requirements were established to be flexible enough to allow each manufacturer to decide individually how to best implement the necessary controls by using scientifically sound design, processing methods and testing procedures. The flexibility in these regulations allows companies to use modern technologies and innovative approaches to achieve higher quality through continual improvement. Accordingly, the "C" in CGMP stands for "current," requiring companies to use technologies and systems that are up-to-date to comply with the regulations.

The philosophy in GMP regulations and in the principles of modern quality systems applicable for both drugs and medical devices is: "Quality should be built into the product, and testing alone cannot be relied on to ensure product quality." This fundamental concept speaks to the basic intent of the drug and medical device GMP regulations and guidances, which is to provide a flexible framework for making a product that is "fit for its purpose."

CGMP principles can be summarized as:
- Build quality in—you cannot test or inspect quality in to a product.
- Put controls in place at each step of the process to increase the likelihood the product is safe and fit for its intended use.
- Protect the product from contamination and cross-contamination and prevent mix-ups.
- Know what you are doing in advance and document what really happened.
- Work toward consistency and control and monitor your systems.
- Have an independent quality group making decisions.

Testing to show that a product meets specifications is part of GMP, but GMP involves much more than just testing. GMP takes the approach of regulating the manufacturing and laboratory testing environment itself. An extremely important part of GMP is the documentation of every aspect of the process, activities and operations involved in the manufacture of drugs and medical devices. Additionally, GMP requires all manufacturing and testing equipment to be qualified as suitable for use, and all operational methodologies and procedures utilized in the manufacturing process to be validated to demonstrate that they perform as intended.

Basic CGMP requirements applicable to both pharmaceuticals and medical devices can be expressed as:

- quality system—change control, validation, corrective and preventive action (CAPA)
- qualified and trained personnel
- building and facilities are adequate and fit for use
- equipment is suitable, clean, maintained and calibrated
- materials controls are in place to prevent degradation or contamination
- production and (in-)process controls performance monitoring, deviations
- packaging and labeling—identification, protection
- laboratory controls—specifications, sampling, testing

GMP is global and is influenced by international bodies, such as the International Conference on Harmonisation (ICH), International Organization for Standardization (ISO) and mutual recognition agreements between countries. In 2003, FDA created a CGMP Harmonization Analysis working group to analyze internal and external CGMP requirements, including those related to quality systems. Based on the working group's analysis, the agency decided to take an incremental approach to modifying 21 CFR 210 and 211 while pursuing international harmonization. The goals of the revision will be to encourage timely detection of and response to emerging defects; to provide further clarity and modernize the regulations; and to harmonize various aspects of 21 CFR 210 and 211 with international agency regulations.

GMP requirements for nonbiological drug products can be found in Section 501(a)(2)(b) of the *Food, Drug, and Cosmetic Act (FD&C Act)*. The GMP regulations are in place to ensure that drugs are safe and meet quality and purity requirements. It is important to note that the drug GMP regulation, 21 CFR 211, specifically applies to "finished pharmaceuticals." This includes clinical supply dosage forms (including placebos) and commercially marketed final dosage forms. Active pharmaceutical ingredients (APIs) are subject to the general GMP legal concepts. *Guidance for Industry Q7A Good Manufacturing Practice Guidance for Active Pharmaceutical Ingredients* (www.fda.gov/downloads/RegulatoryInformation/Guidances/ucm129098.pdf) describes FDA's current requirements for drug substances.

GMP requirements for biological drug products are defined in 21 CFR Parts 210 and 211, and the biologics regulations, 21 CFR Parts 600–680. Establishments must comply with their Biologics License Application (BLA) commitments and applicable standards, in addition to GMP.

FDA has a number of implementation tools for use by investigators to monitor and inspect CGMP compliance within industry that also can serve as aids to industry to better understand FDA's current thinking and approaches to GMP compliance. As noted previously, guidance documents are one such tool but others include Compliance

Policy Guides and Compliance Program Guidance Manuals (CPGM), which provide detailed guidance and instructions to FDA staff in performing GMP inspections of both pharmaceutical and medical device manufacturers. These documents contain questions and topic areas on which FDA investigators might focus and are not only useful in preparing for inspections, but also serve to augment a company's internal audit program. FDA Guides to Inspection represent FDA's position on a given topic and serve as aids to investigators and, though they do not impose mandatory requirements, they offer guidance and help investigators to determine acceptable approaches to meet CGMP requirements. These guides are written in some detail and are specific to a topic, e.g., cleaning validation, microbiological and quality control (QC) laboratories, water systems, sterile bulk drug substances.

More information on the drug CGMP regulations is available at www.fda.gov/Drugs/DevelopmentApprovalProcess/Manufacturing/ucm090016.htm.

A generic drug is identical or "bioequivalent" to a brand-name drug in dosage form, safety, strength, route of administration, quality, performance characteristics and intended use. Patent laws prohibit competition with the innovator product for a period of time. Through analytical testing, the chemical composition of the generic is determined to be the same as the branded product. Because many of the research goals of *in vivo* testing were completed previously during innovator product development (i.e., safety, therapeutic effectiveness, effective dose, etc.), the generic drug company is only required to verify "bioequivalence." Bioequivalence is often established through smaller scale clinical research studies than those required initially for innovator drug products. Patient samples and the subsequent pharmacokinetic (PK) assessments are used to verify equivalence to the branded product. Consequently, generic drugs are chemically identical to their branded counterparts, but typically are able to be sold at substantial discounts compared to the branded price as a result of these reduced research and development costs.

The requirements for medical devices are found in *FD&C Act* Section 501(h), and are further referenced in 520(f)(1). The requirements were amended in 1976 by the *Medical Device Amendments*. The device GMP was first promulgated in 1978 and was revised and renamed the Quality System Regulation (QSR) in 1996. Human factors techniques and data should be integral considerations in all medical device design control components. Each manufacturer must establish and maintain procedures to ensure design requirements relating to a device are appropriate and address the device's intended use, including the needs of users and patients. Each manufacturer must establish and maintain procedures for verifying the design input. Design validation must ensure devices conform to defined user needs and intended uses, and must include testing of production units under actual or simulated use conditions. Design validation must include risk analysis and use error.

Combination products are recent advancements that utilize the capabilities of two or more different product types to provide more effective healthcare products. They are defined in 21 CFR 3.2(e) and are composed of two or more regulated products, such as drug-device, device-biologic or biologic-drug products. In the 22 January 2013 *Federal Register*, FDA issued a final rule to be effective 22 July 2013, that codifies an approach for the CGMP requirements for combination products and establishes 21 CFR Part 4, Subpart A. The final rule, working from the 2009 proposed rule, embodies the legal framework that, in FDA's view is: Drugs, devices and biological products do not lose their individual regulatory identities when they become constituent parts of a combination product either as single-entity or co-packaged combination products. In other words, a drug-device combination product is both a drug and a device, and both sets of CGMP requirements (21 CFR 210 and 211 for drugs and 21 CFR 820 for devices) apply to the combination product itself. However, the final rule and the requirements under Part 4, Subpart A recognizes that Parts 210 and 211 and Part 820 are similar in many respects. In this context, for single entity and co-packaged combination products, the rule provides a "streamlined approach" as an alternative to fully implementing and complying with both sets of CGMP requirements. Under this streamlined approach, a manufacturer could choose to operate under and comply with Parts 210 and 211 or Part 820, rather than both, provided that additional specific aspects of the other CGMP framework are also incorporated. For more information, see Chapter 25 Combination Products.

FDA's *Guidance for Industry: Current Good Manufacturing Practice for Phase 1 Investigational Drugs* (July 2008) has replaced the guidance issued in 1991, entitled *Preparation of Investigational New Drug Products* (please note, the 1991 guidance still applies for investigational new drug products for Phase 2 and 3). The 2008 guidance states the requirements for manufacture of Phase 1 clinical materials. The guidance redefines CGMP requirements for Phase 1 clinical trial materials as: well-defined and written procedures; adequately controlled equipment and manufacturing environment; and accurately and consistently recorded data. Manufacturers of Phase 1 investigational drugs should consider carefully how to best ensure the implementation of standards, practices and procedures that conform to CGMP for their specific product and manufacturing operations. At the same time, the applicability of CGMPs defined under 21 CFR 201.2 was amended stating that drug products used in Phase 1 studies—provided the product was not already lawfully marketed or had been used in Phase 2 or 3 studies—were exempt from the requirements of 21 CFR 211.

The *FD&C Act* specifically declares that a drug or device is deemed to be adulterated unless it is manufactured in conformity with "current good manufacturing practice," which indicates GMPs are constantly changing to meet industry standards.

A robust quality system can provide the necessary framework for implementing Quality by Design, continuous improvement and risk management in the drug manufacturing process. The CGMP regulations are harmonized to the extent possible with other widely used quality management systems, including ISO 9000, non-US pharmaceutical quality management requirements and FDA's own QSR.

There are many different, equally acceptable ways to document that a pharmaceutical or medical device has been manufactured in compliance with all FDA regulations and guidances. The underlying principle, whether the documentation system is paper-based or electronic, is that all data must be able to be traced back to the source and verified. The statement that most aptly sums up pharmaceutical and medical device manufacturing compliance is, "If it wasn't documented, it wasn't done."

This chapter provides a brief overview of the regulations involved in ensuring a drug product or medical device complies with CGMPs, and provides some insight on industry-accepted practical interpretation of these regulations.

Device Quality System Regulation

In the device QSR, FDA defines "quality system" as the organizational structure, responsibilities, procedures, processes and resources for implementing quality management. All domestic or foreign manufacturers must have a quality system in place for the design, manufacture, packaging, labeling, storage, installation and servicing of finished medical devices intended for commercial distribution in the US. Compliance with the QSR requirements for a full quality system helps ensure medical devices are safe and effective for their intended use. The QSR is found in 21 CFR 820.

The QSR applies to quality management and organization, device design, buildings, equipment, purchase and handling of components, production and process controls, packaging and labeling control, device evaluation, distribution, installation, complaint handling, servicing and records. The QSR requires various specifications and controls to be established for devices; devices to be designed under a quality system to meet these specifications; devices to be manufactured under a quality system; finished devices to meet these specifications; devices to be correctly installed, checked and serviced; quality data to be analyzed to identify and correct quality problems; and complaints to be processed.

The QSR states specific requirements for such key elements as management responsibility, quality planning, CAPA, design controls and purchasing control. These requirements are not specifically stated in the drug GMPs as such, although certainly the expectation for management responsibility and CAPA in a drug manufacturer inspection would be to have these in place and operating effectively. However, both FDA's 2006 guidance on the quality systems approach to drug CGMPS and ICH's *Pharmaceutical Quality System Q10* guideline describe management responsibility and corrective and preventive action (CAPA) as key elements.

The additional requirements for devices are:
- Each device manufacturer must maintain a design history file, a device master record and a device history record for each device type.
- Every company must have quality plans and quality system records that define its quality practices.
- Device manufacturers are required to establish purchasing controls and institute post-distribution device failure investigations and corrective and preventive actions for defects or recurring technical problems.

Information on the QSR, medical device GMPs and additional medical device quality system information can be accessed at www.fda.gov/MedicalDevices/DeviceRegulationandGuidance/PostmarketRequirements/QualitySystemsRegulations/default.htm.

The QSR does not apply to manufacturers of finished device components or parts.

The CAPA process is a required element specified by 21 CFR 820.100 for medical devices. A firm is required to establish (define, document and implement) CAPA processes, even if they have not experienced a CAPA event. Depending on the organization, the number and complexity of the established procedures may vary. Review of the CAPA system and supporting documentation is a basic component of each regulatory inspection of medical device manufacturers. A CAPA system evaluates data supplied from a variety of internal and external data sources to monitor the quality of products, problems, processes or people. The basic elements of the CAPA process include data analysis, investigation of root cause, identifying actions, verifying or validating effectiveness of action taken and providing processes for documenting the event. Typical outputs of a CAPA investigation require implementation of change, dissemination of information and management review.

The procedure should clearly define the sources of data, how frequently they will be analyzed and the statistical processes utilized. Examples of data sources include rework, employee feedback, returned goods and audit observations. Typical statistical analyses include Pareto charts, trend analysis, run charts, control charts, etc. Some common errors in effective implementation of the CAPA system that lead to inspectional observations are: not considering all data sources in analysis, e.g., forgetting service or complaint calls or product nonconformances; and vague data sources, e.g., the organization is unable to explain to an inspector how data from the source was collected or analyzed. The CAPA

Figure 10-1. Quality System Elements

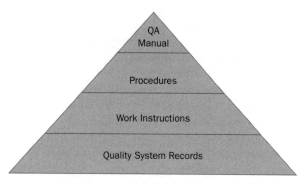

program should be administered by the quality assurance (QA) department rather than the sales team.

Effectively analyzing data is a very important part of ensuring all pharmaceutical systems are operating in a state of control. An annual evaluation of batch trends is required under 21 CFR 211.180(e). However, an annual evaluation is not sufficient to spot potential problem areas early enough to implement a correction. The CAPA system will define frequency of evaluation of data. FDA requires that appropriate statistical methodology be employed where necessary to detect recurring quality problems. The organization should avoid misuse of statistics in an effort to minimize rather than address an identified problem.

The CAPA system offers an avenue for continuous improvement. The following definitions are utilized by FDA to describe corrections and actions:

- "Nonconformity" is non-fulfillment of a specified requirement.
- "(Field) Correction" is repair, rework or adjustment related to the disposition of an existing nonconformity.
- "Corrective Action" is action taken to eliminate the causes of an existing nonconformity, defect or other undesirable situation to prevent recurrence.
- "Preventive Action" is action taken to eliminate the cause of a potential nonconformity, defect or other undesirable situation in order to prevent occurrence.

Approach to a Pharmaceutical Quality System

In August 2002, FDA initiated a new approach to drug product manufacturing and quality regulation. The intent was to harmonize the drug CGMPs with FDA's own medical device QSR and non-US pharmaceutical regulatory systems, taking a science- and risk-based approach that incorporates an integrated pharmaceutical quality system. The new approach was adopted to ensure FDA's regulatory review and inspection polices are up to date scientifically and to encourage adoption of new technological advances.

In addition, as part of this 2002 initiative and to help FDA be more transparent with CGMP policy, FDA developed a question and answer resource on Current Good Manufacturing Practices. This information, which FDA continues to expand and update with new topics and Q&As, provides FDA's thinking on a number of CGMP topics, and is located at www.fda.gov/Drugs/DevelopmentApprovalProcess/Manufacturing/ucm124740.htm.

The 2002 initiative was summarized in the *Guidance for Industry: Quality Systems Approach to Pharmaceutical CGMP Regulations* (September 2006). The guidance is intended to help manufacturers implementing modern quality systems and risk management approaches meet the requirements of the agency's CGMP regulations. The guidance describes a comprehensive quality system model, highlighting the model's consistency with CGMP regulatory requirements for manufacturing human and veterinary drugs, including biological drug products. The guidance also explains how manufacturers implementing such quality systems can fully comply with 21 CFR 210 and 211.

The guidance makes reference to the six-system inspection model described in FDA's Drug Manufacturing Inspection Compliance Program Guidance Manual. The model contains details of six key systems expected to be in place:

1. quality system
2. facilities and equipment system
3. materials system
4. production system
5. packaging and labeling system
6. laboratory control system

In addition, within each system these critical elements would provide the evidence of a robust quality system:

- standard operating procedures (SOPs)
- training
- records and good documentation practice

A structure for Quality System documentation hierarchy is in **Figure 10-1**.

The model FDA describes for use in pharmaceutical manufacturing that is compliant with the CGMP regulations has elements under four major factors: 1) management responsibilities, 2) resources, 3) manufacturing operations and 4) evaluation activities. Within each of these factors, the detailed elements are described to demonstrate how they correlate to specific CGMP requirements under 21 CFR Part 211.

FDA's quality system approach to pharmaceutical GMPs and other quality system standards such as the ISO quality management system guidelines are reflected in the ICH *Pharmaceutical Quality System Q10* guideline. Here again, many similar key elements in Q10 augment the GMPs by describing specific quality system elements and management responsibilities intended to encourage the use of science- and risk-based approaches at each product lifecycle stage. Some of those elements include management responsibility and management review of the quality system, quality risk management and monitoring the improvement of manufacturing processes and product quality. The Q10 model is shown in **Figure 10-2.**

Following this design, FDA employs a six-point inspection model with which industry should become familiar, especially since the eventual preapproval inspection (PAI) of any innovator or generic product being considered for marketing will follow this model. Perhaps just as important as following this six-point inspection model is understanding the philosophy behind it. FDA views the six areas below as related entities, each with a quality component. In other words, the expectation is that quality is built into each area.

The quality unit includes the QC component, which monitors overall compliance with CGMPs and internal procedures and specifications, through its review and approval duties (e.g., change control, reprocessing, batch release, records review, laboratory evaluations, validation protocols, reports, etc.). Also included in the quality unit is the QA component, which provides compliance oversight primarily through conducting auditing functions such as internal system audits, process audits and supplier audits. The QA group would be responsible for product specifications, SOPs, establishment of policy, evaluation of all product defects and returned and salvaged drug products, corrective and preventive action (CAPA) and other trending and metrics evaluations.

For a system to be effective, there should be a distinction between routine QC functions and the oversight responsibilities of the QA group. The terms QA and QC often are used interchangeably; however, they are in fact two distinct functions with equal responsibilities within an effective quality system. The QA department sets the standard, and QC monitors compliance to that standard, e.g., product specification, SOP, etc. Organizations employ a variety of approaches, which can include a combined QA/QC department, or separate dedicated units for QC and QA or building QC responsibilities into the operational functions. The organizational architecture (organizational charts, job descriptions, job specifications, etc.) should clearly delineate the responsibilities of the quality group(s). The structure should establish autonomy between operational departments and quality groups to prevent conflict of interest and/or fear of retaliation or retribution when performing essential functions on either side. Generally, QC functions are more resource dependent and, if not structured properly, will detract from the ability of the organization to effectively implement QA functions.

Investigation of out-of-specification (OOS) results, deviations and failures in both production and the analytical laboratory is a critical GMP compliance element. These investigation outcomes often are reviewed during regulatory inspection. It is important to justify retest work and acceptance of retest values as opposed to original data generated. Unless there is a valid reason to replace the original value, it must be included in the dataset. Without valid reasoning, "testing into compliance" can be inferred and the data (and subsequent decisions made with them, i.e., justification to release) are unable to be defended. Investigation of technical complaints and adverse reactions is mandated in the drug and device GMPs and is critical to assure the final product's safety and efficacy.

Internal and supplier audits for drug products are not required by specific GMPs in 21 CFR 211; however, CGMPs require these activities for compliance. The medical device QSR, 21 CFR 820, requires an internal quality audit, which enables the organization to achieve total quality management. Most companies dread internal audits and put them last on their "to do" list. However, the internal audit process need not be painful or difficult to implement. It is best to start with the 21 CFR 210 and 211 regulations and develop an audit checklist for each area. Once the checklist is complete, it should not change much, which allows for trending over time and demonstration of a state of control within established metrics. The audit process can be conducted periodically in smaller segments so as not to overwhelm the organization. A very simple yet effective audit is a spot check of the production line, i.e., line clearance completion, availability of current product specifications, use of proper personal protective equipment (PPE), equipment approval and availability of cleaning and sanitization records, etc. It is often effective to establish "peer group" audit teams with staff members from other disciplines who can assist in conducting the internal audits. The QA department maintains the lead auditor role. For example, when manufacturing is being audited, the audit team should consist of representatives from disciplines such as QA, formulation and analytical. The formulation and analytical personnel will gain greater insight into the manufacturing process while offering their own unique perspectives. Effective and regular internal audits are a key component of the organization's continuous improvement process.

Facilities and Equipment System

Under a quality system, technical experts are responsible for defining specific facility and equipment requirements. A GMP-compliant facility must be of suitable size to perform the required operations, with temperature and humidity controls, adequate lighting and appropriate sewage and sanitation facilities. Areas within the facility should be designated as "clean" and "dirty" areas. Procedures should be in place to specify personal protection equipment (PPE) (hair nets, beard nets, coats, glasses, etc.) required in each area to prevent contamination of the operations by human interaction. One effective technique is to clearly display signage including pictures in the gowning area showing both PPE being worn properly and being worn improperly by staff to demonstrate the concepts. In facilities that intend to have CGMP and non-CGMP operations, additional care must be taken to clearly designate areas of the facility with a physical separation, equipment and staff for each operation, or ensure effective crossover in instances of resource utilization, optimization and changeover. It is not effective to simply use a paint stripe or tape line to delineate two sections, GMP and non-GMP, on the manufacturing floor. Operating to a single standard—either GMP or non-GMP—eliminates this concern.

Materials of construction should be carefully considered with respect to the intended use. Generally, smooth non-porous surfaces, including floors, walls and ceilings, with coping between floors-walls and walls-ceilings, are preferred in aseptic manufacturing environments.

Direction of air handling equipment and fans should be reviewed to ensure it will not introduce microbiological or particulate contamination into the manufacturing process. In some instances, isolated rooms and dedicated air handling equipment are required. Generally, fans and air diffusers should flow from clean to dirty areas, i.e., in a direction away from product contact surfaces. All bay doors, man doors, etc. should contain screens when open to prevent particulate contamination and flying insects or birds from entering the manufacturing areas. Aisleways around equipment should be designed to reduce air turbulence and exhaust discharge around production lines, especially near product contact surfaces, when removing finished product or resupplying components to the line with motorized equipment.

There must be designated areas for quarantined, released and rejected materials. Clearly visible signage should be used to ensure proper disposition of materials by employees. In modern systems, bar codes or other electronic labeling can facilitate this process. Materials are tracked within the system by the code. When an attempt is made to pull a supply from a lot of material, the supply code is scanned, and if the lot is not available for use, the system will block the action.

Warehouse storage facilities must be temperature-controlled, clean and free from pest infestations; separate areas must be maintained for on-test, off-test and rejected raw materials, components and final products.

Distribution records must be maintained as part of GMP compliance to aid recall activities. Environmental control and alert and action limits must be established, monitored and trended for contaminants (particulate and microbiological). The environment must be controlled and monitored to prevent product cross-contamination and contamination by harmful microorganisms or extraneous matter (filth). Support systems are critical and must be properly constructed, maintained and monitored. Equipment must be qualified, calibrated, clearly labeled, cleaned and maintained to prevent contamination and mix-ups.

Microbiological risk awareness is something that should be considered in every manufacturing environment, regardless of the material being manufactured. Microorganisms, in addition to causing illness in humans and animals, have the potential for other deleterious effects on finished products such as:

- discoloration
- production of malodors
- production of gas that can cause packages to bulge or burst
- breakdown in viscosity or elasticity
- otherwise unable to perform as intended

Microorganisms in the manufacturing environment can prove to be formidable opponents. When introduced into a finished product, the resulting product is considered adulterated according to GMP regulations, and both the product and manufacturer are subject to the applicable restrictions and enforcement actions for adulterated product. Below are a few of the challenges presented by microorganisms:

- Microorganisms have two main modes of introduction into a product—contact or airborne. Therefore, many of the processes implemented in a CGMP environment can directly influence and reduce associated microbiological risk, including sanitization of product contact surfaces, use of PPE, effective housekeeping procedures to reduce dust and sampling programs for raw materials, components, water, etc.
- Microorganisms can develop resistance to product preservative systems and certain sanitizers. Similar to antibiotic resistance, microorganisms can develop resistance over time through exposure within the manufacturing environment to diluted product levels in puddles, rinse water, etc. Once the resistance is developed, a product formulation change is often required to eradicate the microorganisms. One microorganism known to exhibit such resistance was *Pseudomonas cepacia*, later renamed to *Burkholderia cepacia*. This organism alone was responsible for a majority of microbiological FDA recalls and product returns in the 1990s and early 2000s.
- Microorganisms have the ability to reproduce very quickly by binary fission. This simple cellular division means they can quickly overwhelm a product preservative system or production environment. In lower numbers, it may not seem possible, as two cells become four, four become eight, etc.; however, in the log phase of growth and rapid enumeration you could have 100 million cells that become 200 million then 400 million, and can quickly overwhelm a product or process.

Current Good Manufacturing Practice and Quality System Design

Figure 10-2. ICH Q10 Pharmaceutical Quality System Model

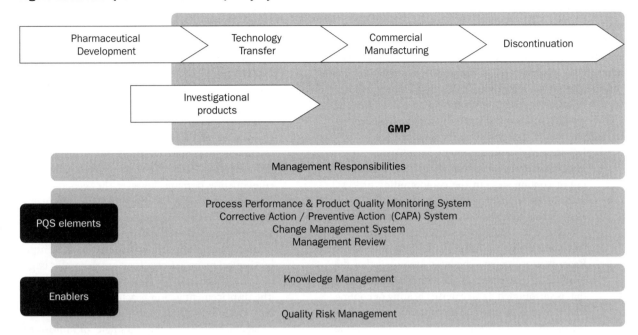

© ICH, November 2010

- Microorganisms are invisible and therefore fall into the "out of sight out of mind" category. No well-intentioned housekeeping staff, compounding or production staff can spot microbiological contamination on a product surface to take action. No line would run with visible filth on contact surfaces, but how do you spot microbiological contamination? A robust GMP program will provide training on microbiological risk awareness and the importance of such items as the use of PPE, keeping tank lids and component hoppers closed, cleaning up spills and puddles, etc. A proactive approach is required to control microorganisms.
- Classic test methods for microorganisms take 48–72 hours for an aerobic plate count and 72–120 hours for a yeast or mold count. Compare this to a routine QC analysis for color, viscosity or pH that could be completed within an hour. Often, the manufacturing and packaging processes are complete by the time results are available. This time-lag significantly increases the risk of product loss if CGMP or sanitary manufacturing practices are not implemented effectively. Rapid identification methods are available that detect the adenosine triphosphate (ATP) present in cells through a chemiluminescent reaction when viewed under ultraviolet light. However, there are limitations with such methods. They have low selectivity for microorganisms relative to biological products, so in instances where natural products are manufactured or natural raw materials are utilized, the ATP in those cells will also give a positive reaction (but this can be used to validate effective cleaning processes). They also do not work well with matrix effects of finished products. In classic microbiological methods, the sample is placed into a dilution fluid that buffers the matrix and neutralizes any preservative system in the product to permit detection of microorganisms. This can be problematic in rapid identification methods. Often, rapid methods are qualitative in nature (presence or absence) as opposed to quantitative, which may further limit applicability in certain applications.

The microorganisms that make up the largest group of human pathogens are the gram negative rods. The term "gram negative" refers to the reaction displayed by the cell wall when viewed under a microscope, during the gram staining process. Within the group of gram negative organisms are two main divisions which include the Enteric (literally "from the gut") and Nonenteric organisms. Typical Enteric species include familiar organisms such as *E. coli* spp., *Salmonella* spp. and *Shigella* spp., and are found in raw foods, including meats and dairy products, as well as human and animal waste. Typical Nonenteric species include the *Pseudomonas* spp. (literally, "false feet") and species such as *Pseudomonas cepacia*, *Pseudomonas aeruginosa*, etc., commonly found in wet environments. The Pseudomonad organisms are non-spore forming, meaning they do not

Regulatory Affairs Professionals Society

form a resting body, and have a thin cell wall that will quickly desiccate in a dry environment. Therefore, they thrive in moist areas within the manufacturing equipment in a typical facility housing water systems, compressed air systems, heat exchangers, pumps, HVAC drain pans, valves, tanks, filling equipment, etc. Initial design, validation and routine preventive maintenance of these systems become critical to lowering overall microbiological risk within the CGMP facility and is an opportunity for the organization to build in quality appropriate to the intended use.

Typical areas of risk in equipment design are:

- Heat exchangers are commonly used for superheating or cooling steps in the compounding process. They often are used for premix applications such as preparing emulsions, opacifiers, waxes, pomades, gelatins, etc. The two most common types are "tube and shell" and "plate frame" heat exchangers. Regardless of the type, the basic premise is that the product stream is circulated within an inner core that is surrounded by an external heating or cooling solution such as glycol. The contamination risk is the potential for a break in the barrier between the cooling fluid and the product.
- Air compressors are commonly used for a variety of applications from manufacturing to maintenance. Many components within the production line—belts, cappers, fillers, label machines, milling machines, sieves/sifts, pumps, etc.—are pneumatically driven by air pressure supplied by the system. Typically, the compressor system design will contain hydrocarbon scrubbers, particulate filters and moisture traps along the system that should be found adjacent to each use point. Additionally, the system will contain a dryer that lowers the system's dew point to eliminate the condensate that forms in the line during the process of condensing the air to create pressure and is worse in pipes that travel through hot and cold areas of the facility. However, should any of the components in the system become clogged or otherwise not function as intended, serious microbiological risk can be introduced. If the system contains condensate water, this will become contaminated with microorganisms that could spray a fine aerosol of bacteria into or over the product at each use point. Compressed air should not be used as a component of the cleaning and sanitization process to dry equipment or parts. In addition to the aerosol risk, spraying the compressed air disturbs dust and other settled debris, including microorganisms, which then settle on the previously cleaned surfaces. Organic solvents such as 70% isopropyl alcohol (IPA) solution are a better option, when able to be used safely, for rapid drying of equipment.
- Pumps are an integral part of the manufacturing process and frequently are used for ancillary support such as water systems, pre-mix operations, cleaning and sanitization processes and, primarily, for circulation and recirculation of product supply, etc. Pumps are of two main types: centrifugal and positive displacement. The design and orientation of the unit, i.e., vertical pump head is nonsanitary vs. horizontal pump head that is sanitary, will impact the degree of clean design. Centrifugal pumps essentially push material to the output by generating centrifugal force. They are often smaller and, consequently, portable; however, they generally have lower flow rates and are infrequently used in manufacturing. The primary designs of centrifugal pumps are radial, mixed and axillary radial flow. Positive displacement pumps move material to the output by displacement action. They are generally larger and, therefore, not portable and more expensive. The displacement action is achieved by two design types: reciprocating via piston-plunger action or diaphragm action, and rotary via single- or multi-rotor action. The type of pump should be selected based on flow rates required, material temperature, pressure requirements, batch size, dispensing accuracy and sanitary design requirements. Replacing pumps within a validated process would require revalidation and approval via the change control system as they are key process components.
- Water systems are major facility components. As indicated, they can pose a significant microbiological risk if not properly maintained. Additionally, they can affect product quality if chemical and physical attributes such as total or dissolved solids, pH, conductivity, etc. are not within specification. Water has two opportunities to negatively affect product attributes as it is often used as a major raw material component and in the cleaning and sanitization process. Frequently, plants establish different grades of water for varying purposes. Water specifications for manufacturing purposes are outlined in the *US Pharmacopeia*. Systems capable of delivering purified water versus sterile water for injection (WFI) would require very different design considerations. The type of treatment system employed would vary depending upon the quality and purity of the local ground water supply. This ranges from raw water to city potable water (generally chlorinated) and well water. Each of these systems will also vary in chemical composition based upon geographic region. A basic first step in system design and planning is to conduct a complete water analysis to determine supply attributes. Based on the results, certain system components can be properly sized and or

excluded as necessary, e.g., a water softener system to remove hardness ions of calcium and magnesium, may or may not be needed. As a design is considered, overall water quality and capacity/flow rate will be key factors. This will determine whether a system to "generate on demand" will be sufficient or if water storage will be necessary, which will require a more complex system design. The system design will determine the most effective methods of cleaning and sanitization such as UV, ozone, thermal, etc. Generally, three main system types are utilized based upon water grade and capacity: vapor compressed distillation, reverse osmosis and resin exchange. In some instances, combination systems are required. Technical experts should be consulted for development of piping diagrams, to ensure pipe angles in turns, Ts, valves, etc. are adequate in relation to system component sizes, e.g., tanks, pipe diameter, pump size, etc.

- Tanks should be of suitable size and materials of construction to sufficiently contain all materials with adequate room for mixing. Design aspects to consider include materials of construction (e.g., polycarbonate, fiber or 316 stainless steel (316 SS)), types of mixers (e.g., internal or external, paddle, side sweeps, etc.), type of outlet and position, thermal requirements and need for jacket, recirculation capabilities, pressure rating, etc. Tanks intended for clean design should be of 316 SS construction, with sterile valves on the inlet and outlet and a conical bottom to permit complete draining. Flat bottom tanks or fiber-bonded, plastic tanks are not appropriate for aseptic applications. Cleaning and sanitization protocols for tanks should be clearly specified. Often large tanks are sanitized via clean-in-place (CIP) through the use of spray balls. This technique should be validated and routine maintenance is required to ensure the ball does not become clogged or does not apply sanitizer to all interior surfaces. In some instances, tanks are entered and cleaned, with the appropriate confined space entry training and safety equipment in place.
- Valves are included throughout the manufacturing environment. In facility design, the type and materials of construction selected should be consistent with intended use. Generally, there are many styles of valves including ball, mixproof, leak protection, diaphragm, check, flush bottom and butterfly. Each is best suited for certain applications. For example, ball valves are essentially a ball bearing with a hole in the middle that rotates. When the valve is in the open position, material is able to flow, and the ball is rotated perpendicular to the product stream to close. In the closed position, material is retained in the ball "dead leg" and is stored for potentially long periods of time. When the valve is opened, the retained material is delivered into the flow, which can potentially contaminate the entire system with microorganisms. Ball valves are best used in unsanitary manufacturing applications or on the exit (discharge to waste) side of tanks, pumps or other equipment. Ball valves, if used, must be sanitized via clean-out-of-place (COP) procedures. The butterfly valve is a sanitary designed valve. This essentially consists of a flat plate that rotates on a pivot point in the center. There is no trapped material on rotation of the plate. This valve type can be sanitized under CIP.
- For design materials of ancillary equipment components, including pipes, clamps, gaskets and O-rings, welds, etc., it is best to "sweat the details" during the design phase. Small differences in these areas can significantly affect the overall clean design of the system, reducing associated microbiological risk, increasing operational effectiveness, reducing down time, leading to longer product life under repeat sanitization, etc. over time. Selection of 316 SS components over plastic, etc. changes the ability of the system to be easily cleaned and sanitized to eliminate harbor points for microorganisms, etc. by reducing porosity of surfaces. Variation in installation techniques will also contribute to a clean design. For example, welds of 316 SS pipe should be orbital welds with complete system passivation prior to system commissioning. Traditional top welding techniques can leave uneven pit marks on the interior of the weld that will be problematic later on.

Effective cleaning and sanitization procedures are essential to batch-to-batch reproducibility within CGMP manufacturing. Processes should be established for all types of equipment design and configurations and include housekeeping standards for each area of the facility. Proper signage should be displayed that shows the location of "clean" and "dirty" parts, equipment and utensils. All staff, including rotations and shifts, who could potentially perform the procedure, must receive adequate training prior to executing a cleaning and sanitization (C&S) event. Often, complete execution of the process may involve multiple functions such as maintenance and sanitization teams when equipment disassembly is required. C&S processes should be fully documented in sufficient detail to permit consistent application of the process, including solution preparation instructions, final strength, contact times, etc.

There are two main approaches to equipment C&S: CIP and COP. Each is specific to the design of the equipment being cleaned and sanitized. CIP refers to C&S procedures that are performed with the equipment fully assembled and in place. This requires draining of product supply from equipment and/or removal of product and visible filth followed by circulation of cleaning and sanitization solutions. This can be effective in equipment of sanitary design that allows for complete removal of all materials without disassembly. When CIP is the primary C&S method, periodic disassembly of equipment sections for visual inspection to verify process effectiveness is suggested. The COP process requires complete disassembly of the equipment for proper cleaning and effective sanitization. Often, the equipment is removed from the production area and taken to a separate designated area for disassembly and C&S. In these cases, longer downtime can be expected, which is another important consideration in the design phase when building quality into the process.

The distinction between cleaning and sanitization should be understood; these terms are often used interchangeably, but they are, in fact, two distinct processes. Cleaning involves removal of all dirt, debris and other organic or inorganic matter from equipment surfaces. The two main methods utilized for cleaning processes are: chemical agents, e.g., detergent solutions; and mechanical action, e.g., brushes or pipe pigging.

Sanitization is the step that removes microorganisms, including bacteria, yeast and molds, viruses, etc., from the equipment surface. The degree to which these are removed may vary from sanitized, which indicates significant reduction in microorganisms (with a baseline level remaining), to sterilized, which indicates complete removal of microorganisms from the surface. The degree of sanitization or sterilization required is dependent upon the intended use of the system. Generally, sanitization is completed by a variety of methods that include chemical agents, e.g., ozone, bleach solutions or 70% IPA; or thermal processes, e.g., circulation of hot water or autoclaving—a sterilization process that uses heat and pressure.

Sanitization cannot begin until effective cleaning has been completed. The sanitizer efficiency is significantly reduced or ineffective on a dirty surface. Most chemical sanitizers are oxidizers that are quickly consumed by organic material on the surface. Thermal sanitization efficiency is reduced as residues insulate the surface being sanitized, thereby increasing contact times (beyond those established in validation) and protecting bacteria from the lethal effects. Generally, cleaning and sanitization procedures should be completed using, and solutions prepared from, purified water grade or above. City water should not be used, as it contains dissolved solids, particulates, chlorine and microorganisms that can interfere with or reduce the overall effectiveness of the process.

The concentration/time relationship is critical when developing the procedure and resulting validation protocols. As concentration increases, the required sanitizer contact time with the equipment surface will decrease. This concept can allow efficient procedures to be established that reduce line downtime, thereby increasing productivity and profitability. The appropriate procedure is established based on materials of construction and corrosiveness to equipment, employee safety considerations and procedure effectiveness based on analytical results, etc.

The procedures should be validated in combination with process validations or as standalone procedures. Validation protocols should include verification of both cleaning and sanitization aspects of the process. The protocol should verify: removal of all residues of prior product, removal of C&S agents from the equipment surfaces in final rinse, exact sanitizer concentrations and contact times with allowable variance, and flow rates and speeds for pumps and valves within the system. It should also confirm the degree of sanitization or sterilization obtained by microbiological swab or contact samples. Protocols should include an adequate number of process replicates, with equipment and staff variations, to ensure repeatability and reproducibility. An effective sampling design should be established that covers the entire system being sanitized. Thermographic cameras, infrared sensors or maximum registering heat tapes are effective for documenting maximum temperatures achieved across a system when conducting thermal validation protocols.

Preparations of chemical sanitizers should be verified by analytical testing during validation. This would include initial concentration, as well as concentration over the duration of the contact time within the equipment during the sanitization cycle. If sanitizers are intended to be stored, validation should include stability data to determine appropriate storage times. Alternatively, procedures should require chemical sanitizers to be made fresh at the point of use.

Materials System

The material system involves measurement and activities to control finished products, components, containers and closures. It includes validation of computerized inventory control processes, drug storage, distribution controls and records. There must be written procedures for the receipt, storage, testing and approval or disapproval of raw materials, components, product and containers and closures.

Production System

In a modern quality system manufacturing environment, significant product characteristics should be defined from design to delivery and control should be exercised over all changes. In addition, quality and manufacturing processes and procedures—and changes to them—must be defined, approved and controlled. It is important to establish responsibility for designing and changing products. Documenting processes, associated controls and changes to these processes helps ensure that sources of variability are identified.

Batch numbering is a key to maintaining proper traceability. Each lot or batch number must be unique and represent the lot's complete history. Batch and equipment use records must show the ingredients, equipment, containers and labeling used and the personnel involved with batch production. Raw materials must be controlled and traceable to products in which they are used. Documentation should support a full "trace back" investigation in case a batch record needs to be completely investigated to determine the root cause of a nonconformance of a product quality attribute (microbiological, chemical or physical).

Verification steps and sign-off are required for critical process steps. All batch-related documents must undergo final review and quality unit approval before products are released.

Packaging and Labeling System

FDA recommends that, as part of the design process and before commercial production, the controls for all processes within the packaging and labeling system be planned and documented with written procedures. Distinct labels with discriminating features for different products, such as a product marketed with different strengths, should be included in the procedure to prevent mislabeling, which could result in product recalls. Approval processes for label format and text should be in place with provisions for variations such as translation and back translation as required for the generation of multilingual labels.

Distribution of approved labels to the manufacturing unit should be controlled, and access to approved labels restricted. A basic process control to have in place in a CGMP environment is a label reconciliation process. Labels should be released to the production line in the exact number required for the run. Labels damaged or destroyed during the run should be accounted for. At the conclusion of the run, a reconciliation is performed between labels issued, applied and returned (including those damaged) to ensure 100% accountability for the quantity issued. A line clearance checklist should include removal of all labels, cartons, neck hangers and other packaging, etc. from a run prior to initiating the next run.

Laboratory Control System

Laboratory controls, including analytical methods validation and laboratory equipment qualification, must be in place. Scientifically sound stability programs must be implemented for each product to support labeled expiration dating.

Important components of effective laboratory control are an adequately designed sampling program and well-trained staff members to collect the samples. Appropriate statistical models should be considered to determine the best sample scheme for a given situation. Traditionally, a $\sqrt{N}+1$ model is used and applies in most situations. In a post-validated system operating in a state of control, a reduced sampling plan could be established that reduces time and cost and improves overall operational efficiency.

Proper training of staff members (generally within the QC unit) who are collecting samples, is critical to ensure the sample is in fact representative of the entire lot. A sample that misrepresents the batch, water system condition, etc., can lead to costly or inaccurate decisions being made regarding the final disposition of the material, e.g., rework, scrap, initiate a C&S and/or line downtime. Staff members collecting microbiological samples require additional training, PPE, sterile sample collection tools and containers, etc., to both ensure aseptic sample collection and protect the bulk material being sampled from contamination during the sampling process.

Procedures should be in place to describe the conditions under which a resample will be collected and/or a retest result is generated or accepted. Unless a valid reason can be identified that would permit resampling or retesting, these should not occur. All data generated must be provided for review, and a written procedure should provide criteria for excluding a result as an "outlier" from a dataset. Failure to consider all data or an ineffective OOS/out-of-limits investigation process that determines the an incorrect root cause of the nonconformance can generate misleading data or the perception of the data "testing into compliance."

Critcal Elements of Subsystems

Standard Operating Procedures (SOPs)

SOPs describe how a company complies with the drug or device regulations and are critical to GMP compliance. They help ensure a consistent operation that reduces variation in finished products and help to ensure compliant practices by all employees. They are also communication tools that can be used for training purposes or to demonstrate to an auditor or inspector the process being performed. Effective SOPs are a great management tool and help build accountability across the organization. Typically, a regulatory inspection will involve an independent review of the organization's SOPs, followed by a series of interviews with key staff members, and then a review of supporting production records and documentation to verify knowledge and compliance to the SOPs reviewed.

There should be a process that clearly defines administration of the SOP infrastructure, typically referred to as the "SOP on SOPs." The procedure will define frequency of review; version control; training requirements; document format and required sections; process for updates and change control; retirement and archive of prior versions; process for management review and approval, etc. The SOP program is traditionally administered by the QA department; however, to be most effective, the content and processes described by each SOP should be developed by the operational groups responsible for performing the procedure. Each SOP should describe a process "actually," not theoretically, as it is being performed within the facility. Documents that simply repeat regulatory requirements but do not reflect the organization's actual practice tend to be difficult to implement, are more open to interpretation by the user, have reduced effectiveness, and are inadequate to demonstrate compliance with supporting documentation.

In addition to an effective system for SOP management, each organization should have a process for managing all other controlled documents, i.e., technical specifications, policies, forms, templates, test methods, etc. Anyone should be able to pick up any document, including a batch record, etc., and learn its version, when it was revised and why.

Each CGMP program requires a robust change control system. Change control exists to prevent unintended consequences to product quality. A proper change control program incorporates systems (document sign-offs) and a committee that oversees all changes likely to affect product quality. All changes are carefully documented in a systematic manner and documentation is stored where it is easily accessible and available for review. Changes could include those to: documentation, i.e., SOPs, technical specifications or test methods; equipment, such as pumps; testing equipment; supplier vendors; a process such as mix time or speed; or to product design or packaging. Each change, if not controlled, has the potential to negatively affect the final product. All changes should be properly evaluated and approved prior to implementation. Unauthorized changes must be strictly prohibited in the CGMP environment.

Training

Each person engaged in the manufacture, processing, packaging or holding of a drug product shall have the appropriate experience, education and training, or a combination thereof, to enable that person to perform the assigned functions. Training could be documented via curriculum vitae, degrees or licenses or internal or external training certificates. Training should encompass general requirements such as SOPs or policies, regulatory training and project-specific aspects as applicable, i.e., on the exact instrument or test method, product compounding specification or production line to which the employee is assigned. Employee GMP training by qualified individuals is required on a continuing basis and with sufficient frequency, as defined by the organization, to ensure employees remain familiar with CGMP requirements applicable to their jobs.

All training must be sufficiently documented to include the topic presented or abstract, name of presenter, date(s) conducted and list of attendees in a format (electronic or print) that is able to be easily retrieved upon request. Training should be adequate to cover any variations in normal routine operations that may have been included in the process validation, e.g., multiple shifts; temporary, part-time or contract workers; variations in equipment components or configurations (changes in pumps or filling equipment); or changes to product supply (tank versus tote, etc.) as applicable.

Records

All GMP activities must be documented in detail. This also includes ancillary support documents such as training records, SOP history files, equipment calibration and maintenance records, cleaning and sanitization logs, etc. All control records—including production, labeling and packaging records—associated with a batch of a drug product are to be retained for at least one year after the batch expiration date or, for certain OTC products exempt from expiration dating, for three years after batch distribution, whichever is longer (21 CFR 211.180). Since this time can be variable, firms often establish a standard document retention period such as 15 or 30 years, and some records are retained permanently depending on their nature. Distribution records must show where products were shipped and a process must be in place to facilitate a recall if necessary.

For medical devices, the record retention period specified in 21 CFR 820.180 requires records to be retained for a period of time equivalent to the design and expected life of the device but no less than two years.

Good documentation practices are essential for the creation and maintenance of records that support CGMP activities. Good documentation principles require that GMP records are permanent, clear, timely, complete, verifiable, correct and traceable.

Documents must be properly secured and archived so as to prevent their accidental loss or destruction for the duration of the required retention period, i.e., protected from damage by fire, water, heat, rodent infestations, etc. Design aspects with regard to record storage should be considered within the facility, such as fire retardant cabinets, shelving to prevent storage directly on the floor, protection from excessive heat and direct sunlight, adequate physical security, no overhead water pipes, etc. If an adequate storage location cannot be established or designed within the facility, there are several vendors with facilities specifically designed for storage of paper records and electronic media according to regulatory requirements. When an offsite location is used, the vendor should be qualified by the QA department to verify the facility has the adequate record retention controls in place.

The record retention system employed by the organization, which includes the combination of format and physical location, should permit easy retrieval upon request by an auditor or regulatory inspector. Records may be retained in the original format or as copies of the original by reduction to electronic media such as microfilm, microfiche, electronic tape, CD, etc. If an electronic source is used, a suitable reader of the electronic format must be available for the duration of the retention period. Appropriate written procedures for disaster recovery as well as routine system backup, restore and archive should be in place for all computerized systems.

Verification, Qualification and Validation

Verification, qualification and validation activities are extremely important compliance elements. Both drug and device GMPs require that all operational methodologies and procedures utilized in manufacturing and testing be validated to demonstrate they can function as intended. Validation activities also include aspects related to batch production such as cleaning and sanitization of production equipment, water systems, etc. Validation activities must be conducted in accordance with approved protocols and follow appropriate guidance.

Process validation is essential in ensuring that product quality, safety and effectiveness are designed and built into, rather than tested into the final product. Establishing batch-to-batch output uniformity is an example of process validation. It is important to develop a written validation protocol that establishes a sufficient number of replicate process runs to demonstrate reproducibility and provide an accurate variability measure across successive runs. Worst-case conditions posing the greatest chance of process or product failure compared to ideal conditions should be included. Factors to include could be variation in raw material suppliers, staff variation in multi-shift operations, changes to equipment components, e.g., pumps, product supply, etc. Design control and process verification are critical elements of the device QSR.

One of the cornerstone guidance documents for process validation for human and veterinary drugs and biologics is *Guidance for Industry: Process Validation: General Principles and Practices* (January 2011), which defines process validation in three stages:
- Stage 1—Process Design: The commercial process is defined during this stage based on knowledge gained through development and scale-up activities.
- Stage 2—Process Qualification: During this stage, the process design is confirmed as being capable of reproducible commercial manufacturing.
- Stage 3—Continued Process Verification: Ongoing assurance is gained that the process remains in a state of control during routine production. An ongoing program to collect and analyze product and process data that relate to product quality must be established (21 CFR 211.180(e)). The data collected should be meaningful and be able to reflect true changes in the process that might affect product quality. An example would be in-process test results. In-process tests results should be monitored closely to detect any trends that could indicate the process may not be as controlled as it should be.

This guidance emphasizes an interdisciplinary team approach in which experts from process engineering, industrial pharmacy, analytical chemistry, microbiology, statistics, manufacturing and quality assurance come together to form the team. Approval of senior management is a requirement of a successful validation program.

The team should consider all factors required for the final system or process being validated in the process design stage. A good motto is "Begin with the End in Mind." For example, a system of plastic piping, diaphragm style pumps, ball valves and polycarbonate tanks may be more cost effective initially than a system of stainless steel pipe, positive displacement pumps, butterfly style valves and stainless steel tanks; however, each will perform differently over time and each has a different intended use. Decisions made solely based upon component cost could quickly be offset by increased sanitization times, increased maintenance times and less up time and, worst case scenario, cost of recall, loss of market share, risk to patient safety or consumer health, or loss of brand recognition.

Each method used to analyze a drug or biological product must have associated validation to support the documentation of drug substance and drug or biological product identity, strength, quality, purity and potency. The primary FDA guidance, *Draft Guidance for Industry: Analytical Procedures and Methods Validation—Chemistry, Manufacturing, and Controls Documentation* (August 2000), is intended to assist applicants in assembling information, submitting samples and presenting data to support analytical methodologies.

Analytical methods for generic or innovator drug compounds frequently are found in the *US Pharmacopeia* (*USP*) or in the published literature, and can serve as a starting point for method validation. If the analytical method used is directly from *USP*, only requalification of the method used on site in the particular laboratory is required, not revalidation. Validation of analytical methods typically starts in the formulation/product development stage. The formulation and analytical groups work as a closely knit team since even slight changes in formulation can necessitate changes to the analytical method. Typically, several formulations are developed, tested against pre-set specifications and stability tested. Any formulations that do not meet the stability requirements are either reformulated or eliminated from the formulation development plan. As with all CGMP processes, in a robust system, method requalification and validation should be carefully documented.

Summary

For repeatable manufacturing results that meet specification, the process model in **Figure 10-3** is recommended. The following list is a general outline of GMP concepts that are among the most important. This outline is not intended to be all-inclusive, but provides some critical points.

Chapter 10

Key GMP Concepts Presented

- GMPs are applicable to preparation of innovator and generic drug products and medical devices administered to humans and animals.
- GMPs are required for both marketed products and clinical supplies, including placebos.
- The fundamental GMP concept is that product quality cannot be "tested into" a product, but must be designed and built into the facility and equipment design and production process through well-defined, written procedures; adequately controlled equipment and manufacturing environment; and accurately and consistently recorded data from manufacturing (including testing).
- GMPs are constantly changing. Current Good Manufacturing Practice represents the "customary practice" or "state-of-the-art" practice used by most companies to ensure that drugs and devices are safe and effective.
- Many international factors influence GMP. The most important are ICH guidelines, ISO standards and mutual recognition agreements with other countries.
- *Guidance for Industry: Quality Systems Approach to Pharmaceutical CGMP Regulations* (September 2006) **and** *Guidance for Industry: Q10 Pharmaceutical Quality System* (April 2009) describe a comprehensive pharmaceutical quality system model. The quality system is similar to FDA's medical device QSR system. The core elements of the quality system model for both pharmaceutical and medical devices are management responsibility, quality risk management and the monitoring and evaluation of the effectiveness of the quality system.
- Product quality must be reviewed annually and a product Annual Report must be compiled for pharmaceutical drug products. However, a robust CAPA process to more frequently evaluate product trends and trends from process performance and product quality monitoring is expected for drugs and biologics and required for medical devices, and is generally more effective.
- Change control and document control concepts are not specifically listed in GMP regulations but are critical to GMP compliance.
- Key differences in the codified regulations between device GMPs and drug GMPs are management responsibility, quality plan, corrective and preventive action, design controls and purchasing control, although management responsibility and CAPA are expected when a drug manufacturer is inspected. Design control is a key element of the device quality system.
- The QSR is intended to ensure that finished devices will be safe and effective and in compliance with the

Figure 10-3. Process Model for Meeting GMP Requirements

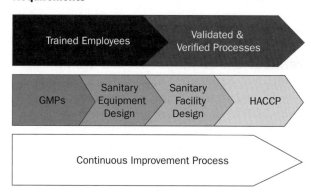

FD&C Act. The regulation does not apply to manufacturers of finished device components or parts.
- GMP compliance is a critical element of new drug and device development and this compliance is verified during FDA's preapproval inspection prior to marketing a new drug or device. Generic drugs (which reduce drug costs to the consumer) are evaluated for "bioequivalence" through testing designed to assess equivalence.
- A focal point of GMP inspections has been the separation of the quality assurance and manufacturing or production functions, while establishing clear responsibilities for decisions affecting the product.
- Validation is an important component of GMP compliance. GMPs require all operational methodologies and procedures utilized in manufacturing and testing to be validated to demonstrate that they can perform their function(s).
- Process validation is the key to ensuring that a product's quality, safety and effectiveness are designed and built into, rather than tested into the final product. Process validation is required by both drug and medical device GMPs. Demonstrating batch-to-batch output uniformity is an example of processes validation.
- Quality risk management is a valuable component of an effective quality system. ICH *Quality Risk Management Q9* (June 2005) provides general guidance on the quality risk management principles that can enable more-effective and consistent risk-based decisions regarding the quality of drug substances and drug products across the product lifecycle. The level of effort, formality and documentation of the quality risk management process should be commensurate with the level of risk and be based upon scientific knowledge.

Chapter 11

Prescription Drug Product Submissions

Updated by Klaus Gottlieb, MD, MS, MBA, RAC, Giuseppe Randazzo, MS and Maria Walsh, RN, MS

OBJECTIVES

❏ Understand the classification of prescription drug products

❏ Provide an overview of the goals and types of applications, as well as FDA's New Drug Application/Biologics License Application review process, content and format (including the Common Technical Document)

❏ Become familiar with presubmission and postapproval activities

❏ Understand the mechanisms to expedite drug development and approval

LAWS, REGULATIONS AND GUIDANCES COVERED IN THIS CHAPTER

❏ *Federal Food, Drug, and Cosmetic Act* of 1938

❏ *Public Health Service Act* of 1944

❏ *Drug Price Competition and Patent Term Restoration Act* of 1984 *(Hatch-Waxman Act)*

❏ *Prescription Drug Marketing Act* of 1987

❏ *Prescription Drug User Fee Act* of 1992

❏ *Federal Advisory Committee Act* of 1972

❏ *Food and Drug Administration Modernization Act (FDAMA)* of 1997

❏ *Food and Drug Administration Amendments Act (FDAAA)* of 2007

❏ *Food and Drug Administration Safety and Innovation Act (FDASIA)* of 2012

❏ 21 CFR 314 Applications for FDA approval to market a new drug

❏ 21 CFR 601 Licensing (biological products)

❏ *Guidance for Industry: Providing Clinical Evidence for Effectiveness for Human Drugs and Biological Products* (May 1998)

❏ *Guidance for Industry on the Disclosure of Materials Provided to Advisory Committees in Connection with Open Advisory Committee Meetings Convened by the Center for Drug Evaluation and Research Beginning on January 1, 2000* (November 1999)

❏ *Guidance for Industry: Reports on the Status of Postmarketing Study Commitments—Implementation of Section 130 of the Food and Drug Administration Modernization Act of 1997* (February 2006)

❏ *Guidance for Industry: Postmarketing Studies and Clinical Trials — Implementation of Section*

- *505(o)(3) of the Federal Food, Drug, and Cosmetic Act (April 2011)*

- *Guidance for Review Staff and Industry: Good Review Management Principles and Practices for PDUFA Products (April 2005)*

- *Guidance for Industry: Fixed Dose Combinations, Co-Packaged Drug Products, and Single-Entity Versions of Previously Approved Antiretrovirals for the Treatment of HIV (October 2006)*

- *Guidance for Industry: Fast Track Drug Development Programs—Designation, Development, and Application Review (January 2006)*

- *Draft Guidance for Industry: Accelerated Approval Products—Submission of Promotional Materials (March 1999)*

- *Guidance for Industry: Formal Meetings with Sponsors and Applicants for PDUFA Products (May 2009)*

- *Draft Guidance for Industry: Applications Covered by Section 505(b)(2) (October 1999)*

- *Manual of Policies and Procedures 6020.3: Review Classification Policy: Priority (P) and Standard (S)*

- *Final Rule for Responding to Drug Applications*

- *Guidance for Industry: Providing Regulatory Submissions in Electronic Format—Human Pharmaceutical Product Applications and Related Submissions Using the eCTD Specifications (October 2005)*

- *Comprehensive Table of Contents Headings and Hierarchy*

- *Guidance for Industry: Providing Regulatory Submissions in Electronic Format—Content of Labeling (April 2005)*

- *Guidance for Industry: Contents for a Complete Submission for the Evaluation of Proprietary Names (February 2010)*

- *Electronic Common Technical Document Specification (ICH)*

- *Guidance for Industry: M4: Organization of the CTD (August 2001)*

- *Draft Guidance for Industry: How to Comply with the Pediatric Research Equity Act (September 2005)*

- *Patient-Reported Outcome Measures: Use in Medical Product Development to Support Labeling Claims (February 2006)*

- *Draft Guidance for Industry: Qualification Process for Drug Development Tools (October 2010)*

- *Draft Guidance for Industry Format and Content of Proposed Risk Evaluation and Mitigation Strategies (REMS), REMS Assessments, and Proposed REMS Modifications (September 2009)*

- *Draft Guidance for Industry and Review Staff: Target Product Profile—A Strategic Development Process Tool (March 2007)*

Introduction

Drugs are regulated under the *Federal Food, Drug, and Cosmetic Act* of 1938 (*FD&C Act*) and its subsequent amendments. The *FD&C Act* also applies to biological products subject to regulation under Section 351 of the *Public Health Service Act* (*PHS Act*).[1] Under the *FD&C Act*, Congress gave the US Food and Drug Administration (FDA) authority and responsibility to oversee public health by regulating and enforcing (among other things):

- human and veterinary drugs and vaccines, blood and other biologics and medical devices intended for human use to ensure they are safe and effective, are manufactured in accordance with specified quality standards and their labeling enables safe use
- food, dietary supplements and cosmetics so they are safe and labeled adequately

Additionally, FDA has other responsibilities, such as protecting the public from electronic product radiation, regulating tobacco products and disseminating science-based information to the public on the products that it regulates.

This chapter provides a broad understanding of FDA's regulations and the regulatory process for obtaining marketing approval for prescription drug products.

A drug is broadly defined as:

- any product (or any component of such product) that is intended for use in the diagnosis, cure, mitigation, treatment or prevention of disease in man
- a product (other than food), or a component of a product, that affects the structure or function of the human body

- a product that is recognized in the *United States Pharmacopoeia* (*USP*), *Homoeopathic Pharmacopoeia of the United States* (*HPUS*) or the *National Formulary* (*NF*) and their supplements

A "new" drug is generally any drug that contains an ingredient, or combination of ingredients, for which the safety and effectiveness under the labeled conditions for use are not previously known. However, a new drug also may be a drug that has a known safety and effectiveness profile under the labeled conditions for use, but has not been in use to a material extent or for a material time under those conditions. Generally, such drugs can be obtained only through a prescription from a healthcare provider. Thus, a prescription drug is any drug that has been approved or licensed for distribution by FDA and requires a healthcare practitioner's authorization before it can be obtained. Prescription drugs are differentiated from over-the-counter (OTC) drugs that may be obtained without a prescription. Prescription drugs are also called Rx-only drugs or "legend" drugs because they bear a legend prohibiting sale without a prescription. Prescription drugs are accompanied by a detailed package insert or prescribing information (PI), which contains specific drug information. The content of the PI is regulated by FDA as it informs both the prescriber and the patient about the drug's intended effects, its mechanism of action (MOA), its side effects, how to take the drug and what to do in case of overdose, and warnings and precautions about using the drug.

Physicians may legally prescribe approved drugs for uses other than those approved by FDA; this is known as off-label use. However, drug companies may not promote or advertise drugs for off-label uses.

The *FD&C Act* prohibits the introduction into interstate commerce of a prescription drug unless the drug's manufacturer has submitted a New Drug Application (NDA) to FDA and obtained agency approval. Likewise, the *PHS Act* prohibits the introduction into interstate commerce of any biologic product unless a biologic license is in effect and each package is plainly and properly marked with specific requirements (e.g., proper name).

The NDA or Biologics License Application (BLA) must contain "substantial evidence" from adequate and well-controlled investigations, including clinical investigations, conducted by qualified experts. These investigations should demonstrate that the drug is safe and effective under conditions for use described in the labeling and that it can be manufactured consistently, in a manner that will preserve its identity, strength, quality and purity.

Manufacturers often strategize how many pivotal (generally Phase 3) clinical trials are needed to provide substantial evidence for a drug's effectiveness. The most widely applied interpretation is that two separate, adequate and well-controlled trials (one investigation confirming the results obtained from a prior/concurrent investigation) are needed to establish effectiveness. However, under certain circumstances, FDA may find data from one well-controlled clinical investigation to be adequate to provide the evidence of effectiveness required to support approval of a new drug, or a new use of the drug.

Aside from effectiveness, the application must provide evidence that the prescription drug is reasonably safe when used under the conditions described in the labeling. Although a new drug's safety is assiduously studied through clinical trials (which often enroll several thousand patients), the reality is that the variables in a clinical trial are specified and controlled, and the results relate only to the populations studied within the trial. Therefore, adverse drug reactions (ADRs) reported to occur less frequently in the trial population become more apparent and sometimes more frequent or severe only after a drug enters the market and is used by millions of people who likely have different demographic profiles than the clinical trial populations. Nevertheless, evidence from clinical trials is critical in identifying ADRs associated with the drug and establishing its benefit:risk profile. The benefit:risk profile evaluates all known data for the drug and attempts to provide answers to such key questions as: does the drug do more good than harm and, if so, how much more good? If the drug has a potential for harm, how probable and how serious is the harm? So, while clinical trials do not tell the whole story of the drug's effects in all populations and all situations, they provide a good indication of the drug's safety that can be extrapolated from the populations studied to larger populations.

To enhance FDA's oversight of drug safety issues, Congress gave the agency new authorities under the *Food and Drug Administration Amendments Act* of 2007 (*FDAAA*). If FDA becomes aware of new safety information about a serious risk associated with a drug's use, the agency can require a manufacturer to implement safety labeling changes, conduct postmarketing studies or clinical trials, or establish Risk Evaluation and Mitigation Strategies (REMS). *FDAAA* also mandated that FDA establish an active, integrated, electronic surveillance system for monitoring the safety of drugs and other medical products continuously and in real-time. FDA is working toward this mandate and in May 2008 launched the FDA Sentinel Initiative to strengthen the agency's ability to track how drugs and other healthcare products perform once they go on the market. While the Sentinel System will be developed and implemented in stages, ultimately it will help monitor healthcare products throughout their entire lifecycle. It will allow FDA to effectively communicate the risks associated with the product to the public, thus better achieving its mission of protecting and promoting public health.

The *Food and Drug Administration Safety and Innovation Act* (*FDASIA*), signed into law in July 2012, includes the reauthorization of the *Prescription Drug User Fee Act*

Table 11-1. Expedited Drug Development

	Accelerated Approval	Fast Track Designation	Priority Review	Breakthrough Designation
Legal Authority	Subpart H (drugs) and Subpart E (biologics) of 21 CFR 314 and 21 CFR 601 of the *FD&C Act*	Section 506 of the *FD&C Act* as added by section 112 of the *Food and Drug Administration Modernization Act* of 1997 (*FDAMA*)	*Prescription Drug User Act* (*PDUFA*) of 1992	Section 506 of the *FD&C Act* as added by section 902 of *Food and Drug Administration Safety and Innovation Act* (*FDASIA*) of 2012
FDA website URL	www.fda.gov/Drugs/DevelopmentApprovalProcess/HowDrugsareDevelopedandApproved/DrugandBiologicApprovalReports/ucm121606	www.fda.gov/downloads/Drugs/GuidanceComplianceRegulatoryInformation/Guidances/UCM079736.pdf	www.fda.gov/downloads/AboutFDA/CentersOffices/CDER/ManualofPoliciesProcedures/ucm082000.pdf	www.fda.gov/RegulatoryInformation/Legislation/FederalFoodDrugandCosmeticActFDCAct/SignificantAmendmentstotheFDCAct/FDASIA/ucm329491.htm
Eligibility	1. Treat serious or life-threatening diseases 2. Provide meaningful therapeutic benefit over existing therapies 3. Surrogate endpoint reasonably likely to predict clinical benefit	1. Intent to treat broad range of serious diseases 2. Potential to fill an unmet medical need	Potential to provide: 1. Safe and effective therapy where no satisfactory alternative therapy exists; or 2. A significant improvement compared to marketed products	1. Treat serious or life-threatening diseases and 2. Early clinical evidence of substantial improvement over existing therapies
Designation	No formal process, however sponsors may request accelerated approval prior to or with NDA/BLA submission	Should be requested by sponsor prior to submission of application. FDA has 60 days to respond	FDA has 60 days to make determination	Should be requested by sponsor prior to submitting application; FDA has 60 days to respond
Clinical Development	Approval granted based on a surrogate endpoint or on an effect on a clinical endpoint other than survival or irreversible morbidity with a post-approval requirement for additional trial(s) to confirm clinical benefit	Earlier and more frequent communication	Not applicable	Abbreviated or condensed development; earlier and more frequent communication; delegation of senior reviewers and cross-disciplinary review team
Review Process	NDA/BLA data submitted in one package; standard 10-month review (12 months if in the "Program")	Option for Rolling NDA/BLA submission. Official review clock begins when last module is submitted	NDA/BLA data submitted in one package; review time shortened to six months (eight months if in the Program)	NDA/BLA data submitted as they are accumulated. Option for Rolling NDA/BLA submission. Official review clock begins when last module is submitted

(*PDUFA V*). While *FDASIA* includes numerous changes that will benefit patients, industry and FDA, a main component affecting the prescription drug review process is the establishment of a new review model referred to as "the Program." This new review model applies to all New Molecular Entity NDAs (NME NDAs) and original BLAs,[2] including applications resubmitted after a refuse-to-file (RTF) action, received from 1 October 2012 through 30 September 2017. Applicants who submit applications in the Program will experience greater transparency, with two meetings to be held during the review process (i.e., the mid-cycle communication and the late-cycle meetings). Additionally, Program applications with a priority review designation have an action goal of eight months, and standard applications have an action goal of 12 months.

Regulatory Responsibility

This chapter covers the review and oversight of small molecule drugs and certain therapeutic biologics regulated by the Center for Drug Evaluation and Research (CDER) that are the subjects of NDAs and BLAs.

On 30 June 2003, the premarket review and oversight of certain therapeutic biologics was transferred from the Center for Biologics Evaluation and Research (CBER)'s Office of Therapeutic Research and Review to CDER's Office of New Drugs (OND). In September 2005, OND was reorganized, and the review of CDER's therapeutic biologics was integrated into OND's review divisions based on indication. As discussed on FDA's website for drugs, while both CDER and CBER have regulatory responsibility for therapeutic biological products, CDER is responsible for monoclonal antibodies for *in vivo* use; cytokines, growth factors, enzymes, immunomodulators and thrombolytics; proteins intended for therapeutic use that are extracted from animals or microorganisms, including recombinant versions of these products (except clotting factors); and other non-vaccine therapeutic immunotherapies. For additional information about therapeutic biological products and each center's regulatory responsibilities, refer to www.fda.gov/Drugs/DevelopmentApprovalProcess/HowDrugsareDevelopedandApproved/ApprovalApplications/TherapeuticBiologicApplications/ucm113522.htm.

Some internal processes utilized by CDER and CBER differ due to historical policies and practices, IT infrastructure and organizational structure. This chapter focuses on the processes followed by CDER.

Regulatory Strategy

Compiling a new marketing application is a highly complex activity that requires much preparation and early and effective communication with FDA. A clear and well-laid-out strategy is essential for navigating the prescription drug submission regulatory process and for ultimately obtaining a timely and smooth FDA approval for the drug product. FDA is, in turn, committed to and responsible for bringing healthcare products, particularly innovative healthcare products, to the market as expeditiously as possible. To achieve this common objective, there are several pathways and tools that should be carefully considered when formulating a regulatory strategy. A sound regulatory strategy should underlie the applicant's drug development program, linking the different activities and drug development phases, assessing the challenges along the way and formulating appropriate risk mitigation activities, all with the ultimate goal of obtaining FDA approval for the desired indications within the desired timeframe. Applicants should develop the regulatory strategy years before the actual application is submitted and as early as Phase 1 of the drug development clinical studies. The strategy is often expanded during Phase 2 or Phase 3 of clinical drug development to a global strategy so approval for the drug may be obtained in the major commercial markets. Throughout the drug development process, applicants are highly encouraged to design trials and collect data to ultimately support planned marketing claims as well as product labeling.

Target Product Profile (TPP)

The Target Product Profile (TPP) was developed in the late 1990s as a joint initiative between FDA and industry to improve sponsor-FDA interactions in the drug development process. Pilots were conducted between 1997 and 2003, and a draft guidance was issued in 2007.[3]

The TPP is a format for a summary of the drug development program described in terms of labeling concepts, i.e., it is organized according to the key sections of the drug's intended labeling. It is prepared by the sponsor, and submission is voluntary.

The TPP links each specific labeling concept to a specific study or other source of data that is intended to support the labeling concept. The TPP is a dynamic summary that will change as knowledge of the drug increases. It is intended to eliminate the need to revisit development issues that have already been discussed with FDA, unless development goals change, and to facilitate final labeling discussions related both to initial approvals and labeling supplements. Moreover, it helps update FDA quickly on revised development goals and facilitates rapid orientation for new personnel. A TPP does not, however, represent a commitment or obligation on the part of either the sponsor or FDA to the drug's development strategy or eventual drug approval.

Drug Development Tools (DDT)

Another critical component of regulatory strategy lies in the use of drug development tools such as animal models, biological markers (biomarkers) and clinical outcomes assessments (COAs) (e.g., patient reported outcome (PRO) measure). A biological marker or biomarker is defined as a characteristic that is objectively measured and evaluated as an indicator of normal biologic processes, pathogenic processes or biological responses to a therapeutic intervention.[4] Thus, a change to a biomarker following treatment with the drug product can predict or identify safety problems related to the drug or reveal a pharmacological activity expected to predict an eventual benefit from treatment. Biomarkers may reduce uncertainty in drug development and evaluation by providing quantitative predictions about drug performance.

While there are several types of COAs, this section will focus on PROs. A PRO is an instrument that captures the outcomes of drug intervention during a clinical trial from the patient's perspective (e.g., change in pain or depression from before the therapy compared over time after therapy). The PRO uses a questionnaire that is self-administered by the patient or through interviews by other parties that report on patient perspectives. The questionnaires measure "characteristics" (or constructs) that should have a sound theoretical basis and be relevant to the patient group in which they are to be used. Questionnaires can be designed to provide data in any disease population and cover a broad aspect of the construct measured, or can be developed specifically to measure those aspects of outcome that are of importance for people with a particular medical condition. In any case, a PRO tool should be thoroughly tested using appropriate methodology and validated in order to justify its use. Results from properly validated PRO instruments can be used to support drug approval and claims in approved medical product labeling. Examples of characteristics that PRO questionnaires can assess include symptoms and other aspects of well-being, functionality (disability) and quality of life (QoL).

In addition to PRO tools, FDA also will consider qualification of other DDTs to support labeling claims, such as clinician rating scales and caregiver rating scales, where a respondent is requested to assign a rating to a concept using a process similar to that used for PROs.

With proper qualification, analytically valid measurements using the DDT can be relied upon to have a specific use and interpretable meaning and can be used broadly in drug development. Once a DDT is qualified for a specific context of use, industry can use the DDT for the qualified purpose during drug development, and reviewers from CDER, and OND's Study Endpoints and Labeling Development Team (SEALD) can be confident in applying the DDT for the qualified use without the need to reconfirm the DDT's utility.

Programs for Expediting Drug Development and Review

FDA currently uses several approaches to expedite the development and review of new drugs: 1) Accelerated Approval; 2) Fast Track Designation; 3) Priority Review; and, since the enactment of *FDASIA*, 4) Breakthrough Therapy Designation. An investigational agent may be eligible for any combination of these programs. For example, approximately 80% of applications that were approved under a Fast Track designation were also Priority Review drugs, and sponsors need to apply for these different programs separately. A novel agent with breakthrough designation is subject to the same drug development and review programs as those agents with Fast Track designation. Priority review will be granted if the breakthrough designation is still in place at the time of NDA or BLA submission. Accelerated Approval will apply if appropriate and all the criteria under 21 CFR 314 Subpart H or Subpart E are met.

As discussed at www.fda.gov under "Expedited Drug Development Pathway" (www.fda.gov/AboutFDA/ReportsManualsForms/Reports/ucm274441.htm), FDA is in the process of developing draft guidance on expedited drug development pathways. **Table 11-1** highlights differences and similarities of the respective programs.[5]

Accelerated Approval

The Accelerated Approval process under Subpart H (drugs, 21 CFR 314) and Subpart E (biologics, 21 CFR 601) was created by FDA in 1992 at the height of the HIV/AIDS crisis. It allows approval of drugs based on surrogate endpoints that are reasonably likely to predict clinical benefit under the following conditions: 1) The disease to be treated must be serious or life-threatening and 2) the treatment must provide meaningful therapeutic benefit over existing treatments. In cancer drug development, a surrogate endpoint could be tumor shrinkage and the clinical benefit increased overall survival.

Approval under these provisions is subject to the requirement that the applicant study the drug further, to verify and describe its clinical benefit, where there is uncertainty as to the relation of the surrogate endpoint to clinical benefit, or of the observed clinical benefit to ultimate outcome.

More than 80 new products have been approved under Accelerated Approval regulations, including 29 drugs to treat cancer, 32 to treat HIV and 20 to treat other conditions, such as pulmonary arterial hypertension, Fabry disease and transfusion-dependent anemia. Two of the 35 NMEs approved in Fiscal 2012 received Accelerated Approval.[6]

Fast Track Designation

Fast Track designation is designed to facilitate the development and expedite the review of drugs to treat serious or life-threatening diseases and that have the potential to address unmet medical needs.[7] Fast Track designation may apply to drugs or biologics intended to treat a broad range of serious diseases, including AIDS, Alzheimer's disease, cancer, epilepsy and diabetes. Addressing an unmet medical need is defined as providing a therapy where none exists or one that may be potentially superior to an existing therapy. Once a drug receives Fast Track designation, FDA offers the sponsor early and frequent communication to facilitate an efficient development program. The frequency of communications ensures that questions and issues are resolved in a timely manner, often leading to earlier drug approval. Fast Track drug sponsors are also eligible for "Rolling Review" of applications, allowing earlier submission and initiation of review. More than a third (12/35) of the 35 NME drugs approved in Fiscal 12 were granted Fast Track designation. Of the 12 drugs that received a Fast Track designation, nine (75%) were approved in the first review cycle. Of the 10 Fast Track designated drugs for which FDA was able to make comparisons to approvals in other countries, 100% were approved in the US first.[8]

Sponsors should submit requests for Fast Track designation to FDA in writing. Supporting documentation should clearly demonstrate that the criteria necessary for designation have been met and that the sponsor has a stage-appropriate clinical development plan in place. Fast Track designation applies to both the product and the specific indication for which it is being studied.

The request for Fast Track designation can be submitted simultaneously with the IND, or at any time thereafter prior to receiving marketing approval. To maximize the use of the Fast Track incentives, it is best to include the designation request in the original IND submission or as soon as possible thereafter. Note that the request for Fast Track designation can be granted by FDA only upon submission of an IND.

FDA will respond to a request for Fast Track designation within 60 days of receipt. If FDA determines that Fast Track criteria have been met, the review division will issue a designation letter that will state that Fast Track designation is granted for development of the product for use in treating the specific serious or life-threatening condition. The letter also will request that sponsors design and perform studies that can show whether the product fulfills unmet medical needs. FDA can issue a non-designation letter either because the Fast Track request package was incomplete or because the drug development program failed to meet the criteria for Fast Track designation. The non-designation letter will explain the reasons for FDA's decision. FDA will respond to a subsequent request for Fast Track designation after a non-designation determination within 60 days of receiving the new request. Sponsors must continue to meet the Fast Track criteria throughout product development to retain the designation. The sponsor should expect the appropriateness of continuing the Fast Track designation for the drug development program to be discussed and evaluated at different times during the drug development process, including at the End-of-Phase 2 meeting and the Presubmission Meeting. If FDA determines that a product is no longer eligible, it will notify the sponsor that the product is no longer part of the Fast Track drug development program. Sponsors can appeal FDA's decision through the dispute resolution process (21 CFR 10.75, 312.48 and 314.103).

Rolling Review

FDA may consider reviewing portions of a marketing application before the complete NDA or BLA is submitted (Rolling Review). To qualify for a Rolling Review, Fast Track designation must have been granted. Furthermore, the pivotal study must be complete or near completion.

A sponsor seeking a Rolling Review may simultaneously submit a Rolling Review request with a request for Fast Track designation. The sponsor should provide a schedule for submission of portions of the application. If the Rolling Review request is granted, FDA may review portions of the application as they become available. However, FDA is not obligated to start the review upon receipt of a portion. The *PDUFA* goal date is determined upon receipt of the final portion of the application, while the user fee is due upon receipt of the first portion. It is recommended that applicants initiate discussion about their plans for submitting a Rolling Review NDA or BLA at the Presubmission Meeting.

Priority Review

In 1992, under *PDUFA*, FDA agreed to specific goals for improving drug review times using a two-tiered system of review times: Priority Review and Standard Review. Priority Review designation is given to drugs that offer major advances in treatment, or provide a treatment where no adequate therapy exists. FDA reviews priority applications more quickly than standard applications, in six months versus 10 months (in eight months versus 12 months for applications in "the Program"). Twelve of the 35 Fiscal 2012 NME drugs received Priority Review. Of those 12, 11 (92%) were approved on the first cycle, and 10 (83%) were approved in the US before any other country.[9] Prior to the enactment of *PDUFA*, application review in CDER was subject to the 180-day review period described in 21 CFR 314.100 (the "regulatory clock") with review extensions allowed for receipt of major amendments. In addition, prior to 1992, CDER used a three-tier therapeutic-potential classification system (Type A—important therapeutic gain; Type B—modest therapeutic gain; and Type C—little or no therapeutic gain) to determine application review priorities. Potentially eligible for Priority Review are drugs that have the potential to provide significant advances in treatment in at least one of the following instances:

- provide evidence of increased effectiveness in treatment, prevention or diagnosis of disease
- eliminate or substantially reduce a treatment-limiting drug reaction
- provide documented evidence of enhanced patient compliance to treatment schedule and dose
- provide evidence of safety and effectiveness in a new subpopulation, such as children

An applicant may submit a request for Priority Review to FDA, providing adequate evidence that its drug product meets one of the criteria listed above. While Fast Track products generally are eligible for Priority Review, as they are intended to treat serious or life-threatening conditions and address unmet medical needs, having a Fast Track designation does not automatically convey a Priority Review; the applicant should request the Priority Review with appropriate justification in the cover letter. CDER currently grants Priority Review for drugs that provide a significant improvement, compared to marketed products, in the treatment, diagnosis or prevention of a disease, i.e., eligibility is not limited to drugs for a serious or life-threatening disease. A Fast Track product ordinarily would meet either center's criteria for Priority Review. However, an applicant need not seek Fast Track designation to be eligible for priority review.

FDA determines within 45 days whether a Priority or Standard Review designation will be assigned. If Priority Review is granted, the applicant still must provide the same amount of scientific and medical evidence as required under Standard Review classification in order for FDA to approve the drug.

Breakthrough Therapy Designation

FDASIA gave FDA a new tool to expedite the development of therapies that show substantial promise in early clinical trials. This new authority arose out of discussions between FDA, the National Institutes of Health (NIH), industry, academia and patient groups on how to create a novel pathway for development of breakthrough therapies. A drug company may seek designation of a drug as a "Breakthrough Therapy" if it is for a serious and life-threatening disease, and preliminary clinical evidence shows the drug may offer substantial improvement over existing therapies. Once FDA designates a drug as a Breakthrough Therapy, it will provide advice and interaction throughout the development process to streamline the drug's clinical trials and review (**Table 11-2**). Not later than 18 months after the date of enactment of *FDASIA*, FDA will issue draft guidance on implementing the requirements with respect to breakthrough therapies,[10] but companies may begin to seek the designation immediately (see Fact Sheet: Breakthrough Therapies, www.fda.gov/RegulatoryInformation/Legislation/FederalFoodDrugandCosmeticActFDCAct/SignificantAmendmentstotheFDCAct/FDASIA/ucm329491.htm).

Risk Evaluation and Mitigation Strategy (REMS)

Title IX, Subtitle A, Section 901 of *FDAAA* amended the *FD&C Act* by creating Section 505-1, which authorizes FDA to require applicants of certain prescription drugs products, to submit a proposed REMS if the agency determines one is necessary to ensure that a drug's benefits outweigh its risks. An applicant also may voluntarily submit a proposed REMS without having been required to do so by FDA. FDA can request the REMS at the time of the initial submission of the original application or at any time after its approval (usually, if FDA becomes aware of new safety information and determines that a REMS is necessary). Once the applicant is notified by FDA that a REMS is necessary, the applicant must submit a proposed REMS within 120 days.

The content of the proposed REMS should adequately describe its proposed goals and the specific elements proposed for inclusion in the drug product's approved REMS. The proposed REMS must include, at a minimum, a timetable for the submission of assessments of the strategy by 18 months, three years and seven years after the REMS is approved by FDA. The proposed REMS also may include one or more of the following elements: Medication Guide (21 CFR 208); patient package insert; communication plan to healthcare providers; and Elements to Assure Safe Use (ETASU). The proposed REMS also should contain a thorough explanation of the rationale for, and supporting information about, the content of the proposed REMS, as well as a timetable by which each of the elements will be implemented.

ETASU may be required if a drug has been shown to be effective but is associated with a serious adverse event. In such a case, the drug can be approved only if, or would be withdrawn unless, such elements are included in the REMS to mitigate the specific serious risks listed in the product's labeling. ETASU may be required for approved products when an assessment and Medication Guide, patient package insert or communication plan are not sufficient to mitigate these risks. An example of an ETASU would be a system or process to ensure that certain laboratory test result outcomes are obtained before a drug may be dispensed.

The applicant must reach agreement with FDA on the elements of a REMS submission and the timelines for implementation. FDA will determine which REMS elements are necessary to ensure that the benefits of the drug outweigh its risks and will determine approvability of the REMS. FDA also must approve REMS that are voluntarily submitted. An approved REMS that is submitted voluntarily is subject to the same requirements and enforcement as a required REMS. FDA will notify applicants who voluntarily submit a proposed REMS whether the REMS will be required. If FDA determines that a REMS is not required, an applicant may undertake voluntary risk management measures that would be performed outside of a REMS.

Once FDA approves the REMS, it will serve as the basis for inspection and enforcement. A drug will be considered to be misbranded if the applicant fails to comply with a requirement of the approved REMS. An applicant that violates a REMS requirement also is subject to civil monetary penalties of up to $250,000 per violation, not to exceed $1 million in a single proceeding. These penalties increase if the violation continues more than 30 days after FDA notifies the applicant of the violation. The penalties double for the second 30-day period, and continue to double for subsequent 30-day periods, up to $1 million per period and $10 million per proceeding. In addition, the sponsor may not introduce into interstate commerce an approved drug that is noncompliant with the conditions of an approved REMS. For additional information on REMS, refer to MaPP 6700.6 REMS Questions and Answers.

Presubmission Activities

Many activities need to be completed by the applicant prior to an application submission, including proprietary name submission and review, establishment registration, labeler code assignment and request for a Presubmission Meeting with the review division.

Proprietary Name Submission and Review

One important activity during the drug development phase is crafting a proprietary name (i.e., "brand name") for the product. The proprietary name is one of the product's critical identifiers for healthcare professionals and consumers. Companies expend a vast amount of resources creating the perfect proprietary name. Equally, FDA allocates many

Table 11-2. Benefits of Breakthrough Designation

Food and Drug Administration Safety and Innovation Act (FDASIA) of 2012
SEC. 902. BREAKTHROUGH THERAPIES. (EXCERPT)

"(B) ACTIONS.—The actions to expedite the development and review of an application under subparagraph (A) may include, as appropriate—
"(i) holding meetings with the sponsor and the review team throughout the development of the drug;
"(ii) providing timely advice to, and interactive communication with, the sponsor regarding the development of the drug to ensure that the development program to gather the nonclinical and clinical
data necessary for approval is as efficient as practicable;
"(iii) involving senior managers and experienced review staff, as appropriate, in a collaborative, cross-disciplinary review;
"(iv) assigning a cross-disciplinary project lead for the Food and Drug Administration review team to facilitate an efficient review of the development program and to serve as a scientific liaison between the
review team and the sponsor; and
"(v) taking steps to ensure that the design of the clinical trials is as efficient as practicable, when scientifically appropriate, such as by minimizing the number of patients exposed to a potentially less efficacious treatment."

resources to review a proposed proprietary name in an attempt to help prevent medication errors.

The applicant must submit proposed proprietary names for FDA review as part of the marketing application. The request for proprietary name approval must be submitted no later than when the application is submitted, although applicants may submit a "request for proprietary name" review prior to application submission (perhaps as early as completion of Phase 2 trials) under the IND. However, to ensure resources are not used to evaluate proposed proprietary names for products that will not be viable candidates for an NDA, ANDA or BLA, or for which proposed indications are not yet sufficiently clear to form the basis of an evaluation of a name for potential medication errors, FDA does not evaluate proprietary names until products have completed Phase 2 trials.

The contents of a proprietary name submission should include the primary and alternate proposed proprietary name, intended pronunciation of the proprietary name, name derivation, intended proprietary name modifier meanings and the name's pharmacologic/therapeutic category.

An FDA review of proprietary names includes an evaluation of both the proposed names' safety and promotional aspects. The safety review focuses primarily on preventing medication errors and evaluating other products that may have similar dosage regimens, overlapping strengths, similar names when said aloud or a similar appearance when written out by hand. The promotional review is to determine whether the name implies superiority, attempts to minimize risk or overstates efficacy.

For a proposed proprietary name submitted during the IND phase, FDA will review and communicate a decision about the name within 180 days of the receipt date of the submission. For a proposed proprietary name submitted with the original NDA or BLA, or as a part of a supplement, FDA will review and communicate a decision within 90 days of the receipt date of the submission. Proprietary names accepted during a pre-review will be re-reviewed 90 days before the action date to ensure they are still acceptable.

Establishment Registration and National Drug Code

A company that manufactures human drugs, certain biological products and animal drugs must register the manufacturing facility before FDA can approve a marketing application. Specifically, owners or operators of all drug establishments, not exempt under Section 510(g) of the act or Subpart B of Part 207, that engage in the manufacture, preparation, propagation, compounding, or processing of a drug or drugs shall register and submit a list of every drug in commercial distribution (21 CFR 207.20(a)).

Prior to 1 June 2009, paper forms for Drug Establishment Registration and Drug Product Listing were completed and submitted to FDA. Changes to the *FD&C Act* from enactment of *FDAAA*, require that drug establishment registration and drug listing information be submitted electronically unless a waiver is granted. Therefore, as of 1 June 2009, FDA only accepts electronic submissions for registration and listing unless a waiver is granted.

The National Drug Code (NDC) system is designed to provide drugs in the US with a specific number that describes the product. Per 21 CFR 207.35, the NDC is limited to 10 digits; however, the passing of the *Health Insurance Portability and Accountability Act* of 1996 (*HIPAA*) propagated more consistent 11-digit codes to allow for proper billing for reimbursement purposes. The first segment of the NDC is assigned by FDA and identifies the vendor (or labeler) involved with the drug's manufacture, packaging or distribution. The second segment conveys the product codes and comprises the entity, strength, dosage form and formulation. The third segment, or package code, indicates

Figure 11-1. The Common Technical Document

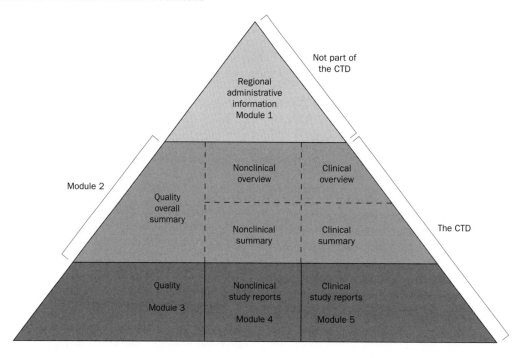

Modified from the International Conference on Harmonisation (ICH) www.ich.org.

the package forms and sizes. The second and third segments of a given product's code are assigned by the manufacturer.

Prior to June 2009, FDA would input the full NDC number and information into a database known as the Drug Registration and Listing System (DRLS). However, with electronic submissions and eDRLS, this is now done automatically. More recently, *FDASIA* amends the *FD&C Act* by requiring additional information to be submitted for the registration of domestic or foreign drug facilities. This additional information includes each drug establishment's unique facility identifier and a point of contact email address. Furthermore, as of 1 October 2012, the re-registration period for domestic and foreign drug manufacturers has been changed to 1 October to 31 December of each year, instead of the previously more open-ended period of on or before 31 December of each year. For more direction on how to properly list and register products, please see the link under "Electronic Drug Registration and Listing Instructions" below.

As of June 2009, eDRLS contains Rx products and OTC products as well as finished and unfinished drug products. FDA utilizes information from the eDRLS database to update the NDC directory on a daily basis (see the NDC Directory at www.accessdata.fda.gov/scripts/cder/ndc/default.cfm). Additionally, FDA relies on establishment registration and drug listing information to administer many of its programs, such as postmarketing surveillance (including risk-based scheduling and planning of inspections), protection against bioterrorism, prevention of drug shortages, management of drug recalls and assessment of user fees.

Presubmission Meeting

Sponsors can request meetings with FDA at various stages during the drug development process. A Presubmission Meeting, considered a Type B meeting (see Chapter 4), is highly recommended prior to NDA or BLA submission. It generally is advisable to hold such a meeting four to six months prior to the anticipated submission date. A request for a Presubmission Meeting should be submitted 60 days prior to the desired date. A briefing package must be submitted for review by FDA attendees and should be received by FDA at least four weeks prior to the scheduled meeting. For additional information on meetings with FDA, refer to *Guidance for Industry: Formal Meetings with Sponsors and Applicants for PDUFA Products*. The Presubmission Meeting allows the sponsor to present data that will be submitted in the application and to provide additional assurance that the sponsor is submitting all the necessary information required by the agency in order to reach a decision on the application's approvability. In addition, for NDAs and BLAs in *PDUFA V*'s "the Program," (i.e., NMEs and original BLAs received on or after 1 October 2012), FDA and the sponsor will agree at the Presubmission Meeting on the content of a complete application for the proposed indication(s) and conduct preliminary discussions on the need for a REMS or other risk management actions.

The NDA or BLA Application

Goals

The goals of the NDA or BLA are to provide enough information to permit FDA reviewers to reach key decisions on whether: the drug is safe and effective when used for the indications described in the labeling; the drug's benefits outweigh its risks; the proposed labeling is appropriate; and the drug's manufacturing methods and the controls used to maintain drug quality are adequate to preserve its identity, strength, quality and purity.

Content and Format

An application must provide all information pertaining to the drug's development. The quantity of information can vary from one application to another; however, the application structure is consistent. Per 21 CFR 314.50 and 601 (NDA and BLA respectively), an application must include an application form, an index, a summary, five or six technical sections, case report forms and tabulations, patent information, financial disclosure or certification and labeling. The technical sections may include product quality, nonclinical pharmacology and toxicology, human pharmacokinetics and bioavailability, microbiology, statistical and clinical data. The product quality section should describe the composition, manufacture and specifications of both the drug substance and the drug product, as well as fairly detailed descriptions of all manufacturing controls and stability data. The nonclinical pharmacology and toxicology section should describe any animal and *in vitro* drug studies that help to define the drug's pharmacologic properties and address toxicity related to its administration. The clinical section should include a description of all clinical investigations completed in support of the drug's efficacy and safety, as well as the study protocols and copies of case report forms for each patient who died during a clinical study or did not complete a study because of an adverse event, regardless of the incident's relationship to the study drug.

Copies of the proposed drug product labeling—including the package insert, carton and container labels and Medication Guide—should be provided in the application. FDA requires that labeling be submitted electronically in a format that the agency can review and process. The content of labeling must utilize the structured product labeling (SPL) format with an extensible markup language (XML) backbone. SPL has several advantages: the exchange of information between computer systems, automation of text comparison by section and exchange of information needed for other submissions (i.e., cross-referencing). SPL allows labeling content to be searched, moved between systems and combined with other data sources and lends itself to the support of electronic healthcare initiatives.

The CTD Format

As outlined above, a huge amount of information is submitted in support of a marketing application. Generally, similar scientific and clinical information is broadly required in countries where a manufacturer (or applicant) plans to market the drug. Because the information is similar—and to allow manufacturers to proceed more quickly and consistently with the submission and application process—the International Conference for Harmonisation (ICH) developed the Common Technical Document (CTD) format. The CTD provides harmonized structure and format for new marketing applications submitted in the US, EU, Japan and to numerous other regulatory authorities.

Per the CTD format, an application is broken up into five modules (**Figure 11-1**). Module 1 contains documents specific to the region where the file is being submitted, and Modules 2–5 are intended to be common across all regions. Module 1 is region-specific and contains administrative and prescribing information (e.g., application forms, proposed labeling and applicable patent information). Module 2 contains CTD summaries (e.g., a quality overall summary and clinical summary). Module 3 contains quality data or product quality information (e.g., drug substance and drug product data). Module 4 contains nonclinical study reports (e.g., pharmacodynamic and pharmacokinetic data). Module 5 contains clinical study reports (e.g., study protocols, case report forms, integrated safety and efficacy summaries and relevant literature references, including FDA meeting minutes and references cited in the Clinical Overview section).

The eCTD Format

Historically, submissions to FDA have been in paper format. Paper submissions not only require many resources for both the sponsor and FDA, but also require a lot of storage space. FDA attempted to address this issue by creating standards that permit electronic submissions (eSubs). FDA started to accept eCTDs in 2003, and it became the recommended standard in 2008.

The value of electronic submissions is well recognized. Under *FDASIA*, FDA, working with stakeholders, will issue draft and final guidance on the standards and format of eSubs. Requirements of eSubs will be phased in over the next few years starting with original NDA and BLA submissions and eventually requiring all original commercial INDs and their amendments to be submitted electronically as well.

The formats of the paper CTD and eCTD submissions are different. With an eCTD submission, each document is separate (granular) and named according to ICH specifications. Each submission has its own eCTD XML backbone file, which allows FDA to receive, archive and review the submission. Once an application is submitted in electronic format, all subsequent submissions to the application are also submitted electronically and should include eCTD backbone files (once eCTD, always eCTD). Without these backbone files, FDA will be unable to process subsequent submissions. FDA also recommends that electronic file cover letters include a description of the submission's approximate size (e.g., 4 gigabytes), the type and number of electronic media used (e.g., two DVDs), a regulatory and technical point of contact and a statement that the submission is virus free, with a description of the software used to virus-check the file.

At any time, a sponsor can decide to convert its paper application to an electronic filing. Should a sponsor decide to do so, it is not necessary to provide all previous submissions in electronic format with eCTD backbone files; instead the electronic filing may begin with the planned submission. For ease of conversion, the Comprehensive Table of Contents Headings and Hierarchy maps the application to the eCTD format. When converting and cross-referencing to past submissions, the applicant should be sure to include specific information, such as the date of the previous submission, document name, page numbers, volume numbers and approval dates, or may consider including any items critical for review of the current submission within the electronic format submission so the reviewer can find it more easily.

Types of Applications

There are several types of drug applications: 1) "Traditional" 505(b)(1) NDA (*FD&C Act* Section 505(b)(1)); 2) 505(b)(2) NDA (*FD&C Act* Section 505(b)(2)); 3) Abbreviated NDA (ANDA) (*FD&C Act* Section 505(j)); 4) Original BLA (*PHS Act* Section 351(a)); and 5) Biosimilar BLA (*PHS Act* Section 351(k)).

505(b)(1) NDA ("traditional" NDA)

A 505(b)(1) application is a complete NDA that contains all the studies conducted by the applicant necessary to demonstrate a drug's safe and effective use. A 505(b)(1) application contains all information as outlined in 21 CFR 314.50.

505(b)(2) NDA

A 505(b)(2) application also contains information required in a 505(b)(1) application necessary to demonstrate safe and effective use of a drug; however, the applicant can provide some of the information required for approval in the application from studies it did not conduct and for which it has not obtained a right of reference.[11]

Section 505(b)(2) was added to the *FD&C Act* by the *Drug Price Competition and Patent Term Restoration Act* of 1984 (*Hatch-Waxman Act*) to allow companies to develop alternative therapies more quickly by relying on existing data. Applicants may rely on published literature that supports approval of an application and/or on FDA's previous finding of safety and effectiveness of an approved drug. For example, a 505(b)(2) application can be submitted if the applicant has changed a product's route of administration from an oral form to an intramuscular injection. In this instance, the applicant can rely on the efficacy data and some of the safety data established for the drug's oral formulation that has already been approved by FDA, but will have to conduct studies showing safety and efficacy that relate to the change to the intramuscular form. In addition, the applicant will have to establish a "bridge" (e.g., via comparative bioavailability data) between the proposed drug and the approved listed drug to demonstrate that reliance on FDA's previous finding of safety and effectiveness is scientifically justified.

Sections 505(b)(2) and 505(j) of the *FD&C Act* together replaced FDA's "paper NDA policy," which had permitted an applicant to rely on studies published in the scientific literature to demonstrate the safety and effectiveness of duplicates of certain post-1962 pioneer drug products.

(505(j)) Abbreviated NDA (ANDA)

A 505(j) application is considered abbreviated because, generally, the applicant is not required to include preclinical and clinical data necessary to demonstrate safety and effectiveness. Instead, it contains chemistry and bioequivalence data to show that the proposed product is identical in active ingredient, dosage form, strength, route of administration, labeling, quality, performance characteristics and intended use to the previously-approved reference listed drug (RLD). More information on ANDAs is provided in Chapter 13.

(351(a)) BLA (Original BLA)

A 351(a) application is a complete BLA that contains all the studies conducted by the applicant necessary to demonstrate a drug's safe and effective use. A 351(a) BLA contains all information as outlined in 21 CFR 601.2.

For additional information, see Therapeutic Biologic Applications at www.fda.gov/Drugs/DevelopmentApprovalProcess/HowDrugsareDevelopedandApproved/ApprovalApplications/TherapeuticBiologicApplications/default.htm.

(351(k)) BLA (Biosimilar BLA)

A 351(k) application is an abbreviated BLA for a biological product that is demonstrated to be "biosimilar" to or "interchangeable" with an FDA-licensed biological product.

For additional information, see Biosimilars at www.fda.gov/Drugs/DevelopmentApprovalProcess/HowDrugsareDevelopedandApproved/ApprovalApplications/TherapeuticBiologicApplications/Biosimilars/default.htm.

This chapter does not discuss the submission or review of ANDAs or Biosimilar BLAs.

Submission of the Marketing Application and Next Steps

Once the application has been compiled and is ready for dispatch, it can be submitted by regular post or express mail to FDA's Document Control Room.

Electronic CTD submissions are submitted either on electronic media or through the FDA Electronic Submissions Gateway (FDA ESG). If submitted on electronic media, it should be sent by regular post or express mail just like the paper submission. The FDA ESG is a centralized, agency-wide communications point for securely receiving electronic regulatory submissions. It electronically receives, acknowledges, routes to and notifies a receiving center of the receipt of an electronic submission. The FDA ESG is a conduit, or "highway," along which submissions travel to reach their final destinations within FDA. FDA ESG staff do not open or review submissions.

Upon receipt of the application, FDA has 60 days to determine whether the application is sufficiently complete to allow for a substantive review. If FDA determines that the application is complete, it will be filed on Day 60. If FDA determines that the application is not complete (see 21 CFR 314.101(d)), FDA may refuse-to-file (RTF) it and, if so, will issue a formal RTF letter by Day 60 that will provide the reasons for the decision. By eliminating incomplete applications from the review queue, FDA is able to focus its resources on complete applications.

Note that FDA tends to be more flexible in accommodating drugs intended for critical diseases, particularly when there is no alternative therapy. In such cases, the agency and applicant will often work together to find a balanced resolution to allow application review to begin as quickly as possible. Note also that FDA may accept some parts of an application and RTF others (e.g., file one of two proposed indications for use and RTF the other). The applicant may resubmit the application after addressing FDA's RTF issues; FDA then determines whether the resubmitted application can be filed.

If an applicant strongly disagrees with FDA's decision to RTF an application, the applicant is given 30 days after receiving the RTF letter to request a meeting with FDA. Following the meeting, the applicant can request that the agency file the application "over protest." In this event, the date of filing will be 60 days after the date the applicant requested the meeting.

For applications that will be filed, FDA performs an "initial filing review" by Day 60 to identify "filing review issues," which are substantive deficiencies or concerns that may have significant impact on FDA's ability to complete the review of or approve the application. Filing review issues are distinct from application deficiencies that serve as the basis for an RTF action. Note that FDA's initial filing review represents a preliminary review of the application and is not indicative of deficiencies that may be identified later in the review cycle.

FDA will then inform the applicant in writing whether or not there are filing review issues by issuing a letter mandated by *PDUFA* within 14 days of the determination (also called a Day 74 letter). The Day 74 letter states the date the application was received, which is also the date the review clock begins. The Day 74 letter provides the planned review timeline and includes an "action" date, when FDA will provide a decision on the application, as well as dates when the applicant can expect to receive feedback from the review division on proposed labeling and postmarketing requirements/commitments. The Day 74 letter also identifies the review classification granted by FDA (i.e., Standard Review or Priority Review). For applications reviewed under the *PDUFA V* "Program," the Day 74 letter will also state whether the division is considering convening an Advisory Committee meeting.

For additional information on filing review issues and the Day 74 letter, refer to MaPP 6010.5 NDAs: Filing Review Issues.

During the review period, FDA may ask the applicant for additional information ("solicited" information) or the applicant may submit additional information on its own initiative ("unsolicited" information). If the new information constitutes a major amendment, FDA may determine that an extension to the *PDUFA* action date is needed to review the new information. Only one three-month extension can be given per review cycle. For a solicited major amendment that extends the *PDUFA* action date, FDA also will provide a new timeline for feedback on proposed labeling and postmarketing requirements or commitments. Thus, an applicant's strategy for providing information contained in the application should be very carefully planned.

FDA Review Process

Once an application is validated and received, the application is routed to the regulatory project manager (RPM) in the appropriate review division. The RPM will ask supervisory team leaders from appropriate disciplines to assign reviewers. The first review task is to determine, from each specific discipline, whether the application is fileable (see Submission of the Marketing Application and Next Steps above).

The review team consists of various disciplines such as clinical, pharmacology and toxicology, chemistry, clinical pharmacology, etc.

Each disciplinary group completes its review and determines whether the data can support the drug's approval. During the review process, a reviewer may identify a minor deficiency, may need a topic clarified or may need additional information in order to facilitate his or her review. These requests for additional information usually are communicated through an information request (IR) or advice letter (AD), and these letters generally are handled via email,

Figure 11-2. Major Steps in the NDA or BLA Review for Applications Not Under the PDUFA V "Program"

Overview of the NDA/BLA Review Process and Major Steps for Completing the Review

| Application Day 0 | Filing/Planning Meetings Day 45 (Day 30 for Priority) | Mid-Cycle Meeting Month 5 (3 for Priority) | Wrap Up Meeting Month 8 (5 for Priority) | Action Date Month 10 (6 for Priority) |

Steps:
1. Presubmission Activities
2. Process Submission
3. Plan Review
4. Conduct Review
5. Take Official Action (Conduct AC Meeting)
6. Post Action Feedback

Timeline: 1 month – 10 months

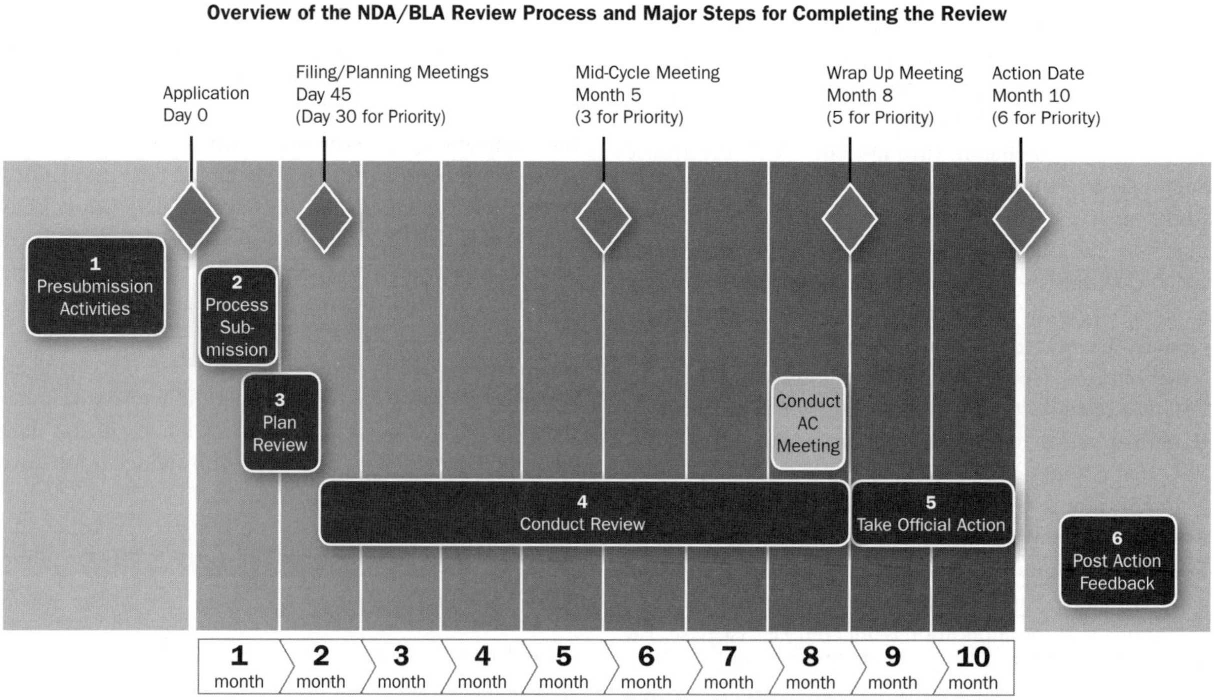

From CDER 21st Century Review Process Desk Reference Guide. Follow this link to see review time lines for applications under the PDUFA V Program.

---

telephone or direct mail. As the regulatory contact for the application, the RPM facilitates these communications. Applicants submit amendments to the application in an attempt to address all additional information requests. If serious deficiencies exist, the review division has the option of notifying applicants via a "discipline review" (DR) letter after each discipline has finished the initial review of its section of the pending application. DR letters had been used sparingly since the release of the 2001 FDA *Guidance for Industry Information Request and Discipline Review Letters Under the Prescription Drug User Fee Act* (2001).

With *PDUFA V*, a renewed focus on DR letters was agreed upon for applications in the "Program" as outlined in the *PDUFA Reauthorization Performance Goals and Procedures Fiscal years 2013 Through 2017*. FDA intends to complete primary and secondary discipline reviews of the application and issue DR letters in advance of the planned late-cycle meeting.

If additional scientific expertise is needed outside the core review team, the review division may consult other parts of the center or beyond (e.g., the Center for Devices and Radiological Health). For certain applications, opinions from outside experts may also be sought through the advisory committee process or by special government employees (SGEs).

As the review proceeds, FDA determines whether any bioresearch monitoring (BIMO) or current Good Manufacturing Practice (CGMP) inspections are required prior to approval. The results of these inspections will allow the agency to determine the credibility and accuracy of the data submitted in the application (see Preapproval Inspections (PAI) below).

FDA will make a determination whether Postmarketing Requirements (PMRs) and/or Postmarketing Commitments (PMCs) are necessary. If so, this is communicated to the applicant, and FDA and the applicant discuss and agree on specific studies, as well as specific milestone dates, including dates for final protocol submission, study or trial completion and final report submission.

In parallel, with PMR and PMC determinations, FDA reviews the product labeling and determines whether it accurately reflects the product's safety and efficacy and allows physicians, healthcare professionals and consumers to determine whether the drug's benefits outweigh its risks. The agency will then decide if it is ready to take action on the application.

Application review consists of several stages and involves a multidisciplinary team (see **Figure 11-2**). The primary review staff summarizes their preliminary review findings at a mid-cycle meeting. Discussions at the mid-cycle meeting can include the need for additional information from the applicant, the need for additional scientific expertise within the center, or the need for a REMS, postmarketing commitments or requirements, if the product is approved. During the review, the applicant's proposed labeling is reviewed, and comprehensive comments are conveyed to the applicant. At the wrap-up meeting, discussions can include issues that preclude approvability of the application, and further discussions involving details of the REMS, or postmarketing commitments or requirements, as needed.

If the product is an NME or an original BLA, the signatory authority for the application is the office director; the signatory authority for all other applications, including efficacy supplements, is usually the division director.

Advisory Committee Meeting

Advisory Committee meetings are discussed in Chapter 5 of this book. Situations that frequently lead FDA to convene an Advisory Committee meeting are described in the relevant draft guidance.[12] According to *FDAAA* (2007), a drug characterized by "…no active ingredient (including any ester or salt of the active ingredient) of which has been approved in any other application under this section or section 351 of the Public Health Service Act" needs[13] to be evaluated by an independent FDA Advisory Committee, unless FDA delineates why such a review will be unnecessary.

FDAAA also amended the *FD&C Act* to limit conflicts of interest and restricted the eligibility criteria for serving on FDA Advisory Committees. It was felt these provisions made the recruitment of suitable individuals for Advisory Committees more difficult. More recently, *FDASIA* largely eliminated those restrictions. Detailed discussions and analysis of the changes can be found in a number of recent third party newsletters.[14]

Preapproval Inspections (PAI)

FDA may approve a drug product if, among other requirements, the methods used in, and the facilities and controls used for, the manufacture, processing, packing and testing of the drug are found adequate, and ensure and preserve its identity, strength, quality and purity.

Prior to approving an application, FDA may inspect manufacturing facilities (CGMP inspections), as well as facilities or sites where the drug was tested in nonclinical or clinical studies (BIMO inspections). A PAI is performed to contribute to FDA's assurance that a manufacturing establishment listed in a drug product application is capable of manufacturing a drug and that data are accurate and complete.

Although the risk-based decision is left to the agency's discretion, BIMO and CGMP inspections generally are conducted for most new NDA and original BLA applications. FDA is likely to conduct PAI inspections in the following instances:

- NMEs or original BLAs
- priority reviews
- the first application filed by an applicant
- for-cause inspections (e.g., if one clinical site had a significantly better trial outcome than other sites)
- original or supplemental applications, if the CGMP status is unknown (e.g., it has been more than two years since the domestic facility was last inspected, or the establishment is new and has yet to be inspected by FDA or another global regulated authority)

CDER evaluates the adequacy of the applicant's data and relies on the facility inspections to verify the authenticity and accuracy of that data. This ensures that applications are not approved if it is determined that the applicant cannot demonstrate the ability to operate with integrity and in compliance with all applicable requirements.

Per *FDASIA*, all applicants are expected to include a comprehensive and readily located list of facilities and establishments. FDA will use this list to facilitate the need for potential inspections of foreign and domestic sites that will manufacture a drug for the US market, or that have completed a study to support the approval of a drug that will be marketed in the US.

FDA Decision on the Application

One of two actions may be taken on an application, namely an approval action or a complete response. The latter lists all review deficiencies identified by FDA and identifies steps the applicant should take to address these deficiencies in a future submission before the application can be approved.

Approval letters are issued when FDA has determined that the drug is safe and effective, can be acceptably manufactured and is appropriately labeled. An approval is effective on the date of approval letter issuance, granting authorization to market the drug for sale in the US.

Postmarketing Requirements and Commitments

The approval letter also stipulates any postmarketing requirements and commitments. A postmarketing requirement is a study (e.g., an observational epidemiologic study, an animal study or a laboratory experiment) or clinical trial that the applicant must conduct after the application is approved. It includes studies that may be required under the *Pediatric Research Equity Act* (*PREA*) (21 CFR 314.55(b)), the *Animal Efficacy Rule* (21 CFR 314.610(b)(1)), Accelerated Approval regulations (21 CFR 314.510 and 601.41) or *FDAAA* (Title IX, Section 901). The applicant must report the status of each postmarketing requirement annually.

A postmarketing commitment is a written commitment by the applicant to FDA to provide additional information after approval of the application. It is not a postmarketing requirement, although 506B-reportable postmarketing commitments require annual status reports to be submitted by the applicant.

(506B is the section of the *FD&C Act* that mandates annual status reports and obligates FDA to make certain information about postmarketing commitments publicly available.)

Maintenance of the Application

After the application is approved, the applicant is expected to continue a number of activities, including the submission of expedited reporting of serious, unexpected adverse events that occur in the postmarketing setting; submission of Periodic Safety Update Reports that provide a review of the drug's safety profile since approval; and submission of Annual Reports. Updated stability data and annual updates to establishment registrations and drug listings also may be necessary. Please refer to Chapter 12 for more information on postmarketing activities.

Special Incentive Programs for Drug Development

Programs under the *Orphan Drug Act* and *PREA* are the most well-known special incentive programs and will be discussed in detail in other chapters of this book. This section briefly introduces programs designed to stimulate the development of new antimicrobial drugs, drugs for certain tropical diseases and the Presidential Emergency Plan for AIDS Relief (PEPFAR).

Antibiotics

FDASIA contains specific provisions to incentivize development of antibiotics known as *Generating Antibiotic Incentives Now* (*GAIN*). *GAIN* is designed to stimulate development of drugs for the treatment of serious or life-threatening infections caused by bacteria or fungi. Eligible drugs must be designated a "qualified infectious disease product" (QIDP). Benefits of QIDP designation include Fast Track designation, FDA Priority Review and a five-year extension to the marketing exclusivity that is granted at the time of NDA approval (e.g., five-year NCE exclusivity, three-year new product exclusivity, seven-year orphan drug exclusivity). CDER has created an Antibacterial Drug Development Task Force (www.fda.gov/Drugs/DevelopmentApprovalProcess/DevelopmentResources/ucm317207.htm). As part of its work, the task force will assist in developing and revising guidance related to antibacterial drug development, as required by *GAIN*.

Tropical Diseases

A guidance that describes the policies and procedures for the tropical disease priority review voucher described in section 524(a)(3) of the *FD&C Act* (21 79 U.S.C. 360n(a)(3)) is available[15] and should be used in conjunction with *Guidance for Industry: Neglected Tropical Diseases of the Developing World: Developing Drugs for Treatment or Prevention*.[16]

Briefly, under the law, a sponsor of certain marketing applications approved for the prevention or treatment of a designated tropical disease (examples include malaria, tuberculosis and cholera) receives a Priority Review Voucher for Priority Review from FDA to be used with a product of its choice. The voucher can be transferred to another developer. A PRV entitles the bearer to Priority Review for a future new drug application that would not otherwise qualify for priority review. The PRV holder must pay FDA an additional user fee ($3,559,000 in Fiscal 2013, reduced from $4,582,000 and $5,280,000 in Fiscal 2011 and 2012, respectively) and provide FDA with a one-year notice before redemption. So far, two manufacturers have been granted PRVs: Novartis for the malaria drug Coartem and Johnson & Johnson for the antimycobacterial drug Sirturo. *FDASIA* includes Section 908, the "Rare Pediatric Disease Priority Review Voucher Incentive Program," which extends the voucher program on a trial basis to rare pediatric diseases.

AIDS Relief

Working with implementing organizations and governments in over 32 countries, PEPFAR has contributed to the rapid acceleration of HIV treatment access, availability of care and support services and HIV prevention interventions. To support PEPFAR's goals, FDA introduced an initiative in 2004 to ensure that antiretroviral drugs produced by manufacturers all over the world could be reviewed rapidly, their quality assessed and their acceptability for purchase with PEPFAR funds supported.

As of 2 July 2012, FDA has approved or tentatively approved a total of 152 antiretroviral drugs in association with PEPFAR. Tentative approval means that although existing patents and/or marketing exclusivity prevent the product from being approved for marketing in the US, FDA has found that the product meets all of the manufacturing quality, safety and effectiveness requirements for marketing in the US.

New Drug Product Exclusivity (Hatch-Waxman Exclusivity)

New Drug Product Exclusivity, under sections 505(c)(3)(E) and (j)(5)(F) of the *FD&C Act* (*Hatch-Waxman Amendments*), provides the holder of an approved NDA limited protection from new competition in the marketplace for the innovation represented by its approved drug product. A five-year period of exclusivity is granted for drugs that contain a new chemical entity (NCE). A new chemical entity[17] means a drug that contains no active moiety that has been approved by FDA in any other application submitted under section 505(b) of the *FD&C Act*. An active moiety means the molecule or ion responsible for the physiological or pharmacological action of the drug substance. Excluded from the concept of "active moiety" are those appended portions of the molecule that cause the drug to be an ester,

Figure 11-3. New Timeline for NMEs and Original BLAs Under *PDUFA V*

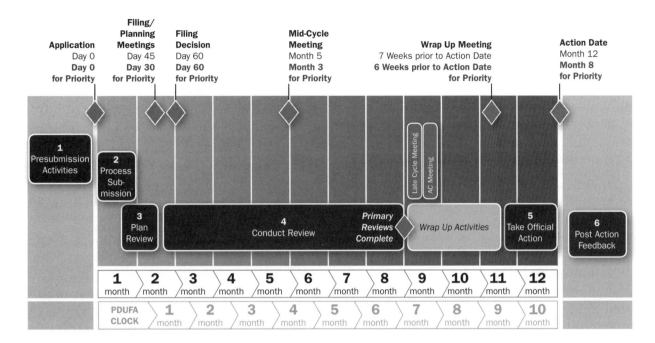

From CDER 21st Century Review Process Desk Reference Guide. Follow this link to see review time lines for applications under the PDUFA V Program.

salt (including a salt with hydrogen or coordination bonds), or other noncovalent derivative (such as a complex, chelate, or clathrate) of the molecule (see 21 CFR 314.108).

A three-year period of exclusivity may be granted for drug products that contain an active moiety that has been previously approved, but the applications contain reports of new clinical investigations (other than bioavailability studies) that were conducted or sponsored by the applicant and were essential to the approval of the application. For example, the changes in an approved drug product that affect its active ingredient, strength, dosage form, route of administration or conditions of use may be granted exclusivity if the application meets the criteria.

Summary

- A prescription drug is any drug approved or licensed for distribution by FDA that requires a healthcare practitioner's authorization before it can be obtained.
- The *FD&C Act* prohibits introduction of a prescription drug product into interstate commerce unless the drug's manufacturer has submitted an application and obtained FDA approval.
- A well-thought-out regulatory strategy is essential to the ultimate success of an applicant's drug development program and could shave months, or even years, off the product launch timeline.
- An application is required to contain all information pertaining to the drug's development, including chemistry, manufacturing and controls, nonclinical and clinical data. The ultimate goal of the application is to provide adequate information to allow FDA to complete its review and provide a decision on the drug's safety, effectiveness and quality.
- There are three different types of NDAs and two different types of BLAs. All of these applications should provide adequate information to allow FDA reviewers to conclude both that the drug is safe and effective when used for the proposed indication and that it can be manufactured consistently under controlled conditions.
- FDA will take action on a submitted application by issuing either a complete response letter or an approval letter, based upon its assessment of the application. Complete response letters are issued when deficiencies are identified. Approval letters are issued once FDA has determined that the drug is safe, effective, can be acceptably manufactured and is appropriately labeled. FDA can require that a REMS be implemented or that postmarketing studies or clinical trials be conducted after approval.
- Ongoing maintenance of the application is required for as long as it is active. Maintenance includes, but is not limited to, adverse event reporting, submission of Annual Reports, submission of advertising and promotional labeling.

- Many incentives and programs are available to expedite drug development, review and approval. Many of these incentives focus on the development, review and approval of drugs intended to treat serious or life-threatening conditions and/or address an unmet medical need.

References

1. All references to "drugs" or "drug products" in this chapter include both human drugs and biological drug products regulated by CDER unless otherwise specified.
2. *PDUFA Reauthorization Performance Goals and Procedures Fiscal Years 2013 Through 2017*. FDA website. www.fda.gov/downloads/forindustry/userfees/prescriptiondruguserfee/ucm270412.pdf. Accessed 26 March 2013.
3. FDA. *Draft Guidance for Industry and Review Staff: Target Product Profile—A Strategic Development Process Tool*. FDA website. www.fda.gov/downloads/Drugs/GuidanceComplianceRegulatoryInformation/Guidances/UCM080593.pdf. Accessed 26 March 2013.
4. Biomarker Definitions Working Group (2001). *Clinical Pharmacology and Therapeutics*, 69, p. 89–95.
5. Table modified from Sawyers CL, Haber DA, Horning SJ, Ivy SP and Selig WKD. "Developing Standards for Breakthrough Therapy Designation." *Cancer Research* (2012). Elsevier website. www.elsevierbi.com/~/media/Supporting%20Documents/The%20Pink%20Sheet/74/48/Breakthrough_therapy_issue_brief_11162012.pdf. Accessed 26 March 2013.
6. FDA. *FY 2012 Innovative Drug Approvals. Bringing Life-saving Drugs to Patients Quickly and Efficiently* (FDA December 2012). FDA website. www.fda.gov/downloads/aboutfda/reportsmanualsforms/reports/ucm330859.pdf. Accessed 26 March 2013.
7. FDA. *Guidance for Industry: Fast Track Drug Development Programs—Designation, Development, and Application Review*. FDA website. www.fda.gov/downloads/Drugs/GuidanceComplianceRegulatoryInformation/Guidances/ucm077104.pdf. Accessed 26 March 2013.
8. Op cit. 6.
9. Ibid.
10. Food and Drug Administration Safety and Innovation Act (FDASIA) of 2012. GPO website. www.gpo.gov/fdsys/pkg/PLAW-112publ144/pdf/PLAW-112publ144.pdf. Accessed 26 March 2013.
11. As defined in 21 CFR 314.3, "right of reference or use" means the authority to rely upon, and otherwise use, an investigation for the purpose of obtaining approval of an application, including the ability to make available the underlying raw data from the investigation for FDA audit, if necessary.
12. FDA. *Guidance for the Public and FDA Staff on Convening Advisory Committee Meetings*. FDA website. www.fda.gov/downloads/RegulatoryInformation/Guidances/UCM125651.pdf. Accessed 26 March 2013.
13. This statutory definition is equivalent to how FDA defines a "New Molecular Entity (NME)." Note that "active ingredient" includes salts and esters. The definition of NME for purposes of convening an Advisory Committee meeting is therefore different from the definition of "New Chemical Entity" for the purpose of determining eligibility for five-year market exclusivity under the *Hatch-Waxman Act*.
14. See for example Covington E-alert 10 August 2012, Covington & Burling LLC website, www.cov.com/files/Publication/0c4b516e-d83a-4f48-9d34-1144bc0e3f90/Presentation/PublicationAttachment/773cafe3-f4c8-48fa-be2b-1fd0a9fcbd11/FDA_Safety&Innovation_Act_2012.pdf, or Hyman,Phelps & McNamara, P.C. 11 July 2012, www.hpm.com/pdf/blog/FDASIA-HP&MSummary&Analysis.pdf. Accessed 26 March 2013.
15. FDA. *Guidance for Industry: Tropical Disease Priority Review Vouchers*. FDA website. www.fda.gov/downloads/Drugs/GuidanceComplianceRegulatoryInformation/Guidances/UCM080599.pdf. Accessed 26 March 2013.
16. FDA. *Guidance for Industry: Neglected Tropical Diseases of the Developing World: Developing Drugs for Treatment or Prevention*. FDA website. www.fda.gov/downloads/Drugs/GuidanceComplianceRegulatoryInformation/Guidances/UCM269221.pdf. Accessed 26 March 2013.
17. The *FD&C Act* uses the term "new chemical entity (NCE)" and clearly refers to small molecules. The terms NCE and "new molecular entity (NME)" have very specific meanings to FDA that are distinct.

Chapter 12

Postapproval Prescription Drug Submissions and Compliance

Updated by Hutch Humphreys, MS, RAC and Brian Miyazaki, RAC

OBJECTIVES

- Understand the role of current Good Manufacturing Practices (CGMP) in ensuring the quality, identity, strength and purity of approved products

- Define and review the postapproval aspects of prescription drugs, including:
  - postapproval reporting requirements for prescription drug marketing applications, including chemistry, manufacturing and controls (CMC) and labeling changes, safety reporting, Annual Reports and Drug Master Files and associated guidance documents
  - postapproval compliance requirements for prescription drugs and associated guidance documents
  - the effect of changes to approved products and applications

- Understand import and export regulations for approved products

- Understand drug establishment registration and drug listing requirements for approved products

LAWS, REGULATIONS AND GUIDANCE DOCUMENTS COVERED IN THIS CHAPTER

- 21 CFR 7.40–7.59 Recalls (Including Product Corrections)—Guidance on Policy, Procedures, and Industry Responsibilities

- 21 CFR 201.122 Exemptions From Adequate Directions for Use—Drugs for processing, repacking, or manufacturing

- 21 CFR 207 Registration of Producers of Drugs and Listing of Drugs in Commercial Distribution

- 21 CFR 210 Current Good Manufacturing Practice in Manufacturing, Processing, Packing, or Holding of Drugs; General

- 21 CFR 211 Current Good Manufacturing Practice for Finished Pharmaceuticals

- 21 CFR 312.32 IND Safety Reports

- 21 CFR 312.110 Import and export requirements

- 21 CFR 314.70 Supplements and other changes to an approved application

- 21 CFR 314.71 Procedures for submission of a supplement to an approved application

- 21 CFR 314.72 Change in ownership of an application

Chapter 12

- 21 CFR 314.80 Postmarketing reporting of adverse drug experiences
- 21 CFR 314.81 Other postmarketing reports
- 21 CFR 314.410 Imports and exports of new drugs
- 21 CFR 314.420 Drug Master Files
- 21 CFR 314.550 Accelerated approval of new drugs for serious or life-threatening illnesses—promotional materials
- *Guidance for Industry: Quality Systems Approach to Pharmaceutical Current Good Manufacturing Practice Regulations* (September 2006)
- *Guidance for Industry: Changes to an Approved NDA or ANDA* (April 2004)
- *Guidance for Industry: Changes to an Approved NDA or ANDA: Questions and Answers* (January 2001)
- *Guidance for Industry: Changes to an Approved NDA or ANDA; Specifications—Use of Enforcement Discretion for Compendial Changes* (November 2004)
- *Guidance for Industry: SUPAC-IR: Immediate-Release Solid Oral Dosage Forms, Scale-Up and Postapproval Changes: Chemistry, Manufacturing, and Controls, In Vitro Dissolution Testing and In Vivo Bioequivalence Documentation* (November 1995)
- *SUPAC-IR: Questions and Answers about SUPAC-IR Guidance* (February 1997)
- *Guidance for Industry: SUPAC-MR: Modified-Release Solid Oral Dosage Forms: Scale-Up and Postapproval Changes: Chemistry, Manufacturing, and Controls, In Vitro Dissolution Testing and In Vivo Bioequivalence Documentation* (September 1997)
- *Guidance for Industry: SUPAC-IR/MR: Immediate-Release and Modified-Release Solid Oral Dosage Forms, Manufacturing Equipment Addendum* (January 1999)
- *Guidance for Industry: SUPAC-SS: Nonsterile Semisolid Dosage Forms; Scale-Up and Postapproval Changes: Chemistry, Manufacturing, and Controls, In Vitro Release Testing and In Vivo Bioequivalence Documentation* (May 1997)
- *Draft Guidance for Industry: SUPAC-SS: Nonsterile Semisolid Dosage Forms, Manufacturing Equipment Addendum* (December 1998)
- *Guidance for Industry: PAC-ATLS: Postapproval Changes—Analytical Testing Sites* (April 1998)
- *Draft Guidance for Industry: Comparability Protocols—Chemistry, Manufacturing, and Controls Information* (February 2003)
- *Guidance for Industry: Format and Content of the CMC Section of an Annual Report* (September 1994)
- *Guidance for Industry: Providing Regulatory Submissions in Electronic Format—Content of Labeling* (April 2005)
- *Draft Guidance for Industry: CMC Postapproval Manufacturing Changes Reportable in Annual Reports* (June 2010)
- *Guidance for Industry: Providing Regulatory Submissions in Electronic Format — Drug Establishment Registration and Drug Listing* (May 2009)
- *Draft Guidance for Industry: Initial Completeness Assessments for Type II API DMFs under GDUFA* (October 2012)
- *Guideline for Drug Master Files* (September 1989)
- ICH, *Good Manufacturing Practice Guidance for Active Pharmaceutical Ingredients Q7A* (August 2001)
- ICH, *Pharmaceutical Development Q8(R2)* (August 2009)
- ICH, *Quality Risk Management Q9* (November 2005)
- ICH *Pharmaceutical Quality System Q10* (April 2009)

- ❑ *Guideline for Postmarketing Reporting of Adverse Drug Experiences (March 1992)*

- ❑ *Guidance for Industry: Postmarketing Adverse Experience Reporting for Human Drugs and Licensed Biological Products: Clarification of What to Report (August 1997)*

- ❑ *Draft Guidance for Industry: Postmarketing Safety Reporting for Human Drug and Biological Products Including Vaccines (March 2001)*

- ❑ *Draft Guidance for Industry: Providing Regulatory Submissions in Electronic Format—Postmarketing Individual Case Safety Reports (June 2008)*

- ❑ *Guidance: Drug Safety Information—FDA's Communication to the Public (March 2007)*

- ❑ *Draft Guidance for Industry: Format and Content of Proposed Risk Evaluation and Mitigation Strategies (REMS), REMS Assessments, and Proposed REMS Modifications (September 2009)*

- ❑ ICH, *Clinical Safety Data Management: Definitions and Standards for Expedited Reporting E2A (October 1994)*

- ❑ ICH, *Draft of the ICH Guideline on Clinical Safety Data Management—Data Elements for Transmission of Individual Case Safety Reports E2B(R3) (October 2005)*

- ❑ ICH, *Clinical Safety Data Management: Periodic Safety Update Reports for Marketed Drugs E2C(R1) (November 1996)*

- ❑ ICH, *Draft Guidance - Periodic Benefit-Risk Evaluation Report (PBRER) E2C(R2) (February 2012)*

- ❑ ICH, *Medical Terminology (MedDRA) M1*

- ❑ ICH, *Electronic Standards for the Transfer of Regulatory Information M2*

Introduction

Prescription drug manufacturers, distributors and marketers are required to remain in compliance with regulations throughout the product lifecycle. This lifecycle starts in early development and extends through the commercial marketing of the product. There are some differences in requirements at the preapproval stage compared with the postapproval stage; however, requirements at both stages are focused on product safety and quality. As in the clinical phases of development, manufacturers of approved products are required to adhere to current Good Manufacturing Practice (CGMP) regulations, and the marketing application sponsor is required to report changes that have a potential effect on the product's safety and quality to the US Food and Drug Administration (FDA). Postapproval requirements for marketing applications, and requirements for the production of commercial products, are similar for products approved under either a New Drug Application (NDA) or an Abbreviated New Drug Application (ANDA).

This chapter focuses on the CGMP manufacturing regulations, postmarketing adverse drug experience reporting requirements and the postapproval maintenance of regulatory applications/files (e.g., NDAs, ANDAs and Drug Master Files (DMFs)). This includes postapproval changes to the manufacturing and labeling of prescription drug products and postapproval requirements of commercial prescription drug manufacturing.

CGMPs for Manufacturing, Processing, Packing or Holding of Drugs and for Finished Pharmaceuticals (21 CFR 210 and 211)

Manufacturers of products undergoing human clinical trials and approved products are required to adhere to CGMP regulations. Title 21 of the US Code of Federal Regulations (CFR) Parts 210 and 211 outline the CGMP regulations for human drugs, including the minimum CGMP requirements for methods to be used in, and facilities or controls to be used for, the manufacture, processing, packing or holding of a drug, including those activities for biological products. Of note, 21 CFR 210.1(b) specifically states that failure to comply with 21 CFR 210 and 211 shall render the drug adulterated. It also provides clarification on how to handle conflicts between applicable regulations in 21 CFR 210 and other parts of the chapter (i.e., the regulation specifically applicable to the drug product in question shall supersede the more general regulation). Finally, 21 CFR 210 sets forth the definitions as used in Section 201 of the *Federal Food, Drug, and Cosmetic Act (FD&C Act)* and 21 CFR 210 and 211.

The CGMP regulations for drugs establish minimum requirements for manufacturing, personnel, equipment, control of product containers/closures, facilities, packaging, holding and distribution procedures and the associated process controls. The intention is to ensure that drugs are safe and that requirements are met for quality, identity, strength and purity. Additionally, CGMP regulations require all manufacturing and testing equipment to be qualified as suitable for use and for all operational methodologies and procedures (such as manufacturing, cleaning and analytical testing) utilized in the drug manufacturing process to be validated (according to predetermined specifications) to demonstrate that they can perform their purported function(s) in a reliable and consistent manner.

Active pharmaceutical ingredients (APIs) are subject to the adulteration provisions of Section 501(a)(2)(B) of the *FD&C Act*, which requires all drugs to be manufactured in conformance with CGMPs. The act makes no distinction between an API and a finished pharmaceutical, and failure of either to comply with CGMPs constitutes a violation of the act. FDA has not promulgated CGMP regulations specifically for APIs or drug components (as it has for finished pharmaceuticals).

FDA has long recognized that the requirements in the CGMP regulations for finished pharmaceuticals (21 CFR 210 and 211) are valid and applicable in concept to API manufacturing. These concepts include building quality into the drug by using suitable equipment and employing appropriately qualified and trained personnel, establishing adequate written procedures and controls designed to ensure manufacturing processes are valid, establishing a system of in-process material testing and final drug tests, and ensuring stability of drugs for their intended period of use. In 2001, FDA adopted an internationally harmonized guidance for industry on API CGMPs in conjunction with regulatory partners in the International Conference on Harmonisation (ICH). This guidance is *Good Manufacturing Practice Guidance for Active Pharmaceutical Ingredients Q7A*. ICH Q7 (as it now is commonly called) represents FDA's current thinking on CGMPs for APIs. Thus, API and related manufacturing and testing facilities that follow this guidance generally will be considered to comply with the statutory CGMP requirements.

CGMP Guidance

In September 2006, FDA published *Guidance for Industry: Quality Systems Approach to Pharmaceutical Current Good Manufacturing Practice Regulations* to help manufacturers implement modern quality systems and risk management approaches to meet the requirements of the agency's CGMP regulations (21 CFR 210 and 211).

The overarching philosophy articulated in both the CGMP regulations and in robust, modern quality systems is:

"Quality should be built into the product, and testing alone cannot be relied on to ensure product quality." The four major sections of the quality systems model include management responsibilities, resources, manufacturing operations and evaluation activities.

This guidance is intended to serve as a bridge between the 1978 CGMP regulations and the agency's current understanding of quality systems. In addition to being part of FDA's CGMP initiative, this guidance was issued for a number of reasons:

- to facilitate the development of a quality system that addresses the public and private sectors' mutual goal of providing a high-quality drug product to patients and prescribers that can eventually reduce the number of recalls and returned or defective products
- to harmonize CGMP regulations, to the extent possible, with other widely used quality management systems
- to reduce the number of prior-approval type regulatory submissions through the use of modern quality systems when coupled with manufacturing process and product knowledge and the use of effective risk management practices
- to require a quality system that can provide the necessary framework for implementing Quality by Design (QbD) (building in quality from the development phase and throughout a product's lifecycle), continuous improvement and risk management in the drug manufacturing process

FDA's *Compliance Program Manual*, which contains instructions to FDA personnel for conducting inspections, provides a systems-based approach and is consistent with the robust quality system model presented in this guidance. The six interrelated systems are the quality system and the five manufacturing systems (facilities and equipment, materials, production, packaging and labeling and laboratory controls). The quality system provides the foundation for the manufacturing systems that are linked and function within it. The quality system model described in this guidance does not consider the five manufacturing systems as discrete entities, but instead integrates them into appropriate sections of the model. Those familiar with the six-system inspection approach will see organizational differences in this guidance; however, the interrelationship should be readily apparent. One of the important themes of the systems-based inspection compliance program is that the applicant must have the ability to assess whether each of the systems is in a state of control. The quality system model presented in this guidance also serves to help firms achieve this state of control.

Pharmaceutical Quality System

In April 2009, FDA published the harmonized (ICH) *Guidance for Industry: Pharmaceutical Quality System Q10*, to assist pharmaceutical manufacturers by describing a model for an effective quality management system for the industry. ICH Q10 describes one comprehensive model for an effective pharmaceutical quality system that is based on International Organization for Standardization (ISO) quality concepts, including applicable GMP regulations and complements ICH *Pharmaceutical Development Q8* and *Quality Risk Management Q9*. Q10 is a model for a pharmaceutical quality system that can be implemented throughout the different product lifecycle stages (i.e., pharmaceutical development, technology transfer, commercial manufacturing and product discontinuation). Much of the content of Q10 applicable to manufacturing sites currently is specified by regional GMP requirements. Q10 is not intended to create any new expectations beyond current regulatory requirements. Consequently, the content of the guidance that exceeds current regional GMP requirements is optional. Q10 demonstrates industry and regulatory authorities' support of an effective pharmaceutical quality system to enhance the quality and availability of medicines around the world in the interest of public health. Implementation of Q10 throughout the product lifecycle should facilitate innovation and continual improvement, set the conditions for achieving product realization and establishing and maintaining a state of control, as well as strengthen the link between pharmaceutical development and manufacturing activities.

Changes to an Approved Application

Almost all changes to an approved marketing application, either NDA or ANDA, are required to be reported to FDA under the *FD&C Act*. Procedural aspects associated with supplementing an approved application are discussed in 21 CFR 314.71, including:

- Only the sponsor, or its designated agent, can supplement the application.
- Only information related to the proposed change(s) is required to be submitted.
- Requirements for archival, review and field copies are the same as for original applications.

Changes and the reporting of changes to the chemistry, manufacturing and controls (CMC) and labeling sections of approved applications are discussed in 21 CFR 314.70. The regulations within 314.70 require reporting CMC changes to the drug substance and drug product that may affect the marketed product's identity, strength, quality, purity or potency. Typographical and spelling errors and changes in formatting to standard operating procedures or batch records need not be submitted (21 CFR 314.70(a)(1)).

Three categories of postapproval CMC changes are described in 21 CFR 314.70: major (314.70(b)), moderate (314.70(c)) and minor (314.70(d)). These changes are categorized based on their potential to adversely affect the drug product's identity, strength, quality, purity or potency. Consequently, the reporting categories and the timing of the ability to distribute product that has been produced under these changes also are stratified. A summary of the postapproval reporting categories, their implementation timeframes and several examples are provided in **Table 12-1**.

Changes to approved product labeling also must be evaluated from the perspective of whether a major, moderate or minor change is being proposed. For example, a change to the product's Indication for Use or any change that affects the "Highlights" section of the product labeling would be major changes, requiring submission of a Prior Approval Supplement and FDA approval before distribution of the new labeling, while minor editorial or stylistic changes to product labeling often can be distributed as necessary and reported to FDA in the next NDA Annual Report.

FDA will review each supplement and Annual Report. If FDA determines that a supplement or Annual Report is deficient, the sponsor cannot distribute the product manufactured with that change until the supplement is amended. If the product with the proposed change is already in commercial distribution (e.g., the product was distributed after submission of a Changes Being Effected (CBE)-type supplement), and FDA believes the supplement is deficient, the agency may order the manufacturer to cease distribution of the product until the supplement is appropriately amended.

FDA has issued several guidance documents associated with changes to approved applications that can be found on the Agency's website. A searchable database of FDA's guidance documents for drugs can be found at www.fda.gov/Drugs/GuidanceComplianceRegulatoryInformation/Guidances/default.htm. If there are changes that are not directly addressed by the regulations, in FDA guidance documents or are multifactorial in nature, consulting the agency is recommended.

Several FDA guidance documents supplement the CFR with respect to reporting requirements associated with changes to approved applications. The most comprehensive of these documents is *Guidance for Industry: Changes to an Approved NDA or ANDA* (April 2004). This is supplemented by two additional guidance documents: *Guidance for Industry: Changes to an Approved NDA or ANDA: Questions and Answers* (January 2001) and *Guidance for Industry: Changes to an Approved NDA or ANDA: Specifications—Use of Enforcement Discretion for Compendial Changes* (November 2004). Additional guidance also can be found in the *Draft Guidance for Industry: CMC Postapproval Manufacturing Changes Reportable in Annual Reports (June 2010)* and *Guidance for Industry: PAC-ATLS: Postapproval Changes—Analytical Testing Sites* (April 1998). These five FDA guidance documents provide direction on postapproval changes to:

- components and composition
- manufacturing sites
- analytical testing sites
- manufacturing process
- specifications
- container closure systems
- labeling
- miscellaneous changes
- multiple related changes

Chapter 12

Table 12-1. Postapproval CMC Supplements

Type of Change	Postapproval Reporting Category	Implementation	Examples
Major Change The change has substantial potential to cause an adverse effect on a drug product's identity, strength, quality, purity or potency.	Prior Approval Supplement (PAS)	Approval of the supplement is required prior to distribution of product manufactured using the proposed change(s)	• Establishing a new regulatory analytical procedure including designation of an alternative analytical procedure as a regulatory procedure • A change in qualitative or quantitative formulation
Moderate Change The change has moderate potential to cause an adverse effect on a drug product's identity, strength, quality, purity or potency.	Changes Being Effected in 30 Days Supplement (CBE-30)	Product manufactured using the proposed change(s) may be distributed 30 days after submission of the supplement if the sponsor is not informed otherwise by FDA	• Changes in the size or shape of a container for a sterile drug substance • Relaxing an acceptance criterion or deleting a test to comply with an official compendium that is consistent with FDA statutory and regulatory requirements
Moderate Change The change has moderate potential to cause an adverse effect on a drug product's identity, strength, quality, purity or potency.	Changes Being Effected Supplement (CBE or CBE-0)	Manufacturer can distribute product manufactured using the proposed change(s) immediately following submission of the supplement	• A change in or addition or deletion of a desiccant • Adding or strengthening a contraindication, warning, precaution or adverse reaction on the product labeling
Minor Change The change has minimal potential to cause an adverse effect on the drug product's identity, strength, quality, purity or potency.	Annual Report	Product manufactured using the proposed change(s) can be distributed prior to reporting the change; the change is reported in the next Annual Report	• A move to a different manufacturing site for secondary packaging (manufacturing) • Extension of an expiration date based on full shelf-life data when the data were obtained in accordance with an approved stability protocol

FDA also has issued a number of guidance documents to aid manufacturers in determining the amount and type of information (data) required to be submitted to support certain postapproval changes. The most notable of these with respect to drug products are the Scale-Up and Postapproval Changes (SUPAC) guidance documents. The SUPAC guidance documents were written to reduce the reporting requirements for low-risk postapproval changes and reduce the reviewing burden on FDA. They also detail the chemistry information and potential bioequivalence study requirements associated with postapproval changes. These documents assess the risk level associated with changes (e.g., manufacturing process, manufacturing site, product formula, equipment, batch size, etc.). The SUPAC documents stratify changes into three levels: 1, 2 and 3, which correspond to minor, moderate and major changes, respectively. Level 1 changes are filed in an Annual Report and include, for example, site changes within a single facility and process changes within validated ranges. Level 2 changes, such as composition changes and changes in manufacturing equipment, are filed in a CBE-0 or CBE-30 supplement (Changes Being Effected immediately or in 30 days, respectively). Level 3 changes are filed in a Prior Approval Supplement (PAS) and can range from site changes to the use of a new manufacturer that does not have experience with the product type. The SUPAC guidance documents include:

- *Guidance for Industry: SUPAC-IR: Immediate-Release Solid Oral Dosage Forms, Scale-Up and Postapproval Changes: Chemistry, Manufacturing, and Controls, In Vitro Dissolution Testing and In Vivo Bioequivalence Documentation* (November 1995)
    o *SUPAC-IR: Questions and Answers about SUPAC-IR* (February 1997)
- *Guidance for Industry: SUPAC-MR: Modified-Release Solid Oral Dosage Forms: Scale-Up and Postapproval Changes: Chemistry, Manufacturing, and Controls, In Vitro Dissolution Testing and In Vivo Bioequivalence Documentation* (September 1997)
    o *Guidance for Industry: SUPAC-IR/MR: Immediate-Release and Modified-Release Solid*

Oral Dosage Forms, Manufacturing Equipment Addendum (January 1999)
- *Guidance for Industry: SUPAC-SS: Nonsterile Semisolid Dosage Forms; Scale-Up and Postapproval Changes: Chemistry, Manufacturing, and Controls; In Vitro Release Testing and In Vivo Bioequivalence Documentation* (May 1997)
  o *Draft Guidance for Industry: SUPAC-SS: Nonsterile Semisolid Dosage Forms, Manufacturing Equipment Addendum* (December 1998)

A sponsor can reduce the reporting requirements of a postapproval change if the change is implemented under an approved comparability protocol. A comparability protocol fully describes the proposed change, the data that will be generated to support the change and the acceptability criteria for the change. Unless submitted with the original NDA or ANDA, the comparability protocol must be submitted and approved as a PAS prior to its implementation. FDA has provided guidance associated with comparability protocols in *Draft Guidance for Industry: Comparability Protocols—Chemistry, Manufacturing, and Controls Information* (February 2003). The reporting requirements associated with postapproval changes also may be reduced if the changes were part of a QbD development and validation program as detailed in ICH's *Pharmaceutical Development Q8(R2), Quality Risk Management Q9* and *Pharmaceutical Quality System Q10*.

A supplement or Annual Report must include a list of all the changes that are being proposed or have been implemented, respectively. FDA recommends the applicant describe each change in enough detail to allow the agency to quickly determine whether the appropriate reporting category has been used. If the agency determines that an incorrect reporting category has been assigned to a change, the change will be reclassified, and the sponsor must adhere to the distribution requirements of the new classification. For example, if the agency reclassified a change from a CBE-30 to a PAS, the product incorporating the change cannot be marketed until the change is reviewed and approved by the agency. For supplements, the list of changes must be provided in the cover letter (21 CFR 314.70(a)(6)). In Annual Reports, the list should be included in the CMC summary section (21 CFR 314.81(b)(2)(i)). The applicant must describe each change fully in the body of the supplement or Annual Report (21 CFR 314.70(a)(1)). An applicant making a change to an approved application under Section 506A of the *FD&C Act* also must conform to other applicable laws and regulations, including CGMP requirements of the *FD&C Act* (21 U.S.C. 351(a)(2)(B)) and applicable regulations in 21 CFR 210, 211 and 314.

Other Postapproval Requirements

FDA has the authority to withdraw an application (NDA or ANDA) if a sponsor does not meet the reporting requirements for adverse drug experience (ADE) reports, field events, Annual Reports and advertising and labeling as listed in 21 CFR 314.80 and 314.81 within the required timeframes. FDA withdrawal of an application prevents the sponsor from marketing and distributing the product.

Adverse Drug Experience Reports

Under 21 CFR 314.80, the sponsor is required to review ADE information obtained from all potential sources (foreign and domestic), including:
- marketing experience (e.g., ADE reports from healthcare providers, patients, competitors, etc.)
- scientific literature (peer-reviewed and non-peer-reviewed)
- unpublished reports
- postmarketing clinical investigations
- postmarketing epidemiological/surveillance studies

Furthermore, the sponsor is required to develop written procedures for collecting, evaluating and submitting postapproval ADE reports to FDA and maintaining records of all ADEs known to the applicant for a period of 10 years, including raw data and any correspondence relating to ADEs. Any company (sponsor, manufacturer, distributor or packer) listed on the approved product labeling is held to these ADE reporting requirements. Obligations of a non-sponsor may be met by submitting all reports of serious ADEs to the sponsor. If a non-sponsor elects to submit ADE reports to the sponsor rather than FDA, the non-sponsor shall submit each report to the sponsor within five calendar days of receipt of the report, and the sponsor is then responsible for submitting these ADEs to FDA.

The sponsor is required to submit the following ADE reports to FDA within the specified timeframes:
- Postmarketing 15-Day Alert Reports—A sponsor shall submit any foreign or domestic ADE that is both serious and unexpected (defined below), whether or not it is considered to be drug related, within 15 days following receipt of the information. If additional information is received after an initial report is submitted, the new information also shall be submitted within 15 days of receipt as follow-up reports or as requested by FDA.
- Periodic Adverse Drug Experience Reports (PADER)—For the first three years following a drug's approval, a sponsor shall submit a PADER on a quarterly basis. Unless otherwise requested by FDA, after three years, the sponsor shall submit the PADER at annual intervals. The PADER should contain:

- a narrative summary and analysis of the report's information, including all ADE information obtained during the reporting period
- analysis of the 15-Day Alert Reports submitted during the reporting interval
- any Form FDA 3500A (MedWatch) for an ADE that was not submitted as a 15-Day Alert Report
- any actions taken during the reporting period due to ADEs (e.g., labeling changes or additional studies initiated)

Sponsors with a product that is approved in the US and at least one other ICH region have successfully negotiated with the FDA to manage some of the periodic ADE reporting requirements more efficiently by use of the Periodic Safety Update Report (PSUR) or the emerging Periodic Benefit-Risk Evaluation Report (PBRER). The PSUR, an ICH-driven document created in 1996, was intended to harmonize the periodic safety reporting requirements to regulatory authorities in ICH regions and to provide, in a common format, the worldwide interval safety experience of a medicinal product on a semiannual basis postapproval. Therefore, to meet the FDA requirement for a periodic ADE report, sponsors with a product approved in the US and another ICH region have negotiated with FDA to submit a PSUR on a semiannual basis and a PADER, if necessary, in the intervening quarters between PSUR submissions.

More recently, ICH has recognized that the assessment of the risk of a medicinal product is most meaningful when considered in light of its benefits. Therefore, ICH has proposed the PBRER to replace the PSUR. The PBRER is described in the ICH draft guidance, *Periodic Benefit-Risk Evaluation Report (PBRER) E2C(R2)* (February 2012) (as of December 2012, this guidance had been adopted as final by the EU regulator, but was at ICH Step 4, "recommended for adoption" for the regulatory bodies of Japan and the US). The proposed report would provide greater emphasis on benefit than the PSUR, particularly when risk estimates change significantly. In such cases there will need to be an overall explicit evaluation of the benefit:risk profile. The PBRER also would provide greater emphasis on the cumulative knowledge regarding a medicinal product, while retaining a focus on new information.

As with adverse event reporting during the IND stage of development, a sponsor should protect the privacy of the patient with an ADE by assigning a unique code instead of using the patient's name and address in the reports. A sponsor can include a disclaimer statement in the report indicating that it is not admitting or denying that the ADE report submitted constitutes an admission that the drug caused or contributed to an adverse effect.

An "unexpected" ADE is defined as an ADE not listed in the drug product's current labeling. A "serious" ADE is defined as an experience that results in:

- death
- a life-threatening event
- in-patient hospitalization or prolongation of existing hospitalization
- a persistent or significant disability/incapacity
- a congenital anomaly/birth defect

Other events may be considered serious ADEs if, based on appropriate medical judgment, they may jeopardize the patient or subject and require medical intervention to prevent one of the outcomes listed above.

ADE reports can be submitted via paper or electronically. FDA has provided guidance regarding submission of ADE reports in electronic format in *Draft Guidance for Industry: Providing Regulatory Submissions in Electronic Format—Postmarketing Individual Case Safety Reports* (June 2008).

To encourage healthcare professionals to collect, evaluate and report serious ADEs, FDA developed the MedWatch educational and publicity program in 1993. The MedWatch webpage can be found at www.fda.gov/Safety/MedWatch/default.htm. Sponsors, manufacturers, distributors and user facilities use MedWatch Form 3500A for mandatory reporting of both adverse events and problems with human drugs and other FDA-regulated products. Healthcare professionals, consumers and patients may use MedWatch Form 3500 for spontaneous reporting of ADEs to the sponsor or directly to FDA. Foreign reportable ADEs also may be submitted on forms developed by the Council for International Organizations of Medical Sciences (CIOMS).

FDA tracks adverse drug reaction reports by entering all safety reports for approved drugs and therapeutic biological products into the computerized FDA Adverse Event Reporting System (FAERS) database, which uses standardized international terminology from the Medical Dictionary for Regulatory Activities (MedDRA). FDA uses FAERS to facilitate postmarketing drug surveillance and compliance activities. The goal of FAERS is to improve the public health by providing the best available tools for storing and analyzing safety data and reports. Data and trends from FAERS may lead to FDA action on products, such as safety alerts communicated via FDA's website, "Dear Health Care Professional" letters or requests to a sponsor for additional safety studies. This is part of an FDA initiative to rapidly collect, analyze and disseminate drug safety information. This initiative is highlighted by FDA's *Guidance: Drug Safety Information—FDA's Communication to the Public* (March 2007).

Similar adverse event reporting requirements are associated with the conduct of clinical trials (21 CFR 312.32); these requirements are discussed in "Chapter 9 Clinical Trials: GCPs, Regulations and Compliance."

Risk Evaluation and Mitigation Strategies

The *Food and Drug Administration Amendments Act* of 2007 (*FDAAA*), which included renewal of the *Prescription Drug User Fee Act* (*PDUFA IV*), gave FDA the authority to require a Risk Evaluation and Mitigation Strategy (REMS) from manufacturers to ensure a drug or biological product's benefits outweigh its risks. A sponsor may propose a REMS as part of an application (NDA, ANDA, BLA) if it is deemed necessary. FDA also can require a REMS during initial review of an application, or any time after a drug is approved for marketing if the agency becomes aware of new safety information and determines that a REMS is necessary to ensure that the drug's benefits continue to outweigh its risks. After a REMS is approved by FDA, the sponsor must assess the effectiveness of the REMS in achieving its stated goals. These assessments usually are conducted at 18 months, three years and seven years after approval of the REMS. Elements that might be part of a REMS include:

- A Medication Guide and/or a patient package insert—materials written for the patient to help ensure safe use of the drug
- A Communication Plan to healthcare providers—an explanation of the strategy being employed to ensure that the benefits of the drug outweigh its risks
- Elements to Assure Safe Use (ETASU)—e.g., requiring healthcare providers who prescribe the drug to have particular training or experience, or be specially certified; only dispensing the drug to patients in certain healthcare settings, such as hospitals; making each patient using the drug subject to certain monitoring

More information on REMS can be found in FDA's *Draft Guidance for Industry: Format and Content of Proposed Risk Evaluation and Mitigation Strategies (REMS), REMS Assessments, and Proposed REMS Modifications (September 2009)*. A list of approved REMS is located at http://www.fda.gov/Drugs/DrugSafety/PostmarketDrugSafetyInformationforPatientsandProviders/ucm111350.htm.

Reporting Field Events

The sponsor of an approved application is required by 21 CFR 314.81(b)(1) to report any of the following incidents or occurrences to the appropriate FDA district office within three working days of becoming aware of the event:

- incidents causing the drug product or its labeling to be mistaken for, or applied to, another article
- any bacteriological contamination; any significant chemical, physical or other change or deterioration in the distributed drug product; or any failure of one or more distributed batches of the drug product to meet the specifications established for it in the application

The information may be provided to the appropriate FDA district office by telephone or other rapid means of communication but should be promptly followed by a written Field Alert Report. Two hard copies of the report are required, and the report and its mailing cover must be plainly marked "NDA-Field Alert Report."

Annual Reports

Sponsors of approved applications are required by 21 CFR 314.81(b)(2) to submit an Annual Report within 60 days of the anniversary date of the approval of the NDA or ANDA. If submitting in paper format, two copies of the report should be sent to the FDA division responsible for reviewing the application. Each copy must be accompanied by a completed Form FDA 2252 (Transmittal of Periodic Reports for Drugs for Human Use). The period covered in the report is defined as one full year from the anniversary date.

Following is the type of information that should be reported:

Summary (21 CFR 314.81(b)(2)(i))

- summary of significant new information that might affect the drug product's safety, effectiveness or labeling and a description of actions the sponsor has taken or intends to take as a result of this new information
- indication whether labeling supplements for pediatric use have been submitted and whether new studies in the pediatric population have been initiated to support appropriate labeling for the pediatric population

Distribution Data (21 CFR 314.81(b)(2)(ii))

- distribution data for the commercial drug product, including the National Drug Code (NDC) number and the total number of dosage units of each strength or potency
- quantities distributed for domestic and foreign use

Labeling (21 CFR 314.81(b)(2)(iii))

- current professional labeling, patient brochures or package inserts, and representative samples of the package labels
- content of labeling required under 21 CFR 201.100(d)(3) (i.e., the package insert or professional labeling), including all text, tables and figures in electronic format
- summary of any changes in labeling that have been made since the last report, listed by date in the order in which they were implemented or, if no changes, a statement of that fact

Chemistry, Manufacturing and Controls (21 CFR 314.81(b)(2)(iv))

- CMC changes: reports of experiences, investigations, studies or tests involving physicochemical or any other properties if they affect the drug product's safety or effectiveness
- full description of CMC changes not requiring a supplemental application under 21 CFR 314.70(b) (i.e., "Annual Reportable" changes)
- updated stability data obtained during the reporting period
- list of outstanding regulatory business, if any

Nonclinical Laboratory Studies (21 CFR 314.81(b)(2)(v))

- copies of unpublished reports and summaries of published reports of new toxicological findings in animal studies and *in vitro* studies conducted by the sponsor or found in the public domain

Clinical Data (21 CFR 314.81(b)(2)(vi))

- published clinical trials (or abstracts) of the drug, including clinical trials on safety and effectiveness; clinical trials on new uses; biopharmaceutic, pharmacokinetic and clinical pharmacology studies; and reports of clinical experience related to safety, conducted by the sponsor or found in the public domain
- summaries of completed unpublished clinical trials or prepublication manuscripts
- analysis of available safety and efficacy data in the pediatric population and changes in labeling based on this information

Status Reports of Postmarketing Study Commitments (21 CFR 314.81(b)(2)(vii))

- status report on each postmarketing requirement (PMR) or postmarketing commitment (PMC) concerning clinical safety, clinical efficacy, clinical pharmacology and nonclinical toxicology
  o Following passage of the *FDAAA* in 2007, FDA has the authority to impose PMR's on an approved drug, as well as working with a sponsor to agree on PMC's.
  o PMRs include studies and clinical trials that sponsors are required to conduct under one or more statutes or regulations (examples of PMRs include studies such as pediatric assessment of a drug, or assessment of a known or suspected serious risk related to the use of a drug).
  o PMCs are studies or clinical trials that a sponsor has agreed to conduct, but that are not required by a statute or regulation. Because commitments and requirements are treated differently under the law, terminology is used that distinguishes between studies and clinical trials that are required and those that a sponsor agrees to conduct that are not required.
  o More background on PMRs and PMCs can be found at www.fda.gov/Drugs/GuidanceComplianceRegulatoryInformation/Post-marketingPhaseIVCommitments/default.htm , and a searchable database of PMRs and PMCs for all approved drugs can be found at www.accessdata.fda.gov/scripts/cder/pmc/index.cfm.

Status of Other Postmarketing Studies (21 CFR 314.81(b)(2)(viii))

- status report of any postmarketing study not included in the PMR/PMC section above; primarily relates to CMC postmarketing studies and product stability studies

Log of Outstanding Regulatory Business (21 CFR 314.81(b)(2)(ix))

- provided at the sponsor's discretion; a listing of any open regulatory business with FDA (e.g., a list of unanswered correspondence between the sponsor and FDA, or vice-versa)

Advertising and Labeling

To comply with 21 CFR 314.81(b)(3)(i), the sponsor must submit specimens of mailing pieces and any other labeling or advertising devised for promotion of a drug product at the time of the promotional material's initial use and at the time of initial publication of an advertisement for a prescription drug product. A copy of the current labeling and a completed Form FDA 2253 (Transmittal of Advertisements and Promotional Labeling for Drugs for Human Use) are required with each submission. These submissions are made to the Office of Prescription Drug Promotion (OPDP; formerly known as the Division of Drug Marketing, Advertising and Communications or DDMAC) for products regulated by CDER, and to the Advertising and Promotional Labeling Branch (APLB) for products regulated by CBER.

For new drug products being considered for accelerated approval under 21 CFR 314.550 for treatment of serious or life-threatening illnesses, sponsors must submit copies of all promotional materials, including promotional labeling and advertisements, intended for dissemination or publication within 120 days following marketing approval to FDA for consideration during the preapproval review period. After the first 120 days following marketing approval, the sponsor must submit promotional materials at least 30 days prior to the intended initial dissemination of the promotional labeling or initial publication of the advertisement.

Submission of Patents to the Orange Book for Patent Exclusivity

Following approval of an application under *FD&C Act* Section 505, the product will be listed in FDA's "Approved Drug Products with Therapeutic Equivalence Evaluations" (electronic *Orange Book*, www.accessdata.fda.gov/scripts/cder/ob/default.cfm; so named because the original print book had an orange cover). The electronic *Orange Book* lists patent and marketing exclusivity information associated with each approved drug product (the *Orange Book* does not include biological products). To add patent information to the *Orange Book*, Form FDA 3542a must be submitted with the application, and Form 3542 must be submitted upon or after approval. These forms detail the patent information associated with the product.

Product Complaints

In accordance with CGMP regulations for APIs and finished pharmaceuticals, complaint files are required to be maintained by both sponsors and manufacturing/control sites. Written procedures describing the handling of all written and oral complaints regarding a drug product must be established and followed (21 CFR 211.198). The procedures should include provisions for review by the quality unit of any complaint involving a drug product's possible failure to meet any of its acceptance criteria in the regulatory specification and, for such drug products, a determination of whether there is a need for an investigation in accordance with 21 CFR 211.192.

The established procedures should include provisions for review to determine whether the complaint represents a serious and unexpected ADE. A serious and unexpected ADE is required to be reported to FDA in accordance with 21 CFR 310.305 and 314.80.

A written record of each complaint should be kept in a file(s) designated for drug product complaints. The file(s) should be maintained in a location where it can be easily retrieved for review during a regulatory inspection. Written records involving a drug product should be maintained until at least one year after the expiration date of the drug product or one year after the date that the complaint was received, whichever is longer. In the case of certain over-the-counter (OTC) drug products that lack expiration dating because they meet the criteria for exemption under 21 CFR 211.137, the written records should be maintained for three years after distribution.

Product Recalls

Recalls are actions taken by a firm (e.g., a manufacturer or distributor) to effectively remove from the market, or correct, consumer products that are in violation of laws administered by FDA. Recalls may be conducted on a firm's own initiative, in response to an FDA request or by FDA order under statutory authority. If many lots of product have been widely distributed, a recall is generally more appropriate than seizure and affords better protection for consumers. Seizure, multiple seizure or other court action is indicated when a firm refuses to undertake a recall requested by FDA or when the agency has reason to believe that a recall would not be effective, determines that a recall is ineffective or discovers that a violation is continuing.

There are three classes of recalls:

- Class I Recall—when there is a reasonable probability that the use of or exposure to a suspected product will cause serious adverse health consequences or death
- Class II Recall—when the use of or exposure to a suspected product may cause temporary or medically reversible adverse health consequences, or where the probability of serious adverse health consequences is remote
- Class III Recall—when use of or exposure to a suspected product is not likely to cause adverse health consequences, but the product violates FDA labeling or manufacturing laws

The product recall process should address the following elements:

- depth of the recall (Depending on the product's degree of hazard and extent of distribution, the recall strategy should specify the level in the distribution chain to which the recall is to be extended, e.g., to the consumer or user level, the retail level or the wholesale level.)
- public warnings to alert affected parties in urgent situations
- effectiveness checks to ensure that all affected parties have received the recall notification and have taken appropriate action

In some cases, the following situations also are considered recalls:

- withdrawal from the market, which occurs when a product has a minor violation that would not be subject to FDA legal action and the firm removes the product from the market or corrects the violation
- medical device safety alert, which is issued in situations where a medical device may present an unreasonable risk of substantial harm

Regulations related to recalls are found in 21 CFR 7.40–7.59. There is also a consumer guide to product recalls on FDA's website at www.fda.gov/ForConsumers/ConsumerUpdates/ucm049070.htm.

Drug Master Files (DMFs)

A DMF (21 CFR 314.420) is a voluntary submission to FDA intended to protect the confidentiality of the information submitted. A DMF provides FDA with details regarding proprietary information such as the chemistry, manufacturing and controls for drug substances, drug products, excipients or packaging materials. Initially, there were five types of DMFs; however, FDA eliminated Type I DMFs in 2000 and requested that information regarding manufacturing sites, facilities, operating procedures, personnel and equipment be submitted in one of the remaining four types of DMFs:

- Type II—chemistry, manufacture and control information for drug substances, intermediates and materials used in their preparation or similar information for drug products
- Type III—component, composition, controls for release and intended uses of packaging materials
- Type IV—excipients, colorants, flavors, essences or materials used in their preparation
- Type V—FDA-accepted reference information

A DMF is prepared in accordance with FDA's 1989 *Guideline for Drug Master Files*. A DMF may be submitted in hard copy form (in duplicate) using either the Common Technical Document (CTD) or traditional format. It also may be submitted in electronic CTD (eCTD) format. The DMF is accompanied by a statement of commitment indicating that all information in the DMF is accurate and that any changes will be communicated to FDA. The DMF also includes a list of firms authorized to reference it in other regulatory applications. If the DMF holder restricts the authorization to particular drug products, the list must include the name of each drug product and the application number, if known, to which the authorization applies. A copy of the letter of authorization to reference the DMF is also provided to each of the firms listed.

A DMF may be used to support an Investigational New Drug Application (IND), NDA or ANDA; an amendment or supplement to these; or another DMF. The DMF is a confidential document and is not available for review by the sponsor of the submission in which it is referenced. FDA reviews the DMF only as part of the review of the application that references it and only if the DMF holder supplies the agency with a letter of authorization for that reference. The sponsor's application references the DMF number, and a copy of the letter of authorization is provided. From a regulatory perspective, DMFs are not officially approved by FDA; they are only reviewed. If deficiencies are noted, FDA will provide a list of deficiencies to the DMF holder and notify the application sponsor that such a list has been provided to the DMF holder. FDA will not disclose the deficiencies to the application sponsor. It is the DMF holder's responsibility to provide responses to FDA and supply additional information, if requested.

With passage of the *Generic Drug User Fee Act (GDUFA)* in 2012, a fee now is required for Type II DMFs that relate specifically to APIs and are referenced in an ANDA, an ANDA Prior Approval Supplement (PAS), or amendment to an ANDA or PAS on or after 1 October 2012. This fee is paid only once during the life of the DMF and the fee facilitates an FDA "Completeness Assessment" of the DMF, which then makes the DMF "available for reference" in future ANDA submissions. Details are provided in FDA's *Draft Guidance for Industry: Initial Completeness Assessments for Type II API DMFs under GDUFA* (October 2012).

Annual updates (Annual Reports) to the DMF are required on the anniversary date of the original submission and should include an updated list of firms authorized to reference the DMF and a list of any changes that have taken place and been reported in an amendment since the last Annual Report. Any technical changes to a DMF should be submitted in the form of a DMF amendment.

A DMF holder may close a DMF by submitting a request to the Drug Master File staff stating the reason for the closure. The request should include a statement that the holder's obligations have been fulfilled. The agency may close a DMF that has not been maintained by Annual Reports and/or amendments. The holder will be notified of FDA's intent to close the DMF and will be given 90 days to appropriately update the DMF to prevent closure.

Changes to Drug Master Files Affecting Approved Applications

Changes to DMFs are submitted in the form of DMF amendments, and the firms authorized to reference the DMF are notified of any change. The sponsor of the application assesses the impact of the change to determine the appropriate reporting category (PAS, CBE-30, CBE-0 or Annual Report) and the timing for distribution of a drug product manufactured using the change, as discussed previously. The sponsor reports the change to the marketing application as appropriate and references the DMF amendment.

Imports and Exports

Drug substances and drug products must comply with the *FD&C Act* to be imported into the US (21 CFR 314.410). Specifically, drug products must be the subject of an approved NDA or ANDA or an active IND (21 CFR 312.110) to be imported into the US. Drug substances may be imported if they are in compliance with the labeling exemption (21 CFR 201.122) and the drug substance is intended for further manufacturing, packaging or other processing operations. Other articles that are components of or are related to unapproved drug products may be imported, even though they do not strictly comply with the *FD&C Act,* if they are processed and incorporated into products that will be exported from the US by their initial owner or consignee ("Import for Export").

Companies that wish to import regulated products into the US are required to file entry notices and entry bonds with the US Customs Service. Imported products are subject to customs inspection at the time of entry. A notification of the product's entry is provided to FDA, which then determines whether the shipment can be admitted through the issuance of a "May Proceed Notice" or "Release Notice." Nonconforming shipments are detained and must either be brought into compliance, destroyed or re-exported; otherwise, the importer will receive a "Notice of Refusal." The burden of proof of compliance with the *FD&C Act* is on the importer, and FDA may detain any shipment that it believes may be unapproved, misbranded or adulterated.

Foreign manufacturers of drug substances and drug products that wish to import products must have a US agent and are required to register with FDA under 21 CFR 207.40 (as described in the Drug Establishment Registration and Drug Listing section of this chapter).

A drug substance or drug product that is the subject of an approved application may be exported. A drug substance that is the subject of an NDA or ANDA may be exported if it has been shown to be within the approved specifications and is shipped with the approved labeling. A drug product that is the subject of an approved NDA or ANDA may be exported in accordance with 21 CFR 314.410. A drug product that is the subject of an active IND may be exported in accordance with 21 CFR 312.110.

Drug Establishment Registration and Drug Listing

The owner or operator of an establishment entering into the manufacture, preparation, propagation, compounding, processing, packaging, repackaging or relabeling of a human or veterinary drug, including blood and blood products and biologicals, must register the establishment electronically within five days after beginning to manufacture commercial products or within five days of submitting a marketing application. In addition, each product in commercial distribution should be listed with FDA. The drug listing should also include bulk drugs for commercial distribution, whether or not they are involved in interstate commerce.

Private label distributors are not currently required to register their commercial products. However, if a distributor chooses not to submit drug listing information directly to FDA, the registered manufacturing establishment must submit the drug listing information. If the private label distributor elects to list directly with FDA, a labeler code is obtained and each product is listed using that code.

In accordance with FDA's *Draft Guidance for Industry: Providing Regulatory Submissions in Electronic Format—Drug Establishment Registration and Drug Listing* (July 2008), a voluntary pilot program was initiated to allow firms to transition their submissions from paper to electronic format, i.e., electronic drug registration and drug listing. The pilot program ended 31 May 2009. In May 2009, FDA published *Guidance for Industry: Providing Regulatory Submissions in Electronic Format—Drug Establishment Registration and Drug Listing*, which stated that, effective 1 June 2009, it is a requirement that the information that was traditionally included in Forms FDA 2656, 2657 and 2658 be submitted electronically in Structured Product Labeling (SPL) format.

Registrants also need to submit the following information in their SPL file:
- official contact's name, mailing address, telephone number(s) and email address
- each registered establishment's telephone number
- type of operation(s) performed at each registered establishment

After the initial registration, establishments are required to re-register annually. A schedule for annual re-registration is provided in 21 CFR 207.21, based on the first letter of the company name. Establishments also are required to provide updated drug listings. Owners and operators of all registered establishments need to update their drug listing information every June and December or at the discretion of the registrant when a change occurs. Foreign drug establishments whose drugs are imported or offered for import into the US must also comply with the establishment registration and drug listing requirements. However, if the drugs enter a foreign trade zone and are re-exported from that foreign trade zone without having entered US commerce, compliance is not required. Each foreign drug establishment required to register must submit the name, address and phone number of its US agent (who must reside in the US) as part of its initial and updated registration information. Only one US agent is allowed per foreign drug establishment. The foreign drug establishment or the US agent should report changes in the agent's name, address or telephone number to FDA within 10 business days of any change.

The information required for each establishment, foreign or domestic, includes:
- drug establishment name and full address
- all trade names used by the establishment
- type of ownership or operation (e.g., individually owned, partnership or corporation)
- name(s) of the establishment's owner, operator, partners or officers

For each drug substance (bulk API) and finished dosage form in commercial distribution, the drug listing information should include:
- trade name
- NDA or ANDA number or OTC monograph number
- business type and product type
- packaging type and size
- manufacturing site
- copies of all current labeling and representative sampling of advertising
- quantitative listing of the active ingredients
- National Drug Code (NDC) number
- for each listed drug product subject to the imprinting requirements of 21 CFR 206, a document that provides the product name; its active ingredient(s); dosage strength; NDC number; manufacturer or distributor name; product's size, shape, color and code imprint (if any); and any other characteristic that identifies the product as unique

The NDC number currently contains 10 digits. The first four or five digits identify the manufacturer or distributor and are known as the Labeler Code. FDA will expand the Labeler Code to six digits when all available five-digit code combinations have been exhausted. FDA assigns Labeler Code numbers and provides them to registrants. The last five or six digits, identifying the drug product and trade package size and type, are known as a product and package code and are assigned by the registrant. An NDC number is requested but not required for all OTC products, although most companies list the NDC number on their labels.

If any material change to a product occurs—such as a change in the active ingredient, dosage form or route of administration—a new NDC number must be assigned to the product by the registrant and the information must be submitted.

If the registrant decides to discontinue a product, the drug listing should be updated to reflect the discontinuation. The same NDC number may be assigned to another drug product five years after the expiration date of the discontinued product or, if there is no expiration date, five years after the last shipment of the discontinued product into commercial distribution.

Upon application, each business entity will be assigned a distinct, site-specific, nine-digit Data Universal Numbering System (D-U-N-S) number. If the D-U-N-S number for a location has not been assigned, a firm may obtain one at no cost directly from Dun & Bradstreet (www.dnb.com). A D-U-N-S number should be submitted for each site-specific entity (e.g., registrant, establishment, US agent and importer).

To prevent confusion, a note on drug establishment and product fees is in order, to ensure the reader understands there is a distinction between these fees and the drug establishment registration and drug listing that is discussed above. As part of *PDUFA*, sponsors with approved drug products must pay annual maintenance fees to FDA related to each approved product (product fees), and owners of establishments where approved products are manufactured also must pay annual fees (establishment fees) to remain in compliance. These fees are set on an annual basis and communicated through a notice in the *Federal Register*.

Inactivation/Withdrawal of Approved Applications

Under 21 CFR 314.150, an approved application may be withdrawn voluntarily (by the sponsor) or involuntarily (by FDA). FDA will withdraw approval of an NDA or ANDA at the sponsor's request if the drug covered in the application is no longer being marketed, provided there are no safety or manufacturing issues with the drug. FDA considers a written request for a withdrawal of approval of an NDA or ANDA to be without prejudice to refiling.

Alternatively, FDA will notify a sponsor and, if appropriate, all other persons who manufacture or distribute identical, related or similar drug products, of its intent to withdraw approval of an application. FDA may request that a sponsor withdraw the approved application if, among other reasons, it determines: the drug is unsafe and there is imminent hazard to the public health; the application contains any untrue statement of a material fact; the sponsor deliberately fails to keep adequate records; or the facilities, processes and/or analytical test methods are not suitable for establishing the drug's identity, strength, quality and purity. For a new drug, the agency will give the sponsor the opportunity for a hearing on the proposal to withdraw approval of the application.

FDA may notify a sponsor if it believes a potential problem associated with a drug is sufficiently serious for the drug to be removed from the market. The agency also may ask the sponsor to waive the opportunity for a hearing to permit FDA to withdraw approval of the NDA or ANDA for the product or to voluntarily remove the product from the market. If the sponsor agrees, the agency will not make an official finding as to the reason for withdrawal but will withdraw approval of the NDA or ANDA in a notice published in the *Federal Register* that contains a brief summary of the agency's and the sponsor's reasons for withdrawal.

Change in Sponsor (Ownership) of an Approved Application

A sponsor may transfer ownership of an application (21 CFR 314.72). At the time of transfer, the following information must be submitted to FDA:
- The former owner shall submit a letter or other document that states that all rights to the application

have been transferred to the new owner as of the transfer date.
- The new owner shall submit a signed application form and a letter or other document containing the new owner's commitment to agreements, promises and conditions made by the former owner and contained in the application; the date the change in ownership is effective; and either a statement that the new owner has a complete copy of the approved application, including supplements and records, or has requested a copy of the application from FDA's files. FDA will provide a copy of the application to the new owner under a standard fee schedule for public information.
- The new owner shall advise FDA of any change in the conditions in the approved application under 21 CFR 314.70, except that the new owner may advise FDA in the next Annual Report about a change in the drug product's label or labeling to change the product's brand or the name of its manufacturer, packer or distributor.

Summary

- Sponsors of approved marketing applications are required to report almost all changes to FDA under the *FD&C Act*. The reporting requirements for changes are summarized in various sections of Title 21 of the CFR as well as FDA guidance documents.
- Sponsors of applications are responsible for ensuring drug substances and drug products for human or veterinary use are manufactured in accordance with applicable CGMP regulations.
- When considering changes to CMC or labeling sections of an approved application, sponsors must evaluate whether the change is major, moderate or minor and submit the supplement that corresponds to that level of change (i.e., Prior Approval Supplement, CBE-30, CBE-0 or Annual Reportable change).
- Drug manufacturing and control sites are subject to periodic inspection in accordance with FDA's compliance program and applicable CGMP regulations.
- Sponsors of approved marketing applications are required to review ADE information obtained from all potential sources. Sponsors are required to report postmarketing safety information to FDA in 15-Day Alert Reports and periodic ADE reports.
- Risk Evaluation and Mitigation Strategies (REMS) may be proposed by application holders or required by FDA when deemed necessary to ensure that a drug or biological product's benefits outweigh its risks.
- Sponsors of approved applications are required to submit an Annual Report. Each copy of the report must be accompanied by a completed Form FDA 2252 (Transmittal of Periodic Reports for Drugs for Human Use). The period covered in the report is defined as one full year from the approval anniversary date of the preceding year. The report should include a summary; distribution data; status of labeling; chemistry, manufacturing and controls information; nonclinical laboratory studies; clinical data; status of postmarketing study requirements and commitments; status of other postmarketing studies; and a log of outstanding regulatory business.
- DMFs are voluntary submissions to FDA containing detailed, confidential CMC information about drug substances, intermediates, drug products, excipients or packaging materials that may be used for human drugs.
- Manufacturers are required to register drug establishments on an annual basis and provide a current drug product list to FDA on a semi-annual basis. Effective 1 June 2009, the information that was traditionally included in Forms FDA 2656, 2657, and 2658 is required to be submitted electronically in SPL format.

Recommended Reading
- FDA and ICH guidance documents listed at the beginning of this chapter
- 21 CFR Parts 7.40-7.59, 210, 211, 310, 312 and 314
- *The Pharmaceutical Regulatory Process*. Ira R. Berry (ed.). Marcel Decker, New York, NY (2005)

Chapter 13

Generic Drug Submissions

Updated by Michael A. Swit, Esq.

OBJECTIVES

❑ To gain an understanding of the history of generic drug development in the US

❑ To gain an understanding of FDA's generic drug approval process and requirements, including the various paths to approval

❑ To gain an understanding of the concepts of bioequivalence and therapeutic equivalence

LAWS, REGULATIONS AND GUIDELINES COVERED IN THIS CHAPTER

❑ *Federal Food, Drug, and Cosmetic Act* of 1938

❑ *Drug Efficacy Amendments* of 1962

❑ *Drug Regulation Reform Act* of 1978

❑ *Drug Price Competition and Patent Term Restoration Act* of 1984 (Hatch-Waxman Act)

❑ *Medicare Prescription Drug, Improvement, and Modernization Act* of 2003

❑ *Prescription Drug User Fee Act* of 1992

❑ *Pediatric Research Equity Act* of 2003

❑ *Generic Drug User Fee Amendments of 2012*

❑ 21 CFR 314 Applications for FDA Approval to Market a New Drug

❑ 21 CFR 320 Bioavailability and Bioequivalence Requirements

❑ 43 *Fed. Reg.* 39,126 (1 September 1978), Abbreviated New Drug Applications; Proposed Related Drug Amendments

❑ 44 *Fed. Reg.* 2932 (12 January 1979), Therapeutically Equivalent Drugs; Availability of List

❑ 45 *Fed. Reg.* 72,582 (31 October 1980), Therapeutically Equivalent Drugs; Availability of List

❑ 45 *Fed. Reg.* 82,052 (12 December 1980), Response to Petition Seeking Withdrawal of the Policy Described in the Agency's "Paper" NDA Memorandum of 31 July 1978

❑ 46 *Fed. Reg.* 27,396 (19 May 1981), Publication of "Paper NDA" Memorandum

❑ 54 *Fed. Reg.* 28,872 (10 July 1989), Proposed ANDA Regulations

❑ 74 *Fed. Reg.* 2849 (16 January 2009) Requirements for submission of bioequivalence data

Chapter 13

❑ Manual of Policies and Procedures 5240.3, "Review Order of Original ANDAs, Amendments, and Supplements" (October 2006)

❑ *Guidance For Industry: Bioavailability and Bioequivalence Studies for Orally Administered Drug Products—General Considerations* (March 2003)

❑ *Draft Guidance for Industry: Applications Covered by Section 505(b)(2)* (October 1999)

Introduction

The term "generic drug" is not defined in the *Federal Food, Drug, and Cosmetic Act* of 1938 (*FD&C Act*) or in US Food and Drug Administration (FDA) regulations. It generally is used, however, to refer to a drug product with the same active ingredient, dosage form, strength and route of administration as a brand-name drug and for which FDA has concluded that the generic can be substituted for the brand-name drug. Generic drugs cost less because the brand-name drug company has already done the work necessary to develop the active ingredient and show it is safe and effective.

The first generic drugs were marketed during the period between the enactment of the *FD&C Act* (Pub. L. No. 75-717, 52 Stat 1040 (1938)) and the enactment of the *Drug Efficacy Amendments* of 1962 (Pub. L. No. 87-781, 76 Stat. 780 (1962)). These products were marketed without FDA approval, on the theory that the agency's approval of the brand-name drug under a New Drug Application (NDA) (based only on safety) made the next version an "old" drug.[1] After the 1962 *Drug Efficacy Amendments*, FDA required the submission of an Abbreviated New Drug Application (ANDA) for each generic version of a "pre-62" brand-name drug FDA had found to be effective under the Drug Efficacy Study Implementation (DESI) program. However, the agency did not permit ANDAs to be submitted for brand-name drugs approved after 1962.[2] This meant a second version of a post-1962 brand-name drug had to obtain full NDA approval. A full NDA typically was economically prohibitive.

Competitive pressure drove some generic drug companies to market both pre- and post-1962 drugs without FDA approval, arguing that an active ingredient became available as an "old" drug after initial FDA approval. FDA's attempts to suppress this practice culminated in the 1983 Supreme Court decision in *United States v. Generix Drug Corp.*, 460 U.S. 453 (1983). The court accepted FDA's position that "old drug" status applied not to the active ingredient but to the individual finished product. Hence, each new version of a drug was a "new drug"[3] requiring FDA approval, no matter how many times FDA had approved its active ingredient.

Aware that its own policies and interpretations were preventing generic competition for post-1962 drugs, FDA took two steps during the 1970's to address the need for an ANDA program for post-1962 drugs:
1. development of the so-called "paper NDA" policy
2. development of ANDA regulations for post-1962 drug products

In 1978, FDA adopted the paper NDA policy, under which the agency accepted a combination of product-specific data and published literature about an active ingredient to satisfy the approval requirements for a full NDA.[4] FDA's paper NDA policy essentially permitted the sponsor of an application for a "duplicate" of a post-1962 drug product (i.e., a drug product that contained the same active ingredients as an already marketed product, in a similar or identical dosage form and for the same indications) to submit published studies and bridging data in support of its application.[5] However, because the paper NDA approach required published literature rather than information not publicly available, it had limited utility for most drugs.[6]

In 1978, FDA issued proposed regulations in which it expressed its intent to extend its pre-1962 ANDA regulations to post-1962 drugs.[7] FDA began to develop these regulations in the early 1980s. The agency's initiative was controversial because it reportedly would have required a substantial waiting period after initial approval of the brand-name drug before any ANDA could be approved for a generic version. Congressional interest in FDA's initiative, however, coincided with a broader effort to develop legislation that would promote both competition and innovation in the drug industry.[8]

As pressure was building for an ANDA program for post-1962 brand drugs, the innovative industry had grown frustrated with the impact of FDA's lengthening approval process for branded drugs, asserting that longer approval times undercut the value of drug patents, which are granted early in the development process and whose then 17-year (now 20-year) term was eaten up in large part before marketing approval was granted. Congress engineered a compromise in which brand-name drug companies could obtain a patent term extension and generic drug companies could obtain ANDA approval for pre- and post-1962 drugs. The compromise was enacted in the *Drug Price Competition and Patent Term Restoration Act* of 1984 (*Hatch-Waxman Act*).

The *Hatch-Waxman Act* amended the new drug approval provisions of the *FD&C Act* to add Section 505(j). Section 505(j) formalized the legal structure for generic drugs, under which an ANDA containing bioequivalence data to a brand drug—the "Reference Listed Drug" (RLD)—among other data and information, was sufficient for FDA to consider approval. As explained in "Chapter 14, Patents and Exclusivity," the *Hatch-Waxman Act* also amended the patent laws to authorize a patent term extension that could be as long as five years for time lost during the regulatory review period.[9] The new law also required that brand-name drug firms "list" patents with FDA that they asserted claimed the branded drug (ingredient or product) or a method for using the branded product. FDA lists these patents—and all drug approvals—in a publication known as the *Orange Book* (after its cover's original color), the formal name of which is "Approved Drug Products With Therapeutic Equivalence Evaluations."

Under the *FD&C Act* (as amended by the *Hatch-Waxman Act*), ANDA approval is subject to several restrictions. First, non-patent market exclusivity provisions of three or five years were added by the *Hatch-Waxman Act* to compensate brand-name drug companies for allowing reliance on their proprietary research. Second, an ANDA applicant must notify the NDA holder and patent owner (if different) if an *Orange Book*-listed patent claims the RLD; if the NDA owner files a patent infringement suit, approval of the ANDA is deferred. Third, an ANDA drug product must contain the "same" active ingredient as the brand-name drug and have essentially the same labeling, including indications, warnings, contraindications, etc.

ANDA Approval Process

The premise of *FD&C Act* Section 505(j) is that an ANDA drug is the "same as" the brand-name drug—i.e., the RLD, defined as "the listed drug identified by FDA as the drug product upon which an applicant relies in seeking approval of its abbreviated application" (21 CFR 314.3(b)).[10] However, "same" does not mean "identical." Differences may be allowed in route of administration, dosage form and strength as well as in a single active ingredient in a combination drug product if those differences are first approved by FDA under a suitability petition as not requiring clinical investigations.[11] *FD&C Act* Section 505(j)(2)(A) states that an ANDA (that is not the subject of an approved suitability petition) must contain information to show, among other things, that the active ingredient, "the route of administration, the dosage form, and the strength of the new drug are the same as those of the [RLD]."[12]

An ANDA must contain, among other things identified in the *FD&C Act* and in FDA's ANDA format and content regulations at 21 CFR 314.94, information demonstrating that the generic version is bioequivalent to the RLD.[13] This information may come from *in vivo* (human) and/or *in vitro* (test tube) studies (21 CFR 320). The purpose of demonstrating bioequivalence is to determine whether the inherent changes from the brand-name product that are presented by the proposed generic drug product's formulation or manufacturing affect the rate or extent to which the active ingredient reaches the primary site of action. Although data and information demonstrating *in vivo* bioequivalence often are required, FDA may waive this requirement if *in vivo* bioequivalence is considered self-evident (e.g., in the case of many injectable drugs) or for other reasons (21 CFR 320.22).[14]

A drug product is considered bioequivalent to the RLD if:

(i) the rate and extent of absorption of the drug do not show a significant difference from the rate and extent of absorption of the listed drug when administered at the same molar dose of the therapeutic ingredient under similar experimental conditions in either a single dose or multiple doses

or

(ii) the extent of absorption of the drug does not show a significant difference from the extent of absorption of the listed drug when administered at the same molar dose of the therapeutic ingredient under similar experimental conditions in either a single dose or multiple doses and the difference from the listed drug in the rate of absorption of the drug is intentional, is reflected in its proposed labeling, is not essential to the attainment of effective body drug concentrations on chronic use, and is considered medically insignificant for the drug. (*FD&C Act* Section 505(j)(8)(B); 21 CFR 320.1(e))

The choice of which *in vivo* bioequivalence study design to use is based on the ability of the design to compare the drug delivered by the test (generic) and reference (brand-name) drug products at the drug's particular site of action. In a standard *in vivo* bioequivalence study, single doses of the test and reference drug products are administered to volunteers (usually 24–36 healthy adults), and the rate and extent of absorption of the drug is determined from measured plasma concentrations over time for each subject participating in the study. The extent of absorption (i.e., how much of the drug in the given dose was absorbed) is reflected through various measurements. The preferred study design for oral dosage forms is a single-dose, fasting, two-treatment, two-sequence crossover design with a washout period between treatments.[15] In a crossover study, the subjects receive the test and reference drug products in separate sequences (either test before reference or reference before test), with a period between treatments of no drug administration (the washout period) to ensure the previous dose is cleared from the body before the second dose is administered. To demonstrate *in vitro* bioequivalence, FDA recommends that an applicant use an *in vitro* test (e.g., a dissolution rate test) that has been correlated with *in vivo* data.[16] Over the past couple of years, FDA has begun to publish individual product bioequivalence recommendations on its website. FDA has published almost 850 product-specific bioequivalence recommendations already and the agency's website is regularly updated with new recommendations.

An ANDA for a generic version of a brand-name drug (the RLD) also must contain one of four possible

Figure 13-1. ANDA Backlog

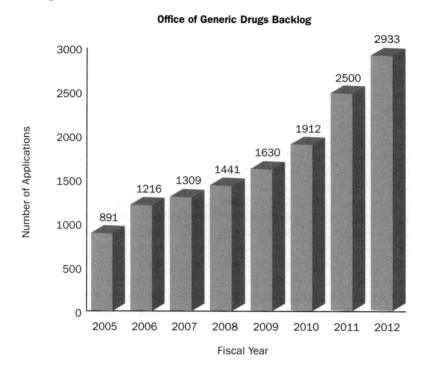

certifications "with respect to each patent which claims the [brand-name] drug...or which claims a use for such listed drug...and for which information is required to be filed" by the NDA holder and that is listed in the *Orange Book* (*FD&C Act* Section 505(j)(2)(A)(vii)). The consequences of the various types of patent certifications are discussed in Chapter 14.

Once an applicant submits an ANDA to FDA, the agency reviews the submission to determine whether the application is sufficiently complete to permit receipt (21 CFR 314.101). FDA generally reviews ANDA submissions within 60 days after they are submitted; however, the agency's decision on whether to receive an ANDA may take longer. If FDA receives an ANDA, the agency performs an in-depth review to determine whether to approve the application. In the past, this review typically took 15–18 months; however, due to a significant backlog of pending ANDAs at FDA—which has increased steadily since 2006 (**Figure 13-1**) and currently stands at about 2,930 original ANDAs—the review process has taken longer in recent years. For example, in Fiscal 2011, the median approval time for an original ANDA was 29.5 months (**Figure 13-2**), and is currently reported to be about 34 months. At the end of its review, the agency either approves or refuses to approve the ANDA (21 CFR 314.127 identifies the reasons for refusing to approve an ANDA). If approved, the generic drug product is listed in the *Orange Book* and may be identified as a "therapeutic equivalent" to the RLD.

Although FDA generally reviews ANDA submissions on a "first in, first reviewed" basis to ensure fair and even-handed treatment of applicants, there are exceptions. For example, an ANDA applicant may qualify for FDA's expedited ANDA review policy:

Certain applications may be identified at the time of submission for expedited review. These include products to respond to current and anticipated public health emergencies, products under special review programs such as the President's Emergency Plan for AIDS Relief (PEPFAR),[17] products for which a nationwide shortage has been identified, and first generic products for which there are no blocking patents or exclusivities on the reference listed drug.[18]

FDA's ANDA approval process is illustrated in **Figure 13-3**.

A Few Words on ANDA Suitability Petitions

Two laws enacted over the past several years have significantly affected suitability petitions with respect to both their availability and their utility.

First, the *Pediatric Research Equity Act* (*PREA*), which was signed into law on 3 December 2003 and amended the *FD&C Act* to add new Section 505B, significantly impacts the economic attractiveness of securing a change to an RLD via an ANDA suitability petition.[19] Under *PREA* and *FD&C Act* Section 505B, Congress granted FDA the statutory authority to require pediatric studies

Figure 13-2. Median ANDA Approval Times

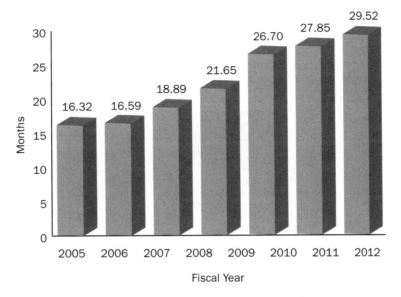

in certain defined circumstances retroactive to 1 April 1999. Specifically, *FD&C Act* Section 505B states that an applicant "that submits an application (or supplement to an application) under section 505 [of the *FD&C Act*] for a new active ingredient, new indication, new dosage form, new dosing regimen, or new route of administration…shall submit with the application" the results of pediatric studies assessing "the safety and effectiveness of the drug…for the claimed indications in all relevant pediatric subpopulations; and to support dosing and administration for each pediatric subpopulation for which the drug…is safe and effective, [unless FDA] concludes that pediatric effectiveness can be extrapolated from adequate and well-controlled studies in adults, usually supplemented with other information obtained in pediatric patients," or unless FDA defers or partially or fully waives this requirement.[20]

An ANDA requiring an approved suitability petition for a change in the RLD with respect to an active ingredient (in a combination drug), route of administration or dosage form meets the criteria of *FD&C Act* Section 505B(1)(A), because it is a type of application submitted under *FD&C Act* Section 505. The only change permitted by a suitability petition that does not trigger the requirements of *FD&C Act* Section 505B is a change in strength from that of the RLD.

FD&C Act Section 505(j)(2)(C)(i) requires FDA to deny a suitability petition if "investigations must be conducted to show the safety and effectiveness of the drug or of any of its active ingredients, the route of administration, the dosage form, or strength which differ from the listed drug." Thus, unless FDA fully waives the *PREA* pediatric studies requirement, the requirement to conduct (or even a deferral from conducting) pediatric studies triggers the statutory requirement to deny a suitability petition.

Second, the *Medicare Prescription Drug, Improvement, and Modernization Act* of 2003 (*MMA*) (Pub. L. No. 108-173, 117 Stat. 2066 (2003)), amended the *FD&C Act* to preclude a generic applicant with a pending ANDA from amending its application to change the RLD. Specifically, *FD&C Act* Section 505(j)(2)(D)(i), the 505(b)(2) application counterpart for which is at *FD&C Act* Section 505(b)(4)(A), states, "[A]n applicant may not amend or supplement an [ANDA] to seek approval of a drug referring to a different listed drug from the listed drug identified in the application as submitted to [FDA]."[21]

FDA recently addressed *FD&C Act* Section 505(j)(2)(D)(i) in a citizen petition response. The agency determined that an applicant with a pending ANDA subject to an approved suitability petition must submit a new application to the agency as the result of the approval of another applicant's NDA for a drug product that is the pharmaceutical equivalent of the drug product described in the pending ANDA, and which is, therefore, the appropriate RLD that should be cited by the applicant.[22] Thus, if at any time before approval of an ANDA subject to an approved suitability petition (or a 505(b)(2) application), another drug product is approved that is the pharmaceutical equivalent—or that is more pharmaceutically similar to the product in a pending 505(b)(2) application—FDA could require the applicant to cite a new RLD to support its petition. And, as a result of the statutory prohibition on amending an ANDA to change the RLD, FDA could require the applicant to submit a new application containing a certification or statement to any relevant *Orange Book*-listed patents (as well as required bioequivalence/bioavailability information).

Figure 13-3. FDA's ANDA Approval Process

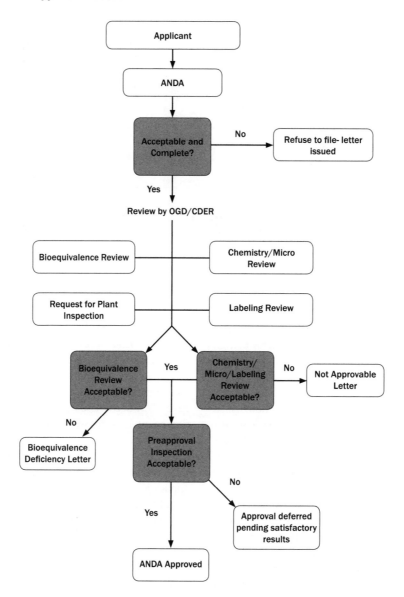

A Few Words on Inactive Ingredients

FD&C Act Section 505(j)(4)(H) states FDA must approve an ANDA unless, among other things:

> (I)nformation submitted in the application or any other information available to [FDA] shows that (i) the inactive ingredients of the drug are unsafe for use under the conditions prescribed, recommended, or suggested in the labeling proposed for the drug, or (ii) the composition of the drug is unsafe under such conditions because of the type or quantity of inactive ingredients included or the manner in which the inactive ingredients are included.

FDA's regulations implementing *FD&C Act* Section 505(j)(4)(H) generally are found in the agency's ANDA content and format regulations at 21 CFR 314.94. Pertinent regulations on inactive ingredient changes for certain types of generic drug products are set forth in 21 CFR 314.94(a)(9). For example, FDA's regulations for parenteral drug products at 21 CFR 314.94(a)(9)(iii) state:

> Generally, a drug product intended for parenteral use shall contain the same inactive ingredients and in the same concentration as the [RLD] identified by the applicant under paragraph (a)(3) of this section. However, an applicant may seek approval of a drug product that differs from the reference listed drug in preservative, buffer, or antioxidant provided that the applicant

identifies and characterizes the differences and provides information demonstrating that the differences do not affect the safety or efficacy of the proposed drug product.

Preservative, buffer and antioxidant changes in generic parenteral drug products are referred to as "exception excipients," which may differ qualitatively or quantitatively from the RLD formulation. Other regulations under 21 CFR 314.94(a)(9)(iv) identify exception excipients for generic ophthalmic and otic drug products (i.e., preservative, buffer, substance to adjust tonicity and thickening agent). Excipients not identified in these regulations are referred to as "non-exception excipients."

FDA's exception excipient regulations under 21 CFR 314.94(a)(9) find their parallel in 21 CFR 314.127(a)(8)(ii), which addresses the grounds for an FDA refusal to approve an ANDA for a parenteral, ophthalmic or otic drug product. For example, one regulation states: "FDA will consider an inactive ingredient in, or the composition of, a drug product intended for parenteral use to be unsafe and will refuse to approve the [ANDA] unless it contains the same inactive ingredients, other than preservatives, buffers, and antioxidants, in the same concentration as the listed drug."[23] Thus, it is important that a company understand the possible implications of changing certain drug product formulations. If such a change is for a non-exception excipient, FDA would, unless under a narrow exception discussed below, refuse to receive or approve an ANDA. Instead a company would need to submit a 505(b)(2) application for the proposed drug product, which, like other NDAs, is subject to much higher user fees under the *Prescription Drug User Fee Act* (*PDUFA*) than those that apply to generic drugs under the *Generic Drug User Fee Amendments* of 2012, which were passed as part of the *Food and Drug Administration Safety and Innovation Act* (*FDASIA*) of 2012 (Pub. L. No. 112-144, 126 Stat. 993 (2012)). For Fiscal 2013, the one-time, full NDA user fee is $1,958,800, and annual product and establishment user fees are $98,380 and $526,500, respectively. In contrast, the ANDA user fee is $51,520 and the establishment fee is $175,389, and no separate product fee exists for generic drugs.

Notwithstanding FDA's exception excipient regulations, the agency has in very limited circumstances, waived these regulations to permit the receipt and approval of an ANDA for a drug product containing a non-exception excipient change from the RLD.

FDA's regulations at 21 CFR 314.99(b) state that a generic applicant "may ask FDA to waive…any requirement that applies to the applicant under 21 CFR 314.92–314.99. The applicant shall comply with the requirements for a waiver under 21 CFR 314.90." 21 CFR 314.90, the parallel waiver regulation for 505(b) applicants, describes the information an applicant must submit to support a waiver request, and states that FDA may grant a waiver if the agency finds: "(1) the applicant's compliance with the requirement is unnecessary for the agency to evaluate the application or compliance cannot be achieved; (2) the applicant's alternative submission satisfies the requirement; or (3) the applicant's submission otherwise justifies a waiver."[24] Pursuant to this regulation, FDA may waive its ANDA exception excipient regulations under 21 CFR 314.99(b) so the agency can receive and approve an ANDA.

FDA has granted a 21 CFR 314.99(b) waiver when an ANDA applicant seeks approval to market a drug product containing a non-exception excipient used in a discontinued RLD formulation that is not used in the currently marketed RLD formulation. For example, FDA has allowed applicants seeking approval to market generic Sandostatin (octreotide acetate) Injection to substitute a different tonicity agent (a non-exception excipient change) and buffer system because "the inactive ingredients (including the buffer system and tonicity agent) used in the discontinued formulation of Sandostatin do not make that formulation unsafe…[and because] the discontinued formulation of Sandostatin is no less safe and effective than the new formulation."[25]

Therapeutic Equivalence

The term "therapeutic equivalence" is not defined in the *FD&C Act* or in FDA's ANDA regulations. However, "[d]rug products are considered to be therapeutic equivalents only if they are pharmaceutical equivalents and if they can be expected to have the same clinical effect and safety profile when administered to patients under the conditions specified in the labeling" (i.e., are bioequivalent).[26] "FDA believes that products classified as therapeutically equivalent can be substituted with the full expectation that the substituted product will produce the same clinical effect and safety profile as the prescribed product."[27]

FDA's regulations define the term "pharmaceutical equivalents" to mean:

> (D)rug products in identical dosage forms that contain identical amounts of the identical active drug ingredient, i.e., the same salt or ester of the same therapeutic moiety, or, in the case of modified release dosage forms that require a reservoir or overage or such forms as prefilled syringes where residual volume may vary, that deliver identical amounts of the active drug ingredient over the identical dosing period; do not necessarily contain the same inactive ingredients; and meet the identical compendial or other applicable standard of identity, strength, quality, and purity, including potency and, where applicable, content uniformity, disintegration times, and/or dissolution rates.[28]

As explained above, the term "bioequivalence" is defined in the *FD&C Act* and FDA's regulations.[29] Because therapeutic equivalence requires two drug products to be pharmaceutically equivalent and bioequivalent in order to be substitutable, "pharmaceutical alternatives" are not therapeutic equivalents and are not substitutable for the RLD relied upon for approval. FDA's regulations define "pharmaceutical alternatives" as:

> (D)rug products that contain the identical therapeutic moiety, or its precursor, but not necessarily in the same amount or dosage form or as the same salt or ester. Each such drug product individually meets either the identical or its own respective compendial or other applicable standard of identity, strength, quality, and purity, including potency and, where applicable, content uniformity, disintegration times and/or dissolution rates.[30]

Thus, products approved pursuant to an approved suitability petition (i.e., a change in strength, route of administration, dosage form or active ingredient in a combination drug) are pharmaceutical alternatives and are not listed in the *Orange Book* as therapeutically equivalent to the RLD. To give one common example, tablets and capsules are considered different dosage forms. Therefore, they are pharmaceutical alternatives, not pharmaceutical equivalents. Consequently, they will not be "A-rated" in the *Orange Book* (described below), even if they are bioequivalent.

Pharmaceutically equivalent prescription drug products (i.e., multisource drug products approved under *FD&C Act* Section 505) usually are identified in the *Orange Book* with either an "A" or "B" therapeutic equivalence code designation, which is further defined by a one-character subcode.[31] (There are six "A" subcodes and 10 "B" subcodes.[32]) The *Orange Book* coding system for therapeutic equivalence evaluations allows users to determine whether FDA has evaluated a particular approved drug product as therapeutically equivalent to other pharmaceutically equivalent drug products (the first character in a code) and provides additional information on the basis of FDA's evaluations (the second character in a code). "A-rated" drug products are considered to be to therapeutically equivalent to other pharmaceutically equivalent products because there are no known or suspected bioequivalence problems or such problems have been resolved with adequate evidence supporting bioequivalence. "B-rated" drug products are not considered to be therapeutically equivalent to other pharmaceutically equivalent drug products because actual or potential bioequivalence problems identified by FDA have not been resolved by adequate bioequivalence evidence.

Drug products assigned an "A" rating fall under one of two categories:

- those active ingredients or dosage forms for which no *in vivo* bioequivalence issue is known or suspected, and for which bioequivalence to the RLD is presumed and considered self-evident based on other data in an application or by a showing that an acceptable *in vitro* dissolution standard is met

- those active ingredients or dosage forms presenting a potential bioequivalence problem, but the applicant's approved application contains adequate scientific evidence establishing (through *in vivo* and/or *in vitro* studies) the bioequivalence of the product to a selected RLD

Drug products that fall under the first category are assigned a therapeutic equivalence code depending upon the dosage form. These codes include AA, AN, AO, AP or AT.[33] Drug products that fall under the second category are coded AB, the most common code assignment.

Drug products assigned a "B" rating fall under one of three categories:

- FDA has documented bioequivalence problems or a significant potential for such problems (and no adequate studies demonstrating bioequivalence have been submitted to the agency)
- FDA has an insufficient basis to determine therapeutic equivalence (e.g., quality standards are inadequate)
- the drug products are under regulatory review

Drug products that fall under these categories are assigned a therapeutic equivalence code largely based upon dosage form. These codes are B*, BC, BD, BE, BN, BP, BR, BS, BT or BX.[34] FDA's assignment of a "B" rating does not mean that a particular drug product is not safe and effective. (Indeed, the applicant has provided sufficient data to meet the statutory and regulatory approval criteria.) Rather, a "B" rating means that FDA has identified unresolved actual or potential bioequivalence problems, and that because of those problems a particular drug product cannot be considered to be therapeutically equivalent to other pharmaceutically equivalent drug products.

A generic drug that is a pharmaceutical alternative to an RLD (e.g., tablet versus capsule) is not assigned a therapeutic equivalence code (such drug products are, by definition, not therapeutic equivalents). Instead, they are listed separately in the *Orange Book* as single-source drug products. However, because each *Orange Book*-listed drug product may be designated as an RLD (pursuant to a request to FDA to assign RLD status), a generic applicant could cite the approved drug as the RLD and obtain approval of an ANDA for a pharmaceutically equivalent drug product. In such a case, if the drug is also shown to be bioequivalent to the RLD, FDA could assign both drug products an "A" therapeutic equivalence code appropriate for such a multisource drug product.

Therapeutic equivalence codes are assigned by FDA based on the agency's scientific and medical evaluations of a marketing application for a generic version of a listed drug. The assignment of a particular therapeutic equivalence code reflects the agency's application of specific criteria to multisource drug products (i.e., those criteria identified in reference 15). As FDA explained in the preamble to the proposal establishing the *Orange Book*:

> The term "therapeutically equivalent drug products" simply means that two such drug products can be expected, in the judgment of FDA, to have equivalent therapeutic effect and equivalent potential for adverse effects when used under the conditions set forth in their labeling. Drug products that are therapeutically equivalent may still vary in certain respects: color, shape, taste, or packaging for example. As a result, patients may not perceive them as identical or equally acceptable. For this reason, it cannot be stated that such drug products are substitutable or interchangeable in all cases. The judgment is not FDA's as to whether different drug products are substitutable or interchangeable for use by a particular patient; rather, it rests with practitioners who, in prescribing and dispensing drug products, can take into consideration the unique characteristics, needs, or problems of individual patients. It is the agency's position, however, that if one therapeutically equivalent drug product is substituted for another under State law, with due professional regard for the individual patient, there is no substantial reason to believe that the patient will receive a drug product that is different in terms of the therapeutic effect intended.[35]

As to the legal status of the *Orange Book*, FDA has commented that it "contain[s] only public information and advice," and that it "[imposes] no requirement or restriction upon any person; it [does] not interpret or apply the [*FD&C Act*] in a manner that creates any obligation on any person; it [makes] no recommendation as to which products persons should purchase, prescribe, or dispense, or conversely, which products should be avoided."[36] However, the criteria FDA uses to assign therapeutic equivalence codes "are regulatory determinations which FDA is statutorily authorized to make."[37]

As to the clinical appropriateness of (and risks associated with) substituting drug products FDA does not consider to be therapeutically equivalent (e.g., a drug product with a two-character "B" therapeutic equivalence code), such issues are generally a matter of state law.[38] FDA emphasized this point in the preamble to the 1979 *Orange Book* proposal: "[A] primary purpose of [the *Orange Book*] is to provide State agencies and officials with information relating to drug products that may be selected for dispensing under applicable State law."[39]

Drug product substitutions must be made in accordance with each individual state's pharmacy practice act. There are, in general, four different approaches taken by such laws:

- the positive formulary approach (requiring that substitution be limited to drugs on a specific list, often the *Orange Book*)
- the negative formulary approach (permitting substitution for all drugs except those prohibited by a particular list—usually drugs for which there are no "A-rated" products listed in the *Orange Book*)
- the combined positive and negative formulary approach
- the "non-formulary" approach (i.e., there is not a clearly defined positive or negative formulary)[40]

In addition, state pharmacy laws may extend the prescribing authority granted to pharmacists beyond substituting a generic drug. For example, pharmacists may be permitted to substitute a product from the same class of drug, even though the drug is not identified in the *Orange Book* as therapeutically equivalent to the prescribed drug product. This procedure is known as "therapeutic interchange." The laws covering therapeutic interchange vary widely from state to state.[41] Thus, the "clinical appropriateness" of substituting drug products FDA does not consider to be therapeutically equivalent is handled on a state-by-state basis. The consequences for violating a particular state substitution law are governed by the laws of that state.

User Fees

With the backlog of unapproved ANDAs reaching over 2,900 by the end of Fiscal 2011 and reportedly not reduced since (see **Figure 13-2**), FDA, Congress and the generic industry realized that historic industry resistance to user fees had to yield to the vital need to markedly increase human resources within the Office of Generic Drugs (OGD) to tackle the backlog. Thus, in 2012, Congress—in addition to addressing the need to re-authorize user fees for innovative drugs, biologics and medical device every-five years—enacted, as Title III of *FDASIA*, the *Generic Drug User Fee Amendments* of 2012 (*GDUFA*).

GDUFA contains a number of provisions aimed at reducing the backlog. First, it established user fees for the review of newly-submitted ANDAs and supplements requiring prior FDA approval (PAS) to cover changes to a previously-approved ANDA. For Fiscal 2013, those fees are $51,250 and $25,760, respectively. Second, to address the backlog of existing ANDAs, *GDUFA* created a "backlog" fee of $17,434 applicable to all ANDAs pending as of 1 October 2012. Third, *GDUFA* mandated that facilities involved in the generic drug process had to pay a "facility" fee that varies depending on the nature of the facility, as follows:

- domestic finished dosage form facility: $175,389
- foreign finished dosage form facility: $190,389
- domestic active pharmaceutical ingredient facility: $26,458
- foreign active pharmaceutical ingredient facility: $41,458

Note that the fees for finished dosage form facilities are due in full even if the facility only is involved in making a single generic drug product; no "small business" or similar waiver or reduction is available.

Finally, any active pharmaceutical ingredient manufacturer whose drug master file (DMF) is referenced in a "generic drug submission" on or after 1 October 2012 must pay a fee of $21,340 the first time their DMF is referenced. The DMF fee is assessed only once and is not charged if the DMF is referenced in later generic drug submissions. For purposes of the DMF fee, a submission triggering the fee includes an ANDA, an amendment to an ANDA or a prior approval supplement. As with many FDA initiatives, a number of guidances have been issued relating to GDUFA.

At this writing, it is too early to tell how GDUFA will impact FDA's processing of ANDAs. Indeed, organizational changes also have been implemented at FDA, including elevating OGD to "super office" status, reporting directly to Center for Drug Evaluation and Research (CDER) Director Janet Woodcock, which will affect the handling of ANDAs. In addition, the resignation in March 2013 of Gregory Geba, MD, as director of OGD and the shifting of OGD's chemistry reviewers from OGD to the newly-formed CDER Office of Pharmaceutical Quality have raised issues over the management of the generic drug review process that readers will need to track carefully going forward.

Summary

The term "generic drug" is not defined in the *FD&C Act* or in FDA regulations. It generally is used, however, to refer to a drug product that is the same as a brand-name drug in these key aspects: active ingredient, dosage form, route of administration and strength, and for which FDA has determined that the generic version is therapeutically equivalent to the branded drug. As a result of these "sameness" aspects, state law typically allows a pharmacist to substitute the generic for a branded drug in filling a prescription. When combined with the lower costs of a generic drug—because the brand-name drug company has already done the work necessary to develop the active ingredient and show that it is safe and effective for its indications—the generic can be sold for a fraction of the brand-name price. The approval of generic drugs in the US is governed by a tapestry of laws, regulations and FDA policies developed over the past few decades. While a complex regime, the generic drug approval process has allowed the use of generic drugs to rise to a level of more than 80% of all prescriptions filled in the US and is estimated to have saved Americans close to a billion dollars over the past 10 years.

References

1. Karst KR. "Marketed Unapproved Drugs–Past, Present and Future?" *Regulatory Affairs Focus*, Vol. 12, No. 2, pp 37–42 (February 2007).
2. ANDAs were permitted under FDA regulations for duplicates (i.e., generic versions). The term "duplicate" applied to a drug product that was the same as an already approved drug product in dosage form, route of administration, kind and amount of active ingredient, indication(s) and any other conditions of use. FDA regulations permitted ANDAs for "similar" and "related" products only if the agency had made a separate finding (following a firm's petition) that an ANDA was appropriate for that drug product.
3. A product that is a "new drug" within the meaning of *FD&C Act* Section 201(p) may not be introduced into interstate commerce unless there is an approved marketing application (e.g., an NDA), or unless an exemption has been granted permitting the introduction of the drug into interstate commerce (e.g., an effective Investigational New Drug Application (IND)).
4. The "paper NDA" policy is described in a 31 July 1978 FDA staff memorandum. The policy was not originally published in the *Federal Register* because FDA determined that rulemaking procedures were not required because "the policy is a lawful exercise of FDA's statutory authority…" 45 *Fed. Reg.* 82,052 (12 December 1980). FDA was challenged on this issue in court and won. See *Burroughs Wellcome Co. v. Schweiker*, 649 F.2d 221, 225 (4th Cir. 1981). Subsequently, in separate litigation, the US District Court for the Northern District of Illinois ruled that upon publication of FDA's policy in the *Federal Register*, the agency could implement it without rulemaking procedures. See *American Critical Care v. Schweiker*, Food, Drug, Cosm. L. Rep. (CCH) 1980-81 Transfer Binder ¶ 38, 110 (N.D. Ill. 1981).
5. The published studies requirement could be met by referencing data available in published literature, laboratory reports, physician evaluation forms and even unpublished reports when available and necessary. However, the underlying data did not have to be included or referenced, as was required under FDA's old interpretation of "full reports" in *FD&C Act* Section 505(b)(1). Reference to information not publicly available was not permitted, including information in the brand-name product's NDA. The "bridging" data requirement could be met by submitting data from a bioavailability/bioequivalence study comparing the drug that was the subject of the "paper NDA" to the approved drug "to show that the drug is comparable in blood levels (or dissolution rate, as required) to the innovator's product." 46 *Fed. Reg.* at 27,397.
6. FDA revoked the "paper NDA" policy in 1989 when the agency proposed regulations implementing the *Drug Price Competition and Patent Term Restoration Act*, Pub. L. No. 98-417, 98 Stat. 1585 (1984) (*Hatch-Waxman Act*). See FDA, Proposed Rule, ANDA Regulations, 54 *Fed. Reg.* 28,872, 28, 890 (10 July 1989).
7. 43 *Fed. Reg.* 39126, 39128 (1 September 1978).
8. *Drug Regulation Reform Act*, 95th Cong., 2d Sess. (1978); *Drug Regulation Reform Act*, 96th Cong., 1st Sess. (1979).
9. The *Hatch-Waxman Act* also replaced the "paper NDA" with the 505(b)(2) application. The *FD&C Act* describes a 505(b)(2) application as an application "for a drug for which the investigations… relied upon by the applicant for approval of the application were not conducted by or for the applicant and for which the applicant has not obtained a right of reference or use from the person by or for whom the investigations were conducted." *FD&C Act* Section 505(b)(2). A 505(b)(2) application differs from a "paper NDA" in that it permits the sponsor of a drug that may differ substantially from a drug listed in FDA's *Approved Drug Products with Therapeutic Equivalence Evaluations* (commonly referred to as the *Orange Book* because of its bright orange cover) to rely on FDA's determination of the safety and effectiveness of a referenced drug and/or on published studies or studies in an NDA (or NDAs) sponsored by another person, together with studies generated on its own drug product, as a way to satisfy the requirement of "full reports" of safety and effectiveness. As with the old "paper NDA" policy, "bridging" studies to the referenced drug are necessary. An application that is for a duplicate of a drug listed in the *Orange Book* and eligible for approval as a generic drug under the ANDA provisions of *FD&C Act* Section 505(j) may not be submitted as a 505(b)(2) application.

10. While an ANDA applicant must identify an RLD in its application, a 505(b)(2) applicant must identify a "listed drug" (or drugs) in its application if the applicant seeks to rely on FDA's previous finding of safety or efficacy for that listed drug(s). While there are no FDA regulations governing how a 505(b)(2) applicant should choose a listed drug when various options are present, FDA has spoken to the issue in guidance and in citizen petition responses. FDA has stated that "[i]f there is a listed drug that is the pharmaceutical equivalent of the drug proposed in the 505(b)(2) application, the 505(b)(2) applicant should provide patent certifications for the patents listed for the pharmaceutically equivalent drug." FDA, *Draft Guidance for Industry: Applications Covered by Section 505(b)(2)*, at 8 (October 1999). This serves to "ensure that the 505(b)(2) applicant does not use the 505(b)(2) process to end-run patent protections that would have applied had an ANDA been permitted." FDA, Citizen Petition Response, Docket No. FDA-2004-P-0089 (formerly 2004P-0386), at 9 (30 November 2004) (hereinafter "RLD Choice Petition Response"). Additionally, these provisions "further ensure that the 505(b)(2) applicant (and FDA) can rely, to the maximum extent possible, on what is already known about a drug without having to re-prove (or re-review) what has already been demonstrated." Id.

    "When there is no listed drug that is a pharmaceutical equivalent to the drug product proposed in the 505(b)(2) NDA, neither the statute, the regulations, nor the Draft Guidance directly addresses how to identify the listed drug or drugs on which a 505(b)(2) applicant is to rely." Id. In FDA's RLD Choice Petition Response, however, the agency stated that:

    > it follows that the more similar a proposed drug is to the listed drug cited, the smaller the quantity of data that will be needed to support the proposed change. Accordingly, to avoid unnecessary duplication of research and review, when a section 505(b)(2) application has been submitted and no pharmaceutically equivalent drug product has previously been approved, the 505(b)(2) applicant should choose the listed drug or drugs that are most similar to the drug for which approval is sought. Similarly, if all the information relied on by FDA for approval...is contained in a single previously approved application and that application is a pharmaceutical equivalent or the most similar alternative to the product for which approval is sought, the 505(b)(2) applicant should certify only to the patents for that application. This is the case even when another application also contains some or all of the same information. Id.

    FDA has not defined the factors that should be taken into account when determining "similarity" of drug products; however, FDA likely considers factors such as active ingredient, dosage form, route of administration, and strength. See 21 CFR 320.1(c).

11. See *FD&C Act* Section 505(j)(2)(C); 21 CFR 314.93. As discussed later in this chapter, the *Pediatric Research Equity Act* (*PREA*), Pub. L. No. 108-155, 117 Stat. 1936 (2003), which amended the *FD&C Act* to require that most applications submitted under *FD&C Act* Section 505 include a pediatric assessment (unless otherwise waived or deferred), has significantly restricted FDA's ability to approve suitability petitions. See generally *FD&C Act* Section 505B.

12. FDA has interpreted the term *same as* to mean identical in the context of dosage forms, see 21 CFR 314.92(a)(1), and has used its discretion to interpret the term *identical* to mean products that have the same dosage form identified in the *Orange Book* at Appendix C ("Uniform Terms—Dosage Forms"). See FDA, Citizen Petition Response, Docket No. 1993P-0421, at 3 (12 August 1997) ("[A] proposed drug product has the same dosage form if it falls within the identical dosage form category, as listed in the *Orange Book*, Appendix C.").

13. See *FD&C Act* Section 505(j)(2)(A)(iv).

14. The *FD&C Act* states that an ANDA must include, among other things, "information to show that the new drug is bioequivalent to the [RLD]...," *FD&C Act* Section505(j)(2)(A)(iv), and that FDA must approve an ANDA unless, among other things, "information submitted in the application is insufficient to show that the drug is bioequivalent to the [RLD] . . . ." Id. at Section505(j)(4)(F). However, FDA has discretion to determine how the bioequivalence requirement is met. See *FD&C Act* Section 505(j)(7)(A)(i)(III). FDA's discretion need only be based on a "reasonable and scientifically supported criterion, whether [the agency] chooses to do so on a case-by-case basis or through more general inferences about a category of drugs...." *Bristol-Myers Squibb Co. v. Shalala*, 923 F. Supp. 212, 218 (D.D.C. 1996) (quoting *Schering Corp. v. Sullivan*, 782 F. Supp. 645, 651 (D.D.C. 1992), vacated as moot sub nom, *Schering Corp. v. Shalala*, 995 F.2d 1103 (D.C. Cir. 1993)); see also *Fisons Corp. v. Shalala*, 860 F. Supp. 859, 865 (D.D.C. 1994) (upholding FDA's authority to grant waivers of the requirement for submission of *in vivo* evidence of bioequivalence where bioequivalence can be determined by other available science.).

15. *Guidance for Industry: Bioavailability and Bioequivalence Studies for Orally Administered Drug Products—General Considerations* (March 2003). Although *in vivo* testing is FDA's preferred method for an ANDA applicant to demonstrate bioequivalence, agency regulations state that "bioequivalence may be demonstrated by several in vivo and in vitro methods," which are described at 21 CFR 320.24 in descending order of accuracy, sensitivity, and reproducibility.

16. See 21 CFR 320.24(b)(5). FDA recently amended its ANDA bioequivalence regulations to require applicants to submit data from all bioequivalence studies that the applicant conducts on the "same drug product formulation" submitted for approval. See 21 CFR 314.94(a)(7), 320.21(b)(1); see also FDA, Final Rule, Requirements for Submission of Bioequivalence Data, 74 *Fed. Reg.* 2849 (16 January 2009).

17. The purpose of PEPFAR is to make antiretroviral drug products available to developing countries. The PEPFAR program applies to both NDA and ANDA drug products. In addition to expedited review for PEPFAR ANDAs, the PEPFAR program permits FDA to grant tentative ANDA approval for such applications (if there are *Orange Book*-listed patents covering the RLD) so that such products can be purchased from ANDA applicants with PEPFAR funding.

18. FDA, Manual of Policies and Procedures 5240.3, "Review Order of Original ANDAs, Amendments, and Supplements," at 2 (18 October 2006).

19. Karst KR. "Is the ANDA Suitability Petition Process Dead?" *Regulatory Affairs Focus*, Vol. 10, No. 5, pp 35-6 (May 2005).

20. *FD&C Act* Sections 505B(1)(A), (2)–(4).

21. *FD&C Act* Section 505(b)(4)(A) states that "[a]n applicant may not amend or supplement an application referred to in [*FD&C Act* Section 505(b)(2)] to seek approval of a drug that is a different drug than the drug identified in the application as submitted to [FDA]."

22. FDA, Citizen Petition Response, Docket No. FDA-2008-P-0329, at 16 n. 30 (25 November 2008). FDA also noted that the agency's: interpretation of § 505(b)(4)(A) of the Act . . . for 505(b)(2) applications is influenced by and intended to be consistent with section 505(j)(2)(D)(i) regarding ANDAs. Accordingly, a 505(b)(2) applicant may not amend or supplement a 505(b)(2) application to seek approval of a drug that relies on the Agency's finding of safety and/or effectiveness for a drug that is different from the drug identified in a previous submission of the application.

23. 21 CFR 314.127(a)(8)(ii)(B).

24. 21 CFR 314.90(b).

25. FDA, Citizen Petition Response, Docket No. FDA-2005-P-0370, at 6 (25 March 2005).

26. *Orange Book* Preface, 29th ed. (2009), at vii. The *Orange Book* Preface further states:

    > FDA classifies as therapeutically equivalent those products that meet the following general criteria: (1) they are approved as safe and effective; (2) they are pharmaceutical equivalents in that they (a) contain identical amounts of the same active drug ingredient in the same dosage form and route of administration, and (b) meet compendial or other applicable standards of strength, quality, purity, and identity; (3) they are bioequivalent in that (a) they do not present a known or potential bioequivalence problem, and they meet an acceptable *in vitro* standard, or (b) if they do present such

a known or potential problem, they are shown to meet an appropriate bioequivalence standard; (4) they are adequately labeled; [and] (5) they are manufactured in compliance with Current Good Manufacturing Practice regulations.
27. Ibid.
28. 21 CFR 320.1(c).
29. *FD&C Act* Section 505(j)(8)(B); 21 CFR 320.1(e).
30. 21 CFR 320.1(d).
31. The *Orange Book*, which is published annually and updated monthly, only identifies therapeutic equivalence codes for multisource prescription drug products. Therefore, neither single-source prescription drugs—e.g., a brand-name drug product without generic competition—nor over-the-counter drug products are assigned a therapeutic equivalence code. Once a therapeutically equivalent generic drug is approved, it is listed in the *Orange Book* with a particular therapeutic equivalence code. The RLD and generic equivalent are differentiated from one another by a "+" sign, which denotes the RLD. FDA assigns RLD status to single-source prescription drugs.
32. In certain instances, a number is added to the end of an AB code to make a three character code (e.g., AB1, AB2, etc.).
    Three-character codes are assigned only in situations when more than one [RLD] of the same strength has been designated under the same heading.... For example, Adalat® CC (Miles) and Procardia XL® (Pfizer), extended-release tablets, are listed under the active ingredient nifedipine. These drug products, listed under the same heading, are not bioequivalent to each other. Generic drug products deemed by FDA to be bioequivalent to Adalat® CC and Procardia XL® have been approved, Adalat® CC and Procardia XL® have been assigned ratings of AB1 and AB2, respectively. The generic drug products bioequivalent to Adalat® CC would be assigned a rating of AB1 and those bioequivalent to Procardia XL® would be assigned a rating of AB2.
    Orange Book Preface at xv.
33. For example, AO refers to injectable oil solutions, and AT refers to topical products. Some drug products are assigned more than one therapeutic equivalence code. For example, FDA has assigned both AB1 and AB2 codes to several approved levothyroxine sodium drug products because the sponsors conducted studies to establish their drugs' therapeutic equivalence to other RLDs.
34. For example, BT refers to "topical products with bioequivalence issues," and BX refers to "drug products for which the data are insufficient to determine therapeutic equivalence."
35. 44 *Fed. Reg.* 2932, 2937 (12 January 1979); see also *Orange Book* Preface at x–xi.
36. 44 *Fed. Reg.* at 2937; see also *Orange Book* Preface at x.
37. 45 *Fed. Reg.* 72,582, 72,584 (31 October 1980) (*Orange Book* final rule). When Congress amended the *FD&C Act* in 1984, it incorporated the *Orange Book* into the statute as a means of facilitating the approval of generic drugs. See *FD&C Act* Section 505(j)(7). The *Orange Book*'s therapeutic equivalence ratings have been accepted and recognized by the courts. See e.g., *Geneva Pharms. Tech. Corp. v. Barr Labs., Inc.*, 201 F. Supp.2d (S.D.N.Y. 2002) ("The *Orange Book* gives an AB rating to all generic warfarin sodium product[s] available today. Consequently, generic warfarin sodium is eligible for unrestricted substitution for Coumadin under most state pharmacy regulations.").
38. The designation of a drug as "A-rated" to another drug also has been incorporated into the federal Medicaid program. See 42 U.S.C. 1396r-8(e)(4) (setting the standard for upper limits on payment for multi-source drug products based on FDA's therapeutic equivalence evaluations).
39. 44 *Fed. Reg.* at 2938. FDA also commented in the preamble to the agency's final *Orange Book* proposal that:
    one reason FDA is publishing the [*Orange Book*] is in response to requests from several States for assistance in developing their drug product selection legislation. Pharmacies, hospitals, States, and private and public institutions and organizations continue to ask FDA to share its broad knowledge of the safety and effectiveness and quality of drug products, so that they can continue to carry out their duties to protect and promote the public health, both in providing health care services safely and with efficiency and cost-effectiveness, and in advising physicians and pharmacists on drug product selection. 45 *Fed. Reg.* at 72,589.
40. State laws also vary regarding how the final product selection is determined. In the majority of states, prescribers must expressly indicate that substitution is not permitted by writing "Brand Necessary," "Do Not Substitute," "Dispense as Written," "Medically Necessary," or other approved wording on the prescription form. Some states include lines on the prescription form with the phrases "Product Selection Permitted" (or similar wording) and "Do Not Substitute." The prescriber can prevent product substitution by signing on the line. See generally National Association of Boards of Pharmacy, Survey of Pharmacy Law, 2003–2004.
41. Vivian JC. "Legal Aspects of Therapeutic Interchange Programs," *U.S. Pharmacist* (2003).

Helpful References and Resources
- FDA's Office of Generic Drugs – Directory Information. FDA website.
- www.fda.gov/AboutFDA/CentersOffices/OfficeofMedicalProductsandTobacco/CDER/ucm119100.htm. Accessed 18 May 2013.
- *Federal Food, Drug, and Cosmetic Act.* FDA website.
- www.fda.gov/RegulatoryInformation/Legislation/default.htm. Accessed 18 May 2013.
- Generic Drugs: Information for Industry. FDA website.
- http://www.fda.gov/Drugs/DevelopmentApprovalProcess/HowDrugsareDevelopedandApproved/ApprovalApplications/AbbreviatedNewDrugApplicationANDAGenerics/ucm142112.htm. Accessed 18 May 2013.
- Abbreviated New Drug Application (ANDA): Generics. FDA website.
- http://www.fda.gov/Drugs/DevelopmentApprovalProcess/HowDrugsareDevelopedandApproved/ApprovalApplications/AbbreviatedNewDrugApplicationANDAGenerics/default.htm. Accessed 18 May 2013.
- The Electronic *Orange Book*. FDA website.
- www.accessdata.fda.gov/scripts/cder/ob/default.cfm. Accessed 18 May 2013.
- Generic Drug User Fee Amendments of 2012. FDA website.
- http://www.fda.gov/ForIndustry/UserFees/GenericDrugUserFees/default.htm. Accessed 18 May 2013.
- FDA's Paragraph IV Patent Certification List. FDA website. www.fda.gov/Drugs/DevelopmentApprovalProcess/HowDrugsareDevelopedandApproved/ApprovalApplications/AbbreviatedNewDrugApplicationANDAGenerics/ucm047676.htm. Accessed 18 May 2013.
- ANDA Suitability Petition Tracking Reports. FDA website. www.fda.gov/Drugs/DevelopmentApprovalProcess/HowDrugsareDevelopedandApproved/ApprovalApplications/AbbreviatedNewDrugApplicationANDAGenerics/ucm120944.htm. Accessed 18 May 2013.
- CTD Modules/Sections Corresponding to Summary Data Tables in Bioequivalence Submissions to ANDAs. FDA website. www.fda.gov/Drugs/DevelopmentApprovalProcess/HowDrugsareDevelopedandApproved/ApprovalApplications/AbbreviatedNewDrugApplicationANDAGenerics/ucm120962.htm. Accessed 18 May 2013.
- FDA's Individual Product Bioequivalence Recommendations. FDA website. www.fda.gov/Drugs/GuidanceComplianceRegulatoryInformation/Guidances/ucm075207.htm. Accessed 18 May 2013.
- FDA Generic Drug Guidance Documents. FDA website. www.fda.gov/Drugs/GuidanceComplianceRegulatoryInformation/Guidances/ucm064995.htm. Accessed 18 May 2013.

- FDA Generic Drug Manual of Policies & Procedures. FDA website. www.fda.gov/AboutFDA/CentersOffices/CDER/ManualofPoliciesProcedures/default.htm#generic. Accessed 18 May 2013.
- FDA's Dissolution Methods Database. FDA website.
- www.fda.gov/Drugs/InformationOnDrugs/ucm135742.htm. Accessed 18 May 2013.
- FDA's Inactive Ingredients Database. FDA website. www.fda.gov/Drugs/InformationOnDrugs/ucm080123.htm. Accessed 18 May 2013.

Acknowledgements

We acknowledge and thank the contribution of Kurt R. Karst, JD, of Hyman, Phelps & McNamara, whose prior version of this chapter formed the core for this current iteration.

Chapter 13

ANDA FILING CHECKLIST
(CTD or eCTD FORMAT)
FOR COMPLETENESS AND ACCEPTABILITY of an APPLICATION

ANDA:
APPLICANT:
RELATED APPLICATION(S):

DRUG NAME:
DOSAGE FORM:

LETTER DATE:
RECEIVED DATE:

☐ P-IV
☐ FIRST GENERIC
☐ EXPEDITED REVIEW REQUEST (Approved/Denied)
☐ PEPFAR

Electronic or Paper Submission: Type II DMF#

BASIS OF SUBMISSION:
NDA/ANDA:
FIRM:
RLD:

Document Room Note: for New Strength amendments and supplements, if specific reviewer(s) have already been assigned for the original, please assign to those reviewer(s) instead of the default random team(s).

Review Team:

CHEM Team: ☐ Activity	Bio Team: ☐ Activity
CHEM Team Leader: ☐ No Assignment Needed in DARRTS	Bio PM: ☐ FYI
CHEM RPM: ☐ FYI	Clinical Endpoint Team: (No) ☐ Activity
DMF Review Team Leader: Aloka Srinivasan ☐ FYI	
Labeling Reviewer: ☐ Activity	Micro Review: (No) ☐ Activity

Regulatory Reviewer:

Date:

Recommendation:

☐ FILE   ☐ REFUSE to RECEIVE

Comments:
Therapeutic Code:
On Cards:
Archival copy:
Sections:

- For More Information on Submission of an ANDA in Electronic Common Technical Document (eCTD) Format please go to: http://www.fda.gov/cder/regulatory/ersr/ectd.htm
- For a Comprehensive Table of Contents Headings and Hierarchy please go to: http://www.fda.gov/cder/regulatory/ersr/5640CTOC-v1.2.pdf
- For more CTD and eCTD informational links see the final page of the ANDA Checklist
- A model Quality Overall Summary for an immediate release tablet and an extended release capsule can be found on the OGD webpage http://www.fda.gov/cder/ogd/

1. Edit Application Property Type in DARRTS where applicable for

   a. First Generic Received
   ☐ Yes ☐ No
   b. Market Availability
   ☐ Rx ☐ OTC
   c. Pepfar
   ☐ Yes ☐ No
   d. Product Type
   ☐ Small Molecule Drug
   e. USP Drug Product (at time of filing review)
   ☐ Yes ☐ No

2. Edit Submission Patent Records
   ☐ Yes
3. Edit Contacts Database with Bioequivalence Recordation where applicable
   ☐ Yes
4. EER (in Draft)
   ☐ Yes

ADDITIONAL COMMENTS REGARDING THE ANDA:

Chapter 13

MODULE 1: ADMINISTRATIVE

		COMMENT (S)
1.1	**Signed and Completed Application Form (356h)** (Rx/OTC Status) (original signature)	
1.1.2	**Establishment Information:** 1. Drug Substance Manufacturer 2. Drug Product Manufacturer 3. Outside Testing Facility(ies)	
1.2	**Cover Letter**	
1.2.1	**Form FDA 3674** (PDF)	
*	**Table of Contents** (paper submission only)	
1.3.2	**Field Copy Certification** (N/A for E-Submissions) (original signature)	
1.3.3	**Debarment Certification-GDEA** (Generic Drug Enforcement Act)/Other: (no qualifying statement) 1. Debarment Certification (original signature) 2. List of Convictions statement (original signature)	
1.3.4	**Financial Certifications** Bioavailability/Bioequivalence Financial Certification (Form FDA 3454) Disclosure Statement (Form FDA 3455)	

1.3.5	**Patent Information**
	 Patents listed for the RLD in the Electronic Orange Book Approved Drug Products with Therapeutic Equivalence Evaluations
	 Patent Certification
	 1. Patent number(s)
	 2. Paragraph: (Check all certifications that apply)
	    MOU ☐ PI ☐ PII ☐ PIII ☐ PIV ☐ (Statement of Notification) ☐
	 3. Expiration of Patent(s):
	    a. Pediatric exclusivity submitted? Select
	    b. Expiration of Pediatric Exclusivity?
	 4. Exclusivity Statement: State marketing intentions?	

1.4.1	**References**
	 Letters of Authorization
	 1. DMF letters of authorization
	    a. Type II DMF authorization letter(s) or synthesis for Active Pharmaceutical Ingredient
	    b. Type II DMF#
	    c. Type III DMF authorization letter(s) for container closure
	 2. US Agent Letter of Authorization (U.S. Agent [if needed, countersignature on 356h])	

1.12.4	**Request for Comments and Advice** - Proprietary name requested If Yes, did the firm provide the request as a separate electronic amendment labeled "Proprietary Name Request" at initial time of filing 1. Yes 2. No - contact the firm to submit the request as a separate electronic amendment.	
1.12.11	**Basis for Submission** NDA#: Ref Listed Drug: Firm: **ANDA suitability petition required?** If Yes, provide petition number and copy of approved petition **ANDA Citizen's Petition Required?** If Yes, provide petition number and copy of petition	

MODULE 1: ADMINISTRATIVE (Continued)

		COMMENT (S)
1.12.12	**Comparison between Generic Drug and RLD-505(j)(2)(A)** 1. Conditions of use 2. Active ingredients 3. Inactive ingredients 4. Route of administration 5. Dosage Form 6. Strength	
1.12.14	**Environmental Impact Analysis Statement** (cite 21CFR 25.31, if applicable)	
1.12.15	**Request for Waiver** Request for Waiver of In-Vivo BA/BE Study(ies)	
1.14.1	**Draft Labeling** (Multi Copies N/A for E-Submissions) **1.14.1.1** 4 copies of draft for paper submission only (each strength and container) **1.14.1.2** 1 side by side labeling comparison of containers and carton with all differences visually highlighted and annotated **1.14.1.3** 1 package insert (content of labeling) and SPL submitted electronically	
1.14.3	**Listed Drug Labeling** **1.14.3.1** 1 side by side labeling (package and patient insert) comparison with all differences visually highlighted and annotated **1.14.3.3** RLD package insert, 1 RLD label and 1 RLD container label	

Regulatory Affairs Professionals Society

MODULE 2: SUMMARIES

		COMMENT (S)

2.3	**Quality Overall Summary (QOS)**
	E-Submission: PDF
	Word Processed e.g., MS Word
	
	A model Quality Overall Summary for an immediate release tablet and an extended release capsule can be found on the OGD webpage http://www.fda.gov/cder/ogd/
	
	Question based Review (QbR)
	
	2.3.S Drug Substance (Active Pharmaceutical Ingredient)
	    2.3.S.1 General Information
	    2.3.S.2 Manufacture
	    2.3.S.3 Characterization
	    2.3.S.4 Control of Drug Substance
	    2.3.S.5 Reference Standards or Materials
	    2.3.S.6 Container Closure System
	    2.3.S.7 Stability
	
	2.3.P Drug Product
	    2.3.P.1 Description and Composition of the Drug Product
	    2.3.P.2 Pharmaceutical Development
	        2.3.P.2.1 Components of the Drug Product
	            2.3.P.2.1.1 Drug Substance
	            2.3.P.2.1.2 Excipients
	        2.3.P.2.2 Drug Product
	        2.3.P.2.3 Manufacturing Process Development
	        2.3.P.2.4 Container Closure System
	    2.3.P.3 Manufacture
	    2.3.P.4 Control of Excipients
	    2.3.P.5 Control of Drug Product
	    2.3.P.6 Reference Standards or Materials
	    2.3.P.7 Container Closure System
	    2.3.P.8 Stability	

2.7	**Clinical Summary (Bioequivalence)** Model BE Data Summary Tables E-Submission: PDF Word Processed: e.g., MS Word **2.7.1 Summary of Biopharmaceutic Studies and Associated Analytical Methods** **2.7.1.1 Background and Overview** Table 1. Submission Summary Table 4. Bioanalytical Method Validation Table 6. Formulation Data **2.7.1.2 Summary of Results of Individual Studies** Table 5. Summary of In Vitro Dissolution **2.7.1.3 Comparison and Analyses of Results Across Studies** Table 2. Summary of Bioavailability (BA) Studies Table 3. Statistical Summary of the Comparative BA Data **2.7.1.4 Appendix** **2.7.4.1.3 Demographic and Other Characteristics of Study Population** Table 7. Demographic Profile of Subjects Completing the Bioequivalence Study **2.7.4.2.1.1 Common Adverse Events** Table 8. Incidence of Adverse Events in Individual Studies	

MODULE 3: 3.2.S DRUG SUBSTANCE

		COMMENT (S)
3.2.S.1	**General Information** (Do not refer to DMF) **3.2.S.1.1 Nomenclature** **3.2.S.1.2 Structure** **3.2.S.1.3 General Properties**	
3.2.S.2	**Manufacturer** **Drug Substance (Active Pharmaceutical Ingredient)** 1. Name and Full Address(es)of the Facility(ies) 2. Contact name, phone and fax numbers, email address 3. Specify Function or Responsibility 4. Type II DMF number for API 5. CFN or FEI numbers	
3.2.S.3	**Characterization** Provide the following in tabular format: 1. Name of Impurity(ies) 2. Structure of Impurity(ies) 3. Origin of Impurity(ies)	

3.2.S.4	**Control of Drug Substance (Active Pharmaceutical Ingredient)**
	3.2.S.4.1 Specification
	Testing specifications and data from drug substance manufacturer(s)
	3.2.S.4.2 Analytical Procedures
	3.2.S.4.3 Validation of Analytical Procedures
	(API that is USP or reference made to DMF, must provide verification of USP or DMF procedures)
	1. Spectra and chromatograms for reference standards and test samples
	2. Samples-Statement of Availability and Identification of:
	    a. Drug Substance
	    b. API lot number(s)
	3.2.S.4.4 Batch Analysis
	1. COA(s) specifications and test results from drug substance mfgr(s)
	2. Applicant certificate of analysis
	3.2.S.4.5 Justification of Specification	

3.2.S.5	**Reference Standards or Materials** (Do not refer to DMF)	
3.2.S.6	**Container Closure Systems**	
3.2.S.7	**Stability** 1. Retest date or expiration date of API	

MODULE 3: 3.2.P DRUG PRODUCT

		COMMENT (S)
3.2.P.1	**Description and Composition of the Drug Product** 1. Unit composition with indication of the function of the inactive ingredient(s) 2. Inactive ingredients and amounts are appropriate per IIG (per/dose justification) 3. Conversion from % to mg/dose values for inactive ingredients (if applicable) 4. Elemental iron: provide daily elemental iron calculation or statement of adherence to 21CFR73.1200 (calculation of elemental iron intake based on **maximum daily dose (MDD)** of the drug product is preferred if this section is applicable) 5. Injections: If the reference listed drug is packaged with a drug specific diluent then the diluent must be Q1/Q2 and must be provided in the package configuration	
3.2.P.2	**Pharmaceutical Development** Pharmaceutical Development Report	
3.2.P.3	**Manufacture** **3.2.P.3.1 Drug Product** (Finished Dosage Manufacturer and Outside Contract Testing Laboratories) 1. Name and Full Address(es) of the Facility(ies) 2. Contact name, phone and fax numbers, email address 3. Specify Function or Responsibility 4. CGMP Certification (from both applicant and drug product manufacturer if different entities) 5. CFN or FEI numbers **3.2.P.3.2 Batch Formula** **3.2.P.3.3 Description of Manufacturing Process and Process Controls** 1. Description of the Manufacturing Process 2. Master Production Batch Record(s) for largest intended production runs (no more than 10x pilot batch) with equipment specified 3. Master packaging records for intended marketing container(s) 4. If sterile product 5. Reprocessing Statement (cite 21CFR 211.115, submitted by the drug product manufacturer and the applicant, if different entities) **3.2.P.3.4 Controls of Critical Steps and Intermediates** **3.2.P.3.5 Process Validation and/or Evaluation** 1. Microbiological sterilization validation 2. Filter validation (if aseptic fill)	
3.2.P.4	**Controls of Excipients** (Inactive Ingredients) Source of inactive ingredients identified **3.2.P.4.1 Specifications** 1. Testing specifications (including identification and characterization) 2. Suppliers' COA (specifications and test results) **3.2.P.4.2 Analytical Procedures** **3.2.P.4.3 Validation of Analytical Procedures** **3.2.P.4.4 Justification of Specifications:** 1. Applicant COA	

MODULE 3: 3.2.P DRUG PRODUCT (Continued)

		COMMENT (S)

3.2.P.5	**Controls of Drug Product**
	3.2.P.5.1 Specification(s)
	3.2.P.5.2 Analytical Procedures
	3.2.P.5.3 Validation of Analytical Procedures
	(if using USP procedure, must provide verification of USP procedure)
	Samples - Statement of Availability and Identification of:
	   1. Finished Dosage Form
	   2. Lot number(s) and strength of Drug Product(s)
	3.2.P.5.4 Batch Analysis
	   Certificate of Analysis for Finished Dosage Form
	3.2.P.5.5 Characterization of Impurities
	3.2.P.5.6 Justification of Specifications	

3.2.P.7	**Container Closure System** 1. Summary of Container/Closure System (if new resin, provide data) 2. Components Specification and Test Data 3. Packaging Configuration and Sizes 4. Container/Closure Testing (water permeation, light transmission, extractables and leachables when applicable) 5. Source of supply and suppliers address	

3.2.P.8	**3.2.P.8.1 Stability (Finished Dosage Form)**
	1. Stability Protocol submitted
	2. Expiration Dating Period
	3.2.P.8.2 Post-approval Stability and Conclusion
	Post Approval Stability Protocol and Commitments
	3.2.P.8.3 Stability Data
	1. Accelerated stability data
	   a. four (4) time points 0,1,2,3
	          -OR-
	   b. three (3) time points 0,3,6 (if 3 time points for accelerated stability data are submitted then provide 3 exhibit batches along with 12 months of room temperature stability data –Refer to Guidance for Industry Q1A(R2) Stability Testing of New Drug Substances and Products November 2003, Section B)
	2. Batch numbers on stability records the same as the test batch	

MODULE 3: 3.2.R REGIONAL INFORMATION (Drug Substance)

		COMMENT (S)
3.2.R Drug Substance	**3.2.R.1.S Executed Batch Records for drug substance (if available)** **3.2.R.2.S Comparability Protocols** **3.2.R.3.S Methods Validation Package** Methods Validation Package (3 copies for paper and N/A for E-Submissions) (Required for Non-USP drugs)	

MODULE 3: 3.2.R REGIONAL INFORMATION (Drug Product)

		COMMENT (S)

3.2.R Drug Product	**3.2.R.1.P.1**
	Executed Batch Records
	Copy of Executed Batch Record with Equipment Specified, including Packaging Records (Packaging and Labeling Procedures)
	Batch Reconciliation and Label Reconciliation
	   a. Theoretical Yield
	   b. Actual Yield
	   c. Packaged Yield
	3.2.R.1.P.2 Information on Components
	3.2.R.2.P Comparability Protocols
	3.2.R.3.P Methods Validation Package
	Methods Validation Package (3 copies for paper and N/A for E-Submissions)
	(Required for Non-USP drugs)	

MODULE 5: CLINICAL STUDY REPORTS

		COMMENT (S)
5.2	**Tabular Listing of Clinical Studies**	

5.3.1
(complete study data)
	Bioavailability/Bioequivalence
	1. Formulation data same?
	    a. Comparison of all Strengths
	       (check proportionality of multiple strengths)
	    b. Parenterals, Ophthalmics, Otics and Topicals
	       (21 CFR 314.94 (a)(9)(iii)-(v)
	2. Lot Numbers and strength of Products used in BE Study(ies)
	3. Study Type: IN-VIVO PK STUDY(IES)
	    (Continue with the appropriate study type box below)	

	5.3.1.2 Comparative BA/BE Study Reports 1. Study(ies) meets BE criteria (90% CI of 80-125, C max, AUC) 2. Summary Bioequivalence tables: Table 10. Study Information Table 12. Dropout Information Table 13. Protocol Deviations **5.3.1.3 In Vitro-In-Vivo Correlation Study Reports** 1. Summary Bioequivalence tables Table 11. Product Information Table 16. Composition of Meal Used in Fed Bioequivalence Study **5.3.1.4 Reports of Bioanalytical and Analytical Methods for Human Studies** 1. Summary Bioequivalence table: Table 9. Reanalysis of Study Samples Table 14. Summary of Standard Curve and QC Data for Bioequivalence Sample Analyses Table 15. SOPs Dealing with Bioanalytical Repeats of Study Samples **Case Report Forms** should be placed under the study to which they pertain, and appropriately tagged. Refer to The eCTD Backbone File Specification for Study Tagging //www.fda.gov/downloads/Drugs/DevelopmentApprovalProcess/FormsSubmissionRequirements/ElectronicSubmissions/UCM163560.pdf	
5.4	**Literature References**	
	Possible Study Types:	
Study Type	**IN-VIVO BE STUDY(IES) with PK ENDPOINTS** (i.e., fasting/fed/sprinkle) 1. Study(ies) meets BE criteria (90% CI of 80-125, C max, AUC) 2. EDR Email: Data Files Submitted 3. In-Vitro Dissolution	
Study Type	**IN-VIVO BE STUDY with CLINICAL ENDPOINTS** 1. Properly defined BE endpoints (eval. by Clinical Team) 2. Summary results meet BE criteria: 90% CI of the proportional difference in success rate between test and reference must be within (-0.20, +0.20) for a binary/dichotomous endpoint. For a continuous endpoint, the test/reference ratio of the mean result must be within (0.80,1.25) 3. Summary results indicate superiority of active treatments (test & reference) over vehicle/placebo ($p<0.05$) (eval. by Clinical Team) 4. EDR Email: Data Files Submitted	

Chapter 13

Study Type	**IN-VITRO BE STUDY(IES)** (i.e., in vitro binding assays) 1. Study(ies) meets BE criteria (90% CI of 80-125) 2. EDR Email: Data Files Submitted 3. In-Vitro Dissolution	

Study Type	**NASALLY ADMINISTERED DRUG PRODUCTS**
	1. <u>Solutions</u> (Q1/Q2 sameness)
	   a. In-Vitro Studies (Dose/Spray Content Uniformity, Droplet/Drug Particle Size Distrib., Spray Pattern, Plume Geometry, Priming & Repriming)
	2. <u>Suspensions</u> (Q1/Q2 sameness):
	   a. In-Vivo PK Study
	      1. Study(ies) meets BE Criteria (90% CI of 80-125, C max, AUC)
	      2. EDR Email: Data Files Submitted
	   b. In-Vivo BE Study with Clinical End Points
	      1. Properly defined BE endpoints (eval. by Clinical Team)
	      2. Summary results meet BE criteria (90% CI within +/- 20% of 80-125)
	      3. Summary results indicate superiority of active treatments (test & reference) over vehicle/placebo ($p<0.05$) (eval. by Clinical Team)
	      4. EDR Email: Data Files Submitted
	   c. In-Vitro Studies (Dose/Spray Content Uniformity, Droplet/Drug Particle Size Distrib., Spray Pattern, Plume Geometry, Priming & Repriming)	

Study Type	**IN-VIVO BE STUDY(IES) with PD ENDPOINTS** (e.g., topical corticosteroid vasoconstrictor studies) 1. Pilot Study (determination of ED50) 2. Pivotal Study (study meets BE criteria 90%CI of 80-125)	

Study Type	**TRANSDERMAL DELIVERY SYSTEMS**
	1. <u>In-Vivo PK Study</u>
	   a. Study(ies) meet BE Criteria (90% CI of 80-125, C max, AUC)
	   b. In-Vitro Dissolution
	   c. EDR Email: Data Files Submitted
	2. <u>Adhesion Study</u>
	3. <u>Skin Irritation/Sensitization Study</u>	

Updated 03/17/2011

Chapter 14

Patents and Exclusivity

Updated by Karen Jaffe, MS, MBA, MRSc, RAC

OBJECTIVES

- To gain an understanding of the various types of patent and non-patent market exclusivity available to sponsors of brand-name drugs and their effects on generic drug approval

- To gain an understanding of 180-day marketing exclusivity available to certain generic drug sponsors

- To gain an understanding of the various acts that impact pharmaceutical development

LAWS, REGULATIONS AND GUIDELINES COVERED IN THIS CHAPTER

- *Federal Food, Drug, and Cosmetic Act of 1938*

- *Drug Price Competition and Patent Term Restoration Act of 1984 (Hatch-Waxman Act)*

- *Food and Drug Administration Modernization Act of 1997*

- *Orphan Drug Act of 1983*

- *Uruguay Rounds Agreements Act of 1994*

- *Leahy-Smith America Invents Act of 2011*

- *Generating Antibiotics Incentives Now Act (GAIN Act), Food and Drug Administration Safety and Innovation Act (FDASIA) Section VIII*

- Humane Use Device provisions, *FDASIA* Title VI, Part L

- *PDUFA V, FDASIA* Title I

- 21 CFR 314 Applications for FDA Approval to Market a New Drug

- 21 CFR 320 Bioavailability and Bioequivalence Requirements

- 21 CFR 316 Orphan Drugs

- 54 *Federal Register* 28,872 (10 July 1989), Proposed ANDA Regulations

- 59 *Federal Register* 50,338 (3 October 1994), ANDA regulations; patent and exclusivity provisions

- 68 *Federal Register* 36,676 (18 June 2003), Applications for FDA approval to market a new drug: patent submission and listing requirements and application of 30-month stays on approval of Abbreviated New Drug Applications certifying that a patent claiming a drug is invalid or will not be infringed

- *Guidance for Industry: Qualifying for Pediatric Exclusivity Under Section 505A of the Federal Food, Drug, and Cosmetic Act (September 1999)*

Chapter 14

- Manual of Policies and Procedures 5240.3, "Review Order of Original ANDAs, Amendments and Supplements" (October 2006)

- Draft Guidance for Industry: Applications Covered by Section 505(b)(2) (October 1978)

Introduction

As discussed in Chapter 13, the *Drug Price Competition and Patent Term Restoration Act* of 1984 (*Hatch-Waxman Act*) amended the *Federal Food, Drug, and Cosmetic Act* of 1938 (*FD&C Act*) to create the contemporary Abbreviated New Drug Application (ANDA) generic drug approval process under Section 505(j). Under the *FD&C Act*'s ANDA statutory provisions and the US Food and Drug Administration's (FDA) implementing regulations, an application containing bioequivalence data to a Reference Listed Drug (RLD), among other data and information, is sufficient for FDA to consider approval. As part of the *Hatch-Waxman Act* compromise, brand-name drug companies may obtain a patent term extension for time lost during the regulatory review period, can submit to FDA for listing certain types of patents in the *Orange Book*, and may also be eligible for a period of non-patent exclusivity. Certain ANDA sponsors may be eligible for a period of 180-day marketing exclusivity for challenging patents listed in FDA's *Orange Book* for the RLD. Under the current law, an ANDA sponsor's eligibility for a period of 180-day marketing exclusivity can be forfeited under various scenarios.

In addition to the incentives created by the *Hatch-Waxman Act*, new or additional incentives have been created by the enactment of several other laws. These laws include the *Orphan Drug Act*, which rewards sponsors for developing products to treat rare diseases and conditions, and the *Best Pharmaceuticals for Children Act* (*BPCA*), which rewards sponsors for developing products for children. Each of the types of non-patent exclusivities is discussed in this chapter.

Patent-Related Market Exclusivity

Patent Term Extensions

Under Title II of the *Hatch-Waxman Act*, certain patents related to products regulated by FDA are eligible for extension if patent life was lost during a period when the product was undergoing regulatory review.[1] The "regulatory review period" is composed of a "testing phase" and a "review phase." For a drug product, the testing phase begins on the effective date of an Investigational New Drug Application (IND) and ends on the date a New Drug Application (NDA) is submitted to FDA.[2] The review phase is the period between the submission and approval of the NDA.[3] A patent term may be extended for a period of time that is the sum of one-half of the time in the testing phase, plus all the time in the review phase.[4] The regulatory review period must be reduced by any time that the applicant "did not act with due diligence."[5] The total (calculated) regulatory review period may not exceed five years, and the extended patent term may not exceed 14 years after the date of approval of the marketing application.[6]

As applied to drugs, the patent term extension law provides that the term of a patent claiming the drug (or a use of the drug or a method of manufacturing a drug) shall be extended from the original expiration date of the patent if:

1. the term of the patent has not expired
2. the patent has not been previously extended
3. the extension application is submitted by the owner of record within 60 days of NDA approval
4. the product, use, or method of manufacturing claimed has been subject to a "regulatory review period" before it is commercially marketed

and

5. the NDA is the first permitted commercial use of the drug product[7]

Criterion 5 has been the most controversial. Until recently, the US Patent and Trademark Office (PTO) relied on decisions by the US Court of Appeals for the Federal Circuit in *Fisons v. Quigg*, 8 U.S.P.Q.2d 1491 (D.D.C.1988), affirmed 876 F.2d 99 U.S.P.Q.2d 1869 (Fed.Cir.1989), and *Pfizer Inc. v. Dr. Reddy's Labs.*, 359 F.3d 1361 (Fed. Cir. 2004) to support the office's interpretation of the term "product" in 35 U.S.C. §156(a)(5)(A) to mean "active moiety" (i.e., the molecule in a drug product responsible for pharmacological action, regardless of whether the active moiety is formulated as a salt, ester or other non-covalent derivative) rather than "active ingredient" (i.e., the active ingredient physically found in the drug product, which would include any salt, ester or other non-covalent derivative of the active ingredient physically found in the drug product). In contrast, the Federal Circuit's 1990 decision in *Glaxo Operations UK Ltd. v. Quigg*, 894 F.2d 392, 13 USPQ2d 1628 (Fed. Cir. 1990), construed the term "product" in 35 U.S.C. §156(a)(5)(A) to mean "active ingredient." In 2010, the US Court of Appeals for the Federal Circuit ruled in *Photocure ASA v. Kappos*, 603 F.3d 1372, 1375 (Fed. Cir. 2010) that the term "product" in 35 U.S.C. §156(a)(5)(A) means "active ingredient" rather than "active moiety."

In some cases, a patent that is scheduled to expire before a term extension application can be submitted to the PTO (e.g., if the patent will expire before the NDA is approved) may be granted an interim patent extension.[8]

Two types of interim patent extensions are available:
1. interim patent extensions available during the review phase of the statutory regulatory review period[9]
2. interim patent extensions available during the PTO's review of an application for patent term extension[10]

The cumulative patent time granted under either type of interim patent extension cannot exceed the patent term extension that a company could obtain under regular patent extension provisions. The PTO reviews each application for an interim patent extension to ensure that a patent will not be extended longer than its eligibility under the law.

Orange Book Patent Listing

The *FD&C Act* and FDA regulations require each NDA sponsor to submit with its application "the patent number and the expiration date of any patent which claims the drug for which the applicant submitted the [NDA] or which claims a method of using[11] such drug and with respect to which a claim of patent infringement could reasonably be asserted if a person not licensed by the owner engaged in the manufacture, use, or sale of the drug."[12] FDA regulations clarify that "such patents consist of drug substance (active ingredient) patents, drug product (formulation and composition) patents, and method-of-use patents."[13] Thus, in order to list a patent in the *Orange Book*: the patent must claim the drug or a method of using the drug that is the subject of the NDA; and a claim of patent infringement could reasonably be asserted by the NDA holder or patent owner for the unauthorized manufacture, use or sale of the drug that is the subject of the NDA.[14] Once an NDA is approved, FDA is required to publish information in the *Orange Book* on the patents claiming the drug or a method of using it.[15] If a new patent meeting the requirements of *FD&C Act* Section 505(b)(1) and FDA patent listing regulations is issued while an NDA is pending FDA review or has received NDA approval, the NDA sponsor must submit information on the patent to FDA within 30 days of issuance.[16]

An ANDA (or 505(b)(2) application) for a generic version of an innovator drug must contain one of four possible certifications "with respect to each patent which claims the [innovator] drug…or which claims a use for such listed drug…and for which information is required to be filed" by the NDA holder and that is listed in the *Orange Book*.[17] If there are patents on the drug and the ANDA applicant does not want to challenge them, the applicant submits a Paragraph III certification, and FDA cannot approve the application until the patents have expired.[18] If the patents have already expired, or if the required patent information has not been filed, the ANDA applicant submits a Paragraph II or Paragraph I certification, respectively, and FDA can approve the application.[19] If the ANDA applicant does want to challenge a patent listed in the *Orange Book*, the applicant submits a Paragraph IV certification claiming that the patent is "invalid or will not be infringed by the manufacture, use, or sale of the new drug for which the [ANDA] is submitted."[20]

As an alternative to these four certifications, if the listed drug is covered by an *Orange Book*-listed "method of use patent which does not claim a use for which the [ANDA] applicant is seeking approval," the application must contain "a statement that the method of use patent does not claim such a use."[21] This is often referred to as a "section viii statement" and permits a generic applicant to "carve out" a patent-protected use from its proposed labeling, provided the omission of such protected information does not "render the proposed drug product less safe or effective than the listed drug for all remaining, non-protected conditions of use."[22]

An NDA holder or patent owner may choose to sue a generic applicant that submits a Paragraph IV certification. Under certain circumstances, a patent infringement suit may delay ANDA approval for 30 months (i.e., the so-called "30-month stay").[23] If a patent infringement suit is not brought by the NDA holder or patent owner, FDA can approve the ANDA.

Non-patent Statutory Market Exclusivity

Five-Year Exclusivity

Under the *FD&C Act* (as amended by Title I of the *Hatch-Waxman Act*), five-year exclusivity is available to the sponsor of an application (either a full 505(b)(1) NDA or a 505(b)(2) application) for a drug product that does not contain an active moiety previously approved under Section 505(b) of the *FD&C Act* (i.e., an NDA for a New Chemical Entity (NCE)). Five-year exclusivity prevents the submission of an ANDA (and a 505(b)(2) application) that "refers to the drug for which the [approved Section 505(b) NCE NDA] was submitted before the expiration of five years from the date of the approval" of the NCE NDA.[24] Thus, five-year exclusivity is sometimes called "NCE exclusivity." NCE exclusivity prevents the approval of a generic application for the approved active ingredient or any salt or ester of the approved active ingredient for five years. However, five-year exclusivity does not prevent FDA from approving, or a company from submitting, a full Section 505(b)(1) NDA for the same drug.[25]

The *FD&C Act* is ambiguous regarding the meaning of the term "drug" in Sections 505(c)(3)(E)(ii) and 505(j)(5)(F)(ii).[26] Neither provision addresses whether drug means the particular drug product that is the subject of the approved NCE NDA with five-year exclusivity or, more generally, the approved active moiety. FDA identified this ambiguity in the preamble to its proposed rule implementing the exclusivity provisions of the *Hatch-Waxman Act*:

> The language of sections 505(c)(3)[(E)] and 505(j)[(5)(F)][27] of the act is ambiguous as to which ANDAs or 505(b)(2) applications are affected by an innovator's exclusivity. The statutory language allows at least two interpretations. The narrower interpretation of the protection offered by exclusivity is that exclusivity covers only specific drug products and therefore protects from generic competition only the first approved version of

a drug…The broader interpretation of the coverage of exclusivity is that it covers the active moieties in new chemical entities…FDA has concluded that the broader interpretation of the scope of exclusivity should be applied to all types of exclusivity conferred by sections 505(c)(3)[(E)] and 505(j)[(5)(F)] of the act. Therefore, when exclusivity attaches to an active moiety or to an innovative change in an already approved drug, the submission or effective date of approval of ANDAs and 505(b)(2) applications for a drug with that active moiety or innovative change will be delayed until the innovator's exclusivity has expired, whether or not FDA has approved subsequent versions of the drugs entitled to exclusivity, and regardless of the specific listed drug product to which the ANDA or 505(b)(2) application refers.[28]

This policy, known as FDA's Umbrella Policy, effectively replaces the term drug in the statutory text with the term "active moiety."[29]

Three-Year Exclusivity

Under the *FD&C Act* (as amended by Title I of the *Hatch-Waxman Act*), a sponsor may qualify for a three-year period of exclusivity for an application (a full 505(b)(1) NDA, a 505(b)(2) application or a supplement to either) if the application is for an active moiety that FDA has previously approved and if the application contains "reports of new clinical investigations (other than bioavailability studies)" that were "essential to approval" of the application and that were "conducted or sponsored by" the applicant.[30] All three of these criteria must be satisfied in order to qualify for three-year exclusivity.[31] Three-year exclusivity is often referred to as "new clinical investigation" or "new use" exclusivity.

Each criterion is defined in FDA's implementing regulations. A "new clinical investigation" is:

an investigation in humans the results of which have not been relied on by FDA to demonstrate substantial evidence of effectiveness of a previously approved drug product for any indication or of safety for a new patient population and do not duplicate the results of another investigation that was relied on by the agency to demonstrate the effectiveness or safety in a new patient population of a previously approved drug product.[32]

An investigation is "essential to approval" of an application if "there are no other data available that could support approval of the application."[33] FDA explained that if the agency was aware of "published reports of studies other than those conducted or sponsored by the applicant, or other information…sufficient for FDA to conclude that a proposed drug product or change to an already approved drug product is safe and effective," then exclusivity would not be appropriate.[34] The applicant must submit a list of all publicly available reports of clinical investigations "that are relevant to the conditions for which the applicant is seeking approval" and explain why these studies or reports do not provide a sufficient basis for approval.[35]

Finally, an investigation is "conducted or sponsored by the applicant" if:

(B)efore or during the investigation, the applicant was named…as the sponsor of the [IND]…under which the investigation was conducted, or the applicant or the applicant's predecessor in interest, provided substantial support for the investigation. To demonstrate "substantial support," an applicant must either provide a certified statement from a certified public accountant that the applicant provided 50 percent or more of the cost of conducting the study or provide an explanation why FDA should consider the applicant to have conducted or sponsored the study if the applicant's financial contribution to the study is less than 50 percent or the applicant did not sponsor the investigational new drug. A predecessor in interest is an entity, e.g., a corporation, that the applicant has taken over, merged with, or purchased, or from which the applicant has purchased all rights to the drug. Purchase of nonexclusive rights to a clinical investigation after it is completed is not sufficient to satisfy this definition.[36]

Three-year exclusivity prevents FDA from approving[37] an ANDA or a 505(b)(2) application "that relies on the information supporting a change approved in the [NDA or NDA supplement]" until three years after the date FDA approved the application.[38] Although the general rule is that the labeling of a generic drug product approved under an ANDA must have the "same" labeling as the RLD,[39] the sponsor can omit "an indication or other aspect of labeling protected by patent or accorded exclusivity under [505(j)(5)(F)] of the [*FD&C Act*]."[40] FDA can approve an ANDA with labeling "carve outs" if a particular use of the innovator drug is protected by a patent or period of exclusivity, and other uses are not protected. Before approving such a drug, FDA must first determine that the "carve out" of the protected information does not "render the proposed drug product less safe or effective than the listed drug for all remaining, non-protected conditions of use."[41]

Pediatric Exclusivity

The *BPCA* amended the *FD&C Act* to create Section 505A, which provides an additional six months of exclusivity to pharmaceutical manufacturers that conduct acceptable pediatric studies[42] of new and currently marketed drug products identified by FDA in a Pediatric Written Request (PWR) for which pediatric information would be beneficial. An initial grant of pediatric exclusivity extends all other types of *Orange Book*-listed patent[43] and non-patent market exclusivity (e.g., five-year NCE exclusivity, three-year new clinical investigation exclusivity and seven-year orphan drug exclusivity) an application holder may have under the *FD&C Act*. The *Food and Drug Administration Safety and Innovation Act* of 2012 (*FDASIA*) has made the *BPCA* amendments permanent and they are not required to be reauthorized by future user fee negotiations.

An important aspect of an initial grant of pediatric exclusivity is that it provides additional market exclusivity not just for the pediatric indications or formulations, but for all protected indications and formulations of that sponsor's drug. Thus, an initial grant of pediatric exclusivity attaches to the patent and non-patent market exclusivities for any of the sponsor's approved drug products (including certain combination products) that contain the active moiety for which pediatric exclusivity was granted, and not to a specific drug product.[44]

While an initial period of pediatric exclusivity is broad, a second exclusivity period is narrow. Specifically, a second period of pediatric exclusivity attaches only to any period of three-year new clinical investigation exclusivity granted by FDA with respect to a pediatric use supplement containing studies submitted in response to a second PWR issued by FDA.[45] A second period of pediatric exclusivity does not apply to any existing *Orange Book*-listed patent exclusivity or to any existing periods of five-year NCE exclusivity or orphan drug exclusivity. FDA's September 1999 guidance document further explains the scope of a second period of pediatric exclusivity:

> Pediatric studies submitted in a supplemental application for a drug that has already received one period of pediatric exclusivity may qualify the drug to receive a different 6-month period of pediatric exclusivity if submitted in response to a [PWR]. The different 6-month period of pediatric exclusivity will attach only to any exclusivity period under sections 505(c)(3)(D)(iv) and 505(j)(5)(D)(iv) [(i.e., three-year exclusivity)] granted to the supplemental application for which the studies were completed.[46]

An important exception to the applicability of pediatric exclusivity relative to new PWRs was added to the law in 2007. Under the exception, FDA will not apply a period of pediatric exclusivity to an unexpired period of patent or non-patent exclusivity if the agency's decision to grant pediatric exclusivity "is made later than 9 months prior to the expiration of such period."[47]

Orphan Drug Exclusivity

Under the *Orphan Drug Act* of 1983 (Pub. L. No. 97-414, 96 Stat. 2049 (1983)), as amended, a manufacturer or sponsor may submit a written request for FDA to designate a drug as a drug for a rare disease or condition (i.e., an "orphan drug"). A "rare disease or condition" is one that affects fewer than 200,000 people in the US, or affects more than 200,000 people but for which the sponsor can show that it will be unable to recover its development and marketing costs from sales of the product in the US.[48]

Once FDA approves a marketing application for a drug designated as an orphan drug, the agency may not approve another company's version of the "same drug" for the same disease or condition for seven years, unless the subsequent drug is "different" from the approved orphan drug.[49] In addition, the *FD&C Act* and FDA's orphan drug regulations identify circumstances under which the agency can approve another version of the "same drug" for the same orphan disease or condition during the term of another sponsor's orphan drug exclusivity (e.g., failure to assure a sufficient quantity of the drug).[50]

A drug is "different" from an approved orphan drug if it is chemically or structurally distinct. The degree of chemical or structural similarity that allows FDA to determine whether two drugs are "the same" depends on whether the drugs are small molecules or macromolecules.[51] However, even a drug that is structurally "the same" as an approved orphan drug may be approved for the same condition if it is "clinically superior" to the approved orphan drug. FDA's orphan drug regulations define a "clinically superior" drug as "a drug…shown to provide a significant therapeutic advantage over and above that provided by an approved orphan drug (that is otherwise the same drug)" in one of three ways:

1. greater effectiveness as assessed by effect on a clinically meaningful endpoint in adequate and well-controlled trials
2. greater safety in a substantial portion of the target populations
3. a demonstration that the drug makes a major contribution to patient care[52]

Paragraph IV Litigation and 180-Day Exclusivity

A generic applicant making a Paragraph IV certification must notify the NDA holder and patent owner that an application has been submitted to FDA once the agency determines that the ANDA is substantially complete. If the patent certification is in the ANDA, the applicant must give notice to the NDA holder and patent owner "not later than 20 days after the date of the postmark on the notice with which [FDA] informs the applicant that the application has been filed."[53] If the patent certification is in an amendment or supplement to the ANDA, the applicant must give notice to the NDA holder and patent owner "at the time at which the applicant submits the amendment or supplement, regardless of whether the applicant has already given notice with respect to another such certification contained in the application or in an amendment or supplement to the application."[54] The notice must include a "detailed statement of the factual and legal basis of the applicant's opinion that the patent is not valid or will not be infringed," and must "state that an application that contains data from bioavailability or bioequivalence studies has been submitted…for the drug with respect to which the certification is made to obtain approval to engage in the commercial manufacture, use, or sale of the drug before the expiration of the patent referred to in the certification."[55]

The NDA holder or patent owner has 45 days from the date of receipt of such notice to file a suit for patent infringement.[56] If a patent infringement suit is brought by the NDA holder or the patent owner within the 45-day period, FDA cannot approve the ANDA until the earlier of:
- the expiration of a single 30-month stay of approval, which may be shortened or lengthened by the court if "either party to the action fail[s] to reasonably cooperate in expediting the action"[57]
- the date on which a district court enters judgment in favor of the defendant (i.e., the ANDA applicant) that the patent is invalid or not infringed (or on the date of a settlement order or consent decree signed and entered by the court stating that the patent that is the subject of the certification is invalid or not infringed)
- if the district court enters judgment in favor of the plaintiff (i.e., the NDA holder or patent owner) and that decision is appealed by the ANDA applicant, the date on which the court of appeals enters judgment in favor of the ANDA applicant that the patent is invalid or not infringed (or on the date of a settlement order or consent decree signed and entered by the court of appeals stating that the patent that is the subject of the certification is invalid or not infringed)

If the judgment of the district court is not appealed or is affirmed by the court of appeals, ANDA approval can be made effective. An ANDA applicant also may assert a counterclaim "seeking an order requiring the [NDA] holder to correct or delete the patent information submitted by the [NDA] holder…on the grounds that the patent does not claim either the drug for which the application was approved or an approved method of using the drug."[58] An ANDA counterclaimant is not entitled to damages that result from inappropriate listing of patent information.[59]

If a patent infringement suit is not brought by the NDA holder or the patent owner within the 45-day period, FDA can approve the ANDA. In addition, an applicant whose ANDA contains a Paragraph IV certification may bring an action for declaratory judgment on patent infringement or invalidity if it is not sued within the 45-day period.[60] In order to file a declaratory judgment on non-infringement grounds, an ANDA applicant must provide an offer of confidential access to the ANDA to allow the NDA holder or patent owner the opportunity "of evaluating possible infringement of the patent that is the subject of the [Paragraph IV] certification."[61] An ANDA applicant is not entitled to damages even if it obtains a declaratory judgment in its favor.[62]

FD&C Act Section 505(j)(5)(B)(iv) establishes an incentive for generic manufacturers to submit Paragraph IV certifications and to challenge *Orange Book*-listed patents as invalid or not infringed by providing a 180-day period of market exclusivity.[63] This means that, in certain circumstances, an applicant that submits the ANDA containing the first Paragraph IV certification to an *Orange Book*-listed patent is protected from competition from other generic versions of the same drug product for 180 days.

Prior to the enactment of the *Medicare Prescription Drug, Improvement and Modernization Act* of 2003 (*MMA*), 180-day exclusivity was patent-based, such that a period of 180-day exclusivity could arise from each *Orange Book*-listed patent. Pre-*MMA*, 180-day exclusivity (which applies to a dwindling number of pending ANDAs) begins on the date FDA "receives notice from the applicant…of the first commercial marketing of the drug" under the first ANDA, or "the date of a decision of a court in [a patent infringement action] holding the patent which is the subject of the certification to be invalid or not infringed," whichever is earlier. Post-*MMA*, 180-day exclusivity is generally drug-based, such that there is a single 180-day exclusivity period (that can be shared by multiple first applicants) with respect to each listed drug. Also post-*MMA*, there is a single trigger to 180-day exclusivity—first commercial marketing.

Under changes made to the *FD&C Act* by the *MMA*, the first applicant that qualifies for 180-day exclusivity can forfeit exclusivity under various circumstances. While some of the statutory forfeiture provisions are straightforward—e.g., 180-day exclusivity is forfeited if the ANDA sponsor withdraws its exclusivity-qualifying Paragraph IV certification—others are more complex. In particular, the so-called "failure to market" forfeiture provisions under *FD&C Act* Section 505(j)(5)(D)(i)(I) require FDA to calculate a forfeiture date based on the later of two events. Although FDA has not yet issued proposed regulations implementing the 180-day exclusivity forfeiture provisions added to the *FD&C Act* by the *MMA*, the agency has applied them on a case-by-case basis and has issued several letter decisions describing its interpretation of these provisions. Those letters are posted on FDA's website at www.fda.gov/Drugs/DevelopmentApprovalProcess/HowDrugsareDevelopedandApproved/ApprovalApplications/AbbreviatedNewDrugApplicationANDAGenerics/ucm142112.htm. Congress enacted the forfeiture provisions to "ensure that the 180-day exclusivity period enjoyed by the first generic to challenge a patent cannot be used as a bottleneck to prevent additional generic competition."[64]

Of the six 180-day exclusivity forfeiture provisions created by the *MMA*, the one provision that appears to have been the basis for the greatest number is *FD&C Act* Section

Table 14-1. 180-Day Exclusivity Forfeiture Snapshot

- **"Failure to Market":** A first applicant forfeits exclusivity if it fails to market the drug by the *later of* –
    (1) The *earlier of* 75 days after ANDA *approval*, or 30 months after ANDA *submission*; and
    (2) Either:
        ☐ 75 days after favorable court decision on all qualifying patents (*appeals* court, or unappealed district court, decision); or
        ☐ 75 days after favorable court settlement or consent decree on all qualifying patents; or
        ☐ 75 days after all qualifying patents are delisted from the Orange Book.

- **Immediate Forfeiture:**
    ☐ If the ANDA applicant withdraws the ANDA or the application is withdrawn because the applicant failed to meet approval requirements;
    ☐ If the ANDA applicant amends or withdraws its Paragraph IV certification;
    ☐ If the ANDA applicant fails to obtain tentative approval within 30 months after filing the application (unless the failure is caused by a review of or change in approval requirements imposed after the ANDA is filed or because of a related Citizen Petition);
    ☐ If the ANDA applicant enters into an agreement with another generic applicant, the NDA holder, or patent owner, and the Federal Trade Commission (FTC) files a complaint, and either the FTC or an appeals court rules that the agreement violates antitrust laws; or
    ☐ If all of the patents certified to in the generic applicant's Paragraph IV certification have expired.

505(j)(5)(D)(i)(IV), which states that 180-day exclusivity eligibility is forfeited if:

The first applicant fails to obtain tentative approval of the application within 30 months after the date on which the application is filed, unless the failure is caused by a change in or a review of the requirements for approval of the application imposed after the date on which the application is filed.

The *Food and Drug Administration Amendments Act* of 2007 (*FDAAA*) clarified *FD&C Act* Section 505(j)(5)(D)(i)(IV), such that if "approval of the [ANDA] was delayed because of a [citizen] petition, the 30-month period under such subsection is deemed to be extended by a period of time equal to the period beginning on the date on which the Secretary received the petition and ending on the date of final agency action on the petition (inclusive of such beginning and ending dates) . . . ."[65] The growing number of 180-day exclusivity forfeitures under *FD&C Act* Section 505(j)(5)(D)(i)(IV) is likely due, in part, to the increasing time it takes FDA's Office of Generic Drugs to review and act on ANDAs. *FDASIA* further clarified and modified the timeframe within which an ANDA must receive tentative approval to avoid forfeiting the 180-day marketing exclusivity. *FDASIA* shortened the time for FDA to respond to certain Citizen Petitions related to generic drugs and biologics from 180 to 150 days (see **Table 14-1**).

Exclusivity for Antibiotic Drugs

Until 1997, antibiotic drugs were approved under *FD&C Act* Section 507 and were not entitled to any *Hatch-Waxman* benefits.[66] In 1997, the *Food and Drug Administration Modernization Act* (*FDAMA*) (Pub. L. No. 105-115, 111 Stat. 2295 (1997)), among other things, repealed *FD&C Act* Section 507 and required all NDAs for antibiotic drugs to be submitted under *FD&C Act* Section 505.

FDAMA included a transition provision declaring that an antibiotic application approved under Section 507 before the enactment of *FDAMA* would be considered an application submitted, filed and approved under *FD&C Act* Section 505.[67] Congress created an exception to this transition provision. *FDAMA* Section 125(d)(2) exempted certain applications for antibiotic drugs from those provisions of *FD&C Act* Section 505 that provide patent listing, patent certification and market exclusivity. Specifically, *FDAMA* Section 125(d)(2) exempted an antibiotic application from *Hatch-Waxman* benefits when "the drug that is the subject of the application contains an antibiotic drug and the antibiotic drug was the subject of an application" received by FDA under *FD&C Act* Section 507 before the enactment of *FDAMA* (i.e., 21 November 1997). Thus, applications for antibiotic drugs received by FDA prior to 21 November 1997, and applications submitted to FDA subsequent to that date for drugs that contain an antibiotic drug that was the subject of an application received by FDA prior to 21 November 1997 are within the *FDAMA* Section 125(d)(2) exemption and not eligible for *Hatch-Waxman* benefits. These drugs are referred to as "old antibiotics." Applications for antibiotic drugs not subject to the *FDAMA* Section 125(d)(2) exemption (i.e., so-called "new antibiotics") are eligible for *Hatch-Waxman* benefits.

In October 2008, Congress effectively repealed *FDAMA* Section 125(d)(2) so that old antibiotic drugs are now eligible for some *Hatch-Waxman* benefits. Specifically, Section 4 of the *QI Program Supplemental Funding Act* of 2008 (*QI Act*)—"QI" stands for Qualifying Individual—amended the

Table 14-2. Differences Between Applications Submitted and Approved Under *FD&C Act* Section 505

	505(b)(1) NDA	**505(b)(2) Application**	**ANDA**
DESCRIPTION	An NDA is an application that contains full reports of investigations of safety and effectiveness (typically data from two adequate and well-controlled studies) that support the intended use of the product.	A 505(b)(2) application is an application submitted under *FD&C Act* Section 505(b)(1) for a drug for which the full reports of investigations of safety and effectiveness relied upon by the applicant for approval of the application were not conducted by or for the applicant, and for which the applicant has not obtained a right of reference or use from the person by or for whom the investigations were conducted.	An ANDA relies on FDA's previous finding that the RLD is safe and effective. ANDAs contain bioequivalence (BE) data to show that the generic product is the "same as" the RLD, and when there is a change permitted by an approved suitability petition (i.e., dosage form, strength, route of administration, change in an active ingredient in a combination drug), data to support that change.
APPLICATION CONTENT			
Preclinical Data	X	X The need for preclinical data in addition to those data from studies not conducted by or for the applicant must be made on a case-by-case basis, and will vary depending upon the differences between the listed drug and the 505(b)(2) drug.	Safety and effectiveness presumed based on showing BE to the RLD.
Safety & Effectiveness Data	X	X The applicant must provide any additional clinical data necessary to demonstrate the safety and effectiveness of differences between the original drug and its drug.	Safety and effectiveness presumed based on showing BE to the RLD.
Chemistry, Manufacturing & Controls Data	X	X	X
Pharmacokinetic (PK), Bioavailability (BA), & BE Data	X PK and BA data.	X PK and comparative BA data.	X BE data.
Labeling	X	X Labeling different from listed drug to support approved changes (e.g., new indication); labeling must exclude information in listed drug labeling protected by patent and exclusivity.	X Labeling must be the same as the RLD, except that information protected by patent and exclusivity must be excluded.
Pediatric Use Information	X Data to support pediatric use, unless waived or deferred by FDA.	X Data to support change from listed drug, unless waived or deferred by FDA.	X Pediatric labeling must be the same as the RLD, except that information protected by patent and exclusivity must be excluded.
Patent & Exclusivity Information	X Submit information on patents claiming the drug or a method of use; exclusivity request claiming exclusivity.	X Submit information on patents claiming the drug or a method of use (if any); generally, a patent certification (Paragraph I, II, III or IV) or a "section viii" statement is required; exclusivity request claiming exclusivity and exclusivity statement that the listed drug is subject to exclusivity (if any exists).	X Patent certification (Paragraph I, II, III, or IV) or a "section viii" statement is required; exclusivity statement that the RLD is subject to exclusivity (if any exists).
Financial Disclosure & Debarment Certification	X	X	X

Patents and Exclusivity

	505(b)(1) NDA	505(b)(2) Application	ANDA
MARKET EXCLUSIVITY			
Five-Year Exclusivity	X Prevents the submission of an ANDA or 505(b)(2) application for five years after NDA approval, except that an ANDA or 505(b)(2) application with a Paragraph IV certification to an *Orange Book*-listed patent may be submitted after four years.	X Only for applications for NCEs; prevents the submission of an ANDA or another 505(b)(2) application for five years after application approval, except that an ANDA or other 505(b)(2) application with a Paragraph IV certification to an *Orange Book*-listed patent may be submitted after four years; also subject to NDA holder's exclusivity.	No exclusivity; subject to five-year exclusivity of NDA or 505(b)(2) applicant.
Three-Year Exclusivity	X Only if one or more of the clinical studies, other than BA/BE studies, was essential to the product's approval; prevents FDA from making effective an ANDA or 505(b)(2) application for the conditions of approval of the NDA.	X Only if one or more of the clinical studies, other than BA/BE studies, was essential to the product's approval; prevents FDA from making an ANDA or other 505(b)(2) application effective for the conditions of approval of the 505(b)(2) application; also subject to NDA holder's exclusivity.	Subject to three-year exclusivity of NDA or 505(b)(2) applicant.
Orphan Drug Exclusivity	X Prevents FDA from approving an application for the same drug for the same condition for seven years.	X Prevents FDA from approving an application for the same drug for the same condition for seven years; also subject to NDA holder's exclusivity.	Subject to seven-year exclusivity of NDA or 505(b)(2) applicant.
Antibiotic Exclusivity	X Provides an additional five-year exclusivity for qualified infectious disease products	Not applicable	Not applicable
Pediatric Exclusivity	X Extends by six months all other types of patent and non-patent market exclusivity an NDA holder may have under the *FD&C Act* for a particular active moiety.	X Extends by six months all other types of patent and non-patent market exclusivity an applicant may have under the FDC Act for a particular active moiety; also subject to NDA holder's exclusivity.	Subject to exclusivity of NDA or 505(b)(2) applicant.
180-Day Exclusivity	Not applicable.	Not applicable.	X Available to any "first applicant" who files an ANDA with a Paragraph IV certification; prevents FDA from approving other ANDAs submitted by applicants who are not "first applicants."
OTHER			
Adverse Event Reporting Required	X	X	X
User Fees	X	X	Not applicable, but currently under consideration
***Orange Book* Listing**	X Included in the *Orange Book* as a listed drug; may be identified as a RLD.	X Included in the *Orange Book* as a listed drug; can be identified as a therapeutic equivalent (e.g, "AB-rated") to the listed drug if BE is demonstrated and is also a pharmaceutical equivalent.	X Included in the *Orange Book* as a listed drug; can be identified as a therapeutic equivalent (e.g, "AB-rated") to RLD if BE is demonstrated and is also a pharmaceutical equivalent; listed in the *Orange Book* as a "pharmaceutical alternative" without a therapeutic equivalence evaluation code if approved under an approved suitability petition.

Regulatory Affairs Professionals Society

FD&C Act to add new Section 505(v) "Antibiotic Drugs Submitted Before November 21, 1997," to create certain *Hatch-Waxman* benefits for old antibiotics. The *Generating Antibiotic Incentives Now Act* (*GAIN Act*), which was a part of *FDASIA* Title VIII, adds a new Section 505E (21 U.S.C. 355E), which grants an additional five years of market protection at the end of the existing exclusivity for Qualified Infectious Disease Products (QIDP). This adds to any applicable *Hatch-Waxman* five-year NCE exclusivity, *Hatch-Waxman* three-year new clinical studies exclusivity or seven-year orphan drug exclusivity. The five-year extension is also in addition to any six-month pediatric exclusivity. Under Section 505E(d) of the *FD&C Act*, Section 505E(a) provides an extension of five years of market exclusivity to the exclusivity periods provided by Sections 505(c)(3)(E)(ii)–(c)(3)(E)(iv) (21 U.S.C. 355(c)(3)(E)(ii)–(c)(3)(E)(iv)), 505(j)(5)(F)(ii)–(j)(5)(F)(iv) (21 U.S.C. 355(j)(5)(F)(ii)–(j)(5)(F)(iv)), 505A (21 U.S.C. 355a) and 527 (21 U.S.C. 360cc) of the *FD&C Act*. However, as Section 505E(c) of the *FD&C Act* states, not all applications for a QIDP are eligible for the additional market exclusivity. In addition, an application for a drug designated as a QIDP is eligible for Priority Review and Fast Track designation (*FD&C Act* Sections 524A and 506(a)(1) (21 U.S.C. 356(a)(1))), respectively. The *GAIN Act* grants an additional six months of exclusivity for drugs for which a companion diagnostic test is cleared or approved beyond the cumulative total of other applicable exclusivities.

Exclusivity for Enantiomers of Previously Approved Racemates

FDA has for decades treated single enantiomers of approved racemates as previously approved active moieties not eligible for five-year NCE exclusivity (but eligible for three-year exclusivity).[68] (In chemistry, enantiomers are stereoisomers that are non-superimposable complete mirror images of one another. Enantiomers may be either "right-handed" or "left-handed." A racemic mixture is one that has equal amounts of "left- and right-handed" enantiomers of a particular chiral molecule.) *FDAAA*, however, amended the *FD&C Act* to add Section 505(u), which permits a 505(b)(1) NDA applicant for an enantiomer (that is contained in a previously approved racemic mixture) containing full reports of clinical investigations conducted or sponsored by the applicant to "elect to have the single enantiomer not be considered the same active ingredient as that contained in the approved racemic drug," and thus be eligible for five-year NCE exclusivity.[69] The enantiomer NDA applicant cannot "rely on any investigations that are part of an application submitted under [*FD&C Act* Section 505(b)] for approval of the approved racemic drug."[70]

There are certain limitations under the new *FD&C Act* §505(u). The enantiomer 505(b)(1) NDA must not be for a condition of use "(i) in a therapeutic category in which the approved racemic drug has been approved; or (ii) for which any other enantiomer of the racemic drug has been approved."[71] In addition, if the enantiomer NDA applicant elects to receive exclusivity, FDA may not approve the enantiomer drug for any condition of use in the "therapeutic category" in which the racemic drug is approved until 10 years after approving the enantiomer.[72] The term "therapeutic category" is defined in *FD&C Act* Section 505(u) to mean "a therapeutic category identified in the list developed by the United States Pharmacopeia pursuant to section 1860D-4(b)(3)(C)(ii) of the *Social Security Act* and as in effect on [27 September 2007]," which FDA must publish and that may be amended by regulation.[73] FDA has not yet published the therapeutic category list. *FD&C Act* Section 505(u) sunsets on 30 September 2012 unless reauthorized (presumably under *PDUFA V*).[74]

Patent Filing

The *Leahy-Smith America Invents Act* of 2011 (*AIA*) dramatically modified the process surrounding the filing of patents. While there were many procedural changes, this section covers those elements that significantly impact the drug development process. Under *AIA*, the US has changed the right to a patent from the "first to invent" to the "first to file," which took effect in March 2013, and grants the patent to the first entity that files the application regardless of prior publication. *AIA* also narrowed the one-year grace period to be personal to the inventor with some limited provision for third-party publications. This modification of the grace period gives rise to defensive publication planning by pharmaceutical companies and requires greater diligence of the competitive landscape.

Summary

Brand-name drug sponsors may qualify for various periods of patent and non-patent exclusivities, which could delay the submission or final approval of a marketing application for a generic version of the brand-name drug. In addition, certain generic drug sponsors also may qualify for their own 180-day period of market exclusivity. Each type of exclusivity is different in scope and is subject to different rules and interpretations (see **Table 14-2**).

References

1. Before 8 June 1995, patents typically had 17 years of patent life from the date the patent was issued by the US Patent and Trademark Office (PTO). The *Uruguay Rounds Agreements Act* (*URAA*), Pub. L. No. 103-465, 108 Stat. 4809 (1994), changed the patent term in the US so that patents granted after 8 June 1995 (the effective date of the *URAA*) have a 20-year patent life from the date of the first filing of the patent application with PTO. Under a transition provision in the *URAA*, a patent in effect on 8 June 1995 was awarded a term of the greater of 20 years from the filing of the patent or 17 years from the date of patent issuance. See 35 U.S.C. § 154(c)(1).

Patents and Exclusivity

2. 35 U.S.C. §156(g)(1)(B)(i).
3. 35 U.S.C. §156(g)(1)(B)(ii).
4. 35 U.S.C. §§156(c)(2) and 156(g)(1)(B).
5. 35 U.S.C. §156(c)(1).
6. 35 U.S.C. §§156(g)(6)(A) and 156(c)(3).
7. 35 U.S.C. §156(a)(1)-(5). The patent term extension law defines the term "drug product" to mean "the active ingredient of a new drug [as defined in §201(p) of the *FD&C Act*]...including any salt or ester of the active ingredient, as a single entity or in combination with another active ingredient." Id. §156(f)(2). With respect to the applicability of patent term extensions to combination drugs, the US Court of Appeals for the Federal Circuit ruled in 2004 that "the statute places a drug product with two active ingredients, A and B, in the same category as a drug product with a single ingredient.... To extend the term of a patent claiming a composition comprising A and B, either A or B must not have been previously marketed." *Arnold Partnership v. Dudas*, 362 F.3d 1338, 1341 (Fed. Cir. 2004).
8. 35 U.S.C. §§156(a)(1), 156 (d)(5) and 156 (e)(2).
9. 35 U.S.C. §156(d)(5).
10. 35 U.S.C. §156(e)(2).
11. Method-of-use patents listed in the *Orange Book* are typically assigned a "patent use code." The *Orange Book* contains hundreds of such use codes.
12. *FD&C Act* §505(b)(1).
13. FDA regulations at 21 CFR 314.53(b)(1) further state:

For patents that claim the drug substance, the applicant shall submit information only on those patents that claim the drug substance that is the subject of the pending or approved application or that claim a drug substance that is the same as the active ingredient that is the subject of the approved or pending application... For patents that claim a drug product, the applicant shall submit information only on those patents that claim a drug product, as is defined in [21 CFR 314.3 (i.e., a finished dosage form that contains a drug substance)], that is described in the pending or approved application. For patents that claim a method of use, the applicant shall submit information only on those patents that claim indications or other conditions of use that are described in the pending or approved application.... Process patents, patents claiming packaging, patents claiming metabolites, and patents claiming intermediates are not covered by this section, and information on these patents must not be submitted to FDA.

14. FDA, Final Rule; Applications for FDA Approval to Market a New Drug: Patent Submission and Listing Requirements and Application of 30-Month Stays on Approval of Abbreviated New Drug Applications Certifying That a Patent Claiming a Drug Is Invalid or Will Not Be Infringed, 68 *Fed. Reg.* 36,676 (18 June 2003).
15. *FD&C Act* Sections 505(b)(1) & 505(c)(2).
16. Ibid Section 505(c)(2); see also 21 CFR 314.53(c)(2)(ii).
17. *FD&C Act* Section 505(j)(2)(A)(vii).
18. Ibid Section 505(j)(2)(A)(vii)(III) and Section 505(j)(5)(B)(ii).
19. Ibid Sections 505(j)(2)(A)(vii)(I)-(II) & (j)(5)(B)(i).
20. Ibid Sections 505(j)(2)(A)(vii)(IV) & 505(j)(5)(B)(iii).
21. Ibid Section 505(j)(2)(A)(viii). For a listed drug covered by a period of five-year NCE exclusivity, generally an ANDA and 505(b)(2) applicant may not reference the listed drug until such exclusivity (described in the next sections) applicable to that listed drug has expired. For this reason, the information in the NDA for the listed drug is sometimes said to be under "data exclusivity."
22. 21 CFR 314.127(a)(7). An ANDA applicant must make an additional certification (or submit an additional "section viii statement") as to any new patent listed in the *Orange Book* while its application is pending if the NDA holder submits the new patent to FDA for *Orange Book* listing within 30 days of patent issuance. See 21 CFR 314.94(a)(12)(vi). A Paragraph IV certification to a later-listed patent will not result in an additional 30-month stay of ANDA approval.
23. *FD&C Act* Section 505(j)(5)(B).
24. Specifically, five-year exclusivity prevents the submission of an ANDA or 505(b)(2) application for five years unless the applicant submits a Paragraph IV patent certification. See *FD&C Act* Sections 505(b)(2)(A) and 505(j)(2)(A)(vii). In this case, the ANDA or 505(b)(2) application can be submitted after four years; however, "if an action for patent infringement is commenced during the one-year period beginning [four years] after the date of the approval of the [NCE NDA], the thirty-month [stay] period...shall be extended by such amount of time which is required for seven and one-half years to have elapsed from the date of approval of the [NCE NDA]." *FD&C Act* Sections 505(c)(3)(E)(ii) & 505(j)(5)(F)(ii).
25. In addition, it is FDA's policy that five-year exclusivity is not granted for a combination drug containing a previously approved drug. Thus, an application for a two-drug combination containing two previously approved drugs, or even an NCE plus a previously approved drug, is not eligible for five-year exclusivity.
26. A similar ambiguity exists with regard to the scope of three-year exclusivity in Sections 505(c)(3)(E)(iii) and 505(j)(5)(F)(iii) of the *FD&C Act*
27. The original citations are to Sections 505(c)(3)(D) and 505(j)(4)(D) of the *FD&C Act*. These sections were recodified in the *MMA*.
28. 54 *Fed. Reg.* at 28,897.
29. FDA's regulations define the term "active moiety" to mean "the molecule or ion, excluding those appended portions of the molecule that cause the drug to be an ester, salt (including a salt with hydrogen or coordination bonds), or other noncovalent derivative (such as a complex, chelate or clathrate) of the molecule, responsible for the physiological or pharmacological action of the drug substance." 21 CFR 314.108(a).
30. 21 CFR 314.108(b)(4), (5); see also *FD&C Act* Sections 505(j)(5)(F)(iii) and (iv).
31. 21 CFR 314.50(j)(4).
32. 21 CFR 314.108(a).
33. Ibid.
34. FDA, Final Rule, ANDA Regulations; Patent and Exclusivity Provisions, 59 *Fed. Reg.* at 50,338, 50,357 (3 October 1994).
35. 21 CFR 314.50(j)(4)(ii).
36. 59 *Fed. Reg.* at 50,368-69; see also 21 CFR 314.50(j)(4)(iii).
37. This is an important difference compared to five-year exclusivity, which prevents the submission of a generic application.
38. 21 CFR 314.108(b)(4), (5).
39. *FD&C Act* Section 505(j)(2)(A)(v).
40. 21 CFR 314.94(a)(8)(iv).
41. 21 CFR 314.127(a)(7).
42. The term "pediatric studies" is defined as "at least one clinical investigation (that, at [FDA's] discretion, may include pharmacokinetic studies) in pediatric age groups (including neonates in appropriate cases) in which a drug is anticipated to be used." *FD&C Act* Section 505A(a).
43. *FD&C Act* Section 505A does not extend the term of the patent itself, but only the period during which FDA cannot approve (or accept for review) an ANDA or 505(b)(2) application that includes a Paragraph II or Paragraph III certification, or a Paragraph IV certification that concerns a patent that a court has determined is valid and would be infringed. See *FD&C Act* Section 505A(c)(2).
44. See *National Pharmaceutical Alliance v. Henney*, 47 F. Supp. 2d 37 (D.D.C. 1999); and *Guidance for Industry: Qualifying for Pediatric Exclusivity Under Section 505A of the Food, Drug, and Cosmetic Act* (September 1999).
45. *FD&C Act* Section 505A(g).
46. *Guidance for Industry: Qualifying for Pediatric Exclusivity Under Section 505A of the Food, Drug, and Cosmetic Act*, at 14.
47. *FD&C Act* Sections 505A(b)(2), 505A(c)(2).
48. *FD&C Act* Section 526(a)(2).
49. Orphan drug exclusivity operates independently of patent protection and independently of five- and three-year exclusivity (and therefore, pediatric exclusivity as well).
50. *FD&C Act* Sections 527(b)(1) and (2); see also 21 CFR 316.31(a).
51. 21 CFR 316.3(13).

52. 21 CFR 316.3(b)(3)(i)-(iii).
53. *FD&C Act* Section 505(j)(2)(B)(ii)(I).
54. *FD&C Act* Section 505(j)(2)(B)(ii)(II).
55. *FD&C Act* Sections 505(j)(2)(B)(iv)(I)–(II).
56. *FD&C Act* Section 505(j)(5)(B)(iii).
57. *FD&C Act* Section 505(j)(5)(B)(iii).
58. *FD&C Act* Section 505(j)(5)(C)(ii).
59. *FD&C Act* Section 505(j)(5)(C)(iii).
60. *FD&C Act* Section 505(j)(5)(C)(i).
61. Ibid.
62. *FD&C Act* Section 505(j)(5)(C)(iii).
63. A 505(b)(2) application is not eligible for 180-day exclusivity.
64. 149 Cong. Rec. S15746 (daily ed. Nov. 24, 2003) (statement of Sen. Schumer).
65. *FD&C Act* Section 505(q)(1)(G)
66. *Glaxo, Inc. v. Heckler*, 623 F. Supp. 69 (E.D.N.C. 1985).
67. *FDAMA* Section 125(d)(1).
68. See 54 *Fed. Reg.* at 28,898. "FDA will consider whether a drug contains a previously approved active moiety on a case-by-case basis. FDA notes that a single enantiomer of a previously approved racemate contains a previously approved active moiety and is therefore not considered a new chemical entity."
69. *FD&C Act* Section 505(u)(1).
70. *FD&C Act* Section 505(u)(1)(A)(ii)(II).
71. *FD&C Act* Section 505(u)(1)(B).
72. *FD&C Act* Section 505(u)(2)(A).
73. *FD&C Act* Section 505(u)(3).
74. *FD&C Act* Section 505(u)(4).

Helpful References and Resources
- FDA's Office of Generic Drugs webpage, including exclusivity decisions www.fda.gov/Drugs/DevelopmentApprovalProcess/HowDrugsareDevelopedandApproved/ApprovalApplications/AbbreviatedNewDrugApplicationANDAGenerics/ucm142112.htm
- *Federal Food, Drug, and Cosmetic Act* www.fda.gov/RegulatoryInformation/Legislation/default.htm The Electronic *Orange Book* www.accessdata.fda.gov/scripts/cder/ob/default.cfm.
- FDA's Paragraph IV Patent Certification List www.fda.gov/Drugs/DevelopmentApprovalProcess/HowDrugsareDevelopedandApproved/ApprovalApplications/AbbreviatedNewDrugApplicationANDAGenerics/ucm047676.htm

Chapter 15

Over-the-Counter Drug Products

Updated by Melissa Cavuto, MS, MBA, RAC

OBJECTIVES

- Provide an overview of the criteria for marketing over-the-counter (OTC) drugs
- Discuss the drug product classification and regulations surrounding OTC drugs
- Discuss the regulatory pathways available for marketing OTC drugs
- Provide an overview of OTC drug advertising and compliance regulations

LAWS, REGULATIONS AND GUIDELINES COVERED IN THIS CHAPTER

- *Federal Food, Drug, and Cosmetic Act* of 1938
- *Durham-Humphrey Amendments* of 1951
- *Fair Packaging and Labeling Act* of 1966
- *Kefauver-Harris Amendments* of 1962
- *Federal Anti-Tampering Act* of 1983
- *Poison Prevention Packaging Act* of 1970
- *Dietary Supplement and Nonprescription Drug Consumer Protection Act* of 2006
- OTC Drug Review and monograph system (21 CFR 328-358)
- OTC Drug Product Labeling Format and Content Requirements (21 CFR 201.66)
- *Guidance for Industry: Labeling OTC Human Drug Products—Questions and Answers* (December 2008)
- *Guidance for Industry: Postmarketing Adverse Event Reporting for Nonprescription Human Drug Products Marketed Without an Approved Application* (July 2009)
- *Draft Guidance for Industry: Time and Extent Applications* (February 2004)
- *Guidance for Industry: Label Comprehension Studies for Nonprescription Drug Products* (August 2010)
- *Guidance for Industry: Contents of a Complete Submission for the Evaluation of Proprietary Names* (February 2010)

Introduction

Over-the-counter (OTC) drugs continue to play an increasingly important role in the daily lives of every person in the US and are viewed as a significant component to the overall soundness of our healthcare system. Physicians are prescribing OTC drugs at increasing levels, primarily due to the growing cost of prescription pharmaceuticals. Prior to 1951, there was no legal basis for the designation of what was acceptable as an OTC drug product. The 1951 *Durham-Humphrey Amendment* to the *Federal Food, Drug,*

Chapter 15

and Cosmetic Act (FD&C Act) established three criteria that would limit a drug to prescription status:
- habit forming drugs
- not safe for use unless supervised by a healthcare professional
- limited to prescription use under a New Drug Application (NDA)

All drugs that did not meet these criteria were classified, by default, OTC.

Typically, OTC drugs have the following characteristics:
- benefits clearly outweigh possible risks
- potential for misuse and abuse is low
- public can use them for self-diagnosed conditions
- can be labeled to help assure appropriate use by the average person
- healthcare practitioners are not needed for their safe and effective use

Regulation of OTC Drugs

OTC drugs can receive regulatory approval by submission and approval of a New Drug Application (NDA) or through an OTC Drug Monograph. In most cases, regulations applicable to prescription drugs also apply to OTC drug products. Regulations relating to all aspects of drug manufacture and testing (current Good Manufacturing Practices (CGMPs)), facility listing and inspection, drug registration, clinical trials and safety oversight apply equally to prescription and OTC drug products. There are two main avenues to receive approval for an OTC drug. Both review and approval processes for OTC drugs would be handled by the FDA Center for Drug Evaluation and Research's (CDER) Office of Drug Evaluation IV.

The NDA route would involve submission to the agency by one of the three processes below:
- 505(b)(1) New Drug Application (NDA)
- 505(b)(2) New Drug Application (NDA)
- (505)(j) Abbreviated New Drug Application (ANDA)

A 505(b)(1) application contains full safety and efficacy trial reports. The trials included in this application are conducted either by or for the applicant, or rights have been obtained by the applicant to reference the data. A 505(b)(2) application relies on safety and efficacy data submitted from trials that the applicant did not conduct and did not obtain a right to reference. Essentially, this type of application relies on safety and efficacy data in either the published literature or from data that resulted in an approved NDA previously submitted by another applicant. A (505)(j) application, commonly referred to as an ANDA, is used to gain approval of a generic product.

Table 15-1 summarizes the differences between the NDA/ANDA and OTC drug monograph pathways to market a product.

In addition to the NDA route, OTC drug products are approved for marketing via the OTC monograph system that include OTC-specific regulations on labeling (Title 21 of the Code of Federal Regulations (CFR) Part 201 *Subpart C Labeling Requirements for Over-the-Counter Drugs*), on general and administrative procedures for the classification of OTC drugs (21 CFR 330) and on therapeutic categories and related ingredients that have been classified as safe and effective for OTC use under the OTC drug monograph system (21 CFR 331–358).

OTC Drug Monograph Route

Currently, there are over 300,000 OTC drug products on the market, and many of these products were approved by the OTC monograph route. FDA reviews the active ingredients and the labeling of more than 80 therapeutic classes of drugs, instead of individual drug products. For each category, an OTC drug monograph is developed and published in the *Federal Register*.

In 1972, FDA initiated the OTC drug review process as part of the implementation of the *Kefauver-Harris Amendments* of 1962. The OTC drug review process encompassed review of the safety and efficacy of those products already on the market. The OTC drug monograph provides specific guidance covering generally recognized as safe and effective (GRASE) active ingredients (strength and dosage form) and label requirements (indications, warnings and directions for use). By grouping the products into therapeutic drug categories and evaluating the active ingredients rather than assessing each individual product, FDA was able to make the process more efficient. **Table 15-2** details the more than 80 therapeutic categories that are covered in a process comprised of Advisory Panel expert review and a three-step public rulemaking process (call for information, proposed rules and a codified final rule) published in the *Federal Register*.

Under 21 CFR Part 330.10 data regarding OTC monographs can be submitted by anyone, including a drug company, health professional, consumer or citizen's group. If the submission is a request to amend an existing drug monograph or is an opinion regarding a drug monograph, it needs to be submitted in the form of a citizen petition or as correspondence to an established monograph docket. However, if no monograph exists, data must be submitted in the format as outlined in 21 CFR Section 330.1.

The review process commenced with the creation of therapeutic category-specific Advisory Panels composed of subject matter experts. A call for information was published in the *Federal Register* for the public (i.e., industry, healthcare professionals and consumers) to submit data within a defined time

Table 15-1. NDA vs. OTC Drug Monograph

NDA Route	OTC Monograph route
Premarket approval	No premarket approval (conditions of marketing are codified) • The onus is on the manufacturer/distributor to assure compliance
Confidential filing	Public process
Drug product-specific	Active ingredient-specific • OTC drug therapeutic category
May require a user fee	No user fees
Potential for marketing exclusivity	No marketing exclusivity
Mandated FDA review timelines	No mandated FDA review timelines
May require clinical studies for application • Safety and efficacy • Label comprehension • Actual use • Demonstration of appropriate consumer selection/deselection in OTC setting	Clinical studies for claims support or to amend monograph only

period. Advisory Panels held open meetings and reviewed the data to provide expert recommendations, including categorizing active ingredients into one of three categories:

- Category I—generally recognized as safe and effective and not misbranded
- Category II—not generally recognized as safe and effective or is misbranded
- Category III—insufficient data available to permit classification (This category allows a manufacturer an opportunity to show that the ingredients in a product are effective, and if they are not, to reformulate or appropriately relabel the product.)

Advisory Panel recommendations are published as an Advance Notice of Proposed Rulemaking (ANPR) for public review and comment within a defined time period. After collection of public comments, FDA published its conclusions in the form of Tentative Final Monograph (TFM) (Proposed Rule). The TFM is also published for public review and comment. FDA reviewed any additional information submitted prior to publishing a final monograph (FM) (Final Rule). Once the FM is published, manufacturers of products not complying with FM requirements have a defined timeframe to withdraw the product from the market, bring the product into compliance with the monograph or submit an NDA. FMs are codified in the CFR. Products complying with monographs can be marketed without preapproval by FDA, provided they are appropriately drug listed, compliant with CGMPs and manufactured in a registered facility.

The monograph process can be very lengthy as there are no defined timelines within which FDA must move from a TFM to an FM. Hence, there are still a number of monographs that have not been finalized. For example, the monograph for oral healthcare drug products is not final, even though the original Advisory Panel provided its expert opinion in 1979. Products meeting the conditions of in-process TFMs can be marketed. FDA can amend FMs as new information becomes available. For example, the *OTC Internal Analgesic Drug Products* monograph (21 CFR 343) was amended in 2009 to include an organ-specific warning statement for acetaminophen and NSAIDs. Two regulatory pathways are available for industry to request that an OTC drug monograph be reopened and/or amended:

1. Citizen Petition
2. Time and Extent Application (TEA)

The Citizen Petition process is codified in 21 CFR 10.30. A Citizen Petition can be used to amend an OTC drug monograph at any stage of the process.

The TEA process is codified in 21 CFR 330.14. This process can be used to add an ingredient to an OTC monograph that has been approved under an NDA or has been marketed in another country. This process can be utilized only when the ingredient has been used for a significant time (five or more continuous years in the same country) with a significant marketing distribution (tens of millions of dosage units sold).

NDA Route

Products not covered by the OTC drug monographs are subject to FDA preapproval through the NDA process prior to marketing. There are four NDA routes available for OTC products:

- Direct-to-OTC NDA
- Rx-to-OTC Switch
- NDA Monograph Deviation
- generic (ANDA)

Table 15-2. OTC Monograph Therapeutic Category Subtopics Evaluated* as Part of the OTC Review Process.
Therapeutic category subtopics in **BOLD** are codified in the Final Monographs

Acne	**Callus Remover**	**Nighttime Sleep Aid**
Allergy	**Corn Remover**	**Ophthalmic**
Analgesic, External	**Dandruff**	Oral Health Care
Analgesic, Internal	Daytime Sedative	Oral Wound Healing
Anorectal	**Decongestant, Nasal**	**Otic**
Antacid	**Dental Care**	Overindulgence, Food & Drink
Anthelmintic	**Deodorant, Internal**	Pancreatic Insufficiency
Antibiotic, First Aid	**Diaper Rash**	**Pediculicide**
Anticaries	Digestive Aid	**Poison Oak/Ivy**
Anticholinergic	Drink Overindulgence	Poison Treatment
Antidiarrheal	Exocrine Pancreatic Insufficiency	Prostatic Hypertrophy
Antiemetic	**Expectorant**	**Psoriasis**
Antiflatulent	**External Analgesic**	**Seborrheic Dermatitis**
Antifungal	Fever Blister	Sedative, Daytime
Antihistamine	**First Aid Antibiotic**	Skin Bleaching
Antimalarial	Food Overindulgence	**Skin Protectant**
Antimicrobial	Hair Growth & Loss	**Sleep Aid, Nighttime**
Antiperspirant	Hormone	
Antipyretic	Hypophosphatemia/Hyperphosphatemia	Smoking Deterrent
Antirheumatic	**Ingrown Toenail**	**Stimulant**
Antitussive	Insect Bite & Sting	Stomach Acidifier
Aphrodisiac	Insect Repellent, Oral	**Sunscreen**
Astringent	**Internal Analgesic**	Thumbsucking
Benign Prostatic Hypertrophy	**Internal Deodorant**	**Topical Analgesic**
Boil Treatment	Laxative	Vaginal Contraceptive
Bronchodilator	Leg Muscle Cramps	Vaginal Drug Products
Camphorated Oil	**Male Genital Desensitizers**	Vitamins & Minerals
Cholecystokinetic	Menstrual	**Wart Remover**
Cold & Cough	Nailbiting	Weight Control
Colloidal Silver	**Nasal Decongestant**	

*Therapeutic category subtopic active ingredients have been implemented as part of therapeutic category Final Monograph, are part of a proposed rule or have been designated by FDA as not GRASE and/or misbranded

Direct-to-OTC NDA

A product can be approved by the OTC route even if it was never available as prescription. The same requirements apply for direct-to-OTC NDA products as for new prescription drug products, with the exception that the applicant also needs to prove that the product can be safely used by the wide consumer population without healthcare professional oversight. Colgate Total toothpaste (active ingredients: Sodium Fluoride and Triclosan) and Abreva (active ingredient: docosanol) are examples of direct-to-OTC NDAs.

Rx-to-OTC Switch

This route is used when it can be demonstrated that a prescription product can be used by the wide consumer population without healthcare professional oversight. FDA evaluates the toxicity and safe consumer use of the product as well as whether the condition can be self-diagnosed and recognized without a healthcare professional's intervention. This route has gained popularity because it can be timed to coincide with patent expiry, allowing an innovator company to market a product for a longer period of time without generic competition and to a wider consumer base.

One of the challenges in the switch process is transcribing information from the prescription drug product label to the very limited space of the 'Drug Facts' OTC label format in a manner that consumers comprehend and apply. Some examples of products that were switched are Prilosec OTC (proton pump inhibitor for frequent heartburn), Nicorette (smoking cessation aid), Zyrtec (antihistamine) and Plan B (emergency contraceptive). Several attempts to switch cholesterol-lowering medication to date have failed to meet FDA's criteria for appropriate self-selection.

An Rx-to-OTC switch that creates a new OTC product category is referred to as a first-in-class switch. First-in-class switches are often subject to FDA Advisory Panel review (composed of applicable prescription drug Advisory Committee members and members of the Nonprescription Drug Advisory Committee). Examples of first-in-class switches are Prilosec OTC, Alli (weight loss aid) and Claritin (a non-sedating antihistamine). Rx-to-OTC switches also can be partial or complete. For a complete switch (e.g., Claritin, Nicorette), the full product range and indications are switched. For partial switch, either some product strengths or indications remain prescription (e.g., Prilosec OTC).

To address rules for a partial switch, an ANPR was published in the *Federal Register* in 2005 to elicit comments on whether clarification was necessary in circumstances when an active substance can be marketed simultaneously as OTC and prescription. While the rulemaking process for this issue is not finalized, FDA indicated that it will not allow the same active substance to be marketed in a certain population in prescription status and as an OTC for a subset of that population.

NDA Monograph Deviation
This route can be used when the drug product deviates in any aspect from the OTC drug monograph. The applicant submits an NDA referencing the monograph with data to support the drug product's safety and efficacy with the deviation. This route was utilized to gain approval for a head lice aerosol foam product, Rid Mousse. This drug product met all the conditions of the Pediculicide Final Monograph except for the dosage form.

Generic (ANDA)
The ANDA (505)(j) route can be used when the company intends to market an equivalent OTC drug product to one that is already on the market. The same regulations apply here as in prescription products, however the company must submit bioequivalence data in lieu of the safety and efficacy studies. In addition, the product labeling must be the same as for the original product.

OTC NDA Products and Specific Studies
As with prescription products, manufacturers of OTC products conduct safety, efficacy and preclinical studies. However, there are three additional studies that are specific to OTC products:
- label comprehension
- self-selection
- actual use or OTC simulation trials

Label comprehension studies are used to evaluate the extent to which a consumer can understand the information on the proposed OTC drug label and then apply this information when making drug product use decisions in a hypothetical situation. Label comprehension studies are open label and uncontrolled. No drug product is used in these studies, and they do not have to be conducted under an IND; however, it is recommended that they be submitted under an IND to obtain CDER advice on the protocol. FDA issued a guidance document on design aspects of label comprehension testing in August 2010. The guidance describes test standards, hurdle rates and test population literacy demographics.

Identification of a suitable label may take several iterations and should achieve a satisfactory level of comprehension prior to running self-selection and actual use trials (AUT).

Self-selection studies are used to evaluate whether a consumer can make a correct decision about using or not using a drug product based on reading the information on the drug product label and applying knowledge of his or her personal medical history. Drug product is not used in these studies, although a self-selection measure can be incorporated into the design of AUT.

AUT are used to evaluate consumer behavior—whether a consumer will actually use the product safely without healthcare practitioner supervision and as per the label instructions. These trials are typically designed as "all comers" studies, to measure consumer behavior against the product usage intent described in the product labeling and are conducted under an IND. The product label tested in AUT should have been evaluated previously in the label comprehension study.

The sponsor must follow the same process when selecting the proprietary name for an OTC product as for a prescription drug when using submitting an NDA. Ideally, a primary and alternate proposed proprietary name should be submitted to the Division of Medication Error Prevention and Analysis (DMEPA) for review and approval.

Labeling of OTC Drugs- "Drug Facts" Label
The label of an OTC product must include specific information that will help the consumer understand the usage and safety information without the oversight of a healthcare professional. The final rule on the use of "Drug Facts" became effective in 1999. The rule standardized the format, content, headings, graphics and minimum type size requirements to be used on all OTC drug products.

All OTC medicine labels have detailed usage and warning information to help consumers determine whether the product is appropriate to treat their condition and how to take the product correctly.

Specific information on the OTC label must include:
- active ingredient
- uses
- warnings
- inactive ingredients
- purpose
- directions
- other information

An example of a "Drug Facts" label is provided in **Figure 15-1**. All OTC drug products must bear the "Drug Facts" label in accordance with 21 CFR 201.66, and it must be visible to consumers at the time of purchase.

FDA regulations require OTC labeling to be written and tested for use by ordinary people, including those with low comprehension skills, to ensure product information is easy to find and understand including:
- the product's intended uses and results
- active and inactive ingredients
- adequate directions for proper use
- warnings against unsafe use, side effects and adverse reactions

Some OTC drug monographs also provide professional labeling information that includes specific information for healthcare professionals on uses outside the scope of that permitted by OTC consumer drug labeling.

Packaging Requirements

Tamper-evident packing is becoming the standard for most OTC drug products as required by 21 CFR 211.132. Statements must be included on both outer and inner cartons that clearly describe the tamper-evident features utilized. In addition, OTC drugs must comply with child-resistant packaging requirements as defined in the *Poison Prevention Packaging Act of 1970 (PPPA)*. The US Consumer Product Safety Commission (CPSC) enforces child-resistant packaging requirements. There is a provision in place for one container size to be marketed in non-child-resistant packaging as long as it is adequately labeled and as long as child-resistant packages are also supplied.

FDA Oversight of OTC Drug Products

The Office of Drug Evaluation IV (ODE-IV) has two divisions that have oversight responsibility for OTC drugs. The Division of Nonprescription Clinical Evaluation (DNCE) is responsible for managing INDs and the associated NDAs for those products that are approved under the NDA route. The Division of Nonprescription Regulation Development is responsible for the OTC drug monograph process and the products marketed under the respective monograph.

OTC and prescription drugs generally adhere to the same regulatory requirements. All OTC drug manufacturing activities must comply with 21 CFR 210 and 211, current Good Manufacturing Practices for Pharmaceuticals. Drug substance and drug product manufacturing sites are required to be registered with FDA and are subject to prior approval inspections (PAI) for NDA products and routine FDA inspections. All OTC drug products are required to be drug listed, although the National Drug Code (NDC) is suggested but not required to be displayed on the product label. Medical oversight activities for OTC drug products also mimic those required of prescription products. The *Dietary Supplement and Nonprescription Drug Consumer Protection Act* of 2006 mandated safety reporting requirements for OTC drug products marketed without an NDA. Prior to this act, only NDA products were subject to adverse event reporting requirements.

NDA lifecycle management and maintenance activities are identical to those of their prescription counterparts.

Challenges in Assigning a Product Class

Products are classified as drugs based on their intended use as defined by the *FD&C Act*. Intended use can be determined through the product indications or claims, consumer perception or drug ingredients. Because product positioning can define product classification, some cosmetics can be considered unapproved drugs. This is why some cosmetics making drug claims either on the product labeling or through advertising and promotion have been subject to regulatory actions by FDA. Some OTC drug products that make cosmetic-like claims (cleaning)—such as toothpastes—are considered drugs based on the presence of the anti-caries drug ingredient fluoride. In fact, many OTC products meet the definition within the *FD&C Act* of both a cosmetic and a drug because they have two intended uses. Examples of such products include antidandruff shampoo, deodorants that contain antiperspirant actives and moisturizers and makeup marketed with sun-protection ingredients. These products must comply with requirements for both cosmetics and drugs. One such requirement for drugs that are also cosmetics is to list inactive ingredients in descending order of predominance as required by the cosmetic regulations, rather than in alphabetical order as required by drug regulations.

Advertising

Advertising for OTC drug products is regulated by The Federal Trade Commission (FTC). Since 1971, there has been a Memorandum of Understanding between the FDA and FTC that gives primary responsibility over advertising of OTC drugs to FTC and primary responsibility over

OTC drug labeling to FDA. Unlike prescription products, there is no fair balance requirement for OTC drugs, and promotional material is not required to be submitted to FTC prior to distribution. FTC has a number of policy guides on advertising. The National Advertising Division (NAD) of the Council of Better Business Bureaus also oversees advertising either by directly challenging the advertising or resolving the advertising challenge submitted by a competitor.

In addition, the Consumer Healthcare Product Association (CHPA), a not-for-profit trade association that represents the OTC drug industry, has an advertising code of practice.

The regulatory professional should ensure that the advertising standards, including quality claim support data, are available prior to the initiation of advertising.

Summary

OTC drugs must comply with the same quality standards and regulatory requirements as prescription products. However, unlike prescription products, they must be proven to be safe and effective without healthcare professional supervision. Hence, the information on the label of the OTC drug product is critical. A number of regulatory pathways are available to market OTC drug products in the US. The role of the regulatory professional in creating a strategy for product innovation and product differentiation through claims and/or promotion and advertising, while ensuring compliance with the applicable rules and regulations, is essential in the dynamic and challenging arena of OTC drugs.

Recommended Reading
- FTC, Bureau of Consumer Protection, Business Center. Health Claims. FTC website. http://business.ftc.gov/advertising-and-marketing/health-claims. Accessed 26 April 2013.
- FTC, Bureau of Consumer Protection, Business Center. Advertising FAQ's: A Guide for Small Business. FTC website. http://business.ftc.gov/documents/bus35-advertising-faqs-guide-small-business. Accessed 26 April 2013.
- CHPA website. http://www.chpa-info.org/scienceregulatory/science_regulatory.aspx. Accessed 26 April 2013.
- ODE-IV Presentation of Regulation of Nonprescription Drug Products. FDA website. www.fda.gov/downloads/AboutFDA/CentersOffices/CDER/UCM148055.pdf. Accessed 26 April 2013.
- Is It a Cosmetic, a Drug, or Both? (Or Is It Soap?). FDA website. www.fda.gov/Cosmetics/GuidanceComplianceRegulatoryInformation/ucm074201.htm. Accessed 26 April 2013.
- Drug Applications for Over-the-Counter OTC) Drugs. FDA website. www.fda.gov/Drugs/DevelopmentApprovalProcess/HowDrugsareDevelopedandApproved/ApprovalApplications/Over-the-CounterDrugs/default.htm. Accessed 26 April 2013.
- FAQs About CDER. FDA website. www.fda.gov/AboutFDA/CentersOffices/OfficeofMedicalProductsandTobacco/CDER/FAQsaboutCDER/default.htm. Accessed 26 April 2013.

Figure 15-1. Example of an OTC Drug Facts Label

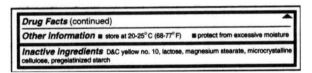

- Development and Approval Process (Drugs). FDA website. www.fda.gov/drugs/developmentapprovalprocess/default.htm. Accessed 26 April 2013.
- FDA MAPP 6020.5R Good Review Practice: OND Review Management of INDs and NDAs for Nonprescription Drug Products. FDA website. www.fda.gov/downloads/AboutFDA/CentersOffices/CDER/ManualofPoliciesProcedures/ucm082003.pdf. Accessed 26 April 2013.
- *Guidance for Industry: Label Comprehension Studies for Nonprescription Drug Products* (August 2010). FDA website. www.fda.gov/downloads/Drugs/GuidanceComplianceRegulatoryInformation/Guidances/UCM143834.pdf. Accessed 26 April 2013.
- *Guidance for Industry: Postmarketing Adverse Event Reporting for Nonprescription Human Drug Products Marketed Without an Approved Application* (July 2009). FDA website. www.fda.gov/downloads/Drugs/.../Guidances/ucm171672.pdf. Accessed 26 April 2013.
- *Guidance for Industry: Time and Extent Applications for Nonprescription Drug Products* (September 2011). FDA website. http://www.fda.gov/downloads/Drugs/Guidances/ucm078902.pdf. Accessed 26 April 2013.
- *Guidance for Industry: Labeling OTC Human Drug Products—Questions and Answers* (December 2008). FDA website. www.fda.gov/downloads/Drugs/GuidanceComplianceRegulatoryInformation/Guidances/ucm078792.pdf. Accessed 26 April 2013.
- *Guidance for Industry: Contents of a Complete Submission for the Evaluation of Proprietary Names* (February 2010). FDA website. www.fda.gov/downloads/Drugs/GuidanceComplianceRegulatoryInformation/Guidances/ucm075068.pdf. Accessed 26 April 2013.

Chapter 16

Prescription Drug Labeling, Advertising and Promotion

By Linda Pollitz, RAC

OBJECTIVES

- Understand the scope of FDA's regulatory authority over prescription drug "labeling"

- Learn the general FDA requirements for the labeling, advertising and promotion of prescription drugs

- Recognize the importance of agency enforcement action in the regulation of promotional materials

LAWS, REGULATIONS AND GUIDELINES COVERED IN THIS CHAPTER

- *Federal Food, Drug, and Cosmetic Act* of 1938

- *Federal Trade Commission Act* of 1914

- *Kefauver-Harris Drug Amendments* of 1962

- 21 CFR 99 Dissemination of information (on unapproved/new uses for marketed drugs, biologics and devices)

- 21 CFR 200.5 Mailing of important information about drugs

- 21 CFR 201 Labeling

- 21 CFR 201.56 Requirements on content and format of labeling for human prescription drug and biological products

- 21 CFR 201.57 Specific requirements on content and format of labeling for human prescription drug and biological products described in 201.56(b)(1).

- 21 CFR 202 Prescription drug advertising

- 21 CFR 203 Prescription drug marketing

- 21 CFR 208 Medication Guides for prescription drug products

- 21 CFR 312.7 Promotion of Investigational Drugs

- 21 CFR 314.50(l) Applications for FDA approval to market a new drug; content and format; labeling

- 21 CFR 314.70 Applications for FDA approval to market a new drug; supplements and other changes to an approved application

- 21 CFR 314.81(2)(iii) Applications for FDA approval to market a new drug; other postmarketing reports; annual report; labeling

- 21 CFR 314.81(b)(3) Other postmarketing reports

- 21 CFR 314.126 Adequate and well-controlled studies

- 21 CFR 314.550 Promotional materials

- 21 CFR 601.12(f)(4) Advertisements and promotional labeling

- 21 CFR 601.45 Accelerated approval of biological products/promotional materials

- *Guidance for Industry: Dosage and Administration Section of Labeling for Human Prescription Drug and Biological Products—Content and Format (March 2010)*

- *Guidance for Industry: Warnings and Precautions, Contraindications, and Boxed Warnings Sections of Labeling for Human Prescription Drug and Biological Products – Content and Format (October 2011)*

- *Guidance for Industry: Adverse Reactions Section of Labeling for Human Prescription Drug and Biological Products—Content and Format (January 2006)*

- *Draft Guidance for Industry: Clinical Pharmacology Section of Labeling for Human Prescription Drug and Biological Products—Content and Format (March 2009)*

- *Guidance for Industry: Clinical Studies Section of Labeling for Human Prescription Drug and Biological Products—Content and Format (January 2006)*

- *Guidance for Industry: Content and Format for Geriatric Labeling (October 2001)*

- *Guidance for Industry: Dosage and Administration Section of Labeling for Human Prescription Drug and Biological Products – Content and Format (March 2010)*

- *Guidance for Industry: Warnings and Precautions, Contraindications, and Boxed Warning Sections of Labeling for Human Prescription Drug and Biological Products—Content and Format (October 2011)*

- *Guidance for Industry and Review Staff: Labeling for Human Prescription Drug and Biological Products — Determining Established Pharmacologic Class for Use in the Highlights of Prescribing Information (October 2009)*

- *Guidance for Industry: Labeling for Human Prescription Drug and Biological Products—Implementing the PLR Content and Format Requirements (February 2013)*

- *Draft Guidance for Industry and Review Staff: Pediatric Information Incorporated Into Human Prescription Drug and Biological Products Labeling (February 2013)*

- *Contents of a Complete Submission for the Evaluation of Proprietary Names (February 2010)*

- *Guidance for Industry: Providing Regulatory Submissions in Electronic Format—Content of Labeling (April 2005)*

- *Guidance: Medication Guides — Distribution Requirements and Inclusion in Risk Evaluation and Mitigation Strategies (REMS) (November 2011)*

- *Draft Guidance for Industry: Public Availability of Labeling Changes in "Changes Being Effected" Supplements (September 2006)*

- *Guidance for Industry: Patient-Reported Outcome Measures: Use in Medical Product Development to Support Labeling Claims (December 2009)*

- *Guidance for Industry: Indexing Structured Product Labeling (June 2008)*

- *Draft Guidance for Industry: SPL Standard for Content of Labeling Technical Qs & As (October 2009)*

- *Draft Guidance for Industry: Providing Regulatory Submissions in Electronic Format—Drug Establishment Registration and Drug Listing (May 2009)*

- *Draft Guidance for Industry: Accelerated Approval Products—Submission of Promotional Materials (March 1999)*

- *Guidance for Industry: Aerosol Steroid Product Safety Information in Prescription Drug Advertising and Promotional Labeling (December 1997)*

- *Draft Guidance for Industry: Brief Summary: Disclosing Risk Information in Consumer-Directed Print Advertisements (January 2004)*

- Guidance for Industry: Consumer-Directed Broadcast Advertisements (August 1999)

- Draft Guidance for Industry and FDA Staff: Dear Health Care Provider Letters: Improving Communication of Important Safety Information (November 2010)

- Draft Guidance for Industry and FDA: Consumer-Directed Broadcast Advertising of Restricted Devices (February 2004)

- Draft Guidance for Industry: "Help-Seeking" and Other Disease Awareness Communications by or on Behalf of Drug and Device Firms (January 2004)

- Guidance for Industry: Industry-Supported Scientific and Educational Activities (November 1997)

- Guidance for Industry: Product Name Placement, Size, and Prominence in Advertising and Promotional Labeling (January 2012)

- Draft Guidance for Industry: Promoting Medical Products in a Changing Healthcare Environment; I. Medical Product Promotion by Healthcare Organizations or Pharmacy Management Companies (PBMs) (December 1997)

- Draft Guidance for Industry: Providing Regulatory Submissions in Electronic Format – Prescription Drug Advertising and Promotional Labeling (January 2001)

- Draft Guidance for Industry: Using FDA-Approved Patient Labeling in Consumer-Directed Print Advertisements (April 2001)

- Guidance for Industry: Good Reprint Practices for the Distribution of Medical Journal Articles and Medical or Scientific Reference Publications on Unapproved New Uses of Approved Drugs and Approved or Cleared Medical Devices (January 2009)

- Draft Guidance for Industry: Presenting Risk Information in Prescription Drug and Medical Device Promotion (May 2009)

- Draft Guidance for Industry: Direct-to-Consumer Television Advertisements – FDAAA DTC Television Ad Pre-Dissemination Review Program (March 2012)

- "PhRMA Code on Interactions with Healthcare Professionals" (July 2008, effective January 2009)

- PhRMA Guiding Principles: Direct to Consumer Advertisements About Prescription Medicines (December 2008)

- OIG Compliance Guidance (see section IV, "Prescription Drug Promotion—Other Considerations")

Introduction

The *Federal Food, Drug, and Cosmetic Act* of 1938 (*FD&C Act*) grants the US Food and Drug Administration (FDA) broad authority over prescription drug "labeling." Beyond the product's "label" (defined in the act as a display of written, printed or graphic material on the immediate container of a drug), "labeling" is a broader term encompassing any written, printed or graphic material on the drug product, any of its containers or wrappers or any material issued in association with the drug.

Therefore, in addition to all product container and packaging labels, the regulatory definition of drug "labeling" includes:

- FDA-approved professional labeling (information for healthcare professionals about approved uses of the drug), also referred to as the prescribing information or the "package insert" (PI)
- FDA-approved patient labeling (drug information directed to patients) for some drug products with serious risk(s) in the form of a Medication Guide
- promotional labeling (any material containing information intended to promote the use of the drug) (Even oral statements by sales representatives are subject to regulation by FDA as "promotional labeling." Unlike the PI and patient labeling, promotional labeling is disseminated by a company without a specific "approval" of the materials by FDA.)

The primary regulations governing FDA-approved prescription drug labeling are in Title 21 of the Code of Federal Regulations (CFR) Part 201. While FDA has issued numerous regulations and guidance documents on the labeling of certain products and within specific therapeutic areas, only the most general labeling requirements are discussed in this chapter. Promotional labeling will be discussed later in this chapter.

General Labeling Requirements (21 CFR 201 Subparts A and B)

The inclusion of certain statements and their appropriate placement and prominence are key concerns in FDA's regulation of drug labeling.

Some of the most broadly applicable requirements are:
- manufacturer, packager or distributor's name and address (21 CFR 201.1)
- location of National Drug Code (NDC) numbers (requested but not required) (21 CFR 201.2) (note: the determination of NDC numbers is included in 21 CFR 207.35)
- statement of ingredients (21 CFR 201.10), including required warning statements for specific ingredients (e.g., FD&C Yellow No. 5 (21 CFR 201.20))
- location of expiration date (21 CFR 201.17) and significance of control numbers (21 CFR 201.18)
- bar code label requirements (21 CFR 201.25)
- statement of identity (21 CFR 201.50)
- declaration of net quantity of contents (21 CFR 201.51)
- statement of dosage (21 CFR 201.55)

Any changes to approved drug product labeling are considered a change to the New Drug Application (NDA) or Biologics License Application (BLA) and are required to be reported to FDA according to the regulations governing supplements to an approved application (21 CFR 314.70). Notably, with the passage of the *Food and Drug Administration Amendments Act* of 2007 (*FDAAA*), FDA was granted new authority to require approved NDA holders to make safety-related labeling changes based on new safety information that becomes available after a drug's approval. Under the new law, NDA holders have a limited time to respond and implement these FDA-requested labeling changes (see Section 505(o)(4) of the *FD&C Act* for details).

Additional labeling requirements for over-the-counter drugs are available at 21 CFR 201 Subpart C. Specific labeling requirements for particular drug products (e.g., estrogenic hormone preparations, pressurized aerosols, nebulizers and powders) are available at 21 CFR 201 Subpart G.

Professional Labeling, Including the 2006 *Physician Labeling Rule* (*PLR*)

The professional labeling, or package insert, for a drug is a compilation of product information based on FDA's comprehensive review of the sponsor's approved NDA/BLA. The package insert is considered "adequate directions for use," written to direct healthcare professionals' use of a drug product.

In 2006, FDA substantially amended its regulations on the content and format of professional labeling (21 CFR 201.56 and 201.57) and issued a final rule. These changes to the regulations, referred to as the *Physician Labeling Rule* (*PLR*), were intended to enhance healthcare professionals' ability to access, read and use the package insert. Unlike the old package insert format (which was less structured and standardized), the PLR format includes three main sections:
- Highlights of Prescribing Information—intended to provide the prescriber with one location to find the information they most commonly refer to and consider most important
- Full Prescribing Information: Contents—a "table of contents" for the Full Prescribing Information (FPI)
- Full Prescribing Information—in fixed numbered sections

The new *PLR* format also requires inclusion of contact information to help make it easier to report adverse events.

In addition to the organizational changes, FDA has issued several guidance documents articulating new standards for the content of professional labeling. As with the rest of the *PLR* initiatives, the goal of these guidance documents is to provide standards for the development of clear, concise and useful prescribing information. In February 2013, FDA published the final *Guidance for Industry: Labeling for Human Prescription Drug and Biological Products—Implementing the PLR Content and Format Requirements* (February 2013). This final guidance takes into consideration comments FDA solicited from the public after publishing the final rule in 2006.

An overview of the *PLR* format, associated regulations and available guidance documents is provided in **Table 16-1**.

Also notable is that the *PLR* regulations established minimum requirements for font size and certain other graphic elements (21 CFR 201.57(d)). These requirements vary depending on the intended use of the labeling (e.g., whether labeling is to accompany the drug product or is for use in accompanying promotional materials). See *Guidance for Industry: Labeling for Human Prescription Drug and Biological Products—Implementing the New Content and Format Requirements* (February 2013) for additional information. The guidance also sets forth requirements for labeling format, including the PI highlights section, when changes or updates to labeling are made. For example, major changes within the past 12 months to boxed warnings, indications and usage, dosage and administration, contraindications, and warnings and precautions must be listed in the Highlights section as well as within the body of the FPI.

Professional labeling for all drugs approved after June 2001 (or for which an efficacy supplement was approved after June 2001) must be converted to the new *PLR* format (21 CFR 201.56(c)). In addition, for drug products approved in June 2006 or later, efficacy supplements may necessitate revisions of the labeling to the *PLR* format; however, as a general rule, bioequivalence or CMC supplements would not trigger a revision. See the February 2013 guidance for a complete list of the types of supplements that would cause a manufacturer to convert to the *PLR* format.

Because converting a product's professional labeling from the old format into *PLR* format is a difficult and time-consuming process, FDA suggests manufacturers develop new sections (being mindful that much of the "old" information gets reorganized); make assessments to determine whether new information warrants a re-analysis of data or new studies to avoid being misleading; and systematically evaluate labeling information to identify and revise and/or remove unsubstantiated claims and outdated information.

FDA has instituted a staggered implementation schedule, prioritizing label revision from the most recently approved products to older products. The deadline for submitting revised labeling to meet the new requirement is based on the date of the most recent NDA efficacy supplement (or the original approval, if there have been no approved efficacy supplements), although manufacturers are encouraged to voluntarily convert product labeling into the *PLR* format. In any case, all label conversions must be submitted as prior approval supplements. A table outlining FDA's implementation schedule is provided in appendix A of the above-mentioned February 2013 guidance.

Patient Labeling, Including Medication Guide

Patient labeling is product information derived from professional labeling, written in consumer-friendly language, that usually focuses on directions for using the product and risks associated with using the drug. For certain products determined by FDA to pose serious and significant risks, the agency may require a patient Medication Guide (21 CFR 208).

All Medication Guides must comply with certain content and format requirements (21 CFR 208.20), including a type size no smaller than 10 points. In addition, Medication Guides must be distributed to patients each time the prescription drug product is dispensed (21 CFR 208.24). Because a manufacturer cannot be present as each prescription is distributed, the manufacturer is required to ensure that adequate means exist for dispensers themselves to comply with the requirement. (This is usually achieved by providing sufficient numbers of printed Medication Guides with each unit of drug product). In February 2011, FDA issued *Draft Guidance for Industry: Medication Guides—Distribution Requirements and Inclusion in Risk Evaluation and Minimization Strategies (REMS)*, clarifying its expectations for the distribution of Medication Guides.

Electronic Labeling, Including Structured Product Labeling (SPL)

Since 2004, FDA has required the submission of "content of labeling" in electronic format for initial NDA submissions (21 CFR 314.50(l)), labeling supplements and Annual Reports for approved NDAs (21 CFR 314.81(b)). "Content of labeling" is defined as the complete professional labeling, including all text, tables and figures.

SPL is the electronic document markup standard adopted by FDA as the mechanism for electronic submission of the content of labeling. The SPL standard uses the extensible markup language (XML) file format with specifications (schema and controlled terminology) as defined by the FDA Data Standards Council. Additional information on SPL, including both technical and nontechnical guidance, can be found on FDA's Structured Product Labeling Resources website (www.fda.gov/ForIndustry/DataStandards/StructuredProductLabeling/default.htm).

Prescription Drug Promotion

Background & Enforcement

FDA has regulatory authority over the advertising and promotion for prescription drugs via the *FD&C Act* and monitors company promotional activity through its Office of Prescription Drug Promotion, or OPDP (formerly the Division of Drug Marketing, Advertising and Communications, or DDMAC). While the language in *FD&C Act* Section 502 is relatively brief and does not specifically define "advertising" or "promotion," FDA has broadly interpreted the act in its regulations and guidances covering drug advertising and promotion. With the passage of the 1962 *Kefauver-Harris Amendments*, the agency gained greater authority over the marketing of prescription drugs. Regulations covering prescription drug promotion are found in 21 CFR 202 and are cross-referenced to 21 CFR 201.

If OPDP finds advertising or promotion to be violative, the agency has both administrative and judicial tools at its disposal for dealing with violations. FDA's administrative tools include issuing Notice of Violation letters (NOV), often referred to as "Untitled Letters;" issuing Warning Letters; ordering a recall; and calling for the delay, suspension or withdrawal of a product approval. Of these, the most common administrative actions taken by FDA are NOVs and Warning Letters.

NOVs are different from Warning Letters in that they typically require the company to stop using the materials that make the claim(s) FDA finds violative. Warning Letters are typically addressed to the company CEO, warn that FDA will take further action if the matter is not immediately addressed and require corrective action by the company. If the subject of the letter is a product advertisement, this correction is typically a remedial advertisement in each of the same venues where the violative advertisement was run. Warning Letters may also require the company to issue a "Dear Doctor" letter to physicians as described in both 21 CFR 200.5(c)(3) and the *Draft Guidance for Industry and FDA Staff: Dear Health Care Provider Letters: Improving Communication of Important Safety Information*

Chapter 16

Table 16-1. PLR Format, Associated Regulations and Guidance Documents

PLR Format	Associated Regulations/Guidance (if any)
Overall	21 CFR 201.56 and 21 CFR 201.57 *Guidance for Industry: Labeling for Human Prescription Drug and Biological Products—Implementing the PLR Content and Format Requirements* (February 2013)
Highlights of Prescribing Information Product Names, Other Required Information Boxed Warning Recent Major Changes Indications and Usage* Dosage and Administration Dosage Forms and Strengths Contraindications Warnings and Precautions Adverse Reactions Drug Interactions Use in Specific Populations	21 CFR 201.57(a) *Guidance for Industry: Labeling for Human Prescription Drug and Biological Products—Implementing the PLR Content and Format Requirements* (February 2013) *Guidance for Industry and Review Staff: Labeling for Human Prescription Drug and Biological Products — Determining Established Pharmacologic Class for Use in the Highlights of Prescribing Information* (October 2009)
Full Prescribing Information: Contents	21 CFR 201.57(b)
Full Prescribing Information	21 CFR 201.57(c)
Boxed Warning (if applicable)	21 CFR 201.57(c)(1) *Guidance for Industry: Warnings and Precautions, Contraindications, and Boxed Warning Sections of Labeling for Human Prescription Drug and Biological Products—Content and Format* (October 2011) *Guidance for Industry: Labeling for Human Prescription Drug and Biological Products—Implementing the PLR Content and Format Requirements* (February 2013)
1 Indications and Usage	21 CFR 201.57(c)(2) *Guidance for Industry: Labeling for Human Prescription Drug and Biological Products—Implementing the PLR Content and Format Requirements* (February 2013)
2 Dosage and Administration	21 CFR 201.57(c)(3) *Guidance for Industry: Dosage and Administration Section of Labeling for Human Prescription Drug and Biological Products —Content and Format* (March 2010) *Guidance for Industry: Labeling for Human Prescription Drug and Biological Products—Implementing the PLR Content and Format Requirements* (February 2013)
3 Dosage Forms and Strengths	21 CFR 201.57(c)(4) *Guidance for Industry: Labeling for Human Prescription Drug and Biological Products—Implementing the PLR Content and Format Requirements* (February 2013)
4 Contraindications	21 CFR 201.57(c)(5) *Guidance for Industry: Warnings and Precautions, Contraindications, and Boxed Warning Sections of Labeling for Human Prescription Drug and Biological Products—Content and Format* (October 2011) *Guidance for Industry: Labeling for Human Prescription Drug and Biological Products—Implementing the PLR Content and Format Requirements* (February 2013)
5 Warnings and Precautions	21 CFR 201.57(c)(6) *Guidance for Industry: Warnings and Precautions, Contraindications, and Boxed Warning Sections of Labeling for Human Prescription Drug and Biological Products—Content and Format* (October 2011) *Guidance for Industry: Labeling for Human Prescription Drug and Biological Products—Implementing the PLR Content and Format Requirements* (February 2013)
6 Adverse Reactions	21 CFR 201.57(c)(7) *Guidance for Industry: Adverse Reactions Section of Labeling for Human Prescription Drug and Biological Products—Content and Format* (January 2006) *Guidance for Industry: Labeling for Human Prescription Drug and Biological Products—Implementing the PLR Content and Format Requirements* (February 2013)
7 Drug Interactions	21 CFR 201.57(c)(8) *Guidance for Industry: Labeling for Human Prescription Drug and Biological Products—Implementing the PLR Content and Format Requirements* (February 2013)
8 Use in Specific Populations	21 CFR 201.57(c)(9) *Guidance for Industry: Content and Format for Geriatric Labeling* (October 2001) *Guidance for Industry: Labeling for Human Prescription Drug and Biological Products—Implementing the PLR Content and Format Requirements* (February 2013) *Draft Guidance for Industry and Review Staff: Pediatric Information Incorporated Into Human Prescription Drug and Biological Products Labeling* (February 2013)
9 Drug Abuse and Dependence	21 CFR 201.57(c)(10)

PLR Format	Associated Regulations/Guidance (if any)
10 Overdosage	21 CFR 201.57(c)(11)
11 Description	21 CFR 201.57(c)(12)
12 Clinical Pharmacology	21 CFR 201.57(c)(13) Draft Guidance for Industry: Clinical Pharmacology Section of Labeling for Human Prescription Drug and Biological Products—Content and Format (March 2009)
13 Nonclinical Toxicology	21 CFR 201.57(c)(14)
14 Clinical Studies	21 CFR 201.57(c)(15) Guidance for Industry: Clinical Studies Section of Labeling for Human Prescription Drug and Biological Products—Content and Format (January 2009)
15 References	21 CFR 201.57(c)(16)
16 How Supplied/Storage and Handling	21 CFR 201.57(c)(17)
17 Patient Counseling Information	21 CFR 201.57(c)(18) Guidance for Industry: Labeling for Human Prescription Drug and Biological Products—Implementing the PLR Content and Format Requirements (February 2013)
Medication Guide (if applicable)	21 CFR 208 Guidance: Medication Guides-Distribution Requirements and Inclusion in Risk Evaluation and Mitigation Strategies (REMS) (November 2011)

(November 2010). All letters issued by OPDP are posted publicly on FDA's "Enforcement Activities" webpage and often include a copy of the violative promotion; this also serves as one of the most important tools in understanding OPDP's position on certain topics.

As in other areas of FDA enforcement, judicial tools at FDA's disposal include injunction, seizure or criminal prosecution. However, OPDP rarely seeks judicial action on its own for promotional violations. FDA is more likely to work with the Office of the Inspector General (OIG), Department of Justice (DOJ), or individual state's attorneys general in pursuing companies for significant promotional violations. Additional information on these agencies beyond FDA is provided at the end of this chapter.

In 2010, DDMAC announced a new program, called Truthful Prescription Drug Advertising and Promotion (or more commonly, the "Bad Ad" program). The stated goal of the Bad Ad program is to educate prescribers about their role in reporting to FDA false or misleading detailing by sales representatives and other forms of drug promotion. Since the inception of the Bad Ad Program, FDA has attended a number of major medical meetings each year and continued to educate attendees about the Bad Ad Program. FDA distributed materials that encouraged prescribers to recognize and report any activities and promotional messages that they believed were false or misleading. OPDP, in turn, has promised to review these reports and issue enforcement letters where appropriate. On 3 December 2010, FDA sent its first Warning Letter referencing the Bad Ad program. In 2012, three letters were generated out of the Bad Ad program.

Summary of Requirements for Advertising and Promotion

No Preapproval Promotion

According to 21 CFR 312.7, sponsors or investigators "shall not represent in a promotional context that an investigational new drug is safe or effective for the purposes for which it is under investigation." The only exceptions to the prohibition on preapproval promotion are disease-state-only promotion, or institutional promotion (which links the name of the drug manufacturer with a field of research); and "Coming Soon" promotions. "Coming Soon" ads reveal only the name of a product that will be available soon, without any written, verbal or graphic suggestions of potential indications or claims of safety or effectiveness. During the preapproval period, a company may choose one of these types of promotional campaigns, but may not switch back and forth between them. The reason is that if a disease awareness campaign is underway for a time (e.g., "Company X is involved in research in the field of diabetes") and then followed by a "Coming Soon" campaign "Coming Soon from Company X: Product Y"), the audience could link the name of the drug with the disease state, which is considered tantamount to preapproval promotion. In January 2004, FDA issued *Draft Guidance for Industry: "Help-Seeking" and Other Disease Awareness Communications by or on Behalf of Drug and Device Firms*, to provide clarification on its thinking about preapproval promotion. In November 2012, OPDP issued an Untitled Letter to a company for preapproval promotion. The letter cited a website and statements made by the company CEO that were available via podcast that suggested the investigational drug was safe and effective for the purposes for which it was being investigated. OPDP asked the company to immediately stop disseminating the violative materials.

Submission and Preclearance of Promotional Materials

With only one exception, all promotional materials must be submitted to OPDP at the time of their initial publication or dissemination using Form FDA 2253 (21 CFR 314.81(b)(i)).

Manufacturers of products approved under Subpart H (Accelerated Approval of New Drugs for Serious or Life-Threatening Illnesses) are required to submit drafts of all promotional labeling for advisory comment at least 30 days prior to dissemination (21 CFR 314.550 and 601.45). Additionally, for products that are anticipated to receive accelerated approval during the NDA preapproval review period, all promotional materials intended to be used in the first 120 days following marketing approval must be submitted to OPDP for advisory review prior to the drug's approval. For additional details about the submission of promotional materials for accelerated approval products, see *Draft Guidance for Industry: Accelerated Approval Products—Submission of Promotional Materials* (March 1999).

For drugs approved under standard conditions, it is common industry practice (although not required) to submit a drug's launch materials to OPDP for advisory comment. OPDP pays careful attention to launch materials during the first year after a drug's approval. In September 2008, DDMAC issued a letter to a company for violations found in a promotional launch journal advertisement, taking issue with included claims such as "novel," "next generation" and "unique." The company was asked to pull the advertisement and run a corrective advertising campaign. In 2012, a company received an untitled letter from OPDP for a branded story that was part of the launch campaign. The branded story included a patient testimonial that overstated efficacy, omitted key information and minimized important risk information. Although a company spokeswoman told the press the patient testimonial was never circulated to the public, this did not stop the company from receiving the FDA letter.

Additionally, while not required, it is common industry practice to send direct-to-consumer television advertisements to OPDP for preclearance prior to dissemination. OPDP's website explains the submission process for preclearance of TV ads and other materials.

Product Name Placement, Size and Prominence

Promotional labeling must include a reference to the established (generic) name of the drug, per 21 CFR 202.1(b)(1). The regulations require the most prominent mention of the brand name to be accompanied by the generic name "in letters at least half as large as the letters comprising the proprietary name or designation with which it is joined."

In January 2012, FDA issued *Guidance for Industry: Product Name Placement, Size, and Prominence in Advertising and Promotional Labeling* to clarify issues in this area.

Fair Balance

All claims of effectiveness in a prescription drug advertisement must be accompanied by information about the product's risks, and the risk information must have comparable prominence to the promotional claims (21 CFR 202.1(e)(5)). This is commonly known as "fair balance." The omission or minimization of risk information is the most commonly cited concern in OPDP's enforcement letters.

OPDP considers many factors when determining fair balance, including whether the safety and efficacy messages have equal prominence, typography and layout, contrast and white space or other methods used to achieve emphasis (21 CFR 202.1(e)(7)(viii)). In addition, if promotional material is directed to a consumer audience, the fair balance information should be written in consumer-friendly language.

In May 2009, FDA issued a draft guidance, entitled *Guidance for Industry: Presenting Risk Information in Prescription Drug and Medical Device Promotion,* to shed more light on the factors the agency considers when evaluating the presentation of risk information in advertisements and promotional labeling. This draft guidance includes many helpful, concrete examples to illustrate FDA's thinking on this important topic.

General Requirements for Promotional Claims/"Substantial Evidence"

Promotional materials may not suggest a use of the product that is not approved or otherwise permitted for use in the FDA-approved labeling (i.e., FPI). This is what is commonly referred to as "off-label" use of a product.

In addition to the "on label" requirement, promotional materials may not suggest that a drug is better, safer or more effective than has been demonstrated by "substantial evidence." Generally, FDA's standard for "substantial evidence" in support of a drug product claim is two adequate and well-controlled clinical trials (21 CFR 314.126). Although certain claims may be allowable based on a single study, OPDP has on numerous occasions articulated the requirement for two studies for claims of product superiority.

Even if product claims are "on-label," if the claims (either overt or implied) are not supported by substantial evidence, FDA will consider the materials to be misleading and therefore violative. Although the regulations in 21 CFR 202.1(e)(6) and (7) detail the general principles by which FDA will evaluate whether or not promotional materials are misleading (e.g., failure to reveal material facts or improper use of graphics or statistics), reviewing OPDP enforcement letters is the best way to learn the agency's expectations in this area.

Pharmacoeconomic Claims and Promotion to Formulary Decision Makers

Pharmaceutical companies not only promote their drug products to prescribers, but also to formularies or other related entities that are primarily responsible for managed care coverage and reimbursement decisions. This kind of promotion often focuses on healthcare economic information (pharmacoeconomic claims).

Section 114 of the *Food and Drug Administration Amendments Act* of 1997 (*FDAAA*) provides for a legal mechanism to allow the promotion of pharmacoeconomic claims using a less-stringent standard for the "substantial evidence" standard described above. The law states that pharmacoeconomic claims may be made based on "competent and reliable" evidence, as long as the information directly relates to an approved indication and is only being provided to formularies or other similar managed care decision makers.

Brief Summary & Accompanying Labeling

The 21 CFR 202(l) regulations differentiate materials that constitute advertising from other forms of promotional labeling. The regulations require that prescription drug advertising contain a "[t]rue statement of information in brief summary relating to side effects, contraindications, and effectiveness" (21 CFR 202.1(e)). Promotional labeling that is not an advertisement (or reminder labeling, as described below) must be disseminated with a copy of the FPI.

In January 2004, FDA issued *Draft Guidance for Industry: Brief Summary: Disclosing Risk Information in Consumer-Directed Print Advertisements*, to explain the agency's expectations regarding the Brief Summary in print advertisements directed to consumers. Like "fair balance," FDA encourages sponsors to write a Brief Summary for consumer pieces in easily understandable language. FDA also recommends that sponsors include a statement in the advertisement reminding consumers the risk information is not comprehensive, and sponsors should provide a toll-free telephone number or website where more information can be found.

Reminder Labeling

An exception to the fair balance and accompanying labeling requirements is reminder labeling (commonly known as "reminder ads"), which, according to 21 CFR 201.100(f), "calls attention to the name of the drug product but does not include indications or dosage recommendations for use… containing no representation or suggestion relating to the drug product." Reminder advertisements are not permitted for products that carry a Boxed Warning in their labeling.

In the past, it was common practice for pharmaceutical companies to give away reminder items. In July 2008, the Pharmaceutical Research and Manufacturers of America (PhRMA) issued an updated PhRMA Code on Interactions with Healthcare Professionals (PhRMA Code) that addressed the topic of reminder items. The Advanced Medical Technology Association (AdvaMed) issued similar guidelines to medical device manufacturers.

The PhRMA Code, which is a voluntary non-regulatory standard, prohibits distribution of non-educational and practice-related promotional materials, including such reminder items as pens, notepads and mugs with product logos on them, even if the item is of minimal value and related to the healthcare professional's work or for the benefit of the patient. Most manufacturers have voluntarily adopted the PhRMA Code and no longer give away reminder items.

Help-seeking, Bulk-sale and Compounding Drug Advertising

Another exception to the Brief Summary requirement includes "help-seeking advertisements" and bulk-sale and compounding drug advertisements. A help-seeking advertisement is intended to inform consumers about a specific medical condition and encourage them to talk to their healthcare professionals about the condition. They must not mention any product name or imply that a certain prescription drug is intended to treat the medical condition. In January 2004, FDA issued *Draft Guidance for Industry: "Help-Seeking" and Other Disease Awareness Communications by or on Behalf of Drug and Device Firms*. Bulk-sale drugs that are intended to be used for further processing or manufacturing are also exempt from the Brief Summary requirement, as are drugs sold to pharmacies for the purpose of compounding. As with help-seeking advertisements, neither bulk-sale drugs nor compounding drugs are permitted to make safety or efficacy claims (21 CFR 202.1(e)(2)(ii) and (iii)).

Direct-To-Consumer (DTC) Advertising

Consumer-directed broadcast advertisements (i.e., television and radio) must include a "major statement" of the product's primary risks, in the audio and, for television, video portion of the advertisement. In addition, the advertisement should make "adequate provision…for dissemination of the approved or permitted package labeling in connection with the broadcast presentation" (21CFR 202.1(e)(1)). This is sometimes referred to as the "adequate provision" requirement and, in August 1999, FDA issued *Draft Guidance for Industry: Consumer-Directed Broadcast Advertisements* to clarify the approach manufacturers may take to fulfill the requirement. A similar guidance is available for restricted medical devices. As noted previously, most companies submit their television advertisements to FDA for advisory comment prior to broadcast. To learn more about submitting DTC television ads for pre-dissemination review, consult the March 2012 *Draft Guidance for Industry:*

Direct-to-Consumer Television Advertisements – FDAAA DTC Television Ad Pre-Dissemination Review Program.

In addition to other requirements, *FDAAA* requires that published DTC advertisements include the following statement printed in conspicuous text: "You are encouraged to report negative side effects of prescription drugs to the FDA. Visit www.fda.gov/Safety/MedWatch/default.htm, or call 1-800-FDA-1088."

Internet and Social Media

The Internet, from specific drug websites to sponsored links to social media sites such as YouTube or Facebook, is commonly used for prescription drug promotion. Although DDMAC issued its first letter regarding a promotional website in 1996, FDA has never issued formal regulations or guidance documents on this topic, citing rapidly changing technology as the reason. However, in response to DDMAC's 14 enforcement letters on 3 April 2009 regarding the sponsored link activities of some 47 drug products, criticism arose that FDA's standards had not been clearly communicated to industry. In response, DDMAC held a public hearing in November 2009 to gather comments from industry, trade organizations, physician and patient groups and others on how to promote medical products appropriately using the Internet and social media. OPDP has expressed strong interest in publishing draft guidances on these topics, but as of March 2013, no guidance documents have been issued. OPDP has said it hopes to meet the *Food and Drug Administration Safety and Innovation Act (FDASIA)* deadline of 9 July 2014 in issuing a social media guidance.

Until such time as guidance is released, regulatory professionals must review the many examples of improper Internet promotion cited in OPDP enforcement letters to develop their own best judgment and practices for online promotion. Some notable examples include a letter for a video posted on YouTube (25 September 2008), a letter for a Facebook widget placed on a product site (29 July 2010) and a video posted on WebMD (20 June 2012). Even an FDA district office issued a Warning Letter in December 2012 to a company over Facebook "likes" that were connected with a company's website for their dietary supplements.

Press Releases

Press releases often cause confusion over where the appropriate regulatory jurisdiction lies. Typically, the Securities and Exchange Commission (SEC) regulates how information is communicated to the investment community. Nevertheless, FDA believes that product-specific press releases fall under FDA promotional regulations, thus requiring fair balance and avoiding false or misleading content or preapproval promotion. Many companies have received Warning Letters and Untitled Letters from OPDP for violative statements in their press releases. In October 2012, a company received an Untitled Letter for a professional pitch letter that included a press release. The press release was cited as making unsupported superiority claims.

Product Promotion vs. Scientific Exchange

FDA does distinguish between drug promotion and the exchange of scientific information. Truly independent and nonpromotional industry-supported activities, where there is an exchange of scientific information—if done properly—may not be deemed promotional labeling, even if the information being exchanged is considered "off-label." Historically, manufacturers were involved in setting up continuing medical education (CME) programs to facilitate an exchange of scientific information. These events and the manufacturers that organized them fell under harsh scrutiny, however, when it was alleged that the CME events were merely "dressed up product promotion."

In December 1997, FDA issued *Guidance for Industry: Industry-Supported Scientific and Educational Activities* to explain its thinking on this topic. This guidance defines what is considered "nonpromotional" and "educational" and places great importance on keeping the scientific activity independent of influence from manufacturers.

Product Detailing

Product detailing, including the oral statements that company representatives make about their prescription drug products, is also considered promotional labeling. While it is difficult for FDA to monitor conversations, there are several examples of OPDP issuing Warning Letters and Untitled Letters to companies for presentations that were made to healthcare professionals by sales representatives.

One company received two different untitled letters—one on 28 April 2011 and the second on 1 August 2012—over oral statements made by a sales representative to a healthcare provider. The 2012 letter states, "On Wednesday, October 12, 2011, two sales representatives… made a call to a physician's office. During this sales call, the sales representative stated in word or substance that…." This letter was notable regarding the stern language used regarding prior advice FDA had given the company, specifically related to its existing Corporate Integrity Agreement (CIA) and expectations around how sales representatives are trained.

Historically, many conversations that have been the subject of enforcement letters have occurred and been overheard at exhibit halls at major medical meetings. This is a key enforcement area for OPDP, and FDA representatives regularly attend major medical meetings and pay close attention to activities in the exhibit halls, including collecting materials passed out at the meetings (see letters dated 30 November 2010, 13 December 2011 and 13 November 2012).

Reprints

FDA-cleared or -approved prescription drugs, biologics and medical devices frequently are the subject of medical research, with study results typically published in medical journals, textbooks and other scientific reference publications. Often these studies describe or suggest uses of the products that go beyond the PI to include "off-label" use. Because manufacturers must limit the promotion of their products to only approved, labeled uses, the promotional use of reprints can be challenging.

In 1997, Section 401 of the *Food and Drug Administration Modernization Act* (*FDAMA*) was written into law in an attempt to address this issue by describing situations where a manufacturer could disseminate reprints containing descriptions of off-label use to healthcare professionals while remaining in a "safe harbor" from being found in violation of the rule against promoting the product for an off-label use. FDA's implementing regulations were codified at 21 CFR 99. On 30 September 2006, *FDAMA* Section 401 ceased to be effective, and the implementing regulations were no longer applicable.

In January 2009, FDA announced the availability of *Guidance for Industry on Good Reprint Practices for the Distribution of Medical Journal Articles and Medical or Scientific Reference Publications on Unapproved New Uses of Approved Drugs and Approved or Cleared Medical Devices* (*Good Reprint Practices Guidance*). This guidance describes the kind of material that FDA considers to be a true reprint (e.g., one that is peer-reviewed vs. a supplement), what information should accompany the reprint and appropriate venues for distribution of these reprints.

Other Agencies Beyond FDA

FDA is not the only agency closely tracking prescription drug advertising and related activities. Many other government agencies, including DOJ, the OIG in the Department of Health and Human Services (DHHS), states' attorneys general, the Federal Trade Commission and Congress, closely monitor drug companies' activities.

Government enforcement efforts against the pharmaceutical industry in the US were greatly enhanced, beginning in 2001. The original focus was suspected kickbacks and violations of the pricing statutes (the *Anti-Kickback Statute*). These laws make it illegal for any person—e.g., healthcare provider, office manager or sales agent—to knowingly and willfully solicit, offer, pay or receive "remuneration" (including kickbacks, bribes, rebates or anything of value) directly or indirectly in cash or in kind to any person to induce or cause that person to prescribe a product for which payment may be made in whole or in part under a federal healthcare program (42 USC 1320a-7b).

More recently, the focus of government agencies has been off-label promotion by pharmaceutical and medical device manufacturers in connection with the *False Claims Act* (*FCA*). The *FCA* was born out of the Civil War when fraud was pervasive, particularly by defense contractors who unscrupulously sold bad goods (defective guns, putrid rations, etc.) to the US government and then sought payment for such goods. Under the *FCA*, an individual who is not affiliated with the government can bring a suit claiming fraud. In such cases, the person filing the claim is known as a "whistleblower," and the reward for a successful prosecution was offered as a *qui tam* provision (meaning "he who brings a case on behalf of our lord the King, as well as himself"). The citizen whistleblower in the case is known as a "relator."

While this legislation has undergone some changes over the years, the tenets remain the same: it is unlawful to knowingly present or cause to be presented to the US government a false claim for payment. Modern-day changes to the laws impose treble (triple) damages and civil fines of $5,000–$10,000 per false claim, among other things. In practical application today, whistleblowers, working with DOJ and states' attorneys general, have investigated and brought many high-profile claims against companies for promoting drugs for off-label uses, resulting in false claims for payment submitted to federal insurance programs such as Medicare and Medicaid, which do not provide coverage for off-label uses. In these cases, each off-label prescription is considered one false claim. Many healthcare product manufacturers that settle *FCA* claims also agree to enter into CIAs with DHHS, placing strict requirements on corporate compliance for a period of years.

In recent years, settlements have reached the billion dollar figure. In July 2012, the largest settlement in history was reached with a manufacturer over allegations the company engaged in unlawful promotion of some of its drugs, failed to report certain safety data and engaged in false price reporting practices. The company agreed to pay $3 billion and plead guilty to charges, which included introducing misbranded drugs into interstate commerce. The company also agreed to enter into a strict five-year CIA with DHHS. The CIA requires individual accountability of the company's executives and board of directors.

In June 2012, another billion dollar settlement with a different manufacturer was announced. That company agreed to pay $1.5 billion to resolve criminal and civil liability arising from unlawful product promotion. The company agreed to be subjected to court-ordered probation and reporting obligations of its CEO and board, along with a five-year CIA.

Prior to these two cases, the two largest settlements were announced in 2009, where one company agreed to pay $1.415 billion to resolve allegations of off-label promotion of its drug. The settlement included a criminal fine of $515 million, and $800 million in a civil settlement with the federal government and a number of states.

The case was brought by four former sales representatives of the company, and the whistleblowers together received more than $78 million as their share of the settlement. The other case involved another large manufacturer accused of off-label promotion of one of its popular drugs. That company settled for $2.3 billion. Although the drug had been removed from the market years before, the company had been plagued by investigations by DOJ and lawsuits from states' attorneys general for alleged off-label promotion tactics connected to the product. These four settlements are the largest to date in any healthcare product cases.

Finally, manufacturers must consider the competition as they develop advertising and promotional materials. Competitors have brought suit against manufacturers for violations of the *Lanham Act*. While this legislation is often thought of in terms of trademark protection, it also allows manufacturers to sue competitors for false advertising. Manufacturers have used courts' interpretations of the act to bring suits charging that comparative claims in advertising are false and misleading, that they deceive a substantial part of the audience viewing the ads and that the deception could influence purchasing decisions. If a plaintiff prevails on a *Lanham Act* false advertising claim, the court can not only bar the advertising, but also can order corrective advertising or a product recall.

Summary

- All drug labeling, including container labels, package inserts, patient labeling, Medication Guides and promotional labeling (including oral statements), is subject to FDA regulation.
- In 2006, FDA issued the *PLR*, affecting the content and format of labeling for new prescription drug products.
- A Medication Guide is a special type of patient labeling for drugs with serious risks and is required to be distributed to the consumer each time a prescription is filled or refilled.
- Structured Product Labeling (SPL) is an electronic document standard adopted by FDA as a mechanism for exchanging drug information.
- FDA monitors prescription drug advertising and promotion through the OPDP. No drug can be promoted until the NDA has been approved by FDA.
- Typical FDA enforcement actions include NOVs and Warning Letters. Although rarely used, the agency has other tools at its disposal to deal with violative advertising and promotional materials.
- All advertising and promotional labeling must be submitted at the time of first use with Form FDA 2253, except for products approved under accelerated approval, which must be submitted for advisory opinion 30 days prior to initial dissemination. Although generally not required, it is strongly recommended that launch materials and new television advertisements be submitted to OPDP for advisory comment prior to dissemination.
- All promotional materials must include a "fair balance" of efficacy and risk information, with the exception of reminder labeling (not allowed for products with a Boxed Warning). Broadcast advertisements must include a "major statement" of risk.
- Promotional materials may not suggest use for the product that is not approved or otherwise permitted for use in the FDA-approved labeling ("off-label" use), and no claims must be made that a product is safer or more effective than has been established by "substantial evidence" (generally, two adequate and well-controlled clinical trials). *FDAMA* Section 114 allows for the distribution of pharmacoeconomic data using a less-stringent standard as long as certain requirements are met.
- All non-reminder promotional materials must be accompanied by the full prescribing information; advertisements require an accompanying "brief summary" of the FPI. Broadcast advertisements must include "adequate provision" for the dissemination of the approved labeling.
- FDA works with other agencies such as the US Attorney's Office and OIG in prosecuting companies alleged to be in violation of the *FCA* or *Anti-Kickback Statute* through off-label promotion. Companies found in violation of the *FD&C Act*, *Anti-Kickback Statute* and/or *FCA* risk disbarment from participation in federal programs (e.g., Medicare) and Corporate Integrity Agreements.

Chapter 17

Pharmacovigilance and Risk Management

By Anne Tomalin

OBJECTIVES

- Understand the reporting requirements for Investigational New Drug (IND) safety data
- Understand the postmarketing requirements for safety data for drugs and biologics
- Understand the postmarketing requirements for safety data for medical devices
- Understand the requirements for Risk Evaluation and Mitigation Strategies (REMS)
- Understand the requirements for proprietary name review of drugs and biologics

LAWS, REGULATIONS AND GUIDELINES COVERED IN THIS CHAPTER

- Center for Drug Evaluation and Research (CDER) Manual of Policies and Procedures (MAPP) 4151.3R3: Drug Safety Oversight Board (DSB)
- CDER MAPP 5240.8: Handling of Adverse Experience Reports and Other Generic Drug Postmarketing Reports
- CDER MAPP 6004.2R: Procedures for Completing and Processing the Form "Annual Status Report Review Form: PMR and PMC Summary"
- CDER MAPP 6010.R: Responsibilities for Tracking and Communicating the Status of Postmarketing Requirements and Commitments
- CDER MAPP 6010.9: Procedures and Responsibilities for Developing Postmarketing Requirements and Commitments
- CDER MAPP 6700.1: Risk Management Plan Activities in OND and ODS
- CDER MAPP 6700.9: FDA Posting of Potential Signals of Serious Risks Identified by the Adverse Event Reporting System
- CDER MAPP 6720.2: Procedures for Handling Requests for Proprietary Name Review
- Center for Biologics Evaluation and Research (CBER) Manual of Regulatory Standard Operating Policies and Procedures (SOPP) 8401.6: The Responsibilities of the Division of Epidemiology (DE/OBE) in the BLA Review Process
- CBER SOPP 8413: Postmarketing Commitment Annual Reports, Final Reports, and Related Submissions—Administrative Handling, Review and CBER Reporting
- CBER SOPP 8415: Procedures for Developing Postmarketing Requirements and Commitments

- CBER SOPP 8420: FDAAA Section 921: Posting of Potential Signals of Serious Risk

- CBER SOPP 8508: Procedures for Handling Adverse Reaction Reports Related to "361" Human Cells, Tissues, and Cellular and Tissue-Based Products (HCT/Ps)

- Compliance Program Guidance Manual 7353.001: Enforcement of the Postmarketing Adverse Drug Experience Reporting Regulations

- *Guidance for Industry Good Pharmacovigilance Practices and Pharmacoepidemiologic Assessment* (March 2005)

- *Guidance for Industry: Postmarketing Adverse Event Reporting for Nonprescription Human Drug Products Marketed Without an Approved Application* (July 2009)

- *Guidance for Industry: Postmarketing Adverse Event Reporting for Medical Products and Dietary Supplements During an Influenza Pandemic* (February 2012)

- *Guidance for Industry: Reports on the Status of Postmarketing Study Commitments—Implementation of Section 130 of the Food and Drug Administration Modernization Act of 1997* (February 2006)

- *Guidance for Industry: Format and Content of Proposed Risk Evaluation and Mitigation Strategies (REMS), REMS Assessments and Proposed REMS Modifications* (September 2009)

- *Guidance for Industry and Investigators: Safety Reporting Requirements for INDs and BA/BE Studies* (December 2012)

- *Guidance for Industry and Investigators: Enforcement of Safety Reporting Requirements for Investigational New Drug Applications and Bioavailability/Bioequivalence Studies* (June 2011)

- *Guidance for Industry: Development and Use of Risk Minimization Action Plans* (March 2005)

- *Guidance: Medication Guides—Distribution Requirements and Inclusion in Risk Evaluation and Mitigation Strategies (REMS)* (November 2011)

- *Draft Guidance for Industry: Providing Regulatory Submissions in Electronic Format—Postmarketing Individual Case Safety Reports* (June 2008)

- *Draft Guidance: Drug Safety Information—FDA's Communication to the Public* (March 2012)

- International Conference on Harmonisation (ICH) *Clinical Safety Data Management: Definitions and Standards for Expedited Reporting E2A* (Final) (1 March 1995)

- ICH *Pharmacovigilance Planning E2E* (Final) (April 2005)

- ICH Electronic Transmission of Individual Case Safety Reports E2B(R2)

- ICH *Periodic Benefit-Risk Evaluation Report E2C(R2)* (17 December 2012)

Introduction

Safety is a key component of investigating and marketing drugs, biologics and medical devices in the US. Reporting requirements are rigorous, and compliance with these requirements is extremely important. When a drug is first approved, not everything is known about it. Additional information is continuously learned about a drug as it is used by more and more individuals. Postmarketing monitoring of safety data is required by both industry and the US Food and Drug Administration (FDA). Other regulatory agencies also require postmarketing follow-up, and safety databases are maintained globally. The International Conference on Harmonisation (ICH) defines safety reporting standards and requirements globally, and US legislation is consistent with these requirements. As new safety signals are detected and validated, labeling is revised, or other health communications are forwarded to healthcare professionals. Regulatory and pharmacovigilance professionals serve a key function in monitoring the safety of the products used by patients and consumers.

Clinical Trials

Definitions of adverse events or suspected adverse reactions are slightly different when used in a clinical trial setting. Definitions are given below and are consistent with ICH definitions used worldwide.

Definitions of Adverse Events in Clinical Studies
Adverse Event
An adverse event is any untoward medical occurrence associated with the use of a drug in humans whether or not considered drug-related.

Life-threatening Adverse Event or Life-threatening Suspected Adverse Reaction

An adverse event or suspected adverse reaction is considered "life-threatening" if, in the view of either the investigator or sponsor, its occurrence places the patient or subject at immediate risk of death. It does not include an adverse event or suspected adverse reaction that, had it occurred in a more severe form, might have caused death.

Serious Adverse Event or Serious Suspected Adverse Reaction

An adverse event or suspected adverse reaction is considered "serious" if, in the view of either the investigator or sponsor, it results in any of the following outcomes: death, a life-threatening adverse event, inpatient hospitalization or prolongation of existing hospitalization, a persistent or significant incapacity or substantial disruption of the ability to conduct normal life functions, or a congenital anomaly/birth defect. Important medical events that may not result in death, be life-threatening, or require hospitalization may be considered serious when, based on appropriate medical judgment, they may jeopardize the patient or subject and may require medical or surgical intervention to prevent one of the outcomes listed in this definition. Examples of such medical events include allergic bronchospasm requiring intensive treatment in an emergency room or at home, blood dyscrasias or convulsions that do not result in inpatient hospitalization, or the development of drug dependency or drug abuse.

Suspected Adverse Reaction

A suspected adverse reaction is any adverse event for which there is a reasonable possibility that the drug caused the adverse event. For the purposes of Investigational New Drug (IND) application safety reporting, "reasonable possibility" means there is evidence to suggest a causal relationship between the drug and the adverse event. Suspected adverse reaction implies a lesser degree of certainty about causality than adverse reaction, which means any adverse event caused by a drug.

Unexpected Adverse Event or Unexpected Suspected Adverse Reaction

An adverse event or suspected adverse reaction is considered "unexpected" if it is not listed in the Investigator Brochure (IB) or is not listed at the specificity or severity that has been observed; or, if an IB is not required or available, is not consistent with the risk information described in the general investigational plan or elsewhere in the current application, as amended. For example, under this definition, hepatic necrosis would be unexpected (by virtue of greater severity) if the IB referred only to elevated hepatic enzymes or hepatitis. Similarly, cerebral thromboembolism and cerebral vasculitis would be unexpected (by virtue of greater specificity) if the investigator brochure listed only cerebral vascular accidents. "Unexpected," as used in this definition, also refers to adverse events or suspected adverse reactions that are mentioned in the IB as occurring with a class of drugs or as anticipated from the pharmacological properties of the drug but are not specifically mentioned as occurring with the particular drug under investigation.

Reporting Requirements for Clinical Trials

The investigator conducting the clinical trial is required to promptly report to the sponsor all adverse events encountered with the drug.[1] The sponsor is responsible for promptly reviewing all information relevant to the drug's safety obtained or otherwise received by the sponsor from any source, foreign or domestic, including information derived from any clinical or epidemiological investigations, animal investigations, commercial marketing experience, reports in the scientific literature and unpublished scientific papers, as well as reports from foreign regulatory authorities that have not already been previously reported to the agency by the sponsor.[2]

The sponsor is responsible for notifying FDA and all participating investigators in a written IND safety report of:
- any adverse experience associated with the use of the drug that is both serious and unexpected

or
- any finding from tests in laboratory animals that suggests a significant risk for human subjects, including reports of mutagenicity, teratogenicity or carcinogenicity

As a result of the New Drug Safety Reporting Requirements for Human Drug and Biological Products and Safety Reporting Requirements for Bioavailability and Bioequivalence studies in Humans,[3] the following information, not previously required by FDA, now must be reported to the agency within 15 days of the sponsor becoming aware of an occurrence:
- findings from clinical or epidemiological studies that suggest a significant risk to study participants
- serious suspected adverse reactions that occur at a rate higher than expected
- serious adverse events from bioavailability studies and bioequivalence studies conducted without an IND

For clinical studies, an adverse experience or fatal outcome need not be submitted to FDA unless the applicant concludes there is a reasonable possibility the product caused the adverse experience or fatal outcome (See 21 CFR 310.305(c)(1)(ii), 314.80(e)(1) and 600.80(e)(1)).

Each written notification may be submitted on Form FDA 3500A or in a narrative format (foreign events may be submitted either on a Form FDA 3500A or, if preferred, on a Council for International Organizations of Medical Sciences (CIOMS) I form). Reports from animal or epidemiological studies should be submitted in a narrative format. All reports should be labeled prominently as "IND Safety Report." Each written notification to FDA should be transmitted to the new drug review division in the Center for Drug Evaluation and Research (CDER) or product review division in the Center for Biologics Evaluation and Research (CBER) that is responsible for the IND.

The sponsor is required to notify FDA by telephone or by facsimile transmission of any unexpected fatal or life-threatening experience associated with the use of the drug as soon as possible, but in no event later than seven calendar days after the sponsor's initial receipt of the information. Each telephone call or facsimile transmission to FDA shall be transmitted to the new drug review division in CDER or product review division in CBER that is responsible for review of the drug.

The sponsor must provide follow-up information for each IND safety report that is submitted. The follow-up information should be submitted as soon as all available information has been gathered. If, upon further investigation into an adverse event, a sponsor establishes that an event not initially determined to be reportable is now reportable, the sponsor shall then report this event as soon as possible but no later than 15 calendar days after the event has been made clear. FDA may require a sponsor to submit IND safety reports in a format or frequency different than those established in the regulations. The sponsor shall provide all additional safety information it has obtained regarding the drug in an information amendment or an annual report.[4]

For bioavailability (BA) and bioequivalence (BE) studies conducted without an IND, the person conducting the study, including any contract research organization (CRO), is required to notify FDA of any serious adverse event within 15 days of its occurrence, and of any fatal or life-threatening adverse event from the study within seven days of its occurrence. Each notification under this paragraph must be submitted to the director, Office of Generic Drugs in CDER. Relevant follow-up information to a BA/BE safety report must be submitted as soon as the information is available and must be identified as such, i.e., "Follow-up BA/BE safety report." Upon request from FDA, the person conducting the study, including any CRO, must submit to FDA any additional data or information that the agency deems necessary within 15 days after receiving the request.

The sponsor's submission of an IND safety report for a drug product under a clinical study does not constitute the sponsor's or FDA's admission that the drug caused or contributed to the adverse event.

Postmarketing Surveillance of Drugs and Biologics

Postmarketing surveillance is the systematic collection, analysis, interpretation and dissemination of health-related data to improve public health and reduce morbidity and mortality. FDA requires manufacturers, packagers and distributors of marketed prescription and nonprescription drug products to establish and maintain records and make reports to the agency of all serious, unexpected adverse drug experiences associated with the use of their drug products. Reporting by healthcare professionals outside industry is voluntary.

Definitions

The following definitions of terms apply to postmarketing reporting of adverse drug experiences.[5]

Adverse Drug Experience
An adverse drug experience is any adverse event associated with the use of a drug, whether or not considered drug related, including the following:
- an adverse event occurring in the course of the use of a drug product in professional practice
- an adverse event occurring from drug overdose whether accidental or intentional
- an adverse event occurring from drug abuse
- an adverse event occurring from drug withdrawal
- any failure of expected pharmacological action

Associated With the Use of the Drug
There is a reasonable possibility that the experience may have been caused by the drug.

Disability
An adverse event that results in a substantial disruption of a person's ability to conduct normal life functions.

Life-threatening Adverse Drug Experience
Any adverse drug experience that places the patient, in the view of the initial reporter, at immediate risk of death from the adverse drug experience as it occurred, i.e., it does not include an adverse drug experience that, had it occurred in a more severe form, might have caused death.

Serious Adverse Drug Experience
Any adverse drug experience occurring at any dose that results in any of the following outcomes: death, a life-threatening adverse drug experience, inpatient hospitalization or prolongation of existing hospitalization, a persistent or significant disability/incapacity, or a congenital anomaly/birth defect. Important medical events that may not result in death, be life-threatening or require hospitalization may be considered a serious adverse drug experience when, based on appropriate medical judgment, they may jeopardize

the patient or subject and may require medical or surgical intervention to prevent one of the outcomes listed in this definition. Examples of such medical events include allergic bronchospasm requiring intensive treatment in an emergency room or at home, blood dyscrasias or convulsions that do not result in inpatient hospitalization or the development of drug dependency or drug abuse.

Unexpected Adverse Drug Experience

An unexpected adverse drug experience is any adverse drug experience that is not listed in the current labeling for the drug product. This includes events that may be symptomatically and pathophysiologically related to an event listed in the labeling, but differ from the event because of greater severity or specificity. For example, under this definition, hepatic necrosis would be unexpected (by virtue of greater severity) if the labeling only referred to elevated hepatic enzymes or hepatitis. Similarly, cerebral thromboembolism and cerebral vasculitis would be unexpected (by virtue of greater specificity) if the labeling only listed cerebral vascular accidents. "Unexpected," as used in this definition, refers to an adverse drug experience that has not been previously observed (i.e., included in the labeling) rather than from the perspective of such experience not being anticipated from the pharmacological properties of the pharmaceutical product.

Authorities

CDER's Office of Surveillance and Epidemiology Divisions consists of three divisions:
- Division of Drug Risk Evaluation (DDRE)
- Division of Medication Errors and Technical Support (DMETS)
- Division of Surveillance, Research, and Communication Support (SRCS)

The DDRE staff are safety evaluators whose primary role is to detect and assess safety signals for all marketed drug products. They work closely with medical reviewers in the Office of New Drugs so potential safety signals are placed in the context of existing preclinical, clinical or pharmacologic knowledge of the drugs in question. The DDRE staff review study protocols that are required of manufacturers as Phase 4 commitments. They evaluate various postmarketing surveillance tools that may be incorporated into risk management strategies, such as patient registries and restricted distribution systems. They estimate the public health impact of safety signals by evaluating computerized databases and the published literature.

The DMETS staff primarily provide premarketing reviews of all proprietary names, labels and labeling in CDER to reduce the medication error potential of a proposed product. DMETS also provides postmarketing review and analysis of all medication errors CDER receives.

SRCS staff handle data resources, risk communication and outcomes and effectiveness research components of drug safety risk management programs. This division oversees MedWatch, risk communication research and activities such as Medication Guides, Patient Package Inserts and pharmacy information surveys, and international regulatory liaison activities for all drug and biologic postmarketing safety issues. SRCS also manages the expansion in the use and number of safety and epidemiologic data resources.

The CDER Drug Safety and Risk Management Advisory Committee advises the Commissioner of Food and Drugs on risk management, risk communication and quantitative evaluation of spontaneous reports for drugs for human use and for any other product for which FDA has regulatory responsibility. The committee also advises regarding the scientific and medical evaluation of all information gathered by the Department of Health and Human Services (DHHS) and the Department of Justice with regard to safety, efficacy and abuse potential of drugs or other substances, and recommends actions to be taken by DHHS with regard to the marketing, investigation and control of such drugs or other substances.

The CDER Drug Safety Oversight Board provides oversight and advice to CDER leadership on managing important drug safety issues and the flow of emerging safety information to healthcare professionals and patients.

Postmarketing Drug/Biologic Surveillance: Individual Case Safety Reports (ICSRs)

Before considering any clinical incident for submission to FDA in an individual case safety report (ICSR), applicants should, at a minimum, have knowledge of the four data elements:
- an identifiable patient
- an identifiable reporter
- a suspect drug or biological product
- an adverse experience or fatal outcome believed to be due to the suspect drug or biological product

If any one of these basic elements remains unknown after being actively sought by the applicant, a report on the incident should not be submitted to FDA because reports without such information make interpretation of their significance difficult, at best, and impossible in most instances. Instead, the applicant should maintain records of its efforts to obtain the basic elements for an individual case in its corporate drug or biological safety files. If an applicant submits a report to FDA that lacks any of the four basic elements, it will be returned to the applicant marked "insufficient data for a report."

An applicant that is actively seeking information on an adverse experience should use direct verbal contact with the initial reporter of the adverse experience (e.g., in person, by telephone or other interactive means, such as a videoconference). The applicant should not merely send the initial reporter a letter requesting information concerning the adverse experience. Applicants should use a healthcare professional (e.g., physician, physician assistant, dentist, pharmacist, nurse) for initial contact with reporters because it is necessary to be able to understand the medical consequences of the case and ask appropriate questions to acquire relevant information rapidly to determine the significance of the case.

With regard to an "identifiable" patient, reports of the type "some patients got anaphylaxis" should be excluded until further information about the patients is obtained. A report stating that "an elderly woman had anaphylaxis" or a "young man experienced anaphylaxis" should be included because there is enough information to suspect that specific patients were involved. Patients should not be identified by name or address. Instead, the applicant should assign a unique code to each report.

For spontaneous reports, the applicant should assume that an adverse experience or fatal outcome was thought to be due to the suspect drug or biological product (implied causality). An adverse experience should, at a minimum, consist of signs (including abnormal laboratory findings, if appropriate), symptoms or disease diagnosis (including any colloquial descriptions) obtained for purposes of reporting. Thus, a report stating that a patient "experienced unspecified injury," or a patient "suffered irreparable damages" should not be included until more specific information about the adverse experience can be determined.

Current regulations dealing with postmarketing reporting of adverse drug experiences (ADEs) include 21 CFR 314.80 and 310.305. US regulations are consistent with ICH and the Council for International Organizations of Medical Sciences (CIOMS) standards.

Under 21 CFR 314.80, the sponsor is required to review ADE information obtained from all potential sources (foreign and domestic), including:
- marketing experience
- scientific literature (peer-reviewed and non-peer-reviewed)
- unpublished reports
- postmarketing clinical investigations
- postmarketing epidemiological or surveillance studies

Furthermore, the sponsor is required to develop written procedures for the surveillance, receipt, evaluation and reporting of postapproval ADE reports to FDA and maintain records of all ADEs known to the applicant for a period of 10 years, including raw data and any correspondence relating to ADEs. Any company (sponsor, manufacturer, distributor or packer) listed on the approved product labeling is held to these ADE reporting requirements. Obligations of a non-sponsor may be met by submitting all reports of serious ADEs to the sponsor. If a non-sponsor elects to submit ADE reports to the sponsor rather than to FDA, the non-sponsor shall submit and report to the sponsor within five calendar days of receipt of the report, and the sponsor would be responsible for submitting ADEs to FDA. The non-sponsor should maintain a record of the submission to the sponsor.

All adverse events (domestic and foreign) that are both serious and unexpected must be submitted within 15 calendar days of initial receipt by anyone in the employ of the applicant. They are submitted on Form FDA 3500A (MedWatch form) with a clearly marked cover letter and separately from other submissions. Foreign reports may use Form FDA 3500A or a CIOMS I form.

Form FDA 3500A should be completed for each report of an adverse drug experience (with the exception that foreign events may be submitted on Form FDA 3500A or a CIOMS I form). Each completed Form FDA 3500A should refer only to an individual patient or a single attached publication.

Instead of using Form FDA 3500A, an applicant may use a computer-generated Form FDA 3500A or other alternative format (e.g., a computer-generated tape or tabular listing) provided that:
- The content of the alternative format is equivalent in all elements of information to those specified in FDA Form 3500A.
- The format is agreed to in advance by the Office of Surveillance and Epidemiology.

Form FDA 3500A and instructions for completing the form are available on the FDA website (www.fda.gov/medwatch/index.html).

ADE reports can be submitted either via paper or electronically. FDA has provided guidance regarding submission of ADE reports in electronic format (see *Draft Guidance for Industry: Providing Regulatory Submissions in Electronic Format – Postmarketing Individual Case Safety Reports*, June 2008).

Unlike IND Safety Reports, causality does not enter into the decision for postmarketing reports, with the exception of postmarketing clinical investigations or studies (whether or not conducted under an IND). In these instances, if the reporter concludes that there is a reasonable possibility that the drug caused the adverse experience, the report is subject to a 15-Day Alert if serious and unexpected. This is the one exception in reporting postmarketing adverse drug experiences where an assessment of causality is required. Reports from postmarketing studies should be separated and identified as coming from postmarketing studies to differentiate them from spontaneous reports.

It should be noted that reports from the scientific literature, i.e., from medical journals, are required to be submitted either as case reports or as the result of a formal clinical trial. Reports based on the scientific literature also should be reported on Form FDA 3500A and should be accompanied by a copy of the published article.

If an adverse event is serious, unexpected and associated with the use of the drug, it must be submitted both as an IND Safety Report and a 15-Day Alert Report.

The sponsor is required to investigate all adverse drug experiences that are the subject of postmarketing 15-Day Alert reports and submit follow-up reports. If additional information is not obtainable, records should be maintained of the number of unsuccessful steps taken to seek additional information. Postmarketing 15-Day Alert Reports and follow-ups to them shall be submitted under separate cover. The mailing label should prominently say "15-Day Alert Report" or "15-Day Alert Report Follow-up."

A sponsor should protect the patient's privacy with an ADE by assigning a unique code instead of using the patient's name and address in the reports. A sponsor can include a disclaimer statement in the report indicating that it is not admitting or denying that the ADE report submitted constitutes an admission that the drug caused or contributed to an adverse effect.

The *Dietary Supplement and Nonprescription Drug Consumer Protection Act* (*DSNDCA*) (PL 109-462) was signed into law in 2006. The *DSNDCA* amended the *Federal Food, Drug, and Cosmetic Act* (*FD&C Act*) to add safety reporting requirements for nonprescription drug products that are marketed without an approved application. Section 760(b) states that the manufacturer, packager or distributor whose name appears on the label of a nonprescription drug marketed in the US without an approved application (referred to as the responsible person) must submit to FDA any report of a serious adverse event associated with such drug when used in the US, accompanied by a copy of the label on or within the retail package of such drug. In addition, the responsible person must submit follow-up reports of new medical information related to a submitted serious adverse event report that is received within one year of the initial report.

Postmarketing Drug/Biologic Surveillance: Periodic Reporting

The sponsor is required to submit the following periodic reports to FDA, for the first three years following approval, on a quarterly, basis. Unless otherwise requested by FDA, after three years, the sponsor shall submit the periodic ADE report at annual intervals. Quarterly reports are required to be filed within 30 days of the close of the quarter, with the first quarter beginning on the date of approval of the application. Annual reports are required to be submitted within 60 days of the close of the year. FDA may extend or re-establish the requirement that an applicant submit quarterly reports after the approval of a major supplement.

The regulations require a postmarketing periodic report to contain:
- a narrative summary and analysis of the information in the report and an analysis of the 15-day Alert Reports submitted during the reporting interval
- a Form FDA 3500A for each spontaneously reported adverse experience occurring in the US that was not reported in a 15-day Alert Report
- a history of actions taken since the last report because of adverse experiences

The information contained within a postmarketing periodic report should be divided into four sections in the order described below and should be clearly separated by an identifying tab. If information for one of these sections is not included, the applicant should simply explain why the information is not provided.

- Section 1: Narrative summary and analysis—A narrative summary and analysis of the information in the postmarketing period report and an analysis of the 15-Day Reports (i.e., serious, unexpected adverse experiences) submitted during the reporting period must be provided.
- Section 2: Narrative discussion of actions taken—A narrative discussion of actions taken must be provided, including any labeling changes and studies initiated since the last periodic report.
- Section 3: Index line listing—An index line listing of Form FDA 3500As or Vaccine Adverse Event Reporting System (VAERS) forms included in Section 4 of the periodic report must be provided.
- Section 4: Form FDA 3500As or VAERS forms—Form FDA 3500As or VAERS forms must be provided for the adverse events that have not already been submitted as 15-Day Alerts for experiences that occurred in the US during the reporting period.

Periodic reporting, except for information regarding 15-Day Alert Reports, does not apply to adverse drug experience information obtained from postmarketing studies (whether or not conducted under an IND), reports in the scientific literature and foreign marketing experience.

An applicant can request a waiver of the requirement to submit postmarketing periodic safety reports in the format described in the regulations. Instead, applicants can prepare these reports using the Periodic Safety Update Report (PSUR) or Periodic Benefit Risk Evaluation Report (PBRER) formats described in ICH E2C. Even if a waiver has been obtained to submit in PSUR format, a separate waiver must be requested to submit in PBRER format.

Chapter 17

Postmarketing Drug/Biologic Surveillance: Safety Monitoring by FDA

FDA tracks adverse drug reaction reports by entering all safety reports for approved drugs and therapeutic biologic products into the computerized FDA Adverse Event Reporting System (FAERS) database, which uses standardized international terminology from the *Medical Dictionary for Regulatory Activities*. FDA uses FAERS to facilitate postmarketing drug surveillance and compliance activities. The goal of FAERS is to improve the public health by providing the best available tools for storing and analyzing safety data and reports. Data and trends from FAERS may lead to FDA action on products, such as "Dear Health Care Professional" letters or requests to a sponsor for additional safety studies. This is part of an FDA initiative to rapidly collect, analyze and disseminate drug safety information. This initiative is highlighted by FDA's *Draft Guidance: Drug Safety Information—FDA's Communication to the Public* (March 2012).

FDA also posts potential signals of serious risks or new safety information identified from FAERS on its website on a quarterly basis. The appearance of a drug on this list does not mean FDA has concluded the drug has this listed risk. It means FDA has identified a potential safety concern, but does not mean the agency has identified a causal relationship between the drug and the listed risk. If, after further evaluation, FDA determines that the drug is associated with the risk, it may take a variety of actions, including requiring changes to the drug's labeling, requiring development of Risk Evaluation and Mitigation Strategies (REMS) or gathering additional data to better characterize the risk. FDA posts these quarterly reports in accordance with Title IX, Section 921 of the *Food and Drug Administration Amendments Act* of 2007 (*FDAAA*). This section in *FDAAA*, among other things, directs FDA to "conduct regular, bi-weekly screening of the Adverse Event Reporting System (AERS) database and post a quarterly report of new safety information or potential signal of a serious risk identified in the last quarter." FDA staff in CDER and CBER regularly examine the FAERS database as part of routine safety monitoring. When a potential serious risk signal is identified from FAERS data, it is entered as a safety issue into CDER's Document Archiving, Reporting and Regulatory Tracking System (DARRTS) or into CBER's Therapeutics and Blood Safety Branch Safety Signal Tracking (SST) system. The table in each quarterly report lists the names of products and potential safety issues that were entered into the above CDER or CBER tracking system where the FAERS database identified (or contributed to identification of) the potential safety issues. Additional information on each issue, such as an FDA Drug Safety Communication, also is provided.

Proprietary Name Review

FDA has considered the role of names and naming processes in medication errors as part of the agency's focus on the safe use of medical products. FDA has developed internal procedures and processes that are part of its marketing application review process for evaluating the potential for a proposed product name (submitted as part of a New Drug Application, Biologics License Application or Abbreviated New Drug Application) to cause or contribute to medication errors. *Guidance for Industry: Contents of a Complete Submission for the Evaluation of Proprietary Names* is intended to assist industry in the submission of a complete package of information for FDA to use in assessing the safety aspects of a proposed proprietary name (to reduce medication errors) and the promotional implications of a proposed name (to ensure compliance with other requirements for labeling and promotion).

Risk Management and REMS

FDAAA created Section 505-1 of the *FD&C Act*, which authorizes FDA to require sponsors of certain applications to submit and implement a REMS. Risk management is defined in FDA's *Guidance for Industry: Good Pharmacovigilance Practices and Pharmacoepidemiologic Assessment* as an iterative process of:
- assessing a product's benefit-risk balance
- developing and implementing tools to minimize a product's risks while preserving its benefits
- evaluating tool effectiveness and reassessing the benefit:risk balance
- making adjustments, as appropriate, to the risk minimization tools to further improve the benefit:risk balance

FDA's *Draft Guidance for Industry: Format and Content of Proposed Risk Evaluation and Mitigation Strategies (REMS), REMS Assessments, and Proposed REMS Modifications* provides guidance to industry on:
- the format and content of a proposed REMS, including REMS supporting documentation
- the content of assessments and proposed modifications of approved REMS
- what identifiers to use on REMS documents
- how to communicate with FDA about REMS

Guidance for Industry: Medication Guides—Distribution Requirements and Inclusion in Risk Evaluation and Mitigation Strategies (REMS) outlines the use of a Medication Guide if required as part of a REMS. The guidance also provides information on enforcement discretion regarding dispensing requirements for Medication Guides.

The *Food and Drug Administration Safety Innovation Act* of 2012 (*FDASIA*) requires an assessment strategy to determine whether a REMS is effective. Under the law, the assessment will determine whether a modification is necessary to maintain an acceptable benefit:risk balance and keep the burden on the healthcare system at an acceptable level. Applicants may propose a modification to a REMS at any time, FDA may propose a modification to a REMS at any time or FDA may request that an applicant submit a modification. If such a request is made by the agency, the applicant must respond within 120 days (or another timeframe agreed upon by FDA and applicant), and the agency must review and act on the submitted strategy within 180 days of the request or within 60 days for minor modifications or modifications based on safety label changes. FDA is required to provide guidance on this process.

Postmarketing Device Surveillance

Medical device postmarketing surveillance presents unique challenges compared to drugs and biologics due to the great diversity and complexity of medical devices, the iterative nature of medical device product development, the learning curve associated with technology adoption and the relatively short product lifecycle. Proper medical device operation depends on optimal device design, the use environment, user training and adherence to directions for use and maintenance. In some cases, these features limit the utility of relying on systems designed for the identification of drug-related adverse events.

The primary regulations that govern postmarketing reporting requirements are included in the following:
- 21 CFR 803: Medical device reporting:
  o Device user facilities must report deaths and serious injuries that a device has or may have caused or contributed to, establish and maintain adverse event files and submit summary annual reports.
  o Manufacturers or importers must report deaths and serious injuries their device has or may have caused or contributed to. In addition, they must report certain device malfunctions. They also must establish and maintain adverse event files. In addition, manufacturers must submit specified follow-up information.
  o Medical device distributors must maintain records of incidents but are not required to file these incidents.
- 21 CFR 806: Medical devices; reports of corrections and removals
- 21 CFR 822: Postmarket surveillance

In 2012, *FDASIA* expanded the Sentinel network to apply to devices. FDA is required to establish procedures for tracking device risk and analyzing public health trends. FDA also was given the ability to require postmarketing studies at any time in the product's marketed lifecycle.

The current US medical device postmarket surveillance system depends primarily on the following:
- Medical Device Reporting (MDR)—See above
- Medical Product Safety Network (MedSun)—MedSun is an enhanced surveillance network comprised of approximately 280 hospitals nationwide that work interactively with FDA to better understand and report on device use and adverse outcomes in the real-world clinical environment. The overall quality of the approximately 5,000 reports received annually via MedSun is significantly higher than those received via MDR. Specialty networks within MedSun focus on device-specific areas such as cardiovascular devices (HeartNet) and pediatric intensive care unit devices (KidNet). In addition, the network can be used for targeted surveys and focused clinical research.
- Postapproval Studies—FDA may order a postapproval study as a condition of approval for a device approved under a Premarket Approval (PMA) application. Typically, postapproval studies are used to assess device safety, effectiveness and/or reliability, including longer-term, real-world device performance. Status updates for the more than 160 ongoing postapproval studies may be found on FDA's website (www.accessdata.fda.gov/scripts/cdrh/cfdocs/cfpma/pma_pas.cfm).
- Postmarket Surveillance Studies—FDA may order a manufacturer of certain Class II or Class III devices to conduct postmarket surveillance studies (often referred to as "522 studies"). Study approaches vary widely and may include nonclinical device testing, analysis of existing clinical databases, observational studies and, rarely, randomized controlled trials. Status updates for ongoing postmarket surveillance studies covering approximately a dozen device types may be found on FDA's website (www.accessdata.fda.gov/scripts/cdrh/cfdocs/cfPMA/pss.cfm).
- FDA Discretionary Studies—In addition to medical device adverse event reports, postapproval and postmarket surveillance studies, FDA also conducts its own research to monitor device performance, investigate adverse event signals and characterize device-associated benefits and risks to patient sub-populations A variety of privacy-protected data sources are used, including national registries, Medicare and Medicaid administrative and claims data, data from integrated health systems, electronic health records and the published scientific literature.
- Other Tools—FDA has other tools it may use in the postmarket setting to track devices, restrict or ban device use and remove unsafe, adulterated or misbranded products from the market.

The Sentinel Initiative in Drug, Biologic and Device Postmarket Surveillance

FDAAA required FDA to collaborate with public, academic and private entities to develop methods for obtaining access to disparate healthcare data sources and to analyze healthcare safety data. In May 2008, the secretary of DHHS and the FDA commissioner announced the Sentinel Initiative, a long-term effort to create a national electronic system for monitoring FDA-regulated medical product safety. The Sentinel System will ultimately expand FDA's existing postmarket safety surveillance systems by enabling the agency to conduct active surveillance and related observational studies on the safety and performance of its regulated medical products once they reach the market.

The Mini-Sentinel is a pilot project sponsored by FDA to create an active surveillance system, the Sentinel System, to monitor the safety of FDA-regulated medical products. It uses pre-existing electronic healthcare data from multiple sources. Collaborating institutions provide access to data as well as scientific and organizational expertise. Mini-Sentinel is exploring a variety of approaches for improving the agency's ability to quickly identify and assess safety issues. The Mini-Sentinel program currently includes data on 126 million individuals.

Conclusion

This chapter has reviewed reporting requirements for manufacturers and distributors of drugs, biologics and medical devices, including reporting requirements under INDs. Periodic update reports also have been discussed. In addition, the activities of FDA in monitoring postmarketing safety of healthcare products through the Sentinel and Mini-Sentinel programs and through other safety monitoring have been addressed. A review of proprietary nomenclature for pharmaceutical products and the need for a REMS have been discussed. Safety is one of FDA's highest priorities and of pharmaceutical companies that have developed products for the benefit of patients and consumers. For regulatory and pharmacovigilance professionals, vigilant attention to product safety is of paramount importance.

References

1. 21 CFR Part 312.64(b) Investigator reports. FDA website. www.accessdata.fda.gov/scripts/cdrh/cfdocs/cfcfr/CFRSearch.cfm?fr=312.64. Accessed 1 May 2013.
2. 21 CFR Part 312.32(b) IND safety reporting. FDA website. www.accessdata.fda.gov/scripts/cdrh/cfdocs/cfcfr/cfrsearch.cfm?fr=312.32. Accessed 1 May 2013.
3. Investigational New Drug Safety Reporting Requirements for Human Drug and Biological Products and Safety Reporting Requirements for Bioavailability and Bioequivalence Studies in Humans, 21 CFR Parts 312 and 320 (Final Rule). *Federal Register*, 29 September 2010. Federal Register website. https://www.federalregister.gov/articles/2010/09/29/2010-24296/investigational-new-drug-safety-reporting-requirements-for-human-drug-and-biological-products-and. Accessed 1 May 2013.
4. 21 CFR Part 312.32(d) IND safety reporting. FDA website. www.accessdata.fda.gov/scripts/cdrh/cfdocs/cfcfr/cfrsearch.cfm?fr=312.32. Accessed 1 May 2013.
5. 21 CFR Part 314.80 Postmarketing reporting of adverse drug experiences. FDA website. www.accessdata.fda.gov/scripts/cdrh/cfdocs/cfcfr/cfrsearch.cfm?fr=314.80. Accessed 1 May 2013

Chapter 18

Medical Device Submissions

Updated by Alay Bhayani, MS, RAC

OBJECTIVES

- Discuss the types of submissions made to the Center for Devices and Radiological Health (CDRH)

- Explain how medical devices are classified and how the classification affects the types of submissions required

- Describe the Investigational Device Exemption (IDE) requirements for clinical device studies

- Review the types of 510(k) Premarket Notification submissions, when 510(k) submissions are needed and what information is required

- Review the types of Premarket Approval (PMA) submissions, when PMA submissions are needed and what information is required

- Explain when a Humanitarian Device Exemption (HDE) is appropriate and what information is required

- Discuss when Expedited Review should be requested

- Provide an overview of the nature and status of current proposals for changes in FDA's decision making

LAWS, REGULATIONS AND GUIDELINES COVERED IN THIS CHAPTER

- *Federal Food, Drug, and Cosmetic Act* of 1938

- 21 CFR 807 Establishment Registration and Device Listing, Premarket Notification

- 21 CFR 812 Investigational Device Exemptions

- 21 CFR 814 Premarket Approval

- 21 CFR 860 Medical Device Classification Procedures

Introduction

Medical devices were first regulated by the *Federal Food, Drug and Cosmetic Act* of 1938 (*FD&C Act*), which is enforced by the US Food and Drug Administration (FDA). Under the act, devices were examined for adulteration and misbranding, but no provision was made for review of their safety or effectiveness prior to marketing. In the late 1960s, FDA started to concentrate on devices that posed problems with safety and effectiveness, requiring recalls and replacements.

The *FD&C Act* was amended in 1976 to include premarket review of medical devices. Under the act's amendments, FDA was authorized to set standards, with premarket clearance for some devices and premarket approval for others. Devices posing little or no risk to users or patients were exempted from standards and premarket clearance, but were not necessarily exempt from complying with parts of the Good Manufacturing Practice requirements for devices under 21 CFR 820, the Quality System Regulation (QSR).

FDA, primarily through the Center for Devices and Radiological Health (CDRH), is responsible for assuring that medical devices are safe and effective. Per the FDA Intercenter Agreement (31 October 1991), the Center for Biologics Evaluation and Research (CBER) has responsibility for devices related to blood and cellular products (see Chapter 22 Biologics Submissions). The agency bears this responsibility through authority granted by the *FD&C Act*, which is carried out in accordance with the regulations found in Title 21 of the Code of Federal Regulations (CFR). Medical devices, referred to as "devices," are defined in Section 201(h) of the *FD&C Act*:

"The term 'device' means an instrument, apparatus, implement, machine, contrivance, implant, in vitro reagent, or other similar or related article, including any component, part, or accessory, which is:
(1) recognized in the official *National Formulary*, or the *United States Pharmacopeia*, or any supplement to them,
(2) intended for use in the diagnosis of disease or other conditions, or in the cure, mitigation, treatment, or prevention of disease, in man or other animals, or
(3) intended to affect the structure or any function of the body of man or other animals, and which does not achieve its primary intended purposes through chemical action within or on the body of man or other animals and which is not dependent upon being metabolized for the achievement of its primary intended purposes."

Medical Device Classification (21 CFR 860)

Medical devices are regulated based on a classification system that evaluates the risk posed by the product and the level of control needed to adequately assure safety. The device classification system has been modified by subsequent amendments but generally remains as originally intended. The act defines three classes of medical devices according to increasing complexity and regulatory control:
- Class I—General Controls
- Class II—General Controls and Special Controls
- Class III—General Controls and Premarket Approval

Class I devices are generally low-risk devices, such as non-prescription sunglasses, for which safety and effectiveness are well established and can be assured by adherence to a set of guidelines or "general controls." General controls include compliance with the applicable portions of the QSR for manufacturing and recordkeeping; requirements for issuing notices about repair; replacing or refunding money for devices presenting an unreasonable risk of substantial harm; facility registration and product listing; adverse event reporting; and appropriate, truthful and non-misleading labeling, advertising and promotional materials. In rare circumstances, some Class I devices also require premarket clearance by FDA through the 510(k) premarket notification process.

Class II devices are intermediate-risk devices, such as blood glucose test systems and infusion pumps, where general controls are not sufficient to ensure their safety and effectiveness. Class II devices are subject to "special controls" in addition to general controls. Special controls may include performance standards, FDA guidance documents, special labeling requirements, tracking of implantable devices and other actions the agency deems necessary to assure safety and effectiveness. Most Class II devices are subject to premarket review and clearance by FDA through the 510(k) premarket notification process. At times, the review and requirements are just as rigorous as those for a Class III device.

FDA considers Class III devices, such as life-sustaining, life-supporting or implantable devices, to pose the greatest risk. Devices that have a new intended use or employ a unique, new technology that is not substantially equivalent to a legally marketed predicate device are also categorized as Class III. Class III devices are subject to the most rigorous controls, including general controls (like Class I and Class II devices), any relevant special controls (like Class II devices) and, in most cases, premarket approval, which requires the submission of evidence to establish reasonable assurance of the device's safety and effectiveness. Detailed manufacturing information also may be required. FDA may request a panel of outside experts to recommend the action to be taken on the Class III device. However, the agency is not compelled to take the panel's advice.

FDA uses Medical Device Classification Procedures described in 21 CFR 860 to determine device classifications. 21 CFR 862–892 contain resulting classification regulations. A device may be classified by its regulation and by a product code. Product codes may provide more specific designations within a classification regulation. Occasionally, FDA assigns a product code to a category of devices prior to the formal assignment of a regulatory classification. CDRH's Product Classification database[1] can be used to help determine classifications.

Reclassification

The rules and procedures for establishing a device's classification and requesting a change in device classification are contained in 21 CFR 860. Advantages of reclassifying a device from a PMA to a 510(k) route to marketing include reduced fees required by FDA to review the submission; often, reduced information requirements; and reduced requirements for submissions for changes. In Fiscal 2013, the PMA review fee is approximately $248,000, while the 510(k) processing fee is approximately $4,900.

Since 1976, the primary reclassification activity has been geared toward down-classifying Class III devices into Class II or I. Generating reclassification data requires considerable effort and resources. If one is successful, the reclassified device and any substantially equivalent device can be cleared for marketing through the less-burdensome 510(k) process.

It was the intent of Congress that reclassification play a potentially significant role in the medical device clearance process, although CDRH's interpretation of its mandate has not permitted the reclassification process to be utilized to a meaningful extent. A primary obstacle has been the high level of scientific information CDRH requires to support a device's reclassification. A second obstacle has been difficulty in obtaining agreement among manufacturers whose products have already been cleared by PMAs. Removal of the PMA requirement may be seen as loss of a barrier to entry that limits competitors.

In 2009, FDA initiated the *515 Program Initiative*[2] to facilitate reclassifications.

513(g) Request for Designation

It is sometimes unclear into which classification a device falls. A provision in Section 513(g) of the *FD&C Act* allows the device sponsor to request a classification determination from FDA. This requires a letter with a description of the device and a fee payment. The agency usually responds within 60 days with a classification assignment based on the material presented. More information is provided in a CDRHLearn training class.[3]

Exemptions

Most Class I devices, and some Class II devices, are exempt from 510(k) premarket notification requirements. However, they are not exempt from general controls. All medical devices must be manufactured under a quality assurance program, proven suitable for their intended use, appropriately packaged and properly labeled. The establishment and device must be registered and listed with FDA. Establishment registrations and listings are in the public domain. Some Class I devices are exempt from most GMP requirements, with the exception of complaint files and general recordkeeping.

Devices exempt from 510(k) requirements are pre-amendment devices not significantly changed or modified and Class I and II devices specifically exempted by regulation.

A "preamendment device is one legally marketed in the US before May 28, 1976 that has not been significantly changed or modified and for which a regulation requiring a PMA application has not been published by FDA." Devices meeting this description are referred to as "grandfathered" and do not require a 510(k).

The *FD&C Act* authorizes FDA to exempt certain generic types of Class I devices from the premarket notification requirement. FDA has exempted more than 800 generic types of Class I devices and 60 Class II devices from the premarket notification requirement. Exemptions occur on a periodic basis and are published in the *Federal Register*. The 510(k) exemption has certain limitations (www.fda.gov/MedicalDevices/DeviceRegulationandGuidance/Overview/ClassifyYourDevice/default.htm), which are covered under 21 CFR XXX.9, where XXX refers to Parts 862-892. Before deciding that a device is exempt, the sponsor must determine the device's classification status and limitations.

De Novo Process

The *Food and Drug Administration Modernization Act* of 1997 (*FDAMA*) created a process for the classification of certain low-risk devices for which there is no predicate. Before *FDAMA*, such a device would automatically be designated Class III. Reclassification would be required to move the device to Class I or II. However, under this process, the sponsor of a low- or a moderate-risk device had to go through a 510(k) review process and receive a Not Substantially Equivalent (NSE) determination before it can apply for a risk-based determination. This process was proving to be unwieldy and redundant.

The *Food and Drug Administration Safety and Innovation Act* (*FDASIA*), signed into law on 9 July 2012, amended, among others, Section 513(f) of the *FD&C Act*. It eliminates the requirement of undergoing a 510(k) review process and allows sponsors to directly request a *de novo* classification.

The guidance entitled *New Section 513(f)(2)—Evaluation of Automatic Class III Designation, Guidance for Industry and CDRH Staff*, issued on 19 February 1998, and the draft guidance, *Draft Guidance for Industry and Food and Drug Administration Staff: De Novo Classification Process (Evaluation of Automatic Class III Designation)*, issued on 3 October 2011, were developed and issued prior to the enactment of *FDASIA*, and certain sections of these guidances may no longer be current as a result of *FDASIA*. CDRH is currently working on a new draft *de novo* guidance, that when finalized, will represent FDA's current thinking on this topic (www.fda.gov/MedicalDevices/DeviceRegulationandGuidance/GuidanceDocuments/ucm080195.htm).

Combination Products

Until 1990 and the introduction of the *Safe Medical Devices Act*, there was no formal process to establish which FDA center would regulate combination products, such as drug-device, device-biologic or biologic-drug products.

Regulations have now established that FDA makes a determination based on the primary mode of action of the combination product. By making this determination, the agency in effect decides whether the item is a drug, a device or a biologic. Then, FDA determines which center (Center for Drug Evaluation and Research (CDER), CBER or CDRH) is the primary reviewer. However, representatives of the other appropriate centers are included on the review committee.

If it is not clear whether the combination product is a device or drug, the manufacturer may file a Request for Designation with FDA. This compels the agency to classify the combination product and indicate which center is the primary review group. The agency must respond within 60 days.

For more information on combination products, see Chapter 25.

Investigational Device Exemption (IDE) (21 CFR 812)

The IDE regulations provide a means of distributing devices that are not cleared or approved to be marketed (i.e., by 510(k), PMA or Class I exemption) for the purposes of clinical research or to gather clinical evidence of safety and effectiveness. Guidance is provided at *Device Advice: Investigational Device Exemption (IDE)*.[4]

Quoting the regulations (21 CFR 812.1):

"An IDE approved under 812.30 or considered approved under 812.2(b) exempts a device from the requirements of the following sections of the Federal Food, Drug, and Cosmetic Act and regulations issued thereunder: Misbranding under section 502 of the act, registration, listing, and premarket notification under section 510, performance standards under section 514, premarket approval under section 515, a banned device regulation under section 516, records and reports under section 519, restricted device requirements under section 520(e), good manufacturing practice requirements under section 520(f) except for the requirements found in 820.30, if applicable (unless the sponsor states an intention to comply with these requirements under 812.20(b)(3) or 812.140(b)(4)(v)) and color additive requirements under section 721."

FDA regulations and guidances often use the terms "significant risk" device and "non-significant risk" (NSR) device. In practice, FDA considers the risk of the study, not of the device. For example, a Class III device, depending on the nature of the study, may be in a significant risk study or a non-significant risk study, or in a study that is exempt from IDE requirements. The rest of this section uses FDA's terminology, e.g., "significant risk device."

A "significant risk device" must comply with full IDE requirements, including FDA approval of an IDE submittal. NSR devices must comply with abbreviated IDE requirements as described in 21 CFR 812.2(b). Abbreviated IDE requirements do not require FDA approval, but do require approval by Institutional Review Boards (IRBs). Abbreviated requirements also include informed consent and some reporting and recordkeeping (see **Table 18-1**). FDA IDE approval is presumed for NSR devices.

A "significant risk" device, per 21 CFR 812.3(m), is:
- intended as an implant and poses a serious risk to patient health
- purported or represented to be of use in supporting or sustaining life and presents a serious risk to patient health
- of substantial importance for diagnosing, curing, mitigating or treating disease or preventing impairment of health and poses a serious risk to patient health
- otherwise presents a potential for serious risk to patient health

A device is exempt from the IDE requirements if it is:
- a device in commercial distribution prior to 28 May 1976
- a device, other than a transitional device, "introduced into commercial distribution on or after May 28, 1976, that FDA has determined to be substantially equivalent to a device in commercial distribution immediately before May 28, 1976, and that is used or investigated in accordance with the indications in the labeling FDA reviewed under subpart E of part 807 in determining substantial equivalence"
- (Note that a "transitional device" is one that FDA considered to be a new drug before 28 May 1976)
- a diagnostic device that:
  o is noninvasive
  o does not require a significant risk invasive sampling procedure
  o does not intentionally introduce energy into a subject
  o is not used for a diagnostic procedure without confirmation by another established procedure
- a device undergoing consumer preference testing, if the testing is not for determining safety and effectiveness or puts the subject at risk
- a device for veterinary use or research on animals
- a custom device unless it is being used to establish safety and efficacy for commercial distribution

An IDE application includes:
1. sponsor name and address
2. a complete report of prior investigations of the device and an accurate summary of those sections of the investigational plan described in 812.25(a)–(e) or, in lieu of the summary, the complete plan; a complete investigational plan and a complete report of prior investigations of the device if no IRB has reviewed them, if FDA has found an IRB's review inadequate or if FDA requests them
3. a description of the methods, facilities and controls used for the manufacture, processing, packing,

Table 18-1. Abbreviated IDE Requirements, per 21 CFR 812.2(b)

Requirements	Additional Reference
An investigation of a device other than a significant risk device, if the device is not a banned device.	
Device is labeled per 21 CFR 812.5.	21 CFR 812.5
IRB approves after sponsor presents the IRB with a brief explanation of why the device is not a significant risk device.	
Investigators obtain informed consent from each subject.	
Sponsor monitors investigators and promptly secures compliance or takes appropriate measures if investigators fail to meet requirements.	21 CFR 812.46(a)
Sponsor immediately evaluates unanticipated adverse device effects and takes appropriate action, including termination of the study if there is an unreasonable risk to subject. A terminated study may not be resumed without IRB approval.	21 CFR 812.46(b)
Sponsor keeps records: • of basic study information per 21 CFR 812.140(b)(4) • of records concerning adverse device effects	21 CFR 812.140(b)(4) and (5)
Investigators keep records: • of each subject's documents evidencing informed consent	21 CFR 812.140(a)(3)(i)
Sponsor reports: • to FDA and IRBs, unanticipated adverse device effects • to FDA and IRBs, any withdrawal of IRB approval • to IRBs, withdrawal of FDA approval • to IRBs, progress reports and final report • to FDA and IRBs, recall and device disposition • to FDA, any report of a failure to obtain informed consent • to FDA, any IRB's determination that a device is a significant risk device • upon request of FDA or IRB, any aspect of the investigation	21 CFR 812 150(b)(1)-(3) and (5)-(10)
Investigator reports: • to sponsor and IRB, unanticipated adverse device effects • to sponsor, withdrawal of IRB approval • to sponsor and IRB, any device use without informed consent • upon request of IRB or FDA, any aspect of the investigation	21 CFR 812.150(a)(1), (2), (5), (7)
Sponsor complies with prohibitions against promotion.	21 CFR 812.7

storage and, where appropriate, installation of the device, in sufficient detail that a person generally familiar with Good Manufacturing Practices can make a knowledgeable judgment about the quality control used in the manufacture of the device

4. an example of the agreements to be entered into by all investigators to comply with investigator obligations, and a list of the names and addresses of all investigators who have signed the agreement
5. a certification that all investigators who will participate in the investigation have signed the agreement, that the list of investigators includes all who are participating in the investigation, and that no investigators will be added to the investigation until they have signed the agreement
6. a list of the name, address and chairperson of each IRB that has been or will be asked to review the investigation and a certification of the action concerning the investigation taken by each such IRB
7. name and address of any institution at which a part of the investigation may be conducted that has not been identified in accordance with the regulations
8. if the device is to be sold, the amount to be charged and an explanation of why sale does not constitute commercialization of the device; the submitter also will need to demonstrate cost recovery if sale is approved
9. a claim for categorical exclusion under 21 CFR 25.30 or 25.34 or an environmental assessment under 25.40
10. copies of all device labeling
11. copies of all forms and informational materials to be provided to subjects to obtain informed consent
12. any other relevant information FDA requests for review of the application
    a. additional information—FDA may request additional information concerning an investigation or revision in the investigational plan. This constitutes a clinical hold. The sponsor may treat

such a request as a disapproval of the application for purposes of requesting a hearing.
b. information previously submitted—Information previously submitted to CDRH need not be resubmitted but may be incorporated by reference.

FDA requires a risk analysis under 21 CFR 812.25 investigational plan. This is a description and analysis of increased risks to which subjects will be exposed by the investigation; the manner in which these risks are minimized; a justification for the investigation; and a description of the patient population, including the number, age, sex and condition.

When considering an IDE application, FDA reviews background information, such as animal testing, bench testing and the clinical protocol, to determine whether the product is safe for testing in humans and whether efficacy can be shown based on the protocol requirements.

Supplemental IDE Submissions

Supplemental submissions are required for changes in the investigational plan, informed consent or other substantive information. Supplemental IDE submissions include:
- an IDE supplement, which is any additional submission to an IDE after approval of the IDE
- an IDE amendment is any additional submissions to an IDE before approval of the IDE

Institutional Review Board (IRB) Approval

Per 21 CFR 812.42, IRB approval is necessary before an investigation begins. For further information on IRB regulations and consent forms, see 21 CFR 50 and 56, respectively.

Pre-IDE Meeting

Sponsors are encouraged to contact FDA to obtain further guidance prior to the submission of an IDE application. (Pre-IDE Meetings also may be used to obtain guidance on 510(k) submissions even though no clinical data are required.) Early interaction with the agency should help increase the sponsor's understanding of FDA requirements, regulations and guidance documents and allows FDA personnel to familiarize themselves with the new technologies. Communication with FDA may take the form of a Pre-IDE Meeting and/or a Pre-IDE Submission.

Informal Guidance Meeting

Sponsors are encouraged to meet with the Office of Device Evaluation (ODE) reviewing division to obtain advice that can be used to develop supporting preclinical data or the investigational plan. These meetings may take the form of telephone conference calls, video conferences or face-to-face discussions. The sponsor should contact the reviewing division directly or may contact the IDE staff for assistance.

Formal Guidance Meetings

There are two types of formal guidance meetings—a Determination Meeting and an Agreement Meeting.

For a Determination Meeting, a sponsor anticipating the submission of a PMA submits a written request to discuss the types of valid scientific evidence necessary to demonstrate the device is effective for its intended use. This meeting focuses on the broad outline of clinical trial design. The request and summary information for a meeting should be submitted as a Pre-IDE Submission and identified as a Determination Meeting request. FDA's determination is provided to the applicant in writing within 30 days following the meeting.

For an Agreement Meeting, a sponsor submits a written meeting request to reach an agreement with FDA regarding the agency's review of an investigational plan (including a clinical protocol). The request and summary information should be submitted as a pre-IDE submission and identified as an Agreement Meeting request. This meeting should take place no later than 30 days after receipt of the request. The written request should include a detailed description of the device, a detailed description of the proposed conditions of use of the device, a proposed plan (including a clinical protocol) for determining whether there is a reasonable assurance of effectiveness, and, if available, information regarding the device's expected performance. If an agreement is reached between FDA and the sponsor or applicant regarding the investigational plan (including a clinical protocol), the terms of the agreement are put into writing and made part of the administrative record by FDA.

To request a formal guidance meeting, use the format in, *Early Collaboration Meetings Under the FDA Modernization Act (FDAMA), Final Guidance for Industry and CDRH Staff*.[5]

It is important to establish a good working relationship with the FDA project officer. The project officer may expedite meeting requests and can also provide clarification, ideas and suggestions.

Pre-Submission Program

In 1995, FDA established a pre-IDE program to allow sponsors to submit preliminary information as a "pre-IDE" submission. Sponsors are encouraged to submit pre-IDE submissions while the sponsor is preparing the formal IDE submission whenever the sponsor requires informal FDA guidance on troublesome parts of the IDE application, e.g., clinical protocol design, preclinical testing proposal, preclinical test results, protocols for foreign studies when the studies will be used to support future marketing applications to be submitted to FDA.

Upon completion of the review of the pre-IDE submission, the reviewing division will issue a response to the sponsor in a timely manner, usually within 60 days of receipt. The response may take the form of a letter or comments provided during a meeting or telephone conference call. If FDA's response is provided via comments during a meeting or a telephone conference call, a memo of the meeting or conference call will be prepared.

Originally, the pre-IDE program was designed to provide applicants a mechanism to obtain FDA feedback on future IDE applications. Over time, the pre-IDE program has evolved to include feedback on other device submissions, such as PMA applications, HDE applications and 510(k) submissions, as well as to address questions related to whether a clinical study requires submission of an IDE. To reflect this broader scope of the pre-IDE program, FDA issued a draft guidance entitled, *Medical Devices: The Pre-Submission Program and Meetings with FDA Staff* on 13 July 2012. This guidance also broadens the program to include devices regulated by CBER and renames the pre-IDE program the Pre-Submission (Pre-Sub) program.

In this draft guidance, FDA provides examples of when a Pre-Sub may be particularly helpful; for example, before conducting a clinical study for a device involving a novel technology or prior to submitting a marketing application to gain insight into potential hurdles for approval or clearance. FDA also provides recommendations for the information that should be included in specific types of Pre-Subs.

One of industry's primary concerns about the pre-IDE program has been that FDA often provides advice and guidance in a pre-IDE meeting and then subsequently changes its position. The sponsor then must decide whether it has sufficient resources to address FDA's newly stated concerns or if it must abandon its efforts due to FDA's new approach. Although the draft guidance clearly states that advice provided in a Pre-Sub is "not decisional or binding on the agency or the applicant," it also states that FDA intends to commit to the advice provided in a Pre-Sub "unless the circumstances sufficiently change such that [the] advice is no longer applicable, such as when a sponsor changes the intended use of [its] device after [FDA] provide[s] feedback" (www.fdalawblog.net/fda_law_blog_hyman_phelps/2012/07/fda-issues-draft-guidance-expanding-pre-ide-to-pre-submission-program.html).

510(k) Premarket Notification

A 510(k) submission is made for a new or modified device for which the product classification requires a 510(k). Some Class I products, most Class II products and a small number of Class III products require a 510(k). Product families, such as catheters of various sizes or patient monitor systems of varying configurations, can be cleared on a single 510(k) if the intended uses, technological characteristics and issues of safety and effectiveness are essentially the same within the family.

The purpose of a 510(k) is to demonstrate that a new or modified device is "substantially equivalent" in intended use, safety and effectiveness as a "predicate device." A predicate device is a legally marketed device that was cleared onto the market by a 510(k). A preamendment device can also be used as a predicate device, but the sponsor may need to provide documentation that it meets the preamendment status criteria. Because medical science has advanced greatly since 1976, it is recommended that a sponsor uses a recently cleared device under 510(k) as a predicate device.

The content of 510(k) premarket notifications, described in 21 CFR 807.87, includes: the device name and class, an establishment registration number, an "Indications for Use Statement," a 510(k) summary, proposed labeling, substantial equivalence comparison with the predicate device, supporting performance data and a statement that all data and information submitted are truthful and accurate and that no material fact has been omitted. In particular, the Indications for Use Statement provides the specific indications, clinical settings, target population, anatomical sites, device configuration and other information critical to how the device is intended to be used clinically.

The format and amount of information in a 510(k) varies depending on the intended use, technology, issues of safety and effectiveness, reliance on standards and special controls and, for modified devices, on the nature of the modification.

For more detail, see *Device Advice: Premarket Notification*.[6] This webpage and three linked guidances provide advice on content and links to required forms. Using the recommended format for 510(k) submissions helps reviewers find required information. Companies preparing 510(k)s help ensure the completeness of the submittal when they combine the preparation guidance with product- and technology-specific guidances.[7] (Note: Refer to the CBER website for guidances specific to 510(k)s reviewed by CBER.[8])

Often, clinical studies are not required for 510(k) devices. However, clinical studies may be necessary if the 510(k) device cannot be shown to be as safe and effective as the predicate device using laboratory tests, such as biocompatibility, engineering, bench performance, design verification and voluntary standards tests.

The required truthful and accurate statement, which must be signed by a designated and accountable person within the company requesting market clearance, is defined in 21 CFR 807.87(k) as:

> "A statement that the submitter believes, to the best of his or her knowledge, that all data and information submitted in the premarket notification are truthful and accurate and that no material fact has been omitted."

The truthful and accurate statement carries significant legal implications and should be taken seriously by the individual signing it. It essentially amounts to a certification and, should FDA subsequently determine that false information or misstatement of material facts were included in the submission, or that material facts were omitted, judicial action could be taken against the person who signed the statement. It is prudent to conduct a formal audit of the information in the 510(k), including pertinent development information, documentation and raw data, prior to signing this statement.

Modifications to 510(k) Devices

As described in 21 CFR 807.81(a)(3), a new 510(k) application is required for changes or modifications to an existing device when the modifications could significantly affect the device's safety or effectiveness, or if the device is to be marketed for a new or different indication.

When a 510(k) holder decides to modify an existing device, it must determine whether the proposed modification(s) requires submission of a new 510(k). Changes in indications for use, including a switch from prescription status to over-the-counter availability, require the submission of a 510(k).

Examples of modifications that may require a 510(k) submission include, but are not limited to:
- sterilization method
- structural material
- manufacturing method
- operating parameters or conditions for use
- patient or user safety features
- sterile barrier packaging material
- stability or expiration claims
- design

More detail is provided in the guidance, *Deciding When to Submit a 510(k) for a Change to an Existing Device (K97-1)*.[9]

Not all changes to a device require a new submission to FDA. The sponsor must determine whether the submission criteria are met and proceed accordingly. It is good practice for a sponsor to document and file the review of the changes and the decision that a 510(k) is not required.

There are no provisions for a 510(k) amendment or supplement to the existing 510(k). If a modification requires a 510(k), but the indication for use and the fundamental technology of the device are not affected, a Special 510(k) may be submitted.

Traditional 510(k)

See the guidance, *How to Prepare a Traditional 510(k)*.[10] The traditional 510(k) format is the default format. Alternatives are the Abbreviated 510(k) and the Special 510(k).

Abbreviated 510(k)

The Special and Abbreviated 510(k) methods were developed under the "New 510(k) Paradigm" to help streamline the 510(k) review process. An Abbreviated 510(k) relies on the use of guidance documents, special controls and standards (particularly FDA-recognized consensus standards). An Abbreviated 510(k) submission must include required elements. Under certain conditions, the submitter may not need to include test data. See the guidance, *How to Prepare an Abbreviated 510(k)*.[11]

Device sponsors may choose to submit an Abbreviated 510(k) when:
- a guidance documents already exists
- a special control already has been established
- FDA has recognized a relevant consensus standard

In an Abbreviated 510(k) submission, sponsors provide summary reports on the use of guidance documents and/or special controls or Declarations of Conformity to recognized consensus standards to expedite submission review.

An Abbreviated 510(k) that relies on a guidance document should include a summary report that describes the way in which the relevant guidance document was employed. It also should note how the guidance was used during device development and testing. The summary report should include information regarding the sponsor's efforts to conform to the guidance and outline any deviations.

Special controls are a way of providing reasonable assurance of a Class II device's safety and effectiveness. Special controls are defined as those controls (such as performance standards, postmarket surveillance, patient registries, development and dissemination of guidelines, recommendations and other appropriate actions) that establish reasonable assurance of the device's safety and effectiveness. The device classification regulations list special controls for the device, if any.

An Abbreviated 510(k) that relies on a special control(s) includes a summary report that describes adherence to the special control(s). It also notes how the special control(s) was used during device development and testing, including how it was used to address a specific risk or issue. The summary report includes information regarding the sponsor's efforts to conform to the special control(s) and should outline any deviations.

Recognized consensus standards may be cited in guidance documents or individual policy statements or established as special controls that address specific risks associated with a type of device. FDA has recognized more than 800 standards to which 510(k) submitters can declare conformity. The current list of FDA-recognized consensus standards is available in CDRH's standards database.[12]

A submitter may suggest a standard that is not yet recognized by FDA. The submitter should discuss such a strategy with FDA prior to submitting an Abbreviated 510(k) based on an unrecognized standard.

An Abbreviated 510(k) that relies on a standard must include a Declaration of Conformity to the standard.

If FDA determines that an Abbreviated 510(k) does not meet eligibility requirements, the reviewer notifies the sponsor of this decision and offers the option of having the document converted to a traditional 510(k) or withdrawing it for future submission. If the 510(k) is withdrawn and a new one submitted, a new user fee applies. If the 510(k) is converted, the original receipt date remains as the start of the review period. Sponsors should be aware that, in most cases, additional information is necessary for converted submissions.

In the Abbreviated 510(k) process, a sponsor must assess the device's conformance to a Recognized Consensus Standard. Once the assessment is satisfactorily completed, the sponsor may submit the Abbreviated 510(k). Under certain conditions, conformance test data are not required to be submitted in the 510(k). To be sure, consult with the reviewing branch.

The sponsor may use a third party to assess conformance to the recognized consensus standard. The third party performs a conformance assessment with the standard for the sponsor and provides the sponsor with a statement to this effect. For example, a third party may be used to assess conformance to the standard for electromagnetic interference testing and shock hazards, IEC 60601-1-2.

The Abbreviated 510(k) should include a Declaration of Conformity signed by the sponsor, while the third party's statement should be maintained in the Device Master Record (DMR) and Design History File (DHF) (21 CFR 820.30).

Declarations of Conformity to recognized consensus standards should include the following:
- identification of applicable recognized consensus standards met
- statement, for each consensus standard, that all requirements were met except inapplicable requirements or deviations
- identification, for each consensus standard, of any way(s) in which it may have been adapted for application to the device under review (e.g., identification of an alternative series of tests that were performed)
- identification, for each consensus standard, of any requirements not applicable to the device
- specification of any deviations from each applicable standard that was applied
- specification of the differences that may exist, if any, between the tested device and the device to be marketed and a justification of the test results in these areas of difference
- name and address of any test laboratory and/or certification body involved in determining the device's conformance with applicable consensus standards and a reference to any of those organizations' accreditations

Special 510(k)

If a 510(k) is needed for a device's modification, and if the modification does not affect the device's intended use or alter its fundamental scientific technology, summary information resulting from the design control process can serve as the basis for clearing the application along with the required elements of a 510(k). See the guidance, *How to Prepare a Special 510(k)*.[13]

Modifications to the indications for use or any labeling change that affects the device's intended use are not accepted as Special 510(k)s. Special 510(k) sponsors should highlight or otherwise prominently identify changes in the proposed labeling that may result from modifications to the legally marketed device. It should be clearly stated in the Special 510(k) that the intended use of the modified device has not changed as a result of the modification(s). Note that a labeling change from prescription to over-the-counter use, or vice versa, is considered a change in intended use and is not eligible for a Special 510(k) submission.

Special 510(k)s are not accepted for modifications that alter the device's fundamental scientific technology. Such changes include modifications to the device's operating principle(s) or mechanism of action. Specific examples that illustrate types of changes that alter the fundamental scientific technology and should not be submitted as Special 510(k)s include:
- a change in a surgical instrument that uses a sharpened metal blade to one that cuts with a laser
- a change in an in vitro diagnostic device (IVD) that uses immunoassay technology to one that uses nucleic acid hybridization or amplification technology
- incorporation of a sensing mechanism in a device to allow it to function "on demand" rather than continuously

Device modifications that should be appropriate for review as Special 510(k)s include:
- energy type
- environmental specifications
- performance specifications
- ergonomics of the patient-user interface
- dimensional specifications
- software or firmware
- packaging or expiration dating
- sterilization

A sponsor may make changes to the device that do not change the intended use or alter the technology and may not require a 510(k) submission. These changes may be minor but do require appropriate change control in the DMR and DHF.

Refuse to Accept Policy for 510(k)s

FDA issued a guidance document, *Refuse to Accept Policy for 510(k)s*, on 31 December 2012 (www.fda.gov/downloads/MedicalDevices/DeviceRegulationandGuidance/GuidanceDocuments/UCM315014.pdf), which supersedes CDRH's *Premarket Notification (510(k)) Refuse to Accept Policy*, dated 30 June 1993, and *510(k) Refuse to Accept Procedures (K94-1) blue book memo*, dated 20 May 1994.

The purpose of this new guidance is to explain the procedures and criteria FDA intends to use in assessing whether a 510(k) submission meets a minimum threshold of acceptability and should be accepted for substantive review. This will enable FDA to focus its resources on completed submissions to provide a more efficient review and faster clearance of new devices. The guidance includes checklists in the appendix that clarify the necessary elements and contents of a complete 510(k) submission to help the sponsor understand the types of information FDA needs to conduct a substantive review.

Once the sponsor submits a 510(k), the acceptance review clock begins and FDA has 15 days to complete this review and let the sponsor know whether the 510(k) is administratively complete. If one or more items are missing in the 510(k), FDA notifies the sponsor of the submission not being accepted and provides a completed checklist indicating which item(s) is the basis for the Refuse to Accept (RTA) designation. The sponsor may respond by submitting the missing information, and FDA then will have another 15 days to perform the acceptance review.

The FDA review (substantive review) clock for the 510(k) start date is the receipt date of the most recent submission or additional information that resulted in an acceptance designation of the 510(k). For example, if the submission is accepted for substantive review on the first acceptance review, the FDA review clock start date is the receipt date of the submission. However, if the submission is designated RTA, the FDA review clock start date is not yet known. In such cases, the clock start date will be the receipt date of the submission including the additional information that results in an acceptance designation (even if FDA later requests information that should have been requested during acceptance review). In the event the acceptance review is not completed within 15 calendar days, the submission will be considered to be under substantive review, and the FDA review clock start date will be the receipt date of the most recently received information for the submission. For more information on the RTA policy, refer to the guidance on FDA's website.

Third Party Review

FDAMA established the Accredited Persons Program. Accredited Persons, which may be companies or individuals, are authorized to perform 510(k) reviews for certain Class II devices. The product classification database includes for each classification the Accredited Persons, if any, that are authorized to perform third-party reviews for the device classification. Third-party reviews are not subject to an FDA user fee. However, the fee paid to the third-party reviewer is usually higher than the FDA 510(k) user fee. Advantages of third-party reviews typically include:
- shorter review times
- responsiveness to questions
- expertise in testing, standards and international requirements
- local service, depending on the location of the third-party reviewer's office

See the "Device Advice" guidance *Third Party Review*.[14]

Premarket Approval (21 CFR 814)

Premarket Approval (PMA) is the FDA process of scientific and regulatory review to evaluate the safety and effectiveness of Class III medical devices. A PMA is the most stringent type of device marketing application required by FDA. PMA approval is based on a determination by FDA that the PMA contains sufficient "valid scientific evidence" to assure the device is safe and effective for its intended use(s).

Essentially, there are two types of PMA Applications:
- Traditional PMA
- Product Development Process

FDAMA introduced other Premarket Approval options:
- Modular PMA
- Streamlined PMA
- Humanitarian Device Exemption

See *PMA Application Methods*.[15]

Traditional PMA

The information required in a PMA is detailed in 21 CFR 814.20(b). In addition to voluntary completion of the applicable sections of a cover sheet, other required information includes:
1. table of contents showing the volume and page number for each item
2. summary of information in the submission, including:
   a. general description of the indications for use
   b. explanation of how the device functions, the scientific concepts upon which the device is based, general physical and performance characteristics

and a brief description of the manufacturing process, if it aids understanding
  c. generic, proprietary and trade name of the device
  d. description of existing alternative practices and procedures for which the device is intended
  e. brief description of the device's foreign and US marketing history by the applicant and/or any other person, including a list of the countries in which it has been marketed and from which marketing was withdrawn because of adverse safety and effectiveness experiences
  f. summary of studies and reports submitted with the PMA, including:
     i. nonclinical laboratory studies
     ii. human clinical investigations, other data, information or reports relevant to an evaluation of the device's safety and effectiveness from any source, known or that reasonably should be known to the applicant
     iii. discussion demonstrating that data and information in the submission constitute valid scientific evidence providing reasonable assurance of the device's safety and effectiveness, and conclusions drawn from the studies with a discussion of risk:benefit considerations and adverse effects
3. complete description of:
  a. device, including photos, drawings and schematics
  b. each functional component and/or ingredient
  c. device properties relative to its specific indications for use
  d. principles of operation
  e. methods, facilities and controls used to manufacture, process, package, store and, if appropriate, install the device
4. references to any performance standard in effect or proposed at the time of submission and any voluntary standard relevant to the device's safety or effectiveness, including adequate information to demonstrate compliance with the applicable standards and an explanation of any deviation from the standards
5. technical sections containing data and information in sufficient detail to enable approval or disapproval of the application, including results of:
  a. nonclinical laboratory studies in a separate section, including a statement that each study was conducted in accordance with Good Laboratory Practices (21 CFR 58)
  b. human clinical investigations in a separate section, including a statement that each study was conducted in accordance with IRB rules (21 CFR 56), informed consent rules (21 CFR 50) and IDE rules (21 CFR 812)
6. bibliography of all published reports that are known or reasonably should be known concerning the device's safety or effectiveness not submitted under number 5 above:
  a. identification, analysis and discussion of any other data, information and reports relevant to the evaluation of the device's safety and effectiveness from any source that are known or reasonably should be known
  b. copies of all reasonably obtainable published and unpublished reports described in 3d and 3e, if requested by FDA or an FDA Advisory Committee
7. samples of the device and its components, if requested by FDA, submitted or available at a named location if impractical to submit
8. copies of all proposed labeling, including labels, instructions for use, installation, maintenance and servicing, and any information, literature and/or advertising that constitutes labeling (Section 201(m) of the *FD&C Act* and 21 CFR 801 or 809)
9. environmental assessment in accordance with 21 CFR 25.20(n) or justification for categorical exclusion under 21 CFR 25.30 and 25.34
10. disclosure of any financial arrangements between the sponsor and clinical investigators who performed studies included in the submission, or a certification on Form FDA 3454 attesting to the absence of any financial arrangements (21 CFR 54)
11. any other information requested by FDA

Omission of any required information must be identified and justified in a statement attached as a separate section of the PMA. A DHF or other applicable information in FDA files may be incorporated by reference. However, if this information was not submitted by the PMA applicant, the applicant must receive permission from the filer of the information for it to be reviewed by FDA.

The sponsor is required to periodically update a pending PMA with new or newly learned safety and effectiveness information that could reasonably affect the device's evaluation and labeling (21 CFR 814.20(e)). To ensure adherence to all content and format requirements, manufacturers should review the regulations in 21 CFR 814.20(a)–(h) carefully, as well as FDA's guideline on the arrangement and format of a PMA.

Traditional PMA Review Process

FDA issued *Acceptance and Filing Reviews for Premarket Approval Applications (PMAs): Guidance for Industry and Food and Drug Administration Staff* on 31 December 2012 (www.fda.gov/downloads/MedicalDevices/

DeviceRegulationandGuidance/GuidanceDocuments/UCM313368.pdf) that identifies the criteria for PMA filing and supersedes the 2003 PMA filing guidance. This guidance separates the PMA filing criteria into two steps; acceptance criteria and filing criteria. The purpose of the PMA acceptance and filing reviews is to make a threshold determination about whether an application is administratively complete enough for the agency to undertake a substantive review. FDA has 15 days to complete the acceptance review and 45 days to complete the filing review. In order to enhance the consistency of FDA's acceptance and filing decisions and to help applicants better understand the types of information FDA needs to conduct a substantive review of a PMA, this guidance and associated checklist clarify the necessary elements and contents of a complete PMA application. For more information, see the guidance.

The PMA review is performed by an FDA team generally consisting of a medical officer, engineer, biologist, statistician, labeling expert and manufacturing expert. A decision to approve or not approve must be made by FDA within 180 calendar days following receipt of a complete PMA, although, in reality, reviews take much longer.

During the review process, FDA will order an inspection of the sponsor's manufacturing facility to provide evidence that the manufacturer complies with GMP requirements set forth in the QSR (21 CFR 820).

Often, PMAs for important or new technologies also will be reviewed by FDA advisory panels consisting of experts in the medical specialty (e.g., MDs, PhDs, engineers) and consumer and industry representatives. Advisory personnel are not FDA employees but are paid as "special government employees" for the days they participate as members of a panel. The panel members' recommendation is not binding; however, FDA generally follows their advice.

FDA issued *Guidance for Industry and Food and Drug Administration Staff: Factors to Consider When Making Benefit-Risk Determination in Medical Device Premarket Approval and De Novo Classifications*, on 28 March 2012, providing greater clarity for FDA reviewers and industry regarding the principal factors FDA considers when making benefit:risk determinations during the premarket review process for certain medical devices. While reviewing PMA or *De Novo* applications, FDA will consider whether the application provides a reasonable assurance of safety and effectiveness by weighing any probable benefit to health from the use of the device against any probable risk of injury or illness from such use. For more information, see the guidance (http://www.fda.gov/MedicalDevices/DeviceRegulationandGuidance/GuidanceDocuments/ucm267829.htm).

FDA's review process can result in the following outcomes:
- Approval—The PMA substantially meets the requirements of the applicable part of the regulations and the device is safe and effective for its intended use(s).
- Not Approvable—The PMA has major deficiencies, and review issues remain that stand in the way of approval (specifically identified in a letter to the applicant). This requires submission of a PMA amendment(s) by the applicant to respond to issues, and results in an additional review cycle.
- Denial—The PMA does not meet the requirements of the applicable part of the regulations and the device is not safe and effective for its intended use(s).

PMA Amendments—21 CFR 814.37

Changes or revisions to the original PMA submission are submitted to FDA in the form of amendments. Amendments are also submitted to FDA for changes to PMA supplements.

PMA Supplements

When a significant change to the device approved under a PMA affects the device's safety or effectiveness, a supplement to the original PMA is required. This became law when the *FD&C Act* was amended by Section 515(d)(6).

PMA supplements are required in situations including:
- new indication for use of the device
- labeling changes
- the use of a different facility or establishment to manufacture, process, sterilize or package the device
- changes in manufacturing facilities, methods or quality control procedures
- changes in sterilization procedures
- changes in packaging
- changes in the performance or design specifications, circuits, components, ingredients, principles of operation or physical layout of the device
- extension of the device's expiration date based on data obtained under a new or revised stability or sterility testing protocol that has not been approved by FDA (If the protocol has been previously approved by FDA, a supplement is not submitted but the change must be reported to FDA in the postapproval periodic reports as described in the Section 814.39(b).)

Supplements that are pending also can be amended with more information.

There are several ways of filing a PMA supplement:

PMA Supplement (180 days)—21 CFR 814.39(a)

The PMA Supplement is for significant changes that affect the device's safety and effectiveness and will require an in-depth review and approval by FDA before implementing the change. This also may require review by an advisory panel.

Special PMA Supplement—Changes Being Effected (CBE)—21 CFR 814.39(d)

The CBE generally is used when the change enhances or increases the device's safety. It does not require FDA approval before making the change. Examples are labeling changes that add more relevant information and increased quality control testing.

30-Day Notice and 135-Day PMA Supplement—21 CFR 814.39(f)

A 30-Day Notice is used for modifications to manufacturing procedures or methods that affect the device's safety and effectiveness. If FDA does not respond within 30 days after notification, the change can be made to the device and it can be marketed accordingly. If FDA finds the 30-Day Notice is not adequate, but contains data meeting appropriate content requirements for a PMA supplement, the 30-Day Notice will become a 135-Day PMA Supplement. For more information, see FDA guidance (www.fda.gov/downloads/MedicalDevices/DeviceRegulationandGuidance/GuidanceDocuments/UCM080194.pdf).

PMA Manufacturing Site Change Supplement

When the manufacturing site is changed, a supplement needs to be filed. The site must have received a Quality System/GMP inspection within the last two years. If requirements are not met, a 180-Day PMA Supplement must be submitted.

Annual (Periodic) Report or 30-Day Supplements—21 CFR 814.39(e)

Changes can also be reported in the Annual Report instead of in a formal supplement. However, to use this approach, a sponsor should seek an advisory opinion from FDA.

"Real-Time" Review Program for PMA Supplements

In April 1996, ODE implemented a pilot program for "Real-Time" reviews of PMA supplements where the sponsor and the FDA review team meet to discuss any concerns FDA may have. Results of the pilot program demonstrated that faster review times for manufacturers and efficient use of FDA staff time were achieved. Because this type of review is not available for all supplements, a sponsor is advised to contact its FDA reviewer to understand the criteria established for the "Real-Time" review program within a particular ODE branch and division.

The Product Development Protocol (PDP)

The PDP was authorized several years ago as an alternative to the IDE and PMA in *FD&C Act* Section 515(f). For Class III devices subject to premarket approval, the successful completion of a PDP results in market clearance and essentially is a PMA approval.

One intent of the *Medical Device Amendments* of 1976 was to create an alternate pathway for device approval and marketing by having the sponsor and FDA agree early in the development process on items needed for the successful analysis of a Class III device's safety and efficacy.

Once agreement is reached, the PDP contains all the information about design and development activities and acceptance criteria. A project timeline is established and information is furnished to FDA to review in a sequential fashion.

The PDP consists of:
- a description of the device and any changes that may be made to the device
- a description of the preclinical trials, if any
- a description of the clinical trials, if any
- a description of the manufacturing methods, facilities and controls
- a description of any applicable performance standards
- samples of proposed labeling
- any other information "relevant to the subject matter of the protocol"

Upon completion of clinical studies, reports are furnished to FDA, which has 120 days to act on a PDP. Currently, the PDP approval approach is rarely utilized.

Modular PMA

The *Medical Device User Fee and Modernization Act* (*MDUFMA*) amended Section 515(c) of the *FD&C Act* to allow early FDA review of PMA information submitted in separate modules. Though the Modular PMA has the same content requirements as the Traditional PMA, the sponsor must meet with FDA to come to an agreement with the agency on the content of the PMA "Shell," a framework of modules that identifies the information necessary to support the filing and approval. Generally, this occurs during a Pre-IDE Submission meeting.

Each module is submitted to FDA as it is completed. The target FDA review period is 90 days for each module or amendment submitted in response to an agency deficiency letter. Upon receipt of the final module, a PMA number is assigned, and a 180-day review clock will start. The entire PMA user fee is due with the submission of the first module.

The Modular PMA is particularly useful for devices at an early stage of development, rather than for devices that are far along in the development process.

Advantages of the Modular PMA may include:
- allows more efficient use of resources
- potentially reduces PMA application review time
- creates ongoing open dialogue between FDA and the sponsor

Disadvantages may include:
- can cost more money and lengthen time to approval
- the need to establish a plan prior to approaching FDA about utilizing the modular approach

To file a Modular PMA, follow FDA's guidance document, *Premarket Approval Application Modular Review* (3 November 2003).[16]

Streamlined PMA

A Streamlined PMA is designed for devices using well-known technologies for well-known disease processes. A PMA may qualify as streamlined if: the device has a review guidance; two or more previous PMAs have been approved for the same type of device; or the device has a study protocol jointly developed by the manufacturer and FDA. The Manufacturing Facility Inspection may be deferred if FDA completed a GMP inspection within the past two years. The review time is the same as for Traditional PMAs (180 days).

Humanitarian Device Exemption (HDE)—21 CFR 814 Subpart H

A Humanitarian Use Device (HUD) is intended to benefit patients by treating or diagnosing a disease or condition that affects or is manifested in fewer than 4,000 individuals in the US per year. The number of patient contacts with a device may exceed one per patient, but the total number of patients treated or diagnosed with the device is fewer than 4,000 per year.

The HUD regulation provides a financial incentive for the development of devices for these small populations because manufacturers' research and development costs far exceed market returns for diseases or conditions affecting small patient populations.

A sponsor must receive Humanitarian Use status by submitting a Request for HUD Designation to FDA's Office of Orphan Products Development (OOPD).

The request should include:
- a statement that the applicant is requesting a HUD designation for a rare disease or condition
- the applicant's name and address
- a description of the rare disease or condition for which the device is to be used
- a description of the device

documentation, with appended authoritative references, to demonstrate that the device is designed to treat or diagnose a disease or condition that affects or is manifested in fewer than 4,000 people in the US per year

FDA issued *Guidance for Industry and Food and Drug Administration Staff: Humanitarian Use Device (HUD) Designations* on 24 January 2013 (www.fda.gov/downloads/ForIndustry/DevelopingProductsforRareDiseasesConditions/DesignatingHumanitarianUseDevicesHUDS/LegislationRelatingtoHUDsHDEs/UCM336515.pdf) to help sponsors further understand how to demonstrate, in HUD requests, that their devices qualify for HUD designation.

A Humanitarian Device Exemption Application (HDE) is similar in both form and content to a Traditional PMA application; however, it is exempt from the effectiveness requirements of a PMA. An HDE is not required to contain the results of scientifically valid clinical investigations demonstrating that the device is effective for its intended purpose. An HDE must contain sufficient information for FDA to determine that the device does not pose an unreasonable or significant risk of illness or injury and that the probable benefit to health outweighs the risk of injury or illness from its use, taking into account the probable risks and benefits of currently available devices or alternative forms of treatment. Finally, the applicant must demonstrate that no comparable devices are available to treat or diagnose the disease or condition and that it could not otherwise bring the device to market.

The agency has 75 days from the date of receipt to review an HDE. This includes a 30-day filing period during which the agency determines whether the HDE is sufficiently complete to permit substantive review. If FDA notifies the sponsor that the HDE is incomplete and cannot be filed, the 75-day timeframe resets upon receipt of any additional information.

When approved by FDA, an HUD may be used only in facilities that have established a local IRB to supervise clinical testing of devices and have obtained IRB approval for the use of the device to treat or diagnose the specific disease.

HDE amendments and supplements are subject to the same regulations as those for Traditional PMAs; however, the review timeframe for HDE amendments and supplements is 75 days, the same as for HDE originals.

Expedited Review

Devices Appropriate for Expedited Review

FDA considers a device or combination product containing a device appropriate for expedited review if the device or combination product:

1. is intended to treat or diagnose a life-threatening or irreversibly debilitating disease or condition
2. addresses an unmet medical need, as demonstrated by one of the following:
   a. The device represents a breakthrough technology that provides a clinically meaningful advantage over existing technology. Breakthrough technologies should be demonstrated to lead to a clinical improvement in the treatment or diagnosis of the life-threatening or irreversibly debilitating condition.

b. No approved alternative treatment or means of diagnosis exists.
c. The device offers significant, clinically meaningful advantages over existing approved alternative treatments. The device should provide a clinically important earlier or more accurate diagnosis, or offer important therapeutic advantages in safety and/or effectiveness over existing alternatives. Such advantages may include demonstrated superiority over current treatments for effects on serious outcomes, the ability to provide clinical benefit for those patients unable to tolerate current treatments, or the ability to provide a clinical benefit without the serious side effects associated with current treatments.
d. The availability of the device is in the best interest of patients. That is, the device provides a specific public health benefit or meets the need of a well-defined patient population. This may also apply to a device that was designed or modified to address an unanticipated serious failure occurring in a critical component of an approved device for which there are no alternatives, or for which alternative treatment would entail substantial risk of morbidity for the patient.

For more information, see the guidance (www.fda.gov/MedicalDevices/DeviceRegulationandGuidance/GuidanceDocuments/ucm089643.htm).

Proposed Submission Changes

The Institute of Medicine (IOM) report on the 510(k) process was released 29 July 2011 and recommended that FDA eliminate the 510(k) process in favor of developing an integrated premarket and postmarket regulatory framework for medium-risk devices. This regulatory framework, IOM believes, should provide a reasonable assurance of safety and effectiveness throughout the device lifecycle. However, FDA has responded that the 510(k) process should not be eliminated, and it is open to proposals for continued improvement of the agency's device review programs.

FDA issued a draft guidance, *510(k) Device Modifications: Deciding When to Submit a 510(k) for a Change to an Existing Device*, on July 27 2011, which, when finalized, was intended to replace the existing guidance of the same name issued in January 1997. But, this guidance received strong resistance from the industry because the changes introduced in this guidance would, in all probability, lead to an increased number of 510(k)s for changes to an existing device. Hence, Congress required FDA to withdraw this guidance in enacting the *FDASIA* in July 2012. On 8 May 2013, FDA announced a public meeting to discuss FDA's interpretation of its regulations regarding when a modification made to a 510(k)-cleared device requires a new 510(k) submission. This meeting was scheduled for 13 June 2013 and FDA was to discuss five policy options on which it is seeking feedback: risk management, reliance on design control activities, critical specifications, risk-based stratification of medical devices for 510(k) modifications purposes and periodic reporting.

Another draft guidance, to address the increasing calls for overhauling the 510(k) process, was issued by FDA on 27 December 2011. This draft guidance, *The 510(k) Program: Evaluating Substantial Equivalence in Premarket Notifications [510(k)]*, is intended to enhance the predictability, consistency and transparency of the 510(k) program by describing in greater detail the regulatory framework, policies and practices underlying FDA's 510(k) review. Among other changes, this guidance proposes a new substantial equivalence decision-making flowchart and removes the provision of using split predicates in a 510(k) submission. The draft guidance also discusses the difference between "indications for use" and "intended use" of a device, the use of multiple predicates and updates to FDA's policies with respect to the Special 510(k) program. Industry has provided much feedback regarding the substantial changes proposed in this guidance, and it remains to be seen whether the final guidance will look anything like the one proposed.

FDA issued a proposed rule and *Draft Guidance for Industry and Food and Drug Administration Staff: Providing Information about Pediatric Uses of Medical Devices Under Section 515A of the Federal Food, Drug, and Cosmetic Act* 19 February 2013 (www.fda.gov/downloads/MedicalDevices/DeviceRegulationandGuidance/GuidanceDocuments/UCM339465.pdf). These describe how to compile and submit—in PMAs, PMA Supplements or HDEs—readily available information about pediatric subpopulations that suffer from a disease or condition the device is intended to treat, diagnose or cure.

Summary

- FDA regulations for devices comprise sets of rules that classify devices that require agency clearance or approval. Devices may be classified into Class I, II or III. Reclassification or the *de novo* process allows classifications to be changed, but this is complex. Classes I and II may require 510(k) Notification or may be 510(k)-exempt. Except for a small and decreasing number, Class III devices require a PMA. The exceptions require a 510(k).
- Significant risk clinical studies require FDA approval of an IDE.
- Pre-IDE meetings provide a mechanism for sponsors to discuss proposals for submission strategies, as well as clinical trials, with FDA.
- CDRH is implementing a large number of changes to the 510(k) and related device approval and business processes.

References

1. CDRH Product Classification Database. FDA website. www.accessdata.fda.gov/scripts/cdrh/cfdocs/cfPCD/PCDSimpleSearch.cfm. Accessed 15 May 2013.
2. 515 Program Initiative. FDA website. www.fda.gov/AboutFDA/CentersOffices/OfficeofMedicalProductsandTobacco/CDRH/CDRHTransparency/ucm240310.htm. Accessed 15 May 2013.
3. CDRHLearn class regarding 513(g) Requests for Determination. FDA website. www.fda.gov/MedicalDevices/ResourcesforYou/Industry/ucm127147.htm. Accessed 15 May 2013.
4. Device Advice: Investigational Device Exemption (IDE). FDA website. www.fda.gov/MedicalDevices/DeviceRegulationandGuidance/HowtoMarketYourDevice/InvestigationalDeviceExemptionIDE/default.htm. Accessed 15 May 2013.
5. *Early Collaboration Meetings Under the FDA Modernization Act (FDAMA); Final Guidance for Industry and CDRH Staff.* FDA website. www.fda.gov/MedicalDevices/DeviceRegulationandGuidance/GuidanceDocuments/ucm073604.htm. Accessed 15 May 2013.
6. Device Advice: Premarket Notification. FDA website. www.fda.gov/MedicalDevices/DeviceRegulationandGuidance/HowtoMarketYourDevice/PremarketSubmissions/PremarketNotification510k/default.htm. Accessed 15 May 2013.
7. Device Advice: Device Regulation and Guidance. FDA website. www.fda.gov/MedicalDevices/DeviceRegulationandGuidance/default.htm. Accessed 15 May 2013.
8. Guidance, Compliance & Regulatory Information (Biologics). FDA website. www.fda.gov/BiologicsBloodVaccines/GuidanceComplianceRegulatoryInformation/default.htm. Accessed 15 May 2013.
9. Deciding When to Submit a 510(k) for a Change to an Existing Device (K97-1). FDA website www.fda.gov/MedicalDevices/DeviceRegulationandGuidance/GuidanceDocuments/ucm080235.htm. Accessed 15 May 2013.
10. How to Prepare a Traditional 510(k). FDA website. www.fda.gov/MedicalDevices/DeviceRegulationandGuidance/HowtoMarketYourDevice/PremarketSubmissions/PremarketNotification510k/ucm134572.htm. Accessed 15 May 2013.
11. How to Prepare an Abbreviated 510(k). FDA website. www.fda.gov/MedicalDevices/DeviceRegulationandGuidance/HowtoMarketYourDevice/PremarketSubmissions/PremarketNotification510k/ucm134574.htm. Accessed 15 May 2013.
12. CDRH's Standards database. FDA website. www.accessdata.fda.gov/scripts/cdrh/cfdocs/cfStandards/search.cfm. Accessed 15 May 2013.
13. How to Prepare a Special 510(k). FDA website. www.fda.gov/MedicalDevices/DeviceRegulationandGuidance/HowtoMarketYourDevice/PremarketSubmissions/PremarketNotification510k/ucm134573.htm. Accessed 15 May 2013.
14. Device Advice: Third Party Review. FDA website. www.fda.gov/MedicalDevices/DeviceRegulationandGuidance/HowtoMarketYourDevice/PremarketSubmissions/ThirdParyReview/default.htm. Accessed 15 May 2013.
15. PMA Application Methods. FDA website. www.fda.gov/MedicalDevices/DeviceRegulationandGuidance/HowtoMarketYourDevice/PremarketSubmissions/PremarketApprovalPMA/ucm048168.htm. Accessed 15 May 2013.
16. Premarket Approval Application Modular Review (3 November 2003). FDA website. www.fda.gov/MedicalDevices/DeviceRegulationandGuidance/GuidanceDocuments/ucm089764.htm. Accessed 15 May 2013.

Chapter 19

Medical Device Compliance and Postmarketing Activities

Updated by Laurence M. Wallman, RAC (US, EU, CAN)

OBJECTIVES

- Develop a basic understanding of FDA regulations that establish compliance and postmarketing requirements for manufacturers and importers of devices marketed in the US

- Learn how to prepare and file establishment registrations and device listings with FDA

- Review FDA's Quality System Regulation (QSR) for medical devices, as well as FDA's approach to medical device manufacturer inspections

- Understand postmarketing requirements for medical device reports (MDRs), corrections and removals (recalls) and medical device tracking

- Review US requirements for importing and exporting devices

LAWS, REGULATIONS AND GUIDELINES COVERED IN THIS CHAPTER

- *Pure Food and Drugs Act* of 1906

- *Federal Food, Drug, and Cosmetic Act* of 1938

- FD&C Act as amended by the *Food and Drug Administration Modernization Act* of 1997

   o   Chapter III—Prohibited Acts and Penalties

   o   Chapter V—Drugs and Devices

   - Section 501—Adulterated Drugs and Devices
   - Section 502—Misbranded Drugs and Devices
   - Section 506A—Manufacturing Changes
   - Section 506B—Reports of Postmarketing Studies
   - Section 518(e)—Recall Authority
   - Section 519(e)—Device Tracking
   - Section 522—Postmarket Surveillance

   o   Chapter VIII—Imports and Exports, Sections 801–803

- 21 CFR Part 7 Enforcement Policy Subpart C Recalls

- 21 CFR Part 803 Medical device reporting

- 21 CFR Part 806 Medical devices; reports of corrections and removals

- 21 CFR Part 807 Establishment registration and device listing for manufacturers and initial importers of devices

Chapter 19

- 21 CFR Part 810 Medical device recall authority
- 21 CFR 814.82(a)(2) Postapproval requirements [Condition of approval studies]
- 21 CFR Part 820 Quality system regulation
- 21 CFR 821 Medical device tracking requirements
- 21 CFR 822 Postmarket surveillance
- *Guidance for Industry and FDA Staff: Implementation of Medical Device Establishment Registration and Device Listing Requirements Established by the Food and Drug Administration Amendments Act of 2007* (October 2009)
- *"How-To" Guide: Device Facility User Fee Process* (October 2008)
- *Frequently Asked Questions on Recognition of Consensus Standards* (September 2007)
- *Guidance for Industry and FDA Staff: Recognition and Use of Consensus Standards* (September 2007)
- *Quality System Information for Certain Various Premarket Application Reviews; Guidance for Industry and FDA Staff* (February 2003)
- *Design Control Guidance for Medical Device Manufacturers* (March 1997)
- *Do It By Design: An Introduction to Human Factors in Medical Devices* (January 1997)
- *Medical Device Quality Systems Manual: A Small Entity Compliance Guide* (December 1996)
- *Guidance for Industry: Process Validation: General Principles and Practices* (January 2011)
- *Comparison Chart: 1996 Quality System Regulation Versus 1978 Good Manufacturing Practices Regulation Versus*
- *ANSI/ISO/ASQ Q9001-9008 Quality management systems—Requirements*
- *ISO 13485:2003 Medical Devices—Quality management systems—Requirements for regulatory purposes*
- *Compliance Program Guidance Manual 7382.845: Inspection of Medical Device Manufacturers* (2 February 2011)
- *Guide to Inspections of Quality Systems: Quality System Inspection Technique* (August 1999)
- *Guidance for Industry, FDA Staff, and Third Parties: Inspection by Accredited Persons Under the Medical Device User Fee and Modernization Act of 2002 and the FDA Amendments Act of 2007; Accreditation Criteria* (August 6, 2009)
- *Guidance for Industry, FDA Staff, and FDA-Accredited Third Parties: Manufacturer's Notification of the Intent to Use an Accredited Person under the Accredited Persons Inspection Program Authorized by Section 228 of the Food and Drug Administration Amendments Act of 2007 (FDAAA)* (March 2, 2009)
- *Draft Guidance for Industry, User Facilities and FDA Staff: eMDR: Electronic Medical Device Reporting* (August 2009)
- *Medical Device Reporting—Remedial Action Exemption; Guidance for FDA and Industry* (September 2001)
- *Medical Device Reporting—Alternative Summary Reporting (ASR) Program* (October 2000)
- *Medical Device Reporting: An Overview* (April 1996)
- *Instructions for Completing FDA Form 3500A (MedWatch)* (July 2009)
- *Regulation of Medical Devices: Background Information for International Officials* (April 1999)
- *Guidance for Industry: Exports and Imports Under the FDA Export Reform and Enhancement Act of 1996* (July 2007)
- *Guidance for Industry: Exports Under the FDA Export Reform and Enhancement Act of 1996* (July 2007)

- *Compliance Policy Guide for FDA Staff*, Section 110.100 Certification of Exports (CPG 7150.01)

- *Medical Device Tracking; Guidance for Industry and FDA Staff* (January 2010)

- *Guidance for Industry: Product Recalls, Including Removals and Corrections* (November 2003)

- *Guidance for Industry and FDA Staff: Procedures for Handling Post-Approval Studies Imposed by PMA Order* (June 2009)

- *Guidance for Industry and FDA Staff: Postmarket Surveillance Under Section 522 of the Federal Food, Drug and Cosmetic Act* (April 2006)

- *General Principles of Software Validation; Final Guidance for Industry and FDA Staff:* (January 2002)

- *Final Guidance for Industry, FDA Reviewers and Compliance on Off-the-Shelf Software Use in Medical Devices* (September 1999)

- *Computerized Devices/Processes Guidance: Application of the Medical Device GMP to Computerized Devices and Manufacturing Processes* (February 1997)

- *Design Control Guidance for Medical Device Manufacturers* (March 1997)

Introduction

History of FDA Medical Device Regulations

All US medical device regulations are codified under 21 CFR Parts 800–899. However, the heritage of these regulations begins with the *Pure Food and Drugs Act* of 1906. This act was the true beginning of federal food and drug legislation intended to protect Americans from harmful substances and the deceptive practices that were becoming more and more common. Medical devices were not represented in the act, in large part because contemporary devices, such as stethoscopes and scalpels, were relatively simple and their corresponding risks, if any, were conspicuous. Although medical devices were considered helpful tools, they bore no significant weight and did not play a crucial role in mediating a caregiver's ability to diagnose or treat patients—medical devices neither gave life nor sustained it. It would soon become apparent, however, that medical devices represented fertile ground for new and far-reaching technological achievements, along with their accompanying risks. Medical device technology would continue to outgrow its regulatory boundaries over the next century, requiring federal regulations to expand and change at a pace commensurate with the industry.

The modernization of the *Pure Food and Drugs Act* was driven, in part, by the recognized need to introduce a definition of medical devices into federal law. This modernization initiative resulted in the enactment of the *Federal Food, Drug, and Cosmetic Act (FD&C Act)* of 1938, which was the first law to mandate requirements for exporting unapproved devices. For the next 25 years, medical devices were subject only to the discretionary vigilance activities of the US Food and Drug Administration (FDA), whose charge it was to unilaterally determine whether a device was safe and effective, in the absence of any premarket testing, review or approval process. Accordingly, the agency was further empowered to bring federal charges against manufacturers of products or materials found to be either adulterated (e.g., defective, unsafe or unsanitary), or misbranded (e.g., false or misleading statements, designs or labeling).

In the early 1960s, President Kennedy advocated changes to the ways medical devices entered the US market; however, the changes he sought were not realized until the mid-1970s. New legislation was enacted in 1976 that established the ground rules and standards to which all US medical device manufacturers and importers must now adhere: the *Medical Device Amendments* to the *FD&C Act*. The new law applied safety and effectiveness safeguards to new devices and required FDA to establish, for the first time: regulations concerning establishment registration and device listing; Good Manufacturing Practices (GMPs) for medical devices; medical device reporting (MDR); and guidelines on policy, procedures and industry responsibilities for field corrections and removals.

Numerous changes to device laws and regulations have been implemented via various amendments to the *FD&C Act* over the years. Three of the most notable changes, mandated by the *Safe Medical Devices Act* of 1990 (*SMDA*) and the *Medical Device Amendments* of 1992, were:

- introduction of the Humanitarian Device Exemption (HDE), the medical device equivalent of orphan drug designation, providing limited exemptions from the law for devices intended to treat or diagnose rare diseases or conditions affecting fewer than 4,000 persons
- promulgation of the Quality System Regulation, resulting in substantial revisions that essentially harmonized US GMPs for medical devices with the European quality system regulations in EN 46001 and ISO 9001,[1] and added design controls to the GMP regulation, bringing product development under FDA scrutiny for the first time

- establishment of a regulatory requirement (previously an FDA request) that manufacturers and distributors promptly report field corrections and removals to FDA within 10 days after their initiation
- promulgation of the first device tracking regulation

The *FD&C Act* underwent additional change and reform as a result of the *Food and Drug Administration Modernization Act* of 1997 *(FDAMA)*. FDAMA empowered FDA to restrict the marketing of products for which the manufacturing processes are so deficient that use of the products could present a serious health hazard. The agency was given authority to take appropriate action if a device manufacturer advocates an off-label use of its product that may be potentially harmful. *FDAMA* further enhanced FDA's risk-based approach to medical device regulation, allocating FDA resources and diligence to the oversight of medical devices presenting the greatest risks to patients. For example, the law exempts Class I devices not intended for a use that is of substantial importance in preventing impairment of human health or that do not present a potential unreasonable risk of illness or injury from premarket notification. The law also directs FDA to focus its postmarket surveillance on higher-risk devices and allows the agency to implement a reporting system that concentrates on a representative sample of user facilities—such as hospitals and nursing homes—where patients may experience deaths and serious illnesses or injuries linked with the use of devices.

In addition, *FDAMA* expanded an ongoing pilot program under which FDA accredits outside (third-party) experts to conduct the initial review of all Class I and low-to-intermediate risk Class II device applications. The act, however, prohibits any accredited person from reviewing devices that are permanently implantable, life-supporting, life-sustaining or for which clinical data are required.

The *Medical Device User Fee and Modernization Act* of 2002 *(MDUFMA)*, signed into law 26 October 2002, further amended the *FD&C Act* to include provisions that affect the compliance regulations. Under *MDUFMA*:

- Establishment inspections may be conducted by accredited persons (third parties) under carefully prescribed conditions.
- New labeling requirements were established for reprocessed single-use devices.
- The submission of validation data for some reprocessed single-use devices is required. On 30 April 2003, FDA identified the types of devices subject to this requirement (see 68 FR 23139).

MDUFMA made several other significant changes to the law that involve FDA postmarket surveillance appropriations, combination product review, electronic labeling, electronic registration, devices intended for pediatric use and breast implant reports. Additionally, it requires manufacturer identification on the device itself, with certain exceptions.

- Background information, reference materials and additional information about *MDUFMA* can be found on the website of FDA's Center for Devices and Radiological Health (CDRH) (www.fda.gov/MedicalDevices/DeviceRegulationandGuidance/Overview/MedicalDeviceUserFeeandModernizationActMDUFMA/default.htm). *MDUFMA* also imposed various user fees.
- On 28 September 2007, as part of the *Food and Drug Administration Amendments Act* (*FDAAA*), user fees were reauthorized through Fiscal 2012.
- *The Food and Drug Administration Safety and Innovation Act* (Public Law 112-144) included the *Medical Device User Fee Amendments* of 2012, or *MDUFA III*. *MDUFA III* took effect on 1 October 2012 and reauthorized user fees through Fiscal 2017. It added additional performance goals for FDA, as well as the issuance of several guidance documents tied to *MDUFA III* provisions including guidance on review actions taken on 510(k) and premarket approval applications.
- New fees include:
  o a fee for each 30-day notice submitted to FDA
  o a fee for each 513(g) request for classification information submitted to FDA
  o an annual fee for periodic reporting made under a condition of approval for a Class III device
  o an annual fee for the registration of each medical device establishment

Small businesses may qualify for reduced fees through an application process. However, there is no discount for small businesses on the annual establishment registration fee.

Establishment Registration and Product Listing

Registration and listing information provides FDA with the locations of medical device establishments and what devices are manufactured at each site. Knowing where devices are manufactured increases FDA's ability to prepare for and respond to public health emergencies.

A US establishment owner or operator that initiates or develops medical device specifications; manufactures, assembles, processes, repackages or relabels medical devices for domestic human use; or is an initial importer of medical devices (distributor for a foreign manufacturer), must register the establishment annually with FDA and submit medical device listing information, including activities performed on those devices, for all such devices in commercial distribution. Note that if a device requires

Medical Device Compliance and Postmarketing Activities

Table 19-1. Domestic Establishment Registration and Listing Requirements

Establishment Activity	Register	List	Pay Fee
Manufacturer	Yes 807.20(a)	Yes 807.20(a)	Yes
Manufacturer of a custom device	Yes 807.20(a)(2)	Yes 807.20(a)(2)	Yes
Manufacturer of accessories or components that are packaged or labeled for commercial distribution for health-related purposes to an end user	Yes 807.20(a)(5)	Yes 807.20(a)(5)	Yes
Manufacturer of components that are distributed only to a finished device manufacturer	No 807.65(a)	No	No
US manufacturer of export-only devices	Yes 807.20(a)(2)	Yes 807.20(a)(2)	Yes
Relabeler or repackager	Yes 807.20(a)(3)	Yes 807.20(a)(3)	No
Contract manufacturer that commercially distributes the device for the specifications developer	Yes 807.20(a)(2)	Yes 807.20(a)(2)	Yes
Contract manufacturer that does not commercially distribute the device for the specifications developer	No	No	No
Contract manufacturer of a subassembly or component, contract packager or labeler	No	No	No
Contract sterilizer that commercially distributes the device	Yes 807.20(a)(2)	Yes 807.20(a)(2)	Yes
Contract sterilizer that does not commercially distribute the device	No	No	No
Kit assembler	Yes 807.20(a)	Yes 807.20(a)	Yes
Domestic distributor	8007.20(c)(3)	No	No
Specification developer	Yes 807.20(a)(1)	Yes 807.20(a)(1)	Yes
Specification consultant only	No	No	No
Initial distributor/importer	Yes 807.40(a)	No Enforcement Discretion Used for 807.22(c)	No
Device being investigated under TDE	No	No 807.40(c)	No
Reprocessor of single-use devices	Yes 807.20	Yes 807.20	Yes
Remanufacturer	Yes	Yes	No

a premarket submission (e.g., 510(k), Premarket Approval (PMA), Product Development Protocol (PDP) or HDE) for clearance, the owner or operator should also submit the FDA premarket submission number.

There is a fee for annual registration for some establishment types. On 1 October 2008, FDA instituted a new payment process for those establishments required to pay the device establishment user fee. This process involves first visiting the Device Facility User Fee website (DFUF) to pay the user fee and obtain a Payment Identification Number (PIN). Once the payment has been received and processed, the owner or operator will be notified by email. The email will include directions to return to the DFUF website to obtain the Payment Confirmation Number (PCN) for the order. The PIN and PCN are required as proof of payment before the facility can be registered using the FDA Unified Registration and Listing System (FURLS). Detailed information regarding registration and listing can be found at www.fda.gov/MedicalDevices/

Regulatory Affairs Professionals Society

Table 19-2. Foreign Establishment Registration and Listing Requirements

Establishment Activity	Register	List	Pay Fee
Foreign manufacturer	Yes 807.40(a)	Yes 807.40(a)	Yes
Foreign exporter of devices located in a foreign country	807.40 (a)	807.40 (a)	No
Contract manufacturer whose device is shipped to US by the contract manufacturer	Yes 807.40(a)	Yes 807.40(a)	Yes
Contract sterilizer whose sterilized device is shipped to the US by the sterilizer	Yes 807.40(a)	Yes 807.40(a)	Yes
Reprocessor of single-use device	807.20(a)	807.20(a)	Yes
Custom device manufacturers	807.20(a)(2)	807.20(a)(2)	Yes
Relabeler or repackager	Yes 807.20(a)(3)	Yes 807.20(a)(3)	No
Kit assembler	Yes 807.20(a)	Yes 807.20(a)	Yes
Device being investigated under IDE	No 812.1(a)	No 812.1(a) 807.40(c)	No
Specification developer	Yes	Yes	Yes
Remanufacturer	Yes	Yes	No
Manufacturer of components that are distributed only by a finished device manufacturer	No 807.65(a)	No	No
Maintains complaint files as required under 21 CFR 820.198 (Note: register as a manufacturer if physical manufacturing taking place at site, Otherwise register as a specification developer)	Yes	Yes	Yes

DeviceRegulationandGuidance/HowtoMarketYourDevice/RegistrationandListing/default.htm.

Changes brought about by *FDAMA* require foreign manufacturers of devices intended for US commercial distribution to register and list their products with FDA. Additionally, foreign manufacturers are required to designate a US agent to act as the official correspondent responsible for, among other things, submitting establishment registration, device listing and medical device reports (MDRs). This requirement had been indefinitely stayed in July of 1996, but was later reinstated effective 11 February 2002.[2]

FDA changed the requirements for medical device registration and listing as a result of the enactment of the *Food and Drug Administration Safety and Innovation Act* of 2012 (*FDASIA*) and the publication of the revised Title 21 CFR, Part 807 on 2 August 2012.

Starting in Fiscal 2013, which began 1 October 2012, all registered medical device establishments are required to pay the annual registration fee, regardless of establishment type or activities conducted there. In addition, certain establishments must comply with additional registration and listing requirements.

These changes are described in http://www.fda.gov/MedicalDevices/ResourcesforYou/Industry/ucm314844.htm.

The responsibilities of US agents are described at http://www.fda.gov/MedicalDevices/DeviceRegulationandGuidance/HowtoMarketYourDevice/RegistrationandListing/ucm053196.htm.

For domestic and foreign registration and listing requirements, see **Tables 19-1** and **19-2**, respectively.

The initial registration and listing must be submitted 30 days prior to starting any operations at the establishment for the production and/or commercial distribution of finished devices (see **Table 19-3**). A device family with variations in physical characteristics should be considered a single device for listing purposes, provided the function or intended use does not differ within the family. All subsequent establishment registration and product listing information must be updated annually between 1 October and 31 December, even if no changes have occurred. Failure of an establishment to register or maintain its registration can render its commercial medical device products misbranded and subject to regulatory actions.

After 30 September 2007, *FDAAA* mandated that all registration and listing information be submitted electronically via the FURLS Device Registration and Listing Module (DRLM), unless a waiver has been granted. This electronic registration and listing process replaced the

Table 19-3. Registration and Listing Timelines

Information	Due Date
Establishment name and address	Annually between 1 October and 31 December, and anytime throughout year, but within 30 days of change
Owner/operator name and address	Annually between 1 October and 31 December, and anytime throughout year, but within 30 days of change
Official correspondent name and address	Annually between 1 October and 31 December, and anytime throughout year, but within 30 days of change
Trading name(s)	Annually between 1 October and 31 December, and anytime throughout year, but within 30 days of change
US agent (see foreign establishments)	Anytime throughout year, but within 30 days of change
Owner/operator	Anytime throughout year, but within 30 days of change
Proprietary name	Anytime throughout year, but within 30 days of change
Premarket submission number (for nonexempt devices)*	Annually between 1 October and 31 December, and anytime throughout year, but within 30 days of change
Product code (for exempt devices only)	Annually between 1 October and 31 December, and anytime throughout year, but within 30 days of change
* =	For devices requiring 510(k) clearance or PMA approval, examples of change to the premarket submission number may be due to a new 510(k) or PMA supplement submitted for design change of a device.

previously used Forms FDA 2891 and 2891a, "Registration of Device Establishment," and Form FDA 2892 "Medical Device Listing." All owners or operators can access FURLS at any time throughout the year to update their registration and listing information as changes occur. Examples of changes to listings include:

- another device being introduced into commercial distribution
- a change to a previously listed device, such as where it is manufactured
- a previously listed device is removed from commercial distribution or commercial distribution is resumed

The information required for registering an establishment and listing medical device products is provided in 21 CFR 807.25 and is clearly cued during the electronic registration process. A permanent establishment registration number will be assigned to each registered device establishment.

FDA requires any person or entity that initiates and develops device specifications and commercially distributes that device to register and list any such medical device products (21 CFR 807.20(a)). A person or entity that only manufactures devices according to another's specifications and does not commercially distribute the devices is not required to register. Registration and listing also are not required of contract sterilizers that do not commercially distribute the devices (21 CFR 807.20 (c)(2)). *FDAMA* repealed the previous requirement in 21 CFR 807.20(c) to eliminate the registration and listing requirements for distributors who are not importers, effective 19 February 1998.

As amended by *FDAMA*, 21 CFR 807 asserts that entities that reprocess single-use devices for reuse in human patients are considered manufacturers; therefore, owners and operators of such establishments also must comply with registration and listing requirements. The FDA guidance, *Enforcement Priorities for Single Use Devices Reprocessed by Third Parties and Hospitals*[3] provides additional information about this requirement. *MDUFMA* added new regulatory requirements for reprocessed single-use devices that primarily affect premarket submissions for reprocessed devices, "Summary of the Medical Device User Fee and Modernization Act (*MDUFMA*) of 2002" (http://www.fda.gov/MedicalDevices/DeviceRegulationandGuidance/Overview/MedicalDeviceUserFeeandModernizationActMDUFMA/ucm109105.htm).

Quality System Regulation

The Quality System Regulation (QSR), codified under 21 CFR Part 820, went into effect on 18 December 1978, and defined FDA current Good Manufacturing Practice (CGMP) requirements for medical devices and in vitro diagnostic products. Accordingly, the QSR and CGMP for medical devices should be regarded as synonymous.

Over the next 18 years, only three minor changes[4] would be made to the QSR. However, a substantive revision of the QSR, as authorized by the *SMDA*, was undertaken to add design controls, and to harmonize CGMP and quality system regulations with applicable international standards, such as the International Organization for Standards (ISO) 9001:1994 *Quality Systems—Model for Quality Assurance in Design, Development, Production, Installation and Servicing*, and, at the time, the ISO committee draft (CD) revision of ISO/CD 13485 *Quality Systems—Medical Devices—Supplementary Requirements to ISO 9001*. These QSR revisions went into effect 1 June 1997.

FDA had long been a staunch advocate of the international harmonization of medical device standards and regulations, with a shared goal of mutual recognition of CGMP inspections among major global medical device regulatory authorities. FDA's movement toward harmonization and mutual recognition of medical device CGMP inspections, or Quality System Conformity Assessments, was further galvanized through its collaboration with the Global Harmonization Task Force (GHTF) and led to the development of a final rule revising the QSR that incorporates the harmonized quality system requirements, which are today recognized around the world.

GHTF was a voluntary, international group of representatives from medical device regulatory authorities and trade associations comprising the EU and European Free Trade Association (EFTA), the US, Canada, Japan and Australia. Since its inception in 1992, GHTF had pursued international consensus on medical device regulatory controls and practices. FDA, as one of the founding members of GHTF, enjoyed a central role in this international collaboration to globally harmonize medical device regulations, standards and practices. This partnership produced more than 30 voluntary guidance documents in pursuit of its pledge to develop a global regulatory model for medical devices. The GHTF Study Groups were focused in these areas: Study Group 1, Premarket Evaluation; Study Group 2, Postmarket Surveillance/Vigilance; Study Group 3, Quality Systems; Study Group 4, Auditing; and Study Group 5, Clinical Safety/Performance.

In March 2011, GHTF announced its decision to reorganize, and in October 2011 became the International Medical Device Regulators Forum (IMDRF). The new entity currently is comprised solely of the regulatory authorities from Australia, Brazil, Canada, Europe, Japan and the US, with the World Health Organization (WHO) as an official observer. IMDRF's focus is on finding the optimum ways to achieve harmonization at an operational level in such areas as new science and technologies, information and resource sharing and increased opportunities for technical expert interchanges. Information on IMDRF can be found at http://www.imdrf.org/index.asp.

The amended QSR also includes:
- management responsibility and review controls (21 CFR 820.20)
- design controls (21 CFR 820.30)
- purchasing controls (21 CFR 820.50)
- process validation requirements (21 CFR 820.75)
- more robust requirements for corrective and preventive action (21 CFR 820.100)
- service recordkeeping and review requirements (21 CFR 820.200)

Although the original medical device GMPs of 1978 distinguished between requirements for critical and non-critical components and devices, this distinction has since disappeared from the QSR, and all medical devices now are subject to common requirements for specifications, acceptance criteria, identification, supplier agreements and records. As stated in 21 CFR 820.30(a), design controls apply to Class III, Class II and certain Class I devices, as listed.

If a device's failure to perform can result in a significant injury, the QSR requires procedures that allow the identification (21 CFR 820.60) and traceability (21 CFR 820.65) of each unit, lot or batch of finished devices and, where appropriate, components, during all stages of receipt, production, distribution and installation. This is accomplished through the use of a control number intended to aid in any necessary corrective action. This medical device identification is to be documented in the Device History Record (DHR). Traceability generally applies to the manufacturing process of all eligible devices. This differs from medical device tracking (21 CFR 821), wherein the manufacturer must be capable of tracking (e.g., locating) certain devices from the device manufacturing facility to the actual person for whom the device was indicated. Effective tracking of devices from the manufacturing facility, through the distributor network, to the patient, is necessary in the event that patient notifications or device recalls are necessary. Device tracking requirements for certain devices are further discussed later in this chapter.

The CDRH *Medical Device Quality Systems Manual: A Small Entity Compliance Guide* contains more than 400 pages of detailed guidance information, illustrations and examples of QSR compliance that manufacturers should consider when designing, manufacturing and distributing medical devices.[5] The manual is available on CDRH's website, and each of the 18 chapters and two appendices is available as a separate document that can be downloaded in text format (www.fda.gov/MedicalDevices/DeviceRegulationandGuidance/PostmarketRequirements/QualitySystemsRegulations/MedicalDeviceQualitySystemsManual/default.htm). The manual explains each of the QSR's major provisions and includes a variety of model procedures and example forms. It can assist manufacturers in establishing or upgrading a quality system that will meet the QSR's intent. Quality system elements are traditionally represented by the following documentation (see **Figure 19-1**):
- The quality manual is a document that states the corporate quality policy, describes quality system

components and how the system is implemented, and assigns authority and responsibilities. Quality system components typically are linked by specific reference to quality procedures.
- Quality procedures describe how specific quality system operating processes and controls are implemented. The strength of a set of quality procedures lies in cross-functional and interdepartmental linkages among associated processes and controls.
- Detailed work instructions specify the individual, intradepartmental steps necessary to consistently and reliably perform specific activities, such as those involved in component procurement, inspections, fabrication, assembly and testing, labeling, final acceptance, packaging, shipping, installation, maintenance and servicing of a device.
- Records, forms and reports provide evidence of how the system is functioning.

An important provision of the QSR requires manufacturers to establish and maintain specific records. These records are subject to the document control provisions of 21 CFR 820.40, including change control. Approved device master records (DMRs), as described in 21 CFR 820.181 and Chapter 8 of the CDRH manual, must be maintained. A DMR is analogous to the master batch record in drug manufacturing, and represents the template or stepwise procedure for manufacturing a medical device in accordance with the regulated and validated environment under which it was cleared. For each member (e.g., significant variant) of a family of medical devices being manufactured, there must be a corresponding DMR. Typically a DMR contains, but is not limited to:
- approved component and finished device specifications and drawings, and a complete printout of approved device software code
- production equipment, process and environmental specifications, methods and procedures
- quality assurance procedures and specifications including acceptance criteria and quality assurance equipment, tools and fixtures
- packaging and labeling specifications
- installation, maintenance and servicing procedures

Ideally, a DMR would comprise all of the aforementioned components localized and maintained in a single, physical repository (e.g., a notebook, a server domain, a file drawer, etc.). Alternatively, the DMR, at the very least, must refer to the individual locations of these informational components.

The QSR (21 CFR 820.184) also requires manufacturers to maintain DHRs. The DHR is simply a copy of the DMR that has been completed (e.g., values entered, process steps checked-off, initials/signatures applied, etc.) during the manufacture of a batch, lot or unit quantity of medical

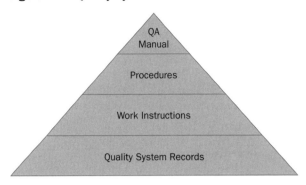

Figure 19-1. Quality System Elements

device product to document the production. The DHR is, therefore, comparable to an individual batch record in drug manufacturing. The DHR includes completed forms and reports for each manufactured batch, lot or unit, and demonstrates that devices were manufactured in accordance with the DMR. The DHR shall include, or refer to the location of, the following information:
- dates of manufacture
- quantity manufactured
- quantity released for distribution
- acceptance records that demonstrate that the device is manufactured in accordance with the DMR
- primary identification label and labeling used for each production unit
- device identification(s) and control number(s) used

The QSR (21 CFR 820.30(j)) also requires manufacturers to establish and maintain a design history file (DHF) for each type of device. The DHF shall contain or reference the records necessary to demonstrate that the design was developed in accordance with the approved design plan and the general requirements of design control. All approved changes to a cleared device should be appropriately chronicled in the DHF.

From a quality perspective, all device properties and specifications, as documented in the DHR representing a specific batch of product, must reconcile with those details as documented in the DMR. Furthermore, all design properties and specifications as documented in the DMR must reside in the DHF (see **Figure 19-2**).

FDA Facility Inspection Programs

A major provision of *MDUFMA* authorizes FDA-accredited third parties to inspect qualified manufacturers of Class II and III devices. This initiative is intended to facilitate a greater focus of FDA's inspectional resources on higher-risk devices and provide greater efficiency in scheduling multiple inspections for medical device firms operating in global markets. Certain conditions must apply for a facility to be eligible for third-party inspections, including:

Figure 19-2. Relationship of Medical Device Records

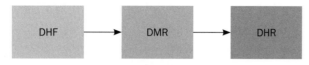

- The most recent inspection must have been classified as "no action indicated" or "voluntary action indicated."
- The establishment must notify FDA of the third party it intends to use, and FDA must agree to the selection.
- The establishment must market a device in the US and must market a device "in one or more foreign countries."
- The third party must be certified, accredited or otherwise recognized by one of the countries in which the device is to be marketed.
- The establishment must submit a statement that one of the countries in which the device is to be marketed "recognizes an inspection of the establishment by FDA."

On 28 April 2003, FDA published a *Federal Register* notice providing criteria for the accreditation of third parties to conduct inspections. Since 26 October 2003, FDA has maintained a list of firms accredited to conduct third-party inspections on its website. FDA published two guidance documents in 2009 on the accredited persons program, and further information on the program and a list of currently accredited persons for inspection is found at http://www.fda.gov/MedicalDevices/DeviceRegulationandGuidance/PostmarketRequirements/ThirdPartyInspection/ucm125410.htm. An establishment is permitted to select any accredited person to conduct an inspection regarding an eligible medical device product in lieu of an FDA inspection.

A Quality Systems Inspection Technique (QSIT) was validated and subsequently implemented by FDA in July 1999, after the agency determined that it allows more focused and efficient inspections of medical device manufacturers. A QSIT inspection handbook was developed and issued in August 1999 and can be downloaded from the FDA website (www.fda.gov/ICECI/Inspections/InspectionGuides/UCM074883).

The QSIT inspectional approach segments the QSR into seven major subsystems:
1. Corrective and Preventive Action
2. Design Controls
3. Production and Process Controls
4. Management Controls
5. Records/Documents/Change Controls
6. Material Controls
7. Facility and Equipment Controls

QSIT inspections focus on the first four subsystems because they are the primary indicators of QSR compliance, and FDA believes discrepancies in the last three subsystems will become evident through diligent review of the first four.

An additional resource is FDA's compliance program, which provides guidance manuals to its FDA field and center staff for inspection, administrative and enforcement activities related to the QSR, MDR, medical device tracking regulation (21 CFR Part 821), corrections and removals regulation (21 CFR Part 806), and the registration and listing regulation (21 CFR Part 807). *Compliance Program Manual 7382.845 Inspection of Device Manufacturers* spans five regulations for inspecting medical device firms and provides specific guidance for each. The relevant CDRH compliance programs manuals can be found at www.fda.gov/MedicalDevices/DeviceRegulationandGuidance/ComplianceActivities/ucm248922.htm.

Medical Device Postmarket Activities

Following market clearance of a medical device, manufacturers and other establishments involved in their commercial distribution must adhere to various postmarketing requirements and applicable regulations. These activities are primarily intended to ensure ongoing monitoring and safety following market approval, and may include a wide array of statutory or voluntary activities for both industry and FDA. These include the use of tracking systems; the reporting of device malfunctions, serious injuries or deaths; and the registration of establishments where devices are produced or distributed.

Some compliance-related activities, such as maintaining quality systems, inspections and import/export, although not strictly postmarket, are regarded as essential to the ongoing safety and effectiveness of marketed devices.

Postmarket requirements also may include postmarket surveillance studies required under Section 522 of the act, as well as postapproval studies required at the time of approval of a PMA, HDE or PDP application. Postmarket activities initiated by FDA may include quality system inspections, monitoring of user reporting and public health notifications. FDA also is involved in disseminating accurate, science-based risk:benefit information for improving the public health.

Medical Device Reporting

Medical device manufacturers and importers were first required to report all device-related deaths, serious injuries and certain malfunctions beginning in 1984. In subsequent years, government studies showed that despite full implementation of the MDR regulation, fewer than 1% of problems occurring in hospitals were being reported to FDA. As a result, the scope of the MDR regulation was extended to require device user facilities to report deaths to both FDA and the manufacturer, and to report serious injuries to the manufacturer. The MDR regulations were amended by the *Medical Device Amendments* of 1992, with a final rule published in 1995, establishing a single reporting standard for device manufacturers, initial importers, domestic distributors and user facilities. The 1995 rule was revised in April 1996 and subsequently amended in March 1997. The *FDAMA* changes to MDR became effective on 19 February 1998. On 26 January 2000,[6] changes to the implementing regulations were published in the *Federal Register*, including:

- Medical device manufacturers, importers and distributors are no longer required to submit an annual certification statement.
- Domestic distributors no longer have to submit MDR reports, but they must continue to maintain records of adverse events and product complaints.
- Importers continue to be subject to the remaining requirements of the MDR regulation, 21 CFR 803.
- User facilities now submit a report annually instead of semi-annually.

The MDR Rule changes became effective 27 March 2000.

The MDR Rule was further amended effective 27 October 2008 to eliminate the requirement for submission of baseline reports and the use of Form FDA 3417, as the information was considered largely redundant with information provided in individual reports.

FDA instituted a voluntary electronic Medical Device Reporting (eMDR) system that provides the capability for electronic data entry and processing of medical device adverse event reports. The project utilizes the Health Level Seven (HL7) Individual Case Safety Report (ICSR) standard to receive medical device adverse events (MDRs). The eMDR application accepts electronic medical device reports via two options, designed for low and high volume reporters.

Further information can be found on the CDRH website at http://www.fda.gov/MedicalDevices/DeviceRegulationandGuidance/ComplianceActivities/ucm248922.htm.

FDA places a high priority on compliance with MDR requirements during manufacturing facility inspections. Observed deficiencies are frequently cited on Form FDA 483 and, depending on their seriousness, can lead to the issuance of a Warning Letter. Adherence to documented procedures that encompass MDR activities, as well as complaints and nonconforming product, is necessary to avoid citations. Information that summarizes reporting, reporting timeframes and recordkeeping requirements for manufacturers, user facilities and initial importers can be found at http://www.fda.gov/MedicalDevices/DeviceRegulationandGuidance/PostmarketRequirements/ReportingAdverseEvents/default.htm. More detailed information regarding reporting requirements is contained in MDR guidance documents, available on CDRH's website (www.fda.gov/MedicalDevices/DeviceRegulationandGuidance/GuidanceDocuments/default.htm).

Recalls, Corrections and Removals

FDA defines a "recall" as the correction or removal of a product that is defective, could be a risk to health or is in violation of the rules administered by the agency. Recalls are classified into a numeric designation (I, II or III) by FDA to indicate the relative degree of health hazard presented by the recalled product. Health hazard evaluation is a key determinant of whether a product should be recalled and includes an assessment of the disease or injury associated with the product, seriousness of the risk posed by the product, likelihood of occurrence and consequences (immediate and long-term). FDA uses the health hazard evaluation as the basis for its recall classification:

- Class I—a situation presenting a reasonable probability that the use of or exposure to a violative product will cause serious adverse health consequences or death
- Class II—a situation in which use of or exposure to a violative product may cause temporary or medically reversible adverse health consequences or where the probability of serious adverse health consequences is remote
- Class III—a situation in which use of or exposure to a violative product is not likely to cause adverse health consequences

On 19 May 1997, FDA issued a final rule implementing provisions under the *SMDA* that made medical device correction and removal (recall) reporting mandatory instead of voluntary. The new rule was applicable to manufacturers, initial importers and domestic distributors but, because of administrative delays in the Office of Management and Budget (OMB), its effective date was delayed until 18 May 1998.[7] A *FDAMA* provision, which was to be effective 19 February 1998, repealed the requirement for reporting any device removal or correction by domestic distributors.[8] However, FDA's final rule eliminating the requirement for distributor reporting did not become effective until 22 February 1999 due to administrative delays. Recall regulations include:

- 21 CFR 7, Enforcement Policy, Subpart C, Recalls—covers voluntary removal of medical device(s)
- 21 CFR 806, Medical Device Corrections and Removals—covers mandatory notification of correction or removal of a medical device(s)
- 21 CFR 810, Medical Device Recall Authority—describes the procedures that FDA will follow in exercising its medical device recall authority under section 518(e) of the *FD&C Act*

Device manufacturers and importers for domestic distribution are required to report to FDA any correction or removal undertaken to reduce the risk to human health posed by a device's use. They also are required to report any action taken to remedy an *FD&C Act* violation caused by a device's risk to human health that would cause FDA to act if the manufacturer did not do so voluntarily. Reports of corrections and removals are required for Class I and Class II recalls. Under 21 CFR 806, Class III recalls need not be reported; only recordkeeping requirements would apply. However, FDA has an expectation that all recalls will be reported so that it may review the risk to health and render a final determination on the most appropriate classification.

Information required in such a report is detailed in 21 CFR 806.10(c)(1)–(13) and includes, but is not limited to:
- recalling firm name, address and telephone number
- batch, lot or unit identification numbers and quantity of affected devices manufactured or distributed
- consignee names, addresses and telephone numbers
- copies of all recall-related communications
- names and addresses of recall information recipients

The report must be submitted to the recalling firm's local FDA district office within 10 working days of initiating the recall. Reporting requirements regarding deaths and serious injury apply in accordance with MDR timeframes. Exemptions from these reporting requirements are provided in 21 CFR 806.1(b) (1)–(4) and include:
- manufacturer's actions to improve a device's performance or quality, which do not reduce a health risk or remedy a violation of the *FD&C Act*
- market withdrawal, defined as a recall of a distributed device that involves a minor or no violation of the *FD&C Act* and would not be subject to legal action by FDA (21 CFR 806.2(h))
- routine servicing, defined as regularly scheduled device maintenance, including the replacement of parts at the end of their normal life expectancy (21 CFR 806.2(k))
- stock recovery, defined as a recall of a device that has not yet been marketed or left the manufacturer's direct control

The recall reporting regulation does not indicate what actions FDA may take upon receiving the report. However, it may be anticipated that the enforcement policy under 21 CFR 7 would apply, involving periodic progress reports and permitting recall termination only when the agency determines that all reasonable efforts have been taken to recall the affected devices in accordance with the recall strategy and plan. The regulation further clarifies which records must be maintained if a recall is not required to be reported (21 CFR 806.20), as well as information about possible FDA actions to publicly disclose submitted recall reports.

Under enforcement, FDA also has the authority to impose a mandatory recall on manufacturers (21 CFR 810).

As noted above, FDA has the authority to impose a mandatory recall on manufacturers under 21 CFR 810. If, after providing the appropriate person with an opportunity to consult with the agency, FDA finds there is a reasonable probability that a device intended for human use would cause serious, adverse health consequences or death, the agency may issue a cease distribution and notification order requiring the person named in the order to immediately:
- cease distribution of the device
- notify healthcare professionals and device user facilities of the order
- instruct these professionals and device user facilities to cease use of the device

The person named in the order will have an opportunity for a regulatory hearing or to provide a written request to FDA asking that the order be modified, vacated or amended. FDA may later amend the order to require a recall of the device.

Additional information concerning recalls, including guidance on recall procedures, effectiveness checks, model press releases, 510(k) requirements during firm-initiated recalls and the FDA recall database, may be found on FDA's website under CDRH Device Advice. In addition, Chapter 7 of the FDA *Regulatory Procedures Manual* provides information on internal FDA procedures used in handling regulatory and enforcement matters for domestic and imported devices.

Exports

Approved or Cleared Devices

There are no export restrictions, approvals, notifications or other requirements for medical devices approved or cleared for marketing in the US, and these may be exported anywhere in the world without prior FDA notification or approval. Although FDA does not place any restrictions on the export of these devices, certain countries may require written certification that a firm or its devices are in compliance with US law. In such instances, FDA will accommodate US firms by providing a Certificate for Foreign Government (CFG). Formerly referred to as a Certificate for Products for Export or Certificate of Free Sale, the CFG uses self-certification to speed the processing of requests, and the certificate is provided on counterfeit-resistant paper bearing an embossed gold foil seal. CDRH requires a fee for the initial certificate and for any additional certificates issued for the same product(s) in the same letter of request.

Requests for a CFG are submitted on Form FDA 3613 and questions regarding the CFG should be directed to the Office of Compliance, Export Certificate Team, at +1 301 796 7400 or via email (exportcert@cdrh.fda.gov). Additional information about certificate fees for device exports can be found at www.fda.gov/MedicalDevices/DeviceRegulationandGuidance/ImportingandExportingDevices/default.htm.

In November 2012 and March 2013, CDRH launched the first two phases of its CDRH Export Certification and Tracking System (CECATS). CECATS is a new voluntary electronic system that allows manufacturers and initial importers to request export documents online as an alternative to paper submissions. CECATS offers several benefits, including a reduction in certificate processing time, savings on material and mailing costs for paper applications, realtime validation of firm-specific data and status updates of the request. During the first phase of the CECATS launch, the system was only available for Certificates for Foreign Governments requests. In March 2013, the second phase of CECATS was launched, making it available for the voluntary submission of requests for certificates of exportability under Sections 801(e)(1) and 802 of the *FD&C Act*.

Unapproved or Uncleared Devices

It is only when a device has not been approved or cleared for domestic marketing and is, hence, considered investigational, that legal export provisions become applicable. The basis for the regulation of imports and exports is contained in Chapter VIII of the *FD&C Act*, because there are no regulations in the Code of Federal Regulations (CFR) that cover export requirements, with the exception of 21 CFR 812.18(b) regarding the export of investigational devices. That provision requires a person exporting an investigational device to obtain prior FDA approval as required by Section 801(e) of the act, or to comply with Section 802 of the act.

The export of devices has been regulated since the *FD&C Act* was enacted in 1938. The 1976 *Medical Device Amendments* tightened the rules, requiring a determination by FDA that exporting the device would not pose a public health and safety hazard (essentially an FDA approval to export) and was approved by the recipient country. Despite US medical device firms' positive balance of trade, industry felt the statute's export approval requirements hindered the ability of US manufacturers to enter and compete in foreign markets. Addressing industry concerns, Congress enacted the *Food and Drug Export Reform and Enhancement Act* of 1996 *(FDERA)*.[9] In contrast to other *FD&C Act* provisions applicable to medical devices, no regulations have been codified to establish how FDA should manage unapproved device export requirements, except 21 CFR 812.18 regarding the export of investigational devices.

Following is a simplified and abridged summary of unapproved device export requirements. The rules are complex, and this summary is not intended to be inclusive of the requirements applicable to all devices or to any specific device. The statute and guidance documents should be consulted for specific requirements (http://www.fda.gov/MedicalDevices/DeviceRegulationandGuidance/ImportingandExportingDevices/ExportingMedicalDevices/ucm346617.htm).

Because the export rules apply to devices that are not approved or cleared for domestic distribution, these devices ordinarily would be considered adulterated, misbranded or both. Essentially, *FDERA* made certain regulatory changes that provide manufacturers with compliance options. When the minimum requirements of Section 801(e)(1) and either Section 801(e)(2) or one or more of the choices under Section 802 of the *FD&C Act* are met, FDA shall deem the devices to be not adulterated or misbranded for the purpose of export.

There are two principal scenarios governing the export of investigational medical devices: a) exportation of Class I and/or Class II devices, and b) the exportation of Class III and/or banned devices. Both scenarios require, at a minimum, that the investigational devices to be exported meet the basic provisions of the *FD&C Act*, as now amended in Section 801(e)(1). These provisions require that the device:

- meet the foreign purchaser's specifications
- not be in conflict with the importing country's laws
- be labeled, "intended for export only" on the outside of the shipping package
- not be sold or offered for sale in domestic commerce

Assuming the device a manufacturer wishes to export complies with these provisions, the remaining regulatory obligations include:

Exportation of Class I and/or Class II Devices

The only additional requirement for exportation is that the manufacturer reasonably believes the device it is to export could obtain 510(k) marketing clearance in the US if reviewed by FDA. If the investigational device represents a Class I device that is exempt from premarket notification, this requirement does not apply. However, if the device represents a Class I or Class II device that is subject to the requirements of premarket notification, the manufacturer's belief that it would be cleared for marketing must be based on it being similar in design, construction and intended use to one or more existing, cleared Class I or Class II devices, or it must be a reasonable belief that the investigational device would be regarded as "substantially equivalent" to one or more existing, cleared Class I or Class II devices. Therefore, if this belief of "approvability" is indeed reasonable, the manufacturer can anticipate securing authorization to export the investigational device solely under Section 801(e)(1) of the *FD&C Act*. Certification is required to complete the process.

FDA has implemented a new certification process referred to as a Certificate of Exportability (COE) in an effort to facilitate the export of a medical device under Section 801(e)(1). Persons exporting an article under Section 801(e)(1) must maintain records demonstrating that the investigational product does indeed comply with the four provisions of Section 801(e)(1) listed above. Retention requirements for these records mirror those for GMP documents, or any such quality systems records that apply to the exported product.

Manufacturers applying for a COE are required to sign a statement attesting they meet the four criteria of Section 801(e)(1). False statements, in such circumstances, are considered violations of United States Code Title 18, Chapter 47, Section 1001. Penalties for a false statement include up to $250,000 in fines and up to five years imprisonment. CDRH requires an initial fee per certificate, and a subsequent nominal fee for each additional certificate issued for the same product(s) in the same letter of request. Original certificates will be provided on special counterfeit-resistant paper with an embossed gold foil seal. CDRH will issue the certification within 20 days upon the firm's demonstration that the product meets the applicable requirements. Requests for a COE are filed on Form FDA 3613a, Supplementary Information Certificate of Exportability Requests. Questions regarding the COE should be directed to the Office of Compliance, Export Certificate Team, at +1 301 796 7400 (email exportcert@cdrh.fda.gov).

By meeting the four provisions of Section 801(e)(1) described above—ensuring that records substantiate that compliance, and obtaining a COE—the manufacturer may legally export the investigational device, without FDA permission, in accordance with Section 801(e)(1).

Exportation of Class III and/or Banned Devices

Along with the four basic requirements of Section 801(e)(1), additional provisions found under either Section 801(e)(2) or Section 802 of the *FD&C Act* allow a manufacturer to export unapproved Class III devices and devices otherwise required to meet a performance standard under Section 514 of the *FD&C Act* (currently, electrode lead wires and patient cables (21 CFR 898) are the only devices with an FDA performance standard under Section 514 of the *FD&C Act*). These devices include investigational devices, that would not be able to obtain Premarket Approval (PMA) or for which a PMA has not been approved, and banned devices (at present, only synthetic hair fibers intended for implant).

A manufacturer electing to comply with Section 801(e)(2) must apply for FDA approval to export and must submit:
- a complete device description
- the device's status in the US
- evidence from the importing foreign governmental authority that the device is not in conflict with its laws (or a notarized certification from a responsible company official in the US that the product is not in conflict with the foreign country's laws),[10] the device's US status is known and the import is permitted
- basic safety data pertaining to the device

Recordkeeping requirements as described above apply for devices exported according to Section 801(e)(2).

An alternative to export under Section 801(e)(2) involves a number of choices under Section 802, which do not require FDA approval but do require the exporter to submit a Simple Notification per 802(g) and maintain substantiating records, should FDA request them. The basic requirements, listed in Section 802(f), call for the devices to:
- satisfy the requirements of Section 801(e)(1)
- be manufactured in acceptable compliance with either the US QSR (no deficiencies or satisfactory correction of deficiencies following the most recent FDA inspection) or an international quality system standard recognized by FDA (currently, none is recognized)
- not be adulterated, other than lack of marketing approval
- not be the subject of a notice by the Department of Health and Human Services that re-importation would pose an imminent hazard or pose an imminent hazard to the receiving country
- not be mislabeled, except that they must meet the importing country's labeling requirements

Records (Section 802(g), in addition to the requirements per Section 801(e)(1)) also must be maintained for devices exported under Section 802, and other requirements may apply. Even though FDA does not require a firm to obtain written permission prior to export under Section 802, a foreign purchaser may request proof of compliance with US law prior to export. FDA will provide a COE to the exporter under Section 802 to facilitate export of a medical device. Exporting manufacturers should consult Section 802 of the *FD&C Act* for further details specific to their devices.

Imports

Foreign establishments that manufacture medical devices and/or products that emit radiation must comply with applicable US regulations before, during and after importing into the US. These products must meet all applicable FDA regulatory requirements, because FDA does not recognize regulatory approvals from other countries.

Foreign Manufacturers

All foreign manufacturers must meet applicable US medical device regulations to import devices into the US, even if the product is authorized for marketing in another country.

These requirements include establishment registration, device listing, manufacturing in accordance with the QSR, medical device reporting of adverse events and a 510(k) or PMA, if applicable. Foreign manufacturing sites are subject to FDA inspection. In addition, the foreign manufacturers must designate a US agent.

Initial Importers

An initial importer is any importer who furthers the marketing of a device from a foreign manufacturer to the person who makes the final delivery or sale of the device to the ultimate consumer or user, but does not repackage or otherwise change the container, wrapper or labeling of the device or device package. The initial importer of the device must register its establishment with FDA. Initial importers also are subject to regulations governing MDR, reports of corrections and removals and medical device tracking, if applicable. Under the MDR regulations, importers are required to report incidents in which a device may have caused or contributed to a death or serious injury, as well as report certain malfunctions. The importers must maintain an MDR event file for each adverse event. All product complaints, MDR and non-MDR events must be forwarded to the manufacturer. Under medical device tracking requirements, certain devices must be tracked through the distribution chain.

Responsibilities of the initial importer, beyond those noted above, may include:[11]

- acting as official correspondent (although this is not required)
- assisting FDA in communications with the foreign establishment and responding to questions concerning the foreign establishment's products that are imported or offered for import into the US
- assisting FDA in scheduling inspections of the foreign establishment if unable to contact the foreign establishment directly or expeditiously; FDA may provide information or documents to the US agent, and such an action shall be considered equivalent to providing the same information or documents to the foreign establishment

All medical devices imported into the US must meet Bureau of Customs and Border Protection (CBP) requirements in addition to those of FDA. A product that does not meet FDA regulatory requirements may be detained upon entry. Additional information about importing medical devices into the US is available at www.fda.gov/MedicalDevices/DeviceRegulationandGuidance/ImportingandExportingDevices/default.htm.

Medical Device Tracking

Medical device tracking is intended to ensure a manufacturer can promptly identify product distribution, notify patients and remove a device from the market if requested by FDA. *SMDA* provided for automatic, mandatory medical device tracking by creating a new Section 519(e) of the *FD&C Act*. Subsequently, the device tracking regulations (21 CFR 821) were amended by *FDAMA*, eliminating mandatory tracking and giving FDA discretion to require a manufacturer to adopt a method of tracking a Class II or Class III device. FDA most recently amended the device tracking regulations, effective 9 May 2002, with changes to 21 CFR 821 as follows:

- revising the existing scope and authority: the types of persons subject to tracking are no longer linked to registration requirements; as amended, the tracking requirements apply only to manufacturers that receive a tracking order from FDA
- modifying existing definitions of "importer" and "permanently implantable device"
- adding new patient confidentiality provisions[12]

Accordingly, the amended regulations specify certain devices to which tracking requirements apply. This includes devices, the failure of which would be reasonably likely to have serious adverse health consequences; devices intended to be implanted in the human body for more than one year; or life-sustaining or life-supporting devices used outside a device user facility. FDA maintains a list of devices subject to tracking regulations.

Manufacturers of a tracked device must establish a written standard operating procedure (SOP) that includes a method for tracking the device throughout distribution and a quality assurance program including audit procedures. Final distributors of these devices will be required to provide manufacturers with patient information. Device tracking is required for the useful life of the device.

Traceability is distinguished from medical device tracking in that traceability involves the identification of one or more device components or a finished device through the use of control numbers that may facilitate any warranted corrective actions. Therefore, traceability generally applies, and is limited to, the manufacturing stage for all devices. Device tracking, on the other hand, alludes to processes and methods that provide for the pursuit and location of devices that have since been distributed away from the manufacturing facility and either may be stored remotely or may have been prescribed and administered to a patient (e.g., implanted). Information to be maintained through tracking activities includes records concerning the patient and his or her whereabouts; the prescribing and treating physician(s); device identification numbers; and device shipment, treatment initiation and termination dates (21 CFR 821.25). For implants, the explant date and explanting physician information must be maintained. The regulation also requires distributors to provide the manufacturer with specified tracking information (21 CFR 821.30).

Device tracking information is available on CDRH's Device Advice website (www.fda.gov/MedicalDevices/DeviceRegulationandGuidance/default.htm). FDA issued *Medical Device Tracking: Guidance for Industry and FDA Staff* (25 January 2010) to provide manufacturers with more detailed information about device tracking requirements. This guidance can be found at www.fda.gov/MedicalDevices/DeviceRegulationandGuidance/GuidanceDocuments/ucm071756.htm.

Medical Device Postmarket Transformation Initiative

CDRH has made significant strides toward more robust monitoring of the safety and effectiveness of medical devices and radiation-emitting products in the postmarketing phase. In January 2006, CDRH created the Postmarket Transformation Leadership Team to evaluate current recommendations and to propose a prioritized implementation plan for a transformed postmarket process. The results of this initiative and the subsequent report published in November 2006 provided a vision and an action plan for changes to the medical devices postmarket program.

A key strategic goal of FDA toward the integration of postmarketing initiatives was the establishment and amplification of the interconnections found at all phases of the total product lifecycle (TPLC) (see **Figure 19-3**). This graphic illustrates the links between and interdependence of the regulatory process and lifecycle steps. The diagram further demonstrates the significance and magnitude of postmarketing activities, which comprise half of the critical steps of the TPLC (i.e., manufacturing, marketing, commercial use and obsolescence), and show the inherent balance and flexibility that exists between premarket and postmarket regulation.

As a result of this initiative, the following areas were designated for improvement. They are:

- Create a Culture of Collaboration—CDRH should transform its operations by adding a permanent matrix of cross-cutting, product-related groups over the current functionally based organizational structure to foster information sharing, collaboration and, ultimately, more effective public health promotion and protection. The cross-cutting matrix is designed to ensure that collaboration occurs not just in crisis situations, but also as a part of routine, day-to-day operations.
- Develop World-class Data Systems—Data input, mining, analysis and tracking systems should be strengthened, improved or created as needed for postmarket issues. Improvements to CDRH's critical medical device data and information systems, including the Manufacturer and User Facility Device Experience database (MAUDE) and the MDR system, are highlighted and additional enhancements to CDRH's analysis and tracking capabilities are being pursued.
- Enhance Benefit:Risk Communication Efforts—CDRH should be a trusted, publicly identifiable source for safety information about medical devices and radiation-emitting products. To that end, an analysis of the communication needs of CDRH stakeholders should be performed. Clinical practitioners and professional communities should collaborate with the agency to develop a process for the dissemination of benefit:risk information.
- Collaborate on Enforcement Strategies and Outcomes—Both the quantity and quality of CDRH/Office of Regulatory Affairs (ORA) interactions should be transformed through increased collaboration among CDRH, ORA and the Office of Chief Counsel. Postmarket data and information should be considered when prioritizing inspections and the inspection preparation process should include a review of recent postmarket data. CDRH should develop ways to leverage the audit results obtained by accredited third-party auditing bodies. Enforcement data systems should be updated and employees trained to use them. All available enforcement tools should be used, including civil money penalties.

Numerous priority actions within these four target areas for improvement were undertaken by FDA and significant accomplishments were realized, including the Medical Product Safety Network (MedSun), Unique Device Identification (UDI), safety news, issues, notifications and alerts.

FDA has continued this initiative with the National Medical Device Postmarket Surveillance Plan. As part of this plan, FDA issued reports in 2012 and 2013 on its efforts to strengthen medical device postmarket surveillance. The reports and further information can be found at www.fda.gov/AboutFDA/CentersOffices/OfficeofMedicalProductsandTobacco/CDRH/CDRHReports/ucm301912.htm.

Medical Product Safety Network (MedSun)

MedSun is an adverse event reporting program launched in 2002 by CDRH. Its primary goal is to work collaboratively with the clinical community to identify, understand and remedy problems associated with the use of medical devices. MedSun also serves as a powerful, two-way communications channel between CDRH and the clinical community.

Figure 19-3. Total Product Lifecycle

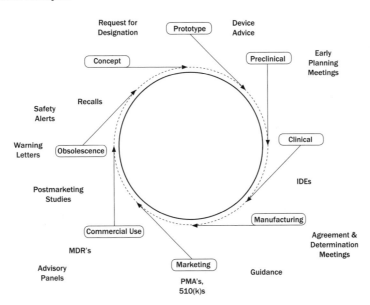

MedSun participants are recruited from all regions of the country using the American Hospital Association (AHA) membership listing. Participants use an Internet-based system as an easy, secure way to report adverse medical device events. Each member facility has online access to the reports submitted to MedSun so they can be tracked and reviewed at any time.

SMDA defines "user facilities" as hospitals, nursing homes and outpatient treatment and diagnostic centers. The facilities that comprise the MedSun participants are required to report medical device problems that result in serious illness, injury or death. They also are encouraged to voluntarily report other problems with devices, such as "close calls;" potential for harm and other safety concerns. By monitoring reports about problems and concerns before a more serious event occurs, FDA, manufacturers and clinicians work together to prevent serious injuries and death.

Once a problem is identified, MedSun researchers work with each facility's representatives to clarify and understand the issue. Reports and lessons learned are shared with the clinical community and the public, without facility and patient identification, so clinicians nationwide may take necessary preventive actions.

Additional information on MedSun can be found at www.fda.gov/MedicalDevices/Safety/MedSunMedicalProductSafetyNetwork/default.htm.

Unique Device Identification

FDAAA contains provisions granting FDA the express authority to propose and ultimately implement regulations requiring medical devices to display a unique device identifier (UDI). This new system, when implemented, will require:

- the label of a device to bear a unique identifier, unless an alternative location is specified by FDA or an exception is made for a particular device or group of devices
- the unique identifier to be able to identify the device through distribution and use
- the unique identifier to include the lot or serial number if specified by FDA

The presence of a UDI on a medical device is intended to improve patient safety by reducing device-related medical errors, improving identification of specific devices in adverse event reports and facilitating more-effective device recalls.

In 2010, FDA continued to explore what the implementation of the UDI system will mean for various stakeholders. Labeling organizations continued to participate in informal feedback sessions, which included teleconference discussions and practical simulation exercises that provided FDA with a range of information that has further elucidated UDI system needs. Pilot activities conducted internally at FDA identified processes that are well equipped to handle UDI requirements, as well as those that will need to be modified. Fewer issues and questions now remain as FDA nears the release of regulations and guidance pertaining to UDI.

FDA issued a proposed rule on a UDI system in July 2012. For more information, see Unique Device Identification at http://www.fda.gov/medicaldevices/deviceregulationandguidance/uniquedeviceidentification/default.htm.

Chapter 19

Safety News, Issues, Notifications, and Alerts

CDRH shares risk communication information with the public primarily through leaflets and Internet sites. Leaflets are mailed to individuals or made available at conferences. The website offers materials on a wide variety of topics of interest to consumers. Information relevant to particular age groups (e.g., children or the elderly) have been developed with those consumers' limitations in mind (e.g., reading level or accessibility needs). These communications are used to inform the public about what to look for in selecting medical devices and products, the availability of new medical devices, product recalls and safety information and how to report adverse events associated with the use of medical devices.

CDRH uses a variety of outreach tools including Urgent Alerts, multimedia outreach, technical publications, presentations and workshops to advise device users about potential risks. These tools utilize a variety of mechanisms, including broadcast media (press releases, talk papers, web-based news programs, websites and television interviews), public health notifications, patient notifications and public meetings to convey risk messages. In addition, staff presentations, CDRH workshops and technical publications, such as standards and guidance documents, convey important safety information to significant stakeholders. FDA's goal is to ensure that healthcare practitioners, industry and the public understand the risks and act appropriately to minimize them.

CDRH staff select risk communication tools depending on the urgency of the message, the intended target audience and the outreach goals. An Urgent Alert mechanism is used when the risk associated with a device problem is greatest. Multimedia outreach tools such as website linkages are readily available to keep the healthcare community informed about public health problems.

Urgent Alerts

When a postmarket assessment determines that a public health problem is an imminent hazard, CDRH utilizes experts from all parts of the center to develop Urgent Alerts to notify healthcare professionals and the affected population.

Preliminary Public Health Notification

The Preliminary Public Health Notification is an early alert issued to healthcare practitioners about a device risk. A key determination triggering the issuance of a Preliminary Public Health Notification is the urgency of providing the healthcare community with existing information to make informed clinical decisions about the use of a device or device type, even though information is often incomplete.

Factors used to determine urgency include the severity of the potential risk, the population likely to be at risk, the likelihood that adverse events may occur and the need for information and feedback from the healthcare community. CDRH experts use their judgment to predict the impact of these factors. Often, the problem is being actively investigated by CDRH, the industry, another agency or some other reliable entity; hence, updates to the Preliminary Public Health Notification are provided when definitive new information becomes available.

The Preliminary Public Health Notification contains:
- current information on the problem
- analysis of the existing data with a preliminary finding
- preliminary or interim recommendations, usually general reminders (e.g., increase observation of the patient, read the device labeling and/or report adverse events)

The decision to issue a Preliminary Public Health Notification often comes from a Postmarket Issue (PMI) action team or as the result of review of a recall by CDRH. CDRH publishes the Preliminary Public Health Notification on the CDRH and FDA websites and advertises on an office listserv, the MedWatch listserv and any other mechanism considered necessary to ensure that the target audience is made aware of its publication.

Preliminary Public Health Notifications are updated as frequently as necessary to keep the healthcare community aware of the problem. When the agency understands the problem and is able to provide recommendations to mitigate the risk, a Preliminary Public Health Notification will be replaced with a Public Health Notification.

Public Health Notification

Public Health Notifications are important messages about risks associated with the use of medical devices. They are placed on the CDRH and FDA websites and may be disseminated in additional ways to ensure the message reaches the target audience. Public Health Notification recommendations usually come from the PMI team, but in unusual circumstances the decision to issue a notification may be made without convening a PMI team.

Public Health Notifications are issued when:
- The information is important in order to make informed clinical decisions about the use of a device or device type.
- The information is not readily available to the affected target.
- CDRH recommendations will help healthcare practitioners mitigate or avoid the risk.

The decision to issue a Public Health Notification is dependent on the quality of the information, the significance of the risk, the population at risk, the nature and frequency of adverse events, the urgency of the situation and the expectations of the public.

Press Releases

Press releases approved by CDRH are issued to the media by FDA's Office of Public Affairs whenever there is a need to alert the broader public to a potential health risk associated with an FDA-regulated product. In addition to Class I recalls, press releases usually are issued for seizures of medical devices. Press releases are distributed to a list of critical media nationwide via a listserv. They also are posted on the FDA and CDRH websites.

Multimedia Outreach

CDRH has established a number of methods for making information about public health concerns readily available to the healthcare community and the general public. For example, the Patient Safety News network disseminates information in video format through one of the center's website links. CDRH also has developed a number of relevant and consumer-friendly webpages addressing issues with commonly used medical devices.

Patient Safety News

CDRH leads the agency's production of FDA Patient Safety News (PSN), a monthly television news show distributed by CDRH. The show is broadcast each month on several medical satellite television networks that bring continuing education for healthcare professionals to more than 4,500 US hospitals and long-term care facilities. FDA PSN is a major vehicle for communicating safety messages about medical products to physicians, nurses, pharmacists, risk managers and educators across the nation. It incorporates stories from FDA's three medical product centers (Center for Drug Evaluation and Research (CDER), CDRH and Center for Biological Evaluation and Research (CBER)) on medical errors, patient safety, recalls and alerts and newly approved drugs, devices and biological products.

The show's website is www.accessdata.fda.gov/scripts/cdrh/cfdocs/psn/index.cfm.

Websites

CDRH communicates postmarket safety information through a variety of public websites.

- Medical Device Safety—This website presents a collection of medical device safety information (e.g., recalls, public health notifications, safety tips, "Dear Doctor" letters, etc.) for healthcare professionals. The site is updated regularly to feature high-priority risk messages. CDRH periodically conducts audience analysis and usability studies of this site to make it more accessible and understandable to practitioners (www.fda.gov/MedicalDevices/Safety/default.htm).
- CDRH Consumer Website—The CDRH consumer website provides information about specific devices and device issues for a patient/consumer audience. It includes links to postmarket safety information (including Class I recalls and Public Health Notifications), as well as information geared toward individuals who use devices in their homes. (www.fda.gov/ForConsumers/ConsumerUpdates/ucm149209.htm).
- Disease-Specific Websites (FDA Diabetes Information, Heart Health Online)—CDRH coordinates FDA's disease-specific websites on diabetes and heart disease. These websites are designed to educate patients and caregivers about the types of interventions involving medical devices that prevent and treat disease. Each includes links to appropriate medical device patient labeling and postmarket safety information.
- Device-Specific and Topic-Specific Websites (i.e., LASIK, Phakic Lenses, Whole Body CT Scanning, Cochlear Implants, etc.)—CDRH's device-specific websites provide coordinated postmarket information about specific types of devices. These websites give patients and healthcare professionals easy access to descriptive information, indications for use, risks and precautions and specific safety information.

Postapproval Studies

A postapproval study (PAS), also known as a Condition of Approval study, under 21 CFR 814.82(a)(2), helps ensure the continued safety and effectiveness of an approved, marketed device. CDRH may require such a study, and FDA will state in the PMA approval order the reason or purpose for the requirement, the number of patients to be evaluated and the subsequent reports that must be submitted.

The last few years have seen a greater focus on PAS for FDA-regulated products. Both CDER and CBER now post the status of certain postmarketing studies on CDER's website (www.accessdata.fda.gov/scripts/cder/pmc/index.cfm). In 2005, the Institute of Medicine (IOM) completed a study entitled, "Safe Medical Devices for Children." Among its recommendations, the report urged FDA to establish a system for monitoring and publicly reporting the status of postmarket study commitments involving medical devices.

The new CDRH Postapproval Studies Program encompasses design, tracking, oversight and review responsibilities for studies mandated as a condition of approval of a PMA application. The program helps ensure that well-designed PAS are conducted effectively and efficiently and in the least burdensome manner. On 1 January 2005, oversight responsibility was transferred to CDRH's Office of Surveillance and Biometrics (OSB) and the PAS review functions were integrated into the medical device epidemiology program. This action enabled epidemiologists on the premarketing review teams to begin early planning regarding postmarketing concerns as the product moves through the approval process. In addition, industry is required to consider the design of its postmarketing studies during the approval process. Postmarketing studies are now a standard part of discussions with advisory panels, and products must have a protocol at the time of approval.

CDRH has an automated tracking system that efficiently identifies the reporting status of active PAS ordered since 1 January 2005. This system represents CDRH's effort to ensure all PAS commitments are fulfilled in a timely manner. The effective tracking system is based on study timelines incorporated in study protocols and agreed to by CDRH and the manufacturer. In addition to this internal tracking system, CDRH launched a publicly available webpage (www.accessdata.fda.gov/scripts/cdrh/cfdocs/cfPMA/pma_pas.cfm?sb=dad) to keep all stakeholders informed of study progress. It displays not only PAS reporting status, but also the status (based upon protocol-driven timelines) of each PAS.

Postmarket Surveillance

Premarket review provides limited information on a device's performance, safety and effectiveness. However, it generally is recognized that quality and/or performance issues, along with newly emergent safety signals or efficacy outcomes, may arise after the device has been utilized by a more diverse population and under more varied conditions.

FDAMA modified postmarket surveillance requirements under Section 522 of the *FD&C Act*. Specifically, under the act, the agency may order a manufacturer to conduct postmarket surveillance for any Class II or Class III device, including a device reviewed under the licensing provisions of Section 351 of the *Public Health Service Act*, which meets any of the following criteria:

- The device's failure would be reasonably likely to have serious adverse health consequences.
- The device is intended to be implanted in the human body for more than one year.
- The device is intended to be a life-sustaining or life-supporting device used outside a device user facility.

There are various considerations in establishing a postmarketing surveillance strategy for a particular device or type of device. A general approach by CDRH is to convene an expert review team within the center to establish the surveillance objective, the information needed to achieve this objective, appropriate sources and mechanisms for obtaining this information and necessary actions needed to address public health concerns. The postmarket surveillance plan will result in the collection of useful data that can reveal unforeseen adverse events, clarify the actual rate of expected adverse events and may provide other information necessary to protect the public health (21 CFR 822.2).

Postmarketing issues or signals may emerge at any point during the device lifecycle and can stem from a variety of sources, such as analysis of adverse event reports, a recall or corrective action, reports from other governmental authorities or the scientific literature. Once such an issue is identified, it is forwarded by the division director to the director of the Issues Management Staff (IMS) in OSB.

An expert review team will consider whether to impose a postmarket surveillance order under Section 522. The expert review team will develop the postmarket surveillance question(s) and the supporting rationale that will be part of the postmarket surveillance order. The questions focus on confirming the nature, severity or frequency of suspected problems. The OSB director will decide whether to order postmarket surveillance. Although postmarket surveillance will not be used in lieu of adequate premarket testing, it can serve to complement premarket studies.

Manufacturers who do not conduct postmarket surveillance in accordance with the approval plan may be subject to FDA enforcement actions, including civil monetary penalties (21 CFR 822.20). The results and status of the postmarket surveillance plan are available under the *Freedom of Information Act* (*FOIA*) and the overall status of the surveillance, along with a brief description of the plan, may be available via the Internet.

Summary

- Both domestic and foreign medical device manufacturers are required to register their establishments with FDA and list the devices they distribute. The regulations are included in 21 CFR Part 807 and described in the FDA guidance, *Implementation of Medical Device Establishment Registration and Device Listing Requirements Established by the Food and Drug Administration Amendments Ace of 2007* (8 October 2009).
- The Quality System Regulation under 21 CFR 820 defines FDA's current GMPs for medical devices. It was substantially augmented in 1996 and now includes premarket product development (design controls), as well as installation and servicing.
- FDA's QSIT is an excellent model on which to base or prepare for quality system audits. The QSIT apportions the quality system into seven core subsystems, as follows:
  1. Corrective and Preventive Action
  2. Design Controls
  3. Production and Process Controls
  4. Management Controls

5. Records, Documents and Change Controls
6. Materials Controls
7. Facility and Equipment Controls

FDA's QSIT inspections generally focus on the first four subsystems because they are primary indicators of compliance.

- Regulations for medical device reporting (MDR) under 21 CFR 803 and corrections and removals (recalls) in 21 CFR 806 require filing timely and accurate reports with FDA. The type and severity of adverse experiences occurring determine the timeframe in which these reports must be submitted.
- There are no restrictions for exporting medical devices already cleared or approved for marketing in the US. However, regulations for exporting unapproved or investigational devices can require careful consideration because they are driven by the device classification, degree of risk and similarity in design, operation and intended use to existing predicate devices in US interstate commerce.
- Device tracking regulations in 21 CFR 821 provide for the post-manufacture identity, distribution, location and patient-specific use of certain eligible significant-risk devices. Traceability requirements in 21 CFR 820 provide for the identity of medical devices or certain components during and throughout the manufacture of the device.

References
1. International Organization for Standardization, ISO 13485:2003 *Medical devices: Quality management systems—Requirements for regulatory purposes.* ISO, Geneva, Switzerland, 2003.
2. FDA. Foreign Establishment Registration and Listing. *Fed Reg* 27 November 2001, 66, 59138.
3. *Enforcement Priorities for Single-Use Devices Reprocessed by Third Parties and Hospitals* (14 August 2000) FDA website. www.fda.gov/MedicalDevices/DeviceRegulationandGuidance/GuidanceDocuments/ucm107164.htm. Accessed 21 May 2013.
4. FDA, *Fed Reg* 21 December 1979, 44, 75628; *Fed Reg* 6 April 1988, 53, 11253; *Fed Reg* 27 March 1990, 55, 11169.
5. Division of Small Manufacturers, International and Consumer Assistance (DSMICA), *Medical Device Quality Systems Manual: A Small Entity Compliance Guide* (1997). FDA website. www.fda.gov/medicaldevices/deviceregulationandguidance/postmarketrequirements/qualitysystemsregulations/medicaldevicequalitysystemsmanual/default.htm. Accessed 21 May 2013.
6. FDA. "Medical Device Reporting: Manufacturer Reporting, Importer Reporting, User Facility Reporting, Distributor Reporting; Final Rule," *Fed Reg* 26 January 2000, 65, 4112.
7. FDA. "Medical Devices; Reports of Corrections and Removals; Final Rule," *Federal Register* 62:27191 (19 May 1997).
8. FDA. "Medical Devices; Reports of Corrections and Removals; Direct Final Rule." *Fed Reg* 7 August 1998, 63, 42232 (7 August 1998).
9. Public Law 104-134, as amended by Public Law 104 180.
10. FDA. "Exports: Notification and Recordkeeping Requirements; Final Rule." *Fed Reg* 19 December 2001, 66, 65429.
11. FDA. "Device Advice: Establishment Registration" (28 February 2002). FDA website. www.fda.gov/MedicalDevices/DeviceRegulationandGuidance/HowtoMarketYourDevice/RegistrationandListing/default.htm. Accessed 21 May 2013.
12. FDA. "Medical Devices; Device Tracking; Final Rule," *Fed Reg* 8 February 2002, 67, 5943.

Recommended Reading
- Device Labeling Guidance # G91-1 (Blue Book Memo) http://www.fda.gov/MedicalDevices/DeviceRegulationandGuidance/GuidanceDocuments/ucm081368.htm.
- FDA. Medical Devices; Current Good Manufacturing Practice Final Rule, Quality System Regulation. *Fed Reg* 7 October 1996, 61, 52602–52662. http://www.fda.gov/medicaldevices/deviceregulationandguidance/postmarketrequirements/qualitysystemsregulations/ucm230127.htm.
- FDA, Medical Devices, Device Tracking, New Orders to Manufacturers. *Fed Reg* 4 March 1998, 63, 10638–10640.
- Garcia DG. "Medtronic v. Lohr Decision Underscores Importance of Regulatory Compliance." *Med Device & Diag Ind.* March 1997, 97–101.
- Gibbs JN. "Treatment IDEs: FDA Proposal Borrows from Treatment INDs." *Reg Aff Focus.* April 1997, 22–23.
- Kahan JS. "FDA's New Approach to Export Regulation." *Med Device & Diag Ind.* September 1996, 68–72.
- Kahan J. "The Reference List: A Legally Suspect, Dying Program." *Reg Aff Focus.* May 1997, 14–15.
- Kingsley PA. (FDA). *Write It Right: Recommendations for Developing User Instruction Manuals for Medical Devices Used in Home Health Care.* FDA, Rockville, MD, FDA, August 1993. http://www.fda.gov/downloads/MedicalDevices/DeviceRegulationandGuidance/GuidanceDocuments/ucm070771.pdf. Accessed 13 April 2011.
- *Medtronic Inc. v. Lohr*, 116 S. Ct. 2240; 1996.
- Spencer RL. Mandatory Device Recall Procedures. *RAPS News.* September 1994, 5–8.
- Webster JL. "Medical Devices, Promotion, Labeling and Advertising." *Reg Aff Focus.* June 1997, 25–27.
- Hooten WF. "FDA Makes Quality the Rule." *Med Device & Diag Ind.* January 1997, 114–128.
- *FDA Regulatory Procedures Manual*, "Chapter 7. Recall Procedures" www.fda.gov/ICECI/ComplianceManuals/RegulatoryProceduresManual/default.htm.
- Recall Procedures and Model Press Releases. www.fda.gov/Safety/Recalls/default.htm.
- 510(k) Requirements During Firm-Initiated Recalls, K95-1—Blue Book Memo. Issued 21 November 1995. www.fda.gov/MedicalDevices/DeviceRegulationandGuidance/GuidanceDocuments/ucm080297.htm .
- FDA Recall Database/Medical Device Class I Recalls. www.fda.gov/MedicalDevices/Safety/ListofRecalls/default.htm.
- FDA Report – Strengthening Our National System for Medical Device Postmarket Surveillance: Update and Next Steps – CDRH/FDA April 2013
- www.fda.gov/downloads/MedicalDevices/Safety/CDRHPostmarketSurveillance/UCM348845.pdf.

Chapter 19

Chapter 20

Advertising, Promotion and Labeling for Medical Devices and In Vitro Diagnostics

Updated by Anthony P. Schiavone, RAC and Andrew P. Zeltwanger

OBJECTIVES

- Understand the difference between "labels" and "labeling"
- Understand the basic regulatory requirements for labels and labeling for medical devices and in vitro diagnostics (IVDs)
- Understand the basic regulatory requirements for promotion and advertising
- Explain the jurisdiction for promotion and advertising
- Understand the submission requirements for advertising and promotional materials
- Explain possible enforcement actions for violations of relevant laws and regulations
- Understand medical device misbranding
- Understand the use of Consensus Standards and the future of graphics and symbols in labeling for medical devices and IVDs

LAWS, REGULATIONS AND GUIDELINES COVERED IN THIS CHAPTER

- Federal Food, Drug, and Cosmetic Act
- 21 CFR 801 (Subpart A) General Labeling Provisions
- 21 CFR 801 (Subpart C) Labeling Requirements for Over-the-Counter (OTC) Devices
- 21 CFR 801.119 In vitro diagnostic products
- 21 CFR 809 In vitro diagnostic products for human use
- 21 CFR 809.10 General labeling requirements on content of labeling for in vitro diagnostic products
- 21 CFR 809.20 General requirements for manufacturers and producers of in vitro diagnostic products
- 21 CFR 809.30 Restrictions on the sale, distribution and use of analyte-specific reagents
- 21 CFR 809.40 Restrictions on the sale, distribution, and use of OTC test sample collection systems for drugs of abuse testing
- 21 CFR 99 Dissemination of information on unapproved/new uses for marketed drugs, biologics, and devices
- 21 CFR 99.103 Mandatory statements and information
- *Guidance for Industry and FDA Staff: Use of Symbols on Labels and in Labeling of In Vitro Diagnostic Devices Intended for Professional Use* (November 2004)

Chapter 20

- *Guidance for Industry: Alternative to Certain Prescription Device Labeling Requirements* (January 2000)

- *Guidance for Industry: User Labeling for Devices that Contain Natural Rubber (21 CFR §801.437); Small Entity Compliance Guide* (April 2003)

- *Guidance on Medical Device Patient Labeling; Final Guidance for Industry and FDA Reviewers* (April 2001)

- *Guidance for Industry: Designation of Special Controls for Male Condoms Made of Natural Rubber Latex (21 CFR 884.5300); Small Entity Compliance Guide* (January 2009)

- *Human Factors Principles for Medical Device Labeling* (September 1993)

- *Labeling Regulatory Requirements for Medical Devices* (August 1989)

- *Device Labeling Guidance #G91-1 (Blue Book Memo)* (March 1991)

- *Write it Right: Recommendations for Developing User Instruction Manuals for Medical Devices Used in Home Health Care* (August 1993)

- *Draft Guidance for Industry: Product Name Placement, Size, and Prominence in Advertising and Promotional Labeling* (January 1999)

- *Draft Guidance for Industry: "Help-Seeking" and other Disease Awareness Communications by or on Behalf of Drug and Device Firms* (January 2004)

- *Draft Guidance for Industry and FDA: Consumer-Directed Broadcast Advertising of Restricted Devices* (February 2004)

- *Guidance for Industry: Good Reprint Practices for the Distribution of Medical Journal Articles and Medical or Scientific Reference Publications on Unapproved New Uses of Approved Drugs and Approved or Cleared Medical Devices* (January 2009)

- *Guidance for Industry: Accelerated Approval Products—Submission of Promotional Materials* (March 1999)

- *Labelling Recommendations for Single-Use Devices Reprocessed by Third Parties and Hospitals; Final Guidance for Industry and FDA* (September 2001)

Label and Labeling

As described in Chapter 16, a "Label," as defined under the *Federal Food, Drug, and Cosmetic Act (FD&C Act)*,[1] is a display of written, printed or graphic material on the immediate container of any article (for the purposes of this chapter, "article" refers to a medical device or IVD). "Labeling" is a broader term and refers to any written, printed or graphic material on any article, on any of its containers or wrappers or on any material accompanying it. It includes any form of publicity such as posters, tags, pamphlets, circulars, booklets, brochures, instruction or direction sheets, fillers, etc., as well as labeling intended to be used in promotional activities, which is sometimes referred to as promotional labeling or marketing literature, for example, on a company's website.

The above phrase "or any material accompanying it" was further defined by the Supreme Court in *Kordel v United States*, 335 U.S. 345 (1948).[2] In this landmark case for the *FD&C Act*, the Supreme Court ruled that the phrase, "accompanying such article" is not restricted or limited to labels that are on or in the article or package that is transported. This more-liberal interpretation meant that a physical association with the device was not necessary. Thus, labeling is considered a wide variety of written, printed or graphic matter such as pamphlets, circulars, booklets, brochures, sales sheets, etc., that bear a textual relationship with the device.

The US Food and Drug Administration (FDA), therefore, recognizes three types of labeling for devices. The first two of these are: FDA-approved labeling and promotional labeling. FDA-approved labeling is part of the submission process with a new drug application (NDA), a biologics license application (BLA) or a premarket approval application (PMA). For prescription medical device products, the FDA-approved labeling must be included in or within the package from which the device is to be dispensed; otherwise, the product is considered misbranded since it lacks adequate directions for use (*FD&C Act* Section 502(f) and 21 CFR 801.109(c)).

The third type of recognized labeling falls under the Premarket Notification or 510(k) process. The 510(k) submission process provides draft labeling to the agency, but since this type of submission receives "clearance," the labeling is not classified as FDA-approved. FDA does provide comment and request revisions to package insert labeling, and it therefore is implied that the labeling is cleared during the submission process. Industry practice refers to this category of labeling as "FDA-cleared." Much in the same manner as FDA-approved labeling above, prescription medical device products cleared under the 510(k) process must be accompanied by the appropriate FDA-cleared labeling or the product is considered misbranded. FDA-cleared labeling is subject to change by manufacturers but, under guidance provided by FDA for the 510(k) process, significant labeling changes can drive the submission of a new 510(k) application for FDA review.

FD&C Act Sections 502(f)(1) and (2) require device labeling to bear adequate directions for use, proper operating and servicing instructions, warnings where a device's use may be dangerous to health or any information necessary to protect the user(s). All devices require directions for use unless specifically exempted by regulation.[3]

The basic outline for labels and/or labeling specific to medical devices includes, but is not limited to:
- manufacturer, packer or distributor name and principal place of business
- device name, other required information
- description
- indications and usage
- contraindications
- warnings
- precautions
- use in specific patient populations (if applicable)
- adverse reactions (if applicable)
- prescription device statement or symbol[4]
- date of issue or latest revision of labeling bearing information for use

Additional labeling requirements for over-the-counter (OTC) devices may be found in 21 CFR 801.60. Label and labeling requirements for Investigational Device Exemption (IDE) medical devices are located in 21 CFR 812.[5]

In vitro diagnostic (IVD) products, according to 21 CFR 809.3, are reagents, instruments and systems intended for use in the diagnosis of diseases or other conditions, including a determination of the state of health, in order to cure, mitigate, treat or prevent disease or its sequelae. IVD products are intended for use in the collection, preparation and examination of specimens taken from the human body. They are considered devices as defined in *FD&C Act* Section 201(h). IVDs also are covered under a separate FDA regulation (21 CFR 809). These devices have their own labels and labeling regulations within that part (809.10).

In addition to some of the basic items outlined above, there are specific requirements determined by the type of IVD:

Label
- proprietary name and established (common or usual) name, if applicable
- indications and usage
- manufacturer, packer or distributor name and place of business
- warnings/precautions per 16 CFR 1500
- IVD use statement and/or reagent use statement
- lot or control number

Reagent Label Requirements
- quantity of contents (i.e., weight or volume, numerical count or any combination of these or accurate indication of the package contents)
- proportion or concentration of each reactive ingredient
- storage conditions such as:
  o temperature
  o light
  o humidity
  o other pertinent factors as applicable
- statement of reagent purity and quality
- if reagent is derived from biological material, the source and a measure of its activity
- expiration date
- statement in reference to any observable indication of an alteration of product

Labeling (i.e., Package Insert, Instruction Manual)
- proprietary name and established (common or usual) name if any
- indication and usage
- type of procedure (qualitative or quantitative)
- warnings/precautions per 16 CFR 1500
- IVD use statement and/or reagent use statement
- summary and explanation of test (history of methodology)
- chemical, physical, physiological or biological principles of the procedure

Reagent Labeling Requirements
- declaration of quantity, proportion or concentration of reactive ingredient
- statement indicating the presence of and characterizing any catalytic or nonreactive ingredients (i.e., buffers, preservatives, stabilizers)
- instructions for reconstitution, mixing, dilution, etc. of reagent, if any
- storage conditions such as:
  o temperature
  o light
  o humidity
  o other pertinent factors as applicable
- statement of any purification or treatment required for use
- physical, biological or chemical indications of instability or deterioration

A labeling outline for an IVD instrument can be found in 21 CFR 809.10(b)(6). Following is an abbreviated list of the basic requirements for instrument labeling:
- use or function
- installation procedures
- principles of operation
- performance characteristics and specifications
- operating instructions
- calibration procedures, including materials and/or equipment to be used
- operational precautions and any limitations
- hazards
- storage, handling or shipping instructions
- list of all materials provided as well as those materials required but not provided
- calibration details
- details of quality control procedures and materials required (i.e., state if there are both positive and negative controls)
- expected values
- specific performance characteristics (i.e., accuracy, precision, specificity and sensitivity)
- bibliography

Additional labeling requirements for OTC IVDs may be found in 21 CFR 801.60. Analyte-specific reagents (ASRs) are considered restricted devices under *FD&C Act* Section 520(e) and are defined and classified in 21 CFR 864.4020. The associated labeling is regulated by FDA (21 CFR 809.10(e) and 809.30). ASRs are defined as antibodies, both polyclonal and monoclonal; specific receptor proteins; ligands; nucleic acid sequences; and similar reagents that, through specific binding or chemical reaction with substances in a specimen, are intended for use in diagnostic application for identification and quantification of an individual chemical substance or ligand in biological specimens.[6] Although most are Class I devices, some more-complex ASRs require submission as Class II or III medical devices.

Unlike drug labels or labeling, there are no specific regulations establishing minimum requirements for key graphic elements such as bold type, bullet points, type size, spacing or use of vertical and horizontal lines for medical devices and IVDs. Within the labeling requirements, it is recommended that instructions or any specific user-related information be clear, concise and understandable by the user—either a healthcare professional or lay person. Although there are no regulations for key graphic elements in medical device labeling, 21 CFR 801.15 does, in fact, reference some specific labeling format requirements for prescription medical devices. Of particular note is the requirement that "[a]ll words, statements, and other information required by or under authority of the act to appear on the label or labeling shall appear thereon in the English language." This particular requirement has led to the interpretation that the use of any graphics, pictures or symbols in labeling that represent required information must be accompanied by explanatory English text adjacent to the symbol in order to "appear thereon in the English language." This has created no small challenge for manufacturers who utilize internationally recognized standards, such as (AAMI)/ANSI/ISO 15223-1:2012, *Medical Devices—Symbols to be Used With Medical Device Labels, Labeling and Information to be Supplied, Part 1, General Requirements*, for the development of their devices, requiring them to develop vastly different labels and labeling for devices to be marketed in the US and on international markets.

In response to industry complaints about this issue, FDA published a proposed rule in the *Federal Register* (Vol. 78, No. 76, Friday, 19 April 2013) concerning the use of symbols and graphic representations. Under this proposal, the regulations (21 CFR 660, 801, and 809) will be amended to explicitly allow the use of symbols under the following conditions:
- the symbol was developed and approved by a nationally or internationally recognized standards development organization
- the symbol is part of a standard recognized by the FDA for use in the labeling of medical devices
- the symbol is explained in a glossary accompanying the device
- additionally, the symbol, "Rx Only" would be officially authorized for medical devices

The comment period for this proposed rule change closed on 18 June 2013.

The labeling format for OTC medical devices is described in 21 CFR 801.60 and 801.61. Additionally, guidance documents are available to assist in developing such labels and labeling:
- *Guidance for Industry: Alternative to Certain Prescription Device Labeling Requirements* (January 2000)
- *Guidance on Medical Device Patient Labeling; Final Guidance for Industry and FDA Reviewers* (April 2001)
- Device Labeling Guidance #G91-1 (Blue Book Memo) (March 1991)
- *Write it Right: Recommendations for Developing User Instruction Manuals for Medical Devices Used in Home Health Care* (August 1993)
- *Human Factors Principles for Medical Device Labeling* (September 1993)
- *Guidance for Industry: User Labeling for Devices that Contain Natural Rubber (21 CFR 801.437); Small Entity Compliance Guide* (April 2003)

For IVDs
- *Guidance for Industry and FDA Staff: Use of Symbols on Labels and in Labeling of In Vitro Diagnostic*

Devices Intended for Professional Use (November 2004)
- *Guidance for Industry and FDA Staff: Commercially Distributed Analyte-Specific Reagents (ASRs): Frequently Asked Questions* (September 2007)

Since most medical device labeling consists of instructions for using the device properly and safely and, where necessary, any care instructions for the device, it would be appropriate to evaluate and include human factors when developing, writing and validating instructional labeling. "Human factors," in this context is the study or evaluation of how people use technology, specifically the interaction of human abilities, expectations and limitations with work environments and system design. FDA's Center for Devices and Radiological Health (CDRH) has a webpage dedicated to human factors (http://www.fda.gov/MedicalDevices/DeviceRegulationandGuidance/HumanFactors/default.htm), which includes links to specific FDA guidance documents.

It is important that all medical devices contain complete and accurate labeling, as it is essential for the device's safe and reliable operation, whether used by a customer in a home or by a professional in a hospital.[7] In addition to reviewing labeling requirements per 21 CFR 801 (medical devices) and 809 (ASRs and IVDs), two FDA guidance documents are available to manufacturers that contain examples of medical device labeling presentation, format and content: *Human Factors Principles for Medical Device Labeling* (September 1993) and *Write It Right, Recommendations for Developing User Instruction Manuals for Medical Devices Used in Home Health Care* (August 1993). These two guidance documents are important reference tools when developing and creating medical device labeling for both home and professional use. With the increased FDA emphasis on risk management and human factors, as evidenced by guidance documents previously referenced and the issuance of recent draft guidance documents such as, *Applying Human Factors and Usability Engineering to Optimize Medical Device Design*, it is clear that integrating label and labeling development into a manufacturer's design control verification and validation process is essential for FDA approval or clearance of medical devices and IVDs.

Furthermore, manufacturers must be aware that if they modify any of their medical devices, the labels and labeling should also be reviewed to ensure that they reflect all current revisions and/or specifications. Therefore, a manufacturer's internal change control process should include a means to capture such label and labeling reviews.

Jurisdiction for Promotional Labeling and Advertising

As noted in Chapter 16, the same agencies have jurisdiction over promotional labeling and advertising of medical devices, including IVDs, as over those for drug products. Healthcare product advertising is regulated by two federal agencies. First, the Federal Trade Commission (FTC), under the *Federal Trade Commission Act (FTC Act)*,[8] utilizes three legal standards (represented as policy statements) related to the regulation of all advertising: substantiation, deception and fairness. The *FTC Act* prohibits advertising that makes deceptive claims, fails to reveal material information, is unfair or makes objective claims for which there is no reasonable basis. FTC has primary responsibility for the advertising of foods, cosmetics, OTC drugs, nonrestricted medical devices and other products whose safety, efficacy and labeling are regulated by FDA.

A Memorandum of Understanding (MOU) between FDA and FTC establishing the division of responsibility between the two agencies with regard to advertising has been in effect since 1971. Although FTC retains legal authority over some aspects of advertising, it generally defers to FDA's more specific authority. Under the MOU, FDA has the primary responsibility for the labeling of foods, drugs, devices and cosmetics.

Each FDA center has its own division responsible for enforcing those regulations. Within the Center for Drug Evaluation and Research (CDER), The Office of Prescription Drug Promotion (OPDP) (formerly DDMAC—the Division of Drug Marketing, Advertising and Communication) is responsible for the regulation of prescription drug promotion (see Chapter 16). In 1993, the Center for Biologics Evaluation and Research (CBER) formed the Advertising and Promotional Labeling Staff (APLS) within the Office of Compliance and Biologics Quality to review and monitor the promotion of biologic products. Because some of the regulations are open to interpretation, this can result in the application of different standards to drug and biologic products competing in the same therapeutic class. In 2003, CDRH's Office of Compliance (OC) assumed responsibility for the review and enforcement of restricted medical device advertising and promotional materials.

CDRH has a webpage with links to all guidance documents covering medical devices and radiation-emitting products (http://www.fda.gov/MedicalDevices/DeviceRegulationandGuidance/GuidanceDocuments/default.htm).

The 1976 *Medical Device Amendments* to the *FD&C Act* gave FDA authority over the promotion of restricted medical devices.[9] As defined in Section 520(e) of the act, "restricted medical devices" have the potential for harmful effect or require collateral measures for use. They have no implementing regulation. However, the approval order for a PMA or FDA's recommendations for many devices cleared for marketing via 510(k) may restrict the device's sale, distribution and use as a condition of approval. Under 21 CFR 801(D)(b)(1), labeling must bear the statement: "Caution: Federal law restricts this device to sale by or on the order of a (indicate type of practitioner and, if applicable, required training/experience, and facilities to which use is restricted)." Promotional labeling cannot make claims beyond the intended use for which the device was cleared. FTC retains authority for nonrestricted medical devices.

It is important to note that while FDA governs the promotion of restricted medical devices, it also maintains authority over unapproved and uncleared devices used in investigational settings (i.e., clinical trials). Within the scope of 21 CFR 812.1, FDA allows the shipment of devices that otherwise would be required to conform with a performance standard or to have premarket approval for the purpose of conducting investigations of the device. Of importance in this section are the labeling requirements set forth in 21 CFR 812.5(a), which mandate the statement: "CAUTION – Investigational device. Limited by Federal (or United States) law to investigational use." Also required on the label or other labeling are descriptions of relevant contraindications, hazards, adverse effects, interfering substances or devices, warnings and precautions. Those placing investigational devices also must refrain from including any false or misleading statements, including those that would lead a user to believe that the device is safe or effective for its investigational purpose.

Promotional Labeling and Advertising

The terms "advertising," "marketing literature," "marketing communications" and the regulations surrounding them are somewhat vague with respect to medical devices and IVDs. Generally, advertising is differentiated from promotional labeling simply by the practicality of supplying a copy of the complete prescribing information versus providing only a brief summary. Even though FDA does not specifically define advertising, the agency's interpretation of labeling, as noted in the sections above, is broad enough to cover most printed materials regardless of media, which include most advertising. FDA's view of advertising also includes virtually all promotional activities including, but not limited to, written pamphlets, letters, websites, social media pages, video content (television, internet, hard disk, etc.), magazine ads, etc.

Unlike FDA regulations for prescription drug advertising and promotional materials (21 CFR 202.1), the agency currently has no specific advertising and promotional regulations for medical devices. However, the medical device labeling regulation (21 CFR 801.109(a)(2)) does discuss "other labeling," which FDA considers to be promotional labeling, and Section 502(r) of the *FD&C Act* addresses advertising for restricted devices.

Three applicable guidance documents provide current FDA thinking on promotional materials and activities: *"Help-Seeking" and Other Disease Awareness Communications by or on Behalf of Drug and Device Firms (Draft)* (January 2004); *Consumer-Directed Broadcast Advertising of Restricted Devices (Draft)* (February 2004); and *Good Reprint Practices for the Distribution of Medical Journal Articles and Medical or Scientific Reference Publications on Unapproved New Uses of Approved Drugs and Approved or Cleared Medical Devices (Final)* (January 2009).

FDA treats press releases, investor relations materials and exhibits as advertising, and therefore, these also are considered labeling by definition. Additionally, information posted on the Internet is considered promotional labeling rather than advertising.

Misbranding

Section 502 of the *FD&C Act* (21 U.S.C. 352) contains misbranding provisions for prescription devices. A device is misbranded and considered in violation of the law if the device labeling:

1. is false or misleading in any way
2. does not contain "adequate directions for use"

In the case of a restricted device, the labeling also must contain:

1. the device's established name printed in type at least half as large as the trade or brand name
2. a brief statement of the intended uses, relevant warnings, precautions, side effects and contraindications

21 CFR 801.125 does provide an exemption from the labeling requirements in 502(f)(1) (21 U.S.C. 352). Under this exemption, medical devices for use in research, analysis, law enforcement and instruction (in pharmacy, chemistry or medicine) need not be shipped with "adequate directions for use." The devices must not, however, be for clinical use. In the case of sale for instruction, these devices must be sold to persons regularly and lawfully engaged in that endeavor.

The *Medical Device Amendments* expanded the authority of the *FD&C Act* over misbranded medical devices. The amendments contain further conditions under which a device is considered misbranded:

- The device's established name (if applicable), name in an official compendium or common or usual name is not printed prominently in type at least half as large as used for any proprietary name.
- The device is subject to a performance standard and it does not bear the labeling requirements prescribed in that standard.
- There is a failure to comply with any requirement prescribed under the *FD&C Act* (Section 518, 21 U.S.C. 36h) on notification and other remedies; failure to furnish material or information requested by or under Section 518; or failure to furnish any materials or information requested by or under Section 519 of the act on records and reports.
- The device is commercially distributed without FDA clearance on a 510(k) premarket notification submission.

Scientific Dissemination of Information

In parallel with the rules for drugs outlined in Chapter 16, FDA traditionally has objected to the dissemination of information that is not supported by the approved product labeling, typically referred to as "off-label" information. FDA does not prohibit physicians from prescribing drugs or devices off label, allowing for the appropriate exchange of scientific information. However, the agency historically has had a restrictive policy on off-label information dissemination, which has been challenged repeatedly.

In response to the provisions outlined in the *Food and Drug Administration Modernization Act* of 1997 (*FDAMA*) regarding dissemination of information, FDA codified regulations under 21 CFR 99 entitled, "Dissemination of Information on Unapproved/New Uses for Marketed Drugs, Biologics, and Devices." These regulations do not apply to a manufacturer's lawful dissemination of information that responds to a healthcare practitioner's unsolicited request for information. The regulations state that off-label information concerning the safety, efficacy or benefit of a use that is not included in the approved labeling for a drug or device approved/cleared by FDA may, conditionally, be disseminated to applicable individuals or institutions (healthcare practitioner, pharmacy benefit manager, health insurance issuer, group health plan or federal or state governmental agency). The information disseminated must:

- be about a drug or device that has been approved, licensed or cleared for marketing by FDA
- be in the form of an unabridged, peer-reviewed journal reprint (does not include letters to the editor or abstracts) or reference publication
- not pose a significant risk to public health
- not be false or misleading
- not be derived from clinical research conducted by another manufacturer without permission

The regulations (21 CFR 99.103) also require that the disseminated off-label information prominently display:

- the statement "This information concerns a use that has not been approved (additionally "or cleared" for devices) by the Food and Drug Administration"
- information on the research funding and the association of the authors and investigators with the manufacturer, and a statement, if applicable, if there are products or treatments that have been approved or cleared for the use being presented in the off-label information
- a copy of the approved labeling
- a bibliography of other relevant articles (supporting and not supporting the off-label information)
- any other information that will provide objectivity and balance to the information being presented

The regulations also require that the manufacturer submit the information 60 days before dissemination and eventually submit a supplemental application for the new use that is the subject of the disseminated information.

The requirements in these regulations have been legally challenged by claiming protection under the First Amendment's provisions for freedom of speech. In response to such challenges, FDA clarified that rather than defining the requirements, these regulations provide sponsors with a "safe harbor" to disseminate information on unapproved new uses for marketed drugs, biologics and devices under specific conditions without threat of enforcement action. This safe harbor allows for the dissemination of information regarding the safety, effectiveness or benefits of new uses of approved or cleared products but does not provide for statements about approved uses that FDA would otherwise find misleading. FDA reserves the right, on a case-by-case basis, to prosecute a manufacturer for misbranding its product if it can be shown that the company was promoting an unapproved use. At least one court has sided with industry, opining that FDA permits physicians to practice medicine and use pharmaceuticals and devices off-label, but "prohibits the free flow of information [from industry] that would inform that outcome" (*United States v. Caronia*, 703 F.3d 149 (2d Cir. 2012). While not the law of the land, this ruling protects this dissemination of information under the auspices of free speech.

In January 2009, the guidance entitled, *Good Reprint Practices for the Distribution of Medical Journal Articles and Medical or Scientific Reference Publications on Unapproved New Uses of Approved Drugs and Approved or Cleared Medical Devices* was issued. Much of this draft guidance originates from the regulations found in 21 CFR 99. It discusses the:

- various types of reprints, articles and reference publications that are permitted to be distributed
- manner of the dissemination of scientific and medical information

Enforcement

FDA can enforce violations of the *FD&C Act* or agency regulations through a variety of mechanisms, including Notices of Violations (NOV) or "untitled letters," Warning Letters and, if the violation warrants, referring the issue for judicial action. With regard to devices, FDA will look at such things as a company website, videos, brochures, flyers/promotional flyers, advertisements in journals, bulk mailings, press releases and newsletters. FDA usually sends an NOV for the least violative practices that, in the agency's opinion, do not greatly jeopardize the public health. An NOV usually requires only that the company stop using materials that contain the claim the agency found to be violative. FDA may also issue a Warning Letter with or without a prior NOV letter. Warning Letters contain stronger language and generally are addressed to the company's CEO. In addition to requiring the company to cease using the violative materials, Warning Letters may require the company to provide corrective actions. For example, a company may be required to run a remedial advertisement to reach the same audience as the original violative advertisement or disseminate corrective information through the issue of a "Dear Healthcare Professional" letter as described in 21 CFR 200.5(c)(3). Warning Letters also frequently direct the sponsor to provide FDA with information on any other promotional items that contain similar messages. All FDA Warning Letters, regardless of issuing center or office, are available at http://www.fda.gov/ICECI/EnforcementActions/WarningLetters/default.htm.

With the advent of social media, a new frontier of advertisement has sprung up within the medical device and pharmaceutical industries. FDA has delayed providing guidance to industry on this topic; therefore, there is no clear direction on proper use of these newer tools. Regardless of its lack of direction, FDA is still taking enforcement actions against companies it deems are breaking the rules in the use of social media. FDA has included "liking" consumer comments on Facebook in a Warning Letter. The agency's apparent rationale is that the "like" by the company is an endorsement of uncleared or unapproved claims (See Amarc Enterprises Warning Letter http://www.fda.gov/ICECI/EnforcementActions/WarningLetters/2012/ucm340266.htm). While this example is for a drug, it shows the agency's thinking with regard to social media, and the care that a company must take with their presence on line.

If FDA is not satisfied by the sponsor's response to the actions, it may choose to recommend enforcement action in the form of injunctions, seizures and/or criminal prosecution. The Department of Justice carries out these activities. One possible outcome is that the company agrees to enter into an arrangement with the government, called a consent decree. A consent decree places severe restrictions on company operations to ensure the firm comes into compliance.

Actions That May be Brought by Competitors

The *Lanham Act*[10] of 1946 (*US Trademark Act*) allows private parties a course of action against false and misleading advertising. Trademarks, themselves, identify the source of a product. The *Lanham Act* prohibits the use of another's mark and false or unfair advertising and is administered by the Patent and Trademark Office (PTO). This act has been amended several times under the *Trademark Law Revision Act* of 1988, which made it easier to register trademarks, and the *Trademark Dilution Act* of 1995, which prohibited the use of terms that would dilute a trademark (e.g., Buick aspirin). Although not often invoked in these cases, state laws covering false advertising, defamation and disparagement also can be applied to comparative advertising. FTC brings cases, primarily before administrative judges, against those companies it believes are making misleading statements in their promotions. In cases of fraud, FTC brings these into federal court. Many companies will settle out of court, agreeing to "cease and desist" while not admitting guilt.

Summary

- Labeling subject to FDA regulations includes the container label, the package insert used by the physician, patient labeling/medication guide and promotional labeling.
- FDA and FTC regulate healthcare product advertising. FDA regulates advertising for drugs (CDER, OPDP) and restricted medical devices (CDRH, OC) under the *FD&C Act* and biologics (CBER, APLS) under the *PHS Act*. FTC regulates food, cosmetics, OTC drugs and nonrestricted medical devices under the *FTC Act*.
- Advertising and promotional materials must not be false or misleading, must present fair balance and must reveal material facts.
- Advertising and promotional labeling are not allowed for unapproved products or unapproved uses of an approved product.
- FDA does, conditionally, allow for the appropriate exchange of scientific materials (unsolicited requests, scientific exhibits).
- FDA can enforce violations through NOVs, Warning Letters or judicial action (consent decrees, injunctions and seizures).

References

1. *Food, Drug, and Cosmetic Act* of 1938 (under Title 21 of the United States Code (U.S.C.)).
2. *Kordel v United States*, 335 U.S. 345 (1948) (available at http://supreme.justia.com/us/335/345/).
3. 21 CFR Part 801 Labeling. FDA website. http://www.accessdata.fda.gov/scripts/cdrh/cfdocs/cfcfr/cfrsearch.cfm?cfrpart=801. Accessed 22 May 2013.
4. *Guidance for Industry: Alternative to Certain Prescription Device Labeling Requirements* (January 2000). FDA website. http://www.fda.gov/downloads/MedicalDevices/DeviceRegulationandGuidance/GuidanceDocuments/ucm072748.pdf. Accessed 22 May 2013.
5. 21 CFR Part 812 Investigational Device Exemptions. FDA website. http://www.accessdata.fda.gov/scripts/cdrh/cfdocs/cfcfr/cfrsearch.cfm?cfrpart=812. Accessed 22 May 2013.
6. 21 CFR 864.4020(a) Analyte specific reagents, Identification. FDA website. http://www.accessdata.fda.gov/scripts/cdrh/cfdocs/cfcfr/cfrsearch.cfm?fr=864.4020. Accessed 22 May 2013.
7. *Human Factors Principles for Medical Device Labeling* (September 1993). FDA website. http://www.fda.gov/downloads/MedicalDevices/.../UCM095300.pdf. Accessed 22 May 2013.
8. *Federal Trade Commission Act* of 1914 (*FTC Act*).
9. *Public Health Service Act* of 1944 (*PHS Act*), 42 USC Section 351 [262].
10. *Trademark Act* of 1946 (*Lanham Act*), 15 USC Chapter 22.

Chapter 21

In Vitro Diagnostics Submissions and Compliance

Updated by Jocelyn Jennings, MS, RAC

OBJECTIVES

- Know the definition of an in vitro diagnostic device (IVD)
- Understand the risk-based classification of IVDs
- Understand the regulatory submission types and their requirements
- Understand the labeling requirements for IVDs
- Know where to find additional information

LAWS, REGULATIONS AND GUIDELINES COVERED IN THIS CHAPTER

- 21 CFR 50, Protection of human subjects
- 21 CFR 54, Financial Disclosure
- 21 CFR 56, Institutional review boards
- 21 CFR 801, Labeling
- 21 CFR 809, In vitro diagnostic products for human use
- 21 CFR 812, Investigational device exemptions
- 21 CFR 814, Premarket approval of medical devices
- 21 CFR 820, Quality system regulation
- 21 CFR 862, Clinical chemistry and clinical toxicology devices
- 21 CFR 864, Hematology and pathology devices
- 21 CFR 866, Immunology and microbiology devices
- 42 CFR 493, Laboratory Requirements
- *Guidance for Industry and FDA Staff: In Vitro Diagnostic (IVD) Device Studies—Frequently Asked Questions* (June 2010)
- *Guidance for Industry and FDA Staff: Administrative Procedures for CLIA Categorization* (May 2008)
- *In Vitro Diagnostic Devices: Guidance for the Preparation of 510(k) Submissions* (January 1997)
- *New Section 513(f)(2)—Evaluation of Automatic Class III Designation, Guidance for Industry and CDRH Staff* (February 1998)
- *Guidance for the Content of Premarket Submissions for Software Contained in Medical Devices* (May 2005)
- *Draft Guidance for Industry and FDA Staff Medical Devices: The Pre-Submission Program and Meetings with FDA Staff* (July 2012)

Definition of an IVD

"In vitro diagnostics" (IVDs) are defined in Title 21 of the Code of Federal Regulations (CFR) Part 809.3 as "those reagents, instruments, and systems intended for use in the diagnosis of disease or other conditions, including a determination of the state of health, in order to cure, mitigate, treat, or prevent disease or its sequelae. Such products are intended for use in the collection, preparation, and examination of specimens taken from the human body."

The definition given in 21 CFR 809.3 also states that IVDs are devices as defined in Section 201(h) of the *Federal Food, Drug, and Cosmetic Act* (*FD&C Act*) and that they also may be biological products regulated under Section 351 of the *Public Health Service Act* (*PHS Act*). IVDs may be considered to be a subset of medical devices, the defining characteristic being the use of specimens taken from the human body. The US Food and Drug Administration's (FDA) classification rules define more than 500 different types of medical devices that meet the definition of an in vitro diagnostic product. Worldwide, the IVD industry accounts for more than $50 billion annually in diagnostic tests alone.

Additionally, the labeling regulation in 21 CFR 809.10 defines two other types of products: Research Use Only (RUO) and Investigational Use Only (IUO). Both RUO and IUO products are considered to be pre-commercial and, under specific circumstances, may be shipped without fully complying with the labeling requirements that apply to commercial IVDs.

RUO products are those "in the laboratory research phase of development, and not represented as an effective in vitro diagnostic product" (21 CFR 809.10(c)(2)(i)). Such products must be prominently labeled with the following statement: "For Research Use Only. Not for use in diagnostic procedures." RUO products are reagents, instruments or test systems that are under development and being evaluated for their potential use as IVDs, or are used in basic life science research and not intended for further development for a clinical diagnostic use.

IUO products are those "being shipped or delivered for product testing prior to full commercial marketing (for example, for use on specimens derived from humans to compare the usefulness of the product with other products or procedures which are in current use or recognized as useful)" (21 CFR 809.10(c)(2)(ii)). IUO products are reagents, instruments or test systems that are being used in a "clinical investigation or research involving one or more subjects to determine the safety and effectiveness of a device" (21 CFR 812.3(h)). Such products must be prominently labeled with the following statement: "For Investigational Use Only. The performance characteristics of this product have not been established."

Finally, the classification rules in 21 CFR 864 define two additional types of specimen preparation reagents: General Purpose Reagents (GPRs), and Analyte Specific Reagents (ASRs).

GPR products are chemical reagents having "a general laboratory application, that is used to collect, prepare, and examine specimens from the human body for diagnostic purposes, and that is not labeled or otherwise intended for specific diagnostic application" (21 CFR 864.4010(a)). Importantly, GPRs are classified as Class I (general controls) and exempt from premarket notification, subject to the limitations described in 21 CFR 864.9. Such products must be labeled in accordance with 21 CFR 809.10(d) with basic identifying information, warnings and precautions and the statement: "For Laboratory Use."

ASR products are "antibodies, both polyclonal and monoclonal, specific receptor proteins, ligands, nucleic acid sequences, and similar reagents which, through specific binding or chemical reaction with substances in a specimen, are intended for use in a diagnostic application for identification and quantification of an individual chemical substance or ligand in biological specimens" (21 CFR 864.4020(a)). Information on the classification of ASRs is given in 21 CFR 864.4020(b). ASRs are Class I and exempt from premarket notification except when they are used in blood banking tests that have been classified as Class II (e.g., cytomegalovirus serological reagents), and when they are intended to be used as components in Class III tests used in contagious fatal diseases (e.g., tuberculosis) or blood donor screening (e.g., blood group typing or hepatitis). ASRs must be labeled in accordance with 21 CFR 809.10(e)(1). Class I ASRs must bear the statement: "Analyte Specific Reagent. Analytical and performance characteristics are not established." Class II and III ASRs must bear the statement: "Analyte Specific Reagent. Except as a component of the approved/cleared test (Name of approved/cleared test), analytical and performance characteristics of this ASR are not established."

FDA Classification and Regulation of IVDs

As with all other medical devices, IVDs are regulated according to a risk-based classification scheme based on their intended use. Factors that determine the classification of IVDs include whether the device is intended for diagnosis, monitoring or screening of a specific disease or condition; the patient population in which it will be used; the type of specimen to be tested; and the consequence of a false test result.

FDA classifies IVD products into Class I, II or III depending upon the level of control necessary to ensure that the devices are reasonably safe and effective when they are placed on the market. The classification determines the regulatory pathway to market. The CFR lists the classification of existing IVDs in 21 CFR 862 (clinical chemistry and toxicology devices), 864 (hematology and pathology devices) and 866 (immunology and microbiology devices).

Class I IVDs are the lowest risk category. Most are exempt from premarket review and are subject to General Controls only. (Some Class I IVDs do require submission of a premarket notification (510(k)). These are termed "Reserved Devices" and include a total of 44 devices in 21 CFR 862, 864 and 866.) General Controls apply to all medical devices, regardless of class, and include establishment registration as a manufacturer, distributor, repackager or relabeler; listing the devices intended to be marketed with FDA; manufacturing in accordance with Good Manufacturing Practices (GMPs) (21 CFR 820), including maintenance of records and providing reports to FDA; and labeling in accordance with 21 CFR 801 and 809.

Approximately 50% of the IVDs currently marketed are regulated as Class I. Some examples of Class I IVDs include clinical chemistry tests for urine pH and osmolality, reagents and kits for immunohistochemistry stains and serological reagents for immunology and microbiology.

Class II IVDs are those products that pose a moderate risk of harm due to a false test result. Their design and mode of operation typically are more complex. Most Class II products require submission of a premarket notification (510(k)) that includes evidence for a determination of "substantial equivalence" to a similar product already on the market. In addition to General Controls, Class II products require "Special Controls" to assure safety and effectiveness. Special Controls include certain mandatory performance standards, special labeling requirements and requirements for postmarket surveillance.

Approximately 42% of the IVDs currently marketed are regulated as Class II. Some examples of Class II IVDs include clinical chemistry tests for newborn screening for metabolic disorders, hematology tests for sickle cell hemoglobin and microbiology tests for pathogenic organisms that cause such diseases as meningitis.

Class III IVDs are those products that present a potential high risk of harm due to a false test result. These typically employ complex methodologies and algorithms for calculating a result and may be intended for diagnosis of serious infectious diseases. Class III products are those for which General Controls and Special Controls alone are not sufficient to provide assurances of safety and effectiveness. They are subject to the most rigorous premarket scrutiny, often requiring extensive clinical data. Class III products require submission of a Premarket Approval application (PMA), which includes a complete description of the manufacturing process and clinical evidence (diagnostic sensitivity and specificity) of safety and effectiveness in the intended use population.

Approximately 8% of the IVDs currently marketed are regulated as Class III. Some examples of Class III IVDs include tests for screening for various cancers (e.g., breast, prostate) and tests for screening the blood supply for infectious agents, such as Hepatitis B and C.

Under an intercenter agreement that became effective in October 1991, two centers within FDA share responsibility for regulating IVDs—the Center for Devices and Radiological Health (CDRH) and the Center for Biologics Evaluation and Research (CBER). CDRH was assigned the lead role for policy development, procedural regulations, regulating all IVDs not assigned to CBER, small business assistance programs, registration and listing, GMP advisory activities and medical device reporting. CBER was assigned the lead role in regulating all IVDs for screening or confirmatory laboratory tests associated with blood banking operations, as well as those medical devices intended for use in collecting, processing, storing and administering blood products and their components. Each center retains authority for surveillance activities and compliance actions, issuing Special Controls guidance documents and performance standards and reviewing IDE, 510(k) and PMA submissions.

The Office of Blood Research and Review (OBRR) within CBER administers the premarket review and postmarket surveillance and compliance programs for IVDs assigned to the center. The Office of In Vitro Diagnostic Device Evaluation and Safety (OIVD) within CDRH administers the premarket review and postmarket surveillance and compliance programs for all other IVDs. OIVD also is responsible for making complexity categorization and waiver determinations under the *Clinical Laboratory Improvement Amendments* (*CLIA*) of 1988, which set standards and certification requirements for clinical laboratory tests. OIVD is organized into three principal divisions: the Division of Chemistry and Toxicology Devices (DCTD), the Division of Immunology and Hematology Devices (DIHD) and the Division of Microbiology Devices (DMD). On an annual basis, OIVD processes more than 1,000 premarket submissions and more than 2,000 *CLIA* determinations and implements more than 150 compliance actions.

The Application of the CLIA to IVDs

As stated above, *CLIA* set standards and certification requirements for clinical laboratory tests. OIVD is responsible for the program for complexity categorization and waiver determinations of commercially marketed *in vitro* diagnostic tests under *CLIA*. Categorization is the process by which FDA assigns IVDs to one of three *CLIA* complexity categories based on the potential risk to the public health. The categories are Waived, Moderate Complexity and High Complexity. FDA evaluates seven criteria to determine the complexity of an IVD and assigns a number score (1 = Low; 2 = Intermediate; 3 = High) to each. The evaluation criteria include: the scientific or technical knowledge required to perform the test; necessary training and experience; the complexity of the preparation of reagents and test materials; characteristics of the operational steps; the need for calibration, QC and proficiency testing; troubleshooting and maintenance; and the difficulty of interpreting the test results. The scores for each criterion are then totaled. Tests receiving scores of 12 or less are assigned Moderate Complexity. Tests receiving scores of 12 or higher are assigned High Complexity. Waived tests are those tests that were specified in the regulations that *CLIA* implemented (42 CFR 493) or tests that are granted a waiver by FDA following review of an application containing valid scientific data that demonstrates the test is simple to use, accurate and unlikely to pose a risk of harm to the patient if performed inaccurately. Manufacturers apply for a *CLIA* categorization during the premarket review process. Further information can be found in *Guidance for Industry and FDA Staff: Administrative Procedures for CLIA Categorization.*

Premarket Submission Types for IVDs

As discussed above, the classification of an IVD determines the regulatory pathway to market. Class II IVDs require submission of a premarket notification (510(k)) at least 90 days prior to placing the device on the market. The 510(k) must contain evidence that the device to be marketed is "substantially equivalent" (SE) to another device that is already legally marketed (i.e., safe and effective). This is termed the "predicate device." A predicate device is one that has a similar intended use and similar technological characteristics. Once FDA has determined that the new device is SE to the predicate device, the new device is "cleared" for marketing in the US. If FDA determines that the new device has no predicate or that its performance is not equivalent to the predicate, then a "not substantially equivalent" (NSE) decision is rendered. The content and format of a 510(k) are given in *In Vitro Diagnostic Devices: Guidance for the Preparation of 510(k) Submissions.* The evidence establishing substantial equivalence to the predicate consists of nonclinical and clinical performance data. This includes analytical sensitivity and specificity, precision, limit of detection, reproducibility and reagent and sample stability. FDA recommends the use of standards published by the Clinical Laboratory Standards Institute (CLSI) to guide the evaluation of analytical performance. Additionally, a method comparison study showing similar clinical performance as the predicate device is also required. This is typically done by calculating the percent agreement between the two methods using retrospectively collected clinical samples. In some cases, a prospective clinical trial using both the predicate and new device is required for Class I and Class II IVDs. OIVD posts a Decision Summary of the 510(k) review on the FDA website that details the basis for the SE determination. These summaries provide manufacturers with valuable information on the choice of likely predicates and data requirements for establishing substantial equivalence to a predicate.

Class III IVDs require submission of a PMA. The required elements of a PMA are given in 21 CFR 814. PMAs are reviewed under a 180-day timeline. For most PMAs, a clinical study using prospectively collected samples is required to establish the device's safety and effectiveness. Such studies must be conducted in accordance with the Informed Consent regulations in 21 CFR 50, the Institutional Review Board regulations in 21 CFR 56 and Financial Disclosure regulations in 21 CFR 54. If the device is the first of its kind, or if FDA's review of the PMA raises significant questions regarding safety and effectiveness, FDA may seek advice or a determination of approvability of a PMA from an advisory panel comprised of external experts. In most cases, an inspection of the manufacturer's facility by FDA is required prior to approval of a PMA. FDA often will add postapproval requirements for manufacturers of Class III devices as a condition of approval. These may include additional studies of safety and effectiveness and periodic reporting of the results of such studies. Once a formal approval order is issued, FDA posts a Summary of Safety and Effectiveness Data (SSED) on its website.

Another important premarket mechanism is the *de novo* reclassification. This was created by the *Food and Drug Administration Modernization Act* of 1997 (*FDAMA*) as a way of classifying new, lower-risk devices that were automatically placed in Class III when the original classification rules were established. Such devices have no predicate, but are devices for which Special Controls would be an appropriate means of controlling risks and ensuring that the devices are reasonably safe and effective. *De novo* allows a manufacturer of an IVD that has been found NSE due to the lack of a predicate device to submit a petition to have a risk-based classification made for the device (often Class II) without submitting a PMA. The petition must include identification of the IVD's risks and benefits, the Special Controls the manufacturer believes will adequately control risks and ensure safety and effectiveness, and a recommendation as to whether the IVD should be placed in Class I or Class II. FDA will make a classification determination within 60 days. If the IVD is placed in either Class I or II, it may be legally marketed and will then become a predicate for any future device having the same intended use and technological characteristics. The *de novo* process is explained in detail in *New Section 513(f)(2)—Evaluation of Automatic Class III Designation, Guidance for Industry and CDRH Staff* (note: this guidance document is being revised by FDA to be in line with *Food and Drug Administration Safety and Innovation Act* of 2012 (*FDASIA*)).

The Pre-Submission

In 1995, FDA issued a memorandum introducing the pre-IDE submission as a mechanism for sponsors of Investigational Device Exemption (IDE) applications under 21 CFR 812 to submit preliminary information to FDA prior to submitting an IDE. Since most IVDs are exempted from the IDE regulations, the pre-IDE has become an informal method for manufacturers to obtain advice and comment on the regulatory pathway and proposed studies prior to submission of a 510(k) or PMA. In fact, OIVD routinely requests that manufacturers submit a pre-IDE when a new device has novel performance characteristics or a new intended use. This is specifically designed for those devices that are likely to require a *de novo* petition, *CLIA* waiver application or complex 510(k) or PMA submission for multiplex tests or companion diagnostics. A pre-IDE also may be useful when a manufacturer is submitting its first premarket application. A pre-IDE should be submitted when the intended use (including the target patient population) has been defined and the manufacturer is ready to discuss the analytical and clinical performance studies that may be required for clearance or approval. *FDASIA* expanded the concept of pre-IDE to include submissions for CBER. The pre-IDE is now known as the pre-Submission (or pre-Sub). The pre-Sub process begins with the submission of a written request to the Document Mail Center. The exchange of information between the submitter of a pre-Sub and FDA may take the form of written memoranda or in-person meetings or teleconferences. An important consideration regarding the pre-Sub is that it is nonbinding on both the manufacturer and FDA.

The pre-Sub package consists of a cover letter with contact information, a brief device description, proposed intended use, predicate device (if known), previous submissions or discussions, overview of product development and any specific questions the manufacturer has regarding the proposed analytical and clinical performance studies or regulatory pathway. Typically, FDA will respond to a pre-Sub submission within 90 days by returning a pre-Sub review memo to the submitter. This document will contain FDA's most current thinking regarding how the device is likely to be regulated and the data likely to be required in a 510(k) or PMA submission. A manufacturer may request a pre-Sub meeting with FDA in person, and vice versa.

Software Considerations for IVDs

Many IVDs employ software to control instrumentation and to calculate complex algorithms prior to providing the test result. As is the case for other medical devices, FDA regulates the software that is integral to the operation and safety of diagnostic test systems. Therefore, a certain amount of information related to the design and development of software must be included in premarket submissions. The extent of the documentation to be included in a 510(k) or PMA is based on the software's "Level of Concern." FDA defines the Level of Concern as Minor, Moderate or Major depending on the role of the software in causing, controlling or mitigating hazards that may result in injury to the patient or device operator. FDA classifies most IVD software as Moderate Level of Concern. Among the software documentation required to be submitted in premarket applications, the most important is a risk analysis. This must include the hardware and software hazards identified in the course of design and development, an assessment of their severity and the mitigations implemented to control them. To the extent that software plays a role in mitigating hazards associated with the laboratory examination of clinical specimens (e.g., user errors; incorrect or delayed diagnostic results), the hazard analysis must address the severity of the harm resulting from software failures. FDA defines these terms and the level of software verification and validation documentation required in *Guidance for the Content of Premarket Submissions for Software Contained in Medical Devices.*

Recent Trends in IVD Compliance—Laboratory Developed Tests (LDTs)

Recently, FDA has begun focusing attention on the marketing of so called "home brew" tests by clinical laboratories that have historically been regulated under *CLIA*. Since the passage of the *CLIA* regulations in 1988, diagnostic tests have reached the market in one of two ways: FDA clearance or approval of a premarket application submitted by a commercial manufacturer, or the offering of such tests directly to clinicians by *CLIA*-licensed laboratories. In a regulatory practice known as "enforcement discretion," FDA allowed the commercialization of such "laboratory developed tests" (LDTs) without premarket review. Over the past decade, FDA has become increasingly concerned with the lack of oversight of such tests, particularly a subset of molecular diagnostic tests that purported to predict the genetic risk of developing clinical diseases that were marketed on direct-to-consumer (DTC) websites. Specifically, FDA cited concerns over the apparent lack of clinical validation, absence of premarket review of diagnostic claims and the lack of postmarket surveillance and reporting. Beginning in 2000, FDA published a number of draft guidance documents related to the use of ASRs in the development of such tests and began exercising its authority over ASRs and ROUs.

In June of 2010, FDA sent a number of regulatory letters to companies operating *CLIA*-certified laboratories offering DTC genetic tests. This was followed on 19–20 July 2010 by an unprecedented two-day public meeting in which FDA, industry and the public gave their perspectives on FDA oversight of LDTs. During the meeting, FDA stated its concerns that the *CLIA* regulations alone were insufficient to evaluate evidence of analytical and clinical validation of test performance of LDTs. FDA was further concerned about the lack of quality system requirements on ASRs, design controls (particularly with regard to validation of software) and postmarket surveillance (e.g., recalls and medical device reporting).

During the course of the FDA public meeting on LDTs, OIVD issued additional regulatory letters to manufacturers of genetic tests. Subsequently, on 22 July 2010, the Subcommittee on Oversight and Investigations of the US House of Representatives Committee on Energy & Commerce held a hearing on "Direct-To-Consumer Genetic Testing and the Consequences to the Public Health," where testimony was provided by representatives of CDRH, the General Accountability Office and several companies offering DTC genetic tests. Since then, FDA has been conducting an internal review prior to preparing further guidance on these matters.

FDA has stated that it will apply a risk-based classification to higher-risk LDTs similar to the current regulations that apply to commercial IVDs. This would bring FDA oversight to tests intended for companion diagnostics associated with drug therapy, screening or diagnosis of cancer and other tests for potentially fatal communicable diseases.

Summary

IVDs are a subset of medical devices that are "intended for use in the collection, preparation, and examination of specimens taken from the human body." FDA's classification rules define more than 500 different types of medical devices that meet the definition of an IVD.

Research Use Only (RUO) and Investigational Use Only (IUO) products are considered to be pre-commercial, and under specific circumstances, may be shipped without fully complying with the labeling requirements that apply to commercial IVDs.

IVDs are regulated according to a risk-based classification scheme as either Class I, II or III, based on their intended use. Factors that determine the classification of IVDs include whether the device is intended for diagnosis, monitoring or screening of a specific disease or condition; the patient population in which it will be used; the type of specimen to be tested; and the consequence of a false test result.

Most Class I IVDs are exempt from premarket review and are subject to General Controls only. Class II IVDs require submission of a premarket notification (510(k)) at least 90 days prior to placing the device on the market. The 510(k) must contain evidence that the device to be marketed is "substantially equivalent" to another device that is already legally marketed (i.e., safe and effective). This is termed the "predicate device." A predicate device is one that has a similar intended use and similar technological characteristics. Class III IVDs require submission of a PMA. For most PMAs, a clinical study using prospectively collected samples is required to establish the device's safety and effectiveness. Such studies must be conducted in accordance with the Informed Consent regulations and the Institutional Review Board regulations.

General Controls apply to all IVD devices, regardless of class, and include establishment registration as a manufacturer, distributor, repackager or relabeler; listing the devices intended to be marketed with FDA; manufacturing in accordance with GMPs (21 CFR 820), including maintenance of records and providing reports to FDA; and labeling in accordance with 21 CFR 801 and 809.

Sources of Additional Information
- The Office of In Vitro Diagnostic Device Evaluation and Safety (OIVD) website (http://www.fda.gov/MedicalDevices/ProductsandMedicalProcedures/InVitroDiagnostics/default.htm) is the primary source of information on IVD regulations, guidance documents, CLIA categorizations, relevant standards, assistance and guidance on pre- and post-market issues and information on cleared/approved IVDs.
- The Association of Medical Diagnostics Manufacturers (AMDM) website (http://amdm.org/) contains archived FDA presentations from public meetings and web links to FDA resources.

Chapter 22

Biologics Submissions

Updated by Linda Yang, PhD, MBA, RAC

OBJECTIVES

- Learn basic concept of biologics

- Understand the organizational structure and responsibilities of the Center for Biologics Evaluation and Research (CBER)

- Understand the changes to biologics regulation resulting from the *Biologics Price Competition and Innovation Act* of 2009

- Understand CBER's Investigational New Drug (IND) process

- Become familiar with US Food and Drug Administration (FDA) recommendations for development of biologics, including requirements for clinical, manufacturing and preclinical development during clinical stages

- Understand the contents of the Biologic License Application (BLA) and BLA review process.

- Become familiar with FDA and sponsor meetings procedure and requirements

- Become familiar with FDA regulations for biologics

LAWS, REGULATIONS AND GUIDELINES COVERED IN THIS CHAPTER

- *Public Health Service Act*, Section 351, including new section (k) Licensure of Biological Products as Biosimilar or Interchangeable

- *Federal Food, Drug, and Cosmetic Act* of 1938

- 21 CFR 210 Current Good Manufacturing Practice in Manufacturing, Processing, Packing, or Holding of Drugs, General

- 21 CFR 211 Good Manufacturing Practice for Finished Pharmaceuticals

- 21 CFR 600 Biological Products: General

- 21 CFR 601 Biologics Licensing

- 21 CFR 610 General Biological Products Standards

- 21 CFR 312 Investigational New Drug Application

- 21 CFR 314 Applications for FDA Approval to Market a New Drug

- 21 CFR 25 Environmental Impact Considerations

- ICH M4: The Common Technical Document

- Administrative Processing of Biologics License Applications (BLA), SOPP 8401

- *Guidance for Sponsors, Industry, Researchers, Investigators, and Food and Drug Administration*

- *Staff: Certifications To Accompany Drug, Biological Product, and Device Applications/ Submissions: Compliance with Section 402(j) of The Public Health Service Act, Added By Title VIII of The Food and Drug Administration Amendments Act of 2007*

- ☐ *Draft Guidance for the Public and the Food and Drug Administration Staff on Convening Advisory Committee Meetings* (August 2008)

- ☐ *Guidance for Industry: Formal Dispute Resolution: Appeals Above the Division Level* (February 2000)

- ☐ *"Intercenter Consultative/Collaborative Review Process"* (August 2002), SOPP 8001.5

- ☐ *Guidance for Industry: Cooperative Manufacturing Arrangements for Licensed Biologics* (November 2008)

- ☐ *Guidance for Industry: Submitting Type V Drug Master Files to the Center for Biologics Evaluation and Research* (August 2001)

- ☐ SOPP 8110, *"Investigational and Marketable Applications: Submission of Regulatory Documents to CBER"* (February 2003)

- ☐ *Draft Guidance for Industry: Investigational New Drugs (INDs)—Determining whether Human Research Studies can be Conducted without an IND* (October 2010)

Introduction

The *Public Health Service Act* (*PHS Act*, 42 United States Code 262), Section 351(i) defines a biological product as "any virus, therapeutic serum, toxin, antitoxin, vaccine, blood, blood component or derivative, allergenic product, protein (except any chemically modified synthetic polypeptide), or analogous product... that is intended for use in the diagnosis, cure, mitigation, treatment, or prevention of disease."

Biological products can be composed of sugars, proteins or nucleic acids, or a combination of these substances. They may also be living entities, such as cells and tissues. Biologics are made from a variety of natural resources—human, animal and microorganism—and may be produced by biotechnology methods.

Most drugs consist of pure chemical substances, and their structures are known. Most biologics, however, are complex mixtures that are not easily identified or characterized. Biological products differ from conventional drugs in that they tend to be heat-sensitive and susceptible to microbial contamination. This requires sterile processes to be applied from initial manufacturing steps.

Pursuant to Section 351(a) of the *PHS Act*, a biologics license must be in effect for any biological product introduced or delivered for introduction into interstate commerce. A submission for a biologic product approval is called a Biologics License Application (BLA). Biological products subject to the *PHS Act* also meet the definition of "drugs" under Sections 201(g) of the *Federal Food, Drug, and Cosmetic Act* of 1938 (*FD&C Act*) and must comply with Title 21 of the Code of Federal Regulations (CFR) Parts 210 and 211, current Good Manufacturing Practices (CGMPs).

Center for Biologics Evaluation and Research

The primary US Food and Drug Administration (FDA) reviewing center for a biological product is the Center for Biologics Evaluation and Research (CBER).

Effective 30 June 2003, oversight responsibility for "well-characterized" or "therapeutic" biological products was transferred from CBER to the Center for Drug Evaluation and Research (CDER). The review of those therapeutic proteins is done by the appropriate therapeutic review division within CDER's Office of New Drugs (OND). These products continue to be regulated as licensed biologics (i.e., BLA) per 21 CFR 601.2(a). CDER also has responsibility for hormone protein products, e.g., insulin, growth hormone and pituitary hormones, as part of an October 1991 Inter-center Agreement between CBER and CDER; however, these products have been regulated as NDAs. However, under the *Biologics Price Competition and Innovation Act* (*BPCI Act*), proteins (with the exception of synthetic polypeptides) that have been approved as NDAs will be considered licensed biologics and will be required to comply with Section 351 of the *PHS Act* by March 2020, 10 years after the date of enactment of the *BPCI Act*.

CBER's regulatory authority is derived from the *PHS Act*, Section 351(a). The first biologics regulation, the *Biologics Control Act*, was approved in 1902. The Division of Biologics Standards (DBS) within the National Institutes of Health (NIH) was responsible for the control and release of biologics until 1972. The DBS was transferred from NIH to FDA and renamed the Bureau of Biologics, which ultimately became CBER. **Table 22-1** lists key milestones in the regulatory oversight of biologics. CBER regulates a wide range of biological products, including:

- allergenic extracts (e.g., for allergy shots and tests)
- blood and blood components
- plasma derivatives
- gene therapy products
- devices and test kits

Table 22-1. History of Biologics Regulation

Year	Regulatory Action
1902	• *Biologics Control Act* (Virus-Toxin Law) later called the *Public Health Service Act*—required regulation of vaccine and antitoxin producers, including licensing and inspections of manufacturers and the interstate sale of serum, vaccines and related products
1903	• First biologics regulations by Public Health Service Hygienic Laboratory—"Poison Squad," effect of food preservatives and artificial colors on public health
1906	• *Pure Food and Drug Act*—Prohibited "misbranding and adulteration"
1930	• PHS Hygienic Lab became National Institutes of Health (NIH)
1937	• NIH reorganized, Hygienic Lab became Division of Biologics Standardization
1938	• *Food, Drug and Cosmetics Act (FD&C Act)*—Products must be shown to be "safe;" authorized factory inspections
1944	• *PHS Act*—Required Product License Application/Establishment License Application (PLA/ELA, precursor to the BLA); gave seizure power
1955	• The Division of Biologics Control became an independent entity within NIH after polio vaccine thought to have been inactivated is associated with about 260 cases of polio
1972	• Division of Biologics Standardization, which was responsible for regulation of biologics, including serums, vaccines and blood products transferred from NIH to FDA; became what is now called CBER
1982	• Bureau of Drugs and Bureau of Biologics combined to form National Center for Drugs and Biologics (ODRR and OBRR)
1988	• FDA becomes part of Department of Health and Human Services (DHHS); Center for Drug Evaluation and Research (CDER) and Center for Biologics Evaluation and Research (CBER) established
1995	• Regulatory Initiative REGO IIb—Eliminated ELA requirement and lot release requirement for specified biotechnology products
1997	• *Food and Drug Administration Modernization Act (FDAMA)*—Revised *PHS Act* and eliminated the ELA for all biologics
2003	• Review of "well-characterized" proteins transferred to CDER
2009	• *Biologics Price Competition and Innovation Act* of 2009 *(BPCI Act)* created an abbreviated approval pathway for biosimilars

- human tissue and cellular products used in transplantation
- vaccines

Within CBER, the responsibility for reviewing the widely diverse range of biological product submissions is divided among three main review offices, which are the Office of Blood Research and Review (OBRR), the Office of Cellular, Tissue and Gene Therapies (OCTGT) and the Office of Vaccine Research and Review (OVRR).

CBER also regulates all medical devices associated with the collection and testing of licensed blood and cellular products through a 31 October 1991 FDA Inter-center Agreement between CBER and CDRH. The devices also must comply with all appropriate medical device laws and regulations.

IND Process for Biologics

21 CFR Part 312 describes three categories of clinical investigations that are exempt from IND requirements: 1) clinical research involving marketed drug products; 2) bioavailability or bioequivalence studies in humans; and 3) radioactive drugs for certain research uses. Clinical investigations that do not meet these three criteria must be conducted under an IND as required by Part 312. Most regulations on IND for small molecular drugs also are applied to biologics, including IND format and content, financial disclosure, special INDs, orphan products, clinical hold and pediatric studies.

An IND for a biologic may be submitted electronically or in paper/CD following Common Technical Document (CTD) format. The IND application must contain:

- administrative information—cover letter and forms, such as Forms FDA 1571, 1572 and 3674 (Certificate of Compliance), should be included in the IND (Form FDA 3674 is an FDA requirement to include clinical trial registration and results on ClinicalTrials.gov.)
- preclinical (animal pharmacology and toxicology) studies—preclinical data to permit an assessment as to whether the product is reasonably safe for initial testing in humans
- previous human experience—any previous experience with the drug in humans, such as results from clinical trials conducted outside of US
- chemistry, manufacturing and control—information pertaining to the composition, manufacturer, testing, stability and controls for the drug substance and the drug product

- clinical protocols and investigator information—study protocols for proposed clinical studies to assess whether the initial clinical trials will expose subjects to unnecessary risks; information on the qualifications of clinical investigators to assess whether they are qualified to fulfill their clinical trial duties; the clinical development plan for the next 12 months, Investigator's Brochure (IB) and commitments to obtain informed consent from the research subjects, to obtain study approval from an institutional review board (IRB), and to adhere to the investigational new drug regulations and study protocols

Once the IND is submitted, the sponsor must wait 30 calendar days before initiating any clinical trials. During this time, FDA has an opportunity to review the IND for safety to ensure research subjects will not be subjected to unreasonable risk.

To accommodate the issues related to biologics, both CDER and CBER have developed a number of guidance documents, including some entitled "Points to Consider," that represent FDA's current thinking on a variety of topics. In addition, guidance from the International Conference on Harmonisation (ICH) is applicable to biologics.

Preclinical Development for Biologics

The preclinical safety package for a biologic can be different from the toxicology package for small molecule drugs. Special considerations for types of toxicological assessments for biologics are described in ICH's *Preclinical Safety Evaluation of Biotechnology-Derived Pharmaceuticals S6*. The important points of S6 are:

- Biological activity—biological activity may be evaluated using in vitro assays to determine which effects of the product may be related to clinical activity. The use of cell lines and/or primary cell cultures can be useful to examine the direct effects on cellular phenotype and proliferation.
- Animal model selection—due to the species specificity of many biotechnology-derived pharmaceuticals, it is important to select relevant animal species for toxicity testing. The biological activity together with species and/or tissue specificity of many biotechnology-derived products often preclude standard toxicity testing designs in commonly used species (e.g., rats and dogs).
- Safety evaluation—safety evaluation normally requires data from two relevant species. However, in certain justified cases, one relevant species may suffice (e.g., when only one relevant species can be identified or where the biological activity of the biopharmaceutical is well understood). In addition, even where two species may be necessary to characterize toxicity in short-term studies, it may be possible to justify the use of only one species for subsequent long-term toxicity studies when the toxicity profile in the two species is comparable in the short term.
- Use analogous products—where there is no animal in which the biologic can function, due to either lack of specificity or anti-drug antibodies, preparing an analogous product, such as an animal homologue of the product intended for humans (e.g., a mouse monoclonal antibody that binds to the same intended target in mouse), can be used to assess potential safety issues.
- Maximum Tolerated Dose (MTD)—because biologics typically are not inherently toxic, it is difficult to provide drug concentrations at high enough levels to induce overt toxicity. Consequently, clinical dosing may be based on the biologically effective dose rather than the MTD. However, an attempt to cover the planned maximum human dose (preferably with up to a 10-fold safety margin) should be assessed in the safety studies.
- Safety pharmacology and acute toxicity studies—safety pharmacology endpoints normally are incorporated into the multiple-dose toxicity testing rather than conducted as separate studies.
- Immunogenicity—many biotechnology-derived pharmaceuticals intended for human are immunogenic in animals. Therefore, measurement of antibodies associated with administration of these types of products should be performed when conducting repeated-dose toxicity studies to aid in the interpretation of these studies. Antibody responses should be characterized, and their appearance should be correlated with any pharmacological and/or toxicological changes.
- Metabolism—the expected consequence of metabolism of biotechnology-derived pharmaceuticals is the degradation to small peptides and individual amino acids. Therefore, the metabolic pathways are generally understood. Classic biotransformation studies as performed for pharmaceuticals are not needed. Instead, understanding the behavior of the biopharmaceutical in the biologic matrix and the possible influence of binding proteins is important.
- Immunotoxicity—many biotechnology-derived pharmaceuticals are intended to stimulate or suppress the immune system and, therefore, may affect not only humoral but also cell-mediated immunity. Inflammatory reactions at the injection site may be indicative of a stimulatory response. Immunotoxicological testing strategies may require screening studies followed by mechanistic studies to clarify such issues. Routine tiered testing approaches

or standard testing batteries are not recommended for biotechnology-derived pharmaceuticals.
- Genotoxicity studies—the range and type of genotoxicity studies routinely conducted for pharmaceuticals are not applicable to biotechnology-derived pharmaceuticals and, therefore, are not needed. Moreover, the administration of large quantities of peptides or proteins may yield uninterpretable results. Studies should be conducted in available and relevant systems.
- Carcinogenicity studies—standard carcinogenicity bioassays are generally inappropriate for biotechnology-derived pharmaceuticals. However, product-specific assessment of carcinogenic potential may still be needed depending on duration of clinical dosing, patient population and/or the product's biological activity of the product. When there is concern about carcinogenic potential, a variety of approaches may be taken to evaluate risk.
- Local tolerance studies—local tolerance should be evaluated using the formulation intended for marketing. The potential adverse effects of the product can be evaluated in single- or repeated-dose toxicity studies, thus obviating the need for a separate local tolerance study.

Clinical Development Considerations for Biologics

Clinical study designs and requirements are similar for biological drugs and small molecule drugs; however, there may be additional safety concerns related to immunogenicity with biological products. Thus, additional testing may be required during the clinical trials to assess immunogenicity and the potential development of autoimmunity. As is the case for NDA drugs, clinical trials for biologics are conducted in phases. Biologics' initial safety is evaluated in Phase 1 trials. Phase 2 trials are performed to assess how well the biologic works in patients and to evaluate safety and dosing assessments in a larger group of subjects. Phase 2 studies sometimes are divided into Phase 2A and Phase 2B. Phase 2A is designed to assess dosing requirements and can also include combination dosing studies if the biologic is to be administered in combination with another therapy. Phase 2B is designed to study efficacy and can include exploratory endpoints to assess other pharmacodynamic markers, safety and efficacy endpoints and patient populations to better design the Phase 3 trial(s). Phase 3 studies typically are randomized controlled studies in larger patient groups and are intended to be the definitive assessment of how effective the drug is, sometimes compared to the current standard of care. Certain Phase 3 trials (Phase 3B) continue while the regulatory submission is being reviewed. This allows patients to continue to receive possibly life-saving drugs until the drug is approved, which allows additional safety and efficacy data to be collected. While not required in all cases, two successful Phase 3 trials demonstrating a drug's safety and efficacy normally are recommended to obtain approval from the appropriate regulatory agencies.

ICH efficacy (E1–E16) and multidisciplinary (M3) guidelines cover topics relevant to the clinical development of biologics. In addition, a number of FDA guidance documents have been issued that provide general guidelines on clinical trial designs. The guidances are selectively listed below:

- *Guidance for Industry: Clinical Pharmacogenomics: Premarket Evaluation in Early-Phase Clinical Studies and Recommendations for Labeling*—This guidance focuses on evaluating how variations in the human genome, specifically DNA sequence variants, could affect a drug's pharmacokinetics (PK), pharmacodynamics (PD), efficacy and/or safety. The guidance provides recommendations on when and how genomic information should be considered to address questions arising during drug development and regulatory review.
- *Guidance for Industry: Enrichment Strategies for Clinical Trials to Support Approval of Human Drugs and Biological Products*—This draft guidance focuses on enrichment strategies that can be used in clinical trials to support effectiveness and safety claims for NDAs and BLAs, including strategies to decrease heterogeneity, prognostic enrichment strategies and predictive enrichment strategies.
- *Draft Guidance for Industry Premarketing Evaluation in Early Phase Clinical Studies*—This draft guidance focuses particularly on use and evaluation of genomic strategies in early drug development and highlights identification of enrichment options for later trials.
- *Draft Guidance for Industry and Food and Drug Administration Staff: In Vitro Companion Diagnostic Devices*—This draft guidance describes FDA's policies for approval for companion diagnostics, concurrently with approval and labeling of the therapeutic product.
- *Draft Guidance for Industry: Adaptive Design Clinical Trials for Drugs and Biologics*—This draft guidance considers the case of enrichment approaches introduced only after randomization and based on interim evaluations. The guidance discusses how to design clinical trials with adaptive features (i.e., changes in design or analyses guided by examination of the accumulated data at an interim point in the trial). These adaptive trial designs may make the studies more efficient (e.g., shorter duration, fewer patients), more likely to demonstrate an effect of the drug if one exists or more informative (e.g., by providing broader

dose-response information). Such retrospective findings would have to be carefully implemented.
- *Guidance for Industry: Providing Clinical Evidence of Effectiveness for Human Drug and Biological Product*—This guidance describes the amount and type of evidence needed to demonstrate effectiveness.
- *Determining the Extent of Safety Data Collection Needed in Late Stage Premarket and Post approval Clinical Investigations*—This draft guidance provides advice on how and when to simplify data collection to maintain a balance between eliminating the collection of data that will not be useful and collecting sufficient data to allow adequate characterization of a drug's safety profile given the potential benefits. The amount and types of safety data collected during clinical trials and safety evaluations vary based on a range of factors, including the disease, patient population, subgroup of interest, preclinical findings, prior experience with the drug, experience with the drug class, phase of development and study design.
- *Draft Guidance for Industry: Non-Inferiority Clinical Trials*—This draft guidance describes the underlying principles involved in the use of non-inferiority (NI) study designs to provide evidence of a drug or biologic's effectiveness. It provides advice on when NI studies can be interpretable, how to choose the NI margin and how to analyze the results.
- *Guidance for Industry: Postmarketing Studies and Clinical Trials—Implementation of Section 505(o)(3) of the Federal Food, Drug, and Cosmetic Act*—The *FD&C Act* was amended in September 2007, adding a new Section 505(o). Section 505(o)(3) authorizes FDA to require certain postmarketing studies and clinical trials for prescription drugs and biological products approved under Section 351 of the *PHS Act*. This guidance provides information about the requirements for postmarketing studies and describes the types of postmarketing studies generally required under the new legislation.
- *Guidance for Industry: Population Pharmacokinetics*—This guidance makes recommendations on the use of population pharmacokinetics in the drug development process to help identify differences in drug safety and efficacy among population subgroups. It summarizes scientific and regulatory issues that should be addressed using population pharmacokinetics.
- *Draft Guidance for Industry: General Considerations for Pediatric Pharmacokinetic Studies for Drugs and Biological Products*—This draft guidance addresses general considerations for conducting such studies so drug and biological products can be labeled for pediatric use.
- *Guidance for Industry: Providing Clinical Evidence of Effectiveness for Human Drug and Biological Products*—This guidance provides FDA's current thinking concerning the quantitative and qualitative standards for demonstrating effectiveness of drugs and biologics.
- *Guidance for Industry: Pharmacokinetics in Patients with Impaired Renal Function—Study Design, Data Analysis, and Impact on Dosing and Labeling*—This guidance focuses on how to conduct studies to assess the influence of renal impairment on the pharmacokinetics of an investigational drug, when PK studies should be conducted with patients with impaired renal function and the design. It also covers the conduct of PK studies in patients with end-stage renal disease.

FDA has issued several guidances on the use of pharmacogenomics (PGx) in the drug development process. PGx studies can contribute to a greater understanding of inter-individual differences in the efficacy and safety of investigational biologics. Across the drug development continuum, genomic data may be used for understanding PK variations and variability in clinical response; elucidating the molecular basis for lack of efficacy or adverse events; and designing clinical trials to test for effects in identified subgroups, possibly for use in study enrichment strategies.

FDA also provides guidance on key safety issues relevant to drug development, such as understanding the risks of prolonged QT interval related to drug treatment or considerations for monitoring a drug's ability to cause drug-induced liver injury. FDA published two guidances: *Draft Guidance for Industry: Immunogenicity, Assay Development for Immunogenicity Testing of Therapeutic Proteins* (December 2009); and *Draft Guidance for Industry: Immunogenicity Assessment for Therapeutic Protein Products* (February 2013). The two guidances are particularly relevant for biologics because treatments with therapeutic proteins frequently stimulate immune responses. The clinical effects of these immune responses to therapeutic proteins, however, have ranged from none to extremely harmful. Such varied immune responses can affect product safety, efficacy and the immunogenicity rates observed during clinical trials, which are included in the product labeling. Thus, the development of a valid, sensitive immune assay is a key aspect of product development. Because immunogenicity poses a high risk, real-time data concerning patient responses are needed. Generally, a preliminary validated assay should be used during clinical studies. Even though immunogenicity in animal models is not predictive of immunogenicity in humans, it may reveal potential antibody-related toxicities that should be monitored in clinical trials. Multiple approaches may be appropriate for immunogenicity testing during clinical trials; however, testing strategies should address sensitivity, interference, functional or physiological consequences and risk-based application. The rationale for the immunogenicity testing paradigm should be provided in the IND.

Chemistry, Manufacturing and Controls for Biologics

Production of investigational biological products are subject to Section 501(a)(2)(B) of the *FD&C Act* (21 U.S.C. 351(a)(2)(B)) and the IND regulations at 21 CFR Part 312. During Phase 1 studies, emphasis generally should be placed on elements to assure the safety of subjects. This should include identification, control and stability of raw materials, drug substances and drug products. In each phase of the investigation, sufficient information is required to assure the proper identification, quality, purity and strength of the investigational drug. The amount of information necessary to make that assurance will vary with the phase of the investigation, proposed duration, dosage form and amount of information known.

In 2008, FDA issued *Guidance for Industry: CGMP for Phase 1 Investigational Drugs*. The guidance recognizes that both manufacturing controls and the extent of such manufacturing controls needed to achieve appropriate product quality differ not only between investigational and commercial manufacture, but also among the various phases of clinical trials.

CBER issued *Guidance for Industry: Chemistry, Manufacturing, and Control Information* in 2012, with recommendations regarding IND submissions for early clinical trials with live biotherapeutic products (LBPs) in the US. An LBP is a biological product that: contains live organisms, such as bacteria; is applicable to the prevention, treatment or cure of a disease or condition of human beings; and is not a vaccine. The guidance describes the requirements for CMC information in the IND. The unique requirements for biologics include:

- Biological name and strain—original source of cells from which the drug substance was derived; product strains with special attention to biological activity; and modifications
- Characterization—description of the acceptable limits and analytical methods used to assure the identity, strength, quality and purity of the drug substance and drug product
- Master cell bank (MCB)—complete history and characterization of the MCB, including the original source of cells used in the establishment of the cell banks; the culture/passage history of the cells; the method used to derive the cell bank; phenotypic and genotypic characterization; purity of culture and a description of all media components
- Working cell banks (WCBs)—description of the cell banking procedures used, including banking system; the size of the cell banks; the methods, reagents and media used for preparation of the cell banks; the conditions employed for cryopreservation and storage; in-process controls; storage conditions; and procedures used to avoid extraneous microbial contamination
- Cell growth and harvesting—step-by-step description from retrieval of the cell bank to culture harvest; the media used at each step with details of their preparation and sterilization; the inoculation and growth of initial and sub-cultures; time and temperature of incubation(s); how transfers are performed; in-process testing conducted to control contamination; the nature of the main culture system, including operating conditions and control parameters
- Purification and downstream processing—step-by-step description of the methods and materials in concentrate intermediate and the final bulk forms (The description of each step in downstream processing also should include the accompanying analytical tests developed or adopted by the manufacturer to show identity, purity and concentration, and the levels of impurities.)

The presence of adventitious agents is of particular concern with biological products, especially vaccines that contain animal materials and/or cellular substrates. An adventitious agent is an infectious agent that is extraneous to the product; potential agents include transmissible spongiform encephalopathy (TSE), viruses and oncogenic agents. Testing and clearance of known agents must be demonstrated to be sufficiently sensitive; testing should also be capable of detecting unsuspected agents. Suitable tests may include techniques such as cell culture, polymerase chain reaction (PCR), electron microscopy and egg or animal inoculation. In addition, sourcing of materials to avoid animal-derived materials can help reduce exposure of materials and substrates to specified risk materials for TSE.

Information amendments are required during the IND stage for significant changes and any changes that are likely to affect safety and efficacy prior to the use of the revised process material in clinical studies. During development through Phase 3, specifications for testing will evolve and become more defined; critical assays will need to be validated and determined to be reproducible, quantitative, sensitive, specific and biologically relevant; and the manufacturing process will be optimized.

Unique requirements for biologics are found in the General Biological Product Standards (21 CFR 610). Under these standards, to receive the BLA or NDA, the product must be shown to be "safe, pure, and potent." In addition, an inspection must confirm the production facility ensures the product meets these standards. The biological standards provide specific tests to be performed on each lot prior to release:

- Potency—ideally, via a product-specific bioassay that correlates with the *in vivo* mechanism of action or is predictive of function
- Sterility—similar to *United States Pharmacopeia* (*USP*) Chapter 71
- Purity—essentially free of extraneous materials, such as residual solvents, antibiotics, animal products, contaminating cell populations and co-purifying proteins; also includes residual moisture and pyrogenic substances (e.g., endotoxin)
- Identity—if product is comprised of multiple components (e.g., cell lines and proteins), the test method should identify all components
- Constituent materials—all ingredients should meet general standards of purity and quality
- Mycoplasma—if applicable

Alternative methods are permitted if they are equal to or greater than the assurances provided by the specified tests and must be validated by the end of Phase 3 to show equivalency to the established tests. The standards also include testing requirements for communicable disease agents, product dating periods and product labeling requirements (i.e., the product package to be labeled with the biologic's proper name; the manufacturer's name, address and applicable license number; and the expiration date).

The amount of information on analytical procedures and methods validation necessary for submissions will vary with the phase of the investigation (21 CFR 312.23(a)(7)). For general guidance on analytical procedures and methods validation information to be submitted for Phase 1 studies, sponsors can refer to FDA's *Guidance for Industry: Content and Format of Investigational New Drug Applications (INDs) for Phase 1 Studies of Drugs, Including Well-Characterized, Therapeutic, Biotechnology-Derived Products* (November 1995). And for Phase 2 or Phase 3 studies, FDA's *Guidance for Industry: INDs for Phase 2 and 3 Studies of Drugs, Including Specified Therapeutic Biotechnology-Derived Products, Chemistry, Manufacturing, and Controls Content and Format* (draft guidance published in April 1999). All analytical procedures should be fully developed and validated when the BLA is submitted. The requested format and content of analytical procedures for the BLA are the same as for an NDA.

A number of guidances for the appropriate development of CMC manufacturing and control are available, including ICH guidelines, CBER Points to Consider and other FDA guidances. Key CMC-related guidances are listed in **Table 22-2**. In addition, there are several general and specific *USP* chapters relevant to biologics, including specific chapters on testing methods and viral safety evaluation.

Drug Master Files

A Drug Master File (DMF) is a submission to FDA, usually concerning confidential CMC information of a drug substance, intermediates, container closures and excipients, which permits FDA to review the confidential information in support of a third party's submission. DMFs are optional and are categorized in 21 CFR 314.420 as follows:

- Type I—reserved, no longer applicable
- Type II—drug substance, drug substance intermediate and material used in their preparation
- Type III—packaging material
- Type IV—excipient, colorant, flavor, essence
- Type V—FDA-accepted reference material

Submitted DMFs are reviewed only in conjunction with a sponsor's IND, NDA or BLA when that DMF is referenced and there is a letter of authorization granting FDA permission to access the DMF in support of the submission. If there are deficiencies in the DMF, the DMF holder will be notified to provide additional information. The sponsor also will be notified in either an Information Request (IR) or Complete Response (CR) letter; however, no confidential details about the deficiency will be included in this communication. If there are no deficiencies, the holder will not receive any communication. DMFs should be updated annually, although FDA does not send reminders. After three years' inactivity (i.e., no annual updates), FDA will notify the holder that the DMF is considered to be inactive; the holder has 90 days to either close the DMF or provide an annual update to keep it open.

A DMF's content should be based on applicable guidance, and the submission should follow the M4Q CTD-Quality format. The submission must also contain a statement of commitment to CGMP compliance. One commonly used DMF submission for CBER is the Type V, under which CBER accepts:

- facility information in support of gene and cell-based therapies (which may be used to support clinical trials and to facilitate IND review)
- production information for a contract manufacturer to confidentially provide a list of other products manufactured in the facility (this information was formerly filed as a Type I DMF)
- submissions from contract testing facilities, such as cell bank testing and viral clearance studies

Before submitting any Type V DMF, a letter of intent should be submitted to FDA to determine the suitability of the DMF submission.

Meetings with FDA

There are three types of meetings that occur between sponsors or applicants and FDA staff: Type A, Type B and Type C. Each meeting type is subject to different procedures:

- Type A—to resolve a clinical hold or Refusal to File, to resolve a dispute or to discuss a special protocol assessment (SPA)
- Type B—key milestone meetings to include Pre-IND, End-of-Phase 1 (for products developed under 21 CFR 601 Subpart E), End-of-Phase 2/Pre-Phase 3 and Pre- BLA
- Type C—for any other purpose

If applicants are considering a request for a Type A meeting, before submitting the request, they should contact the review division in either CBER or CDER to discuss the appropriateness of the request. Type A meetings should be scheduled to occur within 30 days of FDA receipt of a written meeting request.

Type B meetings should be scheduled to occur within 60 days of FDA receipt of the written meeting request. FDA, in general, will not grant more than one of each of the Type B meetings for each potential application.

A Type C meeting is any meeting other than a Type A or Type B meeting between CBER or CDER and a sponsor regarding the development and review of a product. Type C meetings should be scheduled to occur within 75 days of FDA receipt of the written meeting request.

A meeting background package should be submitted to the appropriate review division so that it is received in accordance with the following timeframes:
- Type A meeting—at least two weeks before the formal meeting
- Type B meeting—at least four weeks before the formal meeting
- Type C meeting—at least four weeks before the formal meeting

Animal Rule
FDA's regulations concerning the approval of new drugs or biological products when human efficacy studies are neither ethical nor feasible are based on "the Animal Rule" defined in 21 CFR 601.90. The Animal Rule states that in selected circumstance, when it is neither ethical nor feasible to conduct human efficacy studies, FDA may grant marketing approval based on adequate and well-controlled animal studies when the results of those studies establish that the drug or biological product is reasonably likely to produce clinical benefit in humans. In this case, demonstration of the product's safety in humans is still necessary.

BLA Format and Content
The BLA is regulated under 21 CFR Parts 600–680. A BLA can be submitted by any legal person or entity who takes responsibility for compliance with product and establishment standards. Form FDA 356h specifies the requirements for a BLA. This includes:

- administration information including applicant information
- product and manufacturing (CMC) information including facility information
- preclinical studies
- clinical studies
- labeling

BLAs are required for all biological products submitted to CBER and for well-characterized proteins regulated by CDER. The BLA may be submitted in paper/CD in CTD format or electronically in eCTD format following ICH CTD requirements. Major sections of the NDA and BLA are the same, with a few exceptions. For instance, biologics typically are categorically excluded from requiring an environmental assessment under 21 CFR 25.5(c). In addition, the process needs to be validated for biologics prior to submitting the BLA, which is reviewed as part of the Preapproval Inspection (PAI) requirements for small molecular drugs.

A BLA, similar to an NDA, must provide the multidisciplinary FDA review team (medical officers, microbiologists, chemists, biostatisticians, etc.) with the efficacy and safety information necessary to make a benefit:risk assessment and to recommend or oppose the approval of drug product.

BLA Review Process
The NDA/BLA review process is divided into five phases: 1) filing determination and review planning; 2) review; 3) Advisory Committee meeting preparation and conduct; 4) action; and 5) post-action. **Table 22-3** provides a representative timetable.

Per 21 CFR 601.2, an application for licensure is not considered as filed until CBER has received all pertinent information and data from the applicants. A refuse to file (RTF) decision may be made on applications that contain incomplete or inadequate information required under Section 351 of the *PHS Act*, the *FD&C Act* or in FDA regulations (e.g., 21 CFR 601.2). RTF decisions can be based on:
- administrative incompleteness of an application
- scientific incompleteness of an application (i.e., omission of critical data, information or analyses needed to evaluate safety, purity and potency or provide adequate directions for use (21 CFS 601.2))
- inadequate information content or organization in an application that precludes substantive and meaningful review
- technically deficient electronic submission

In summary, CBER's initial decision on whether to file a BLA will be based on a threshold determination of whether the information submitted to support the license application is sufficiently complete to permit a substantive and

Table 22-2. Key CMC Guidance for Development of Biological Products

ICH Guidelines Specifically Targeted at Biotech Products
• Q5C: Quality of Biotechnological Products: Stability Testing of Biotechnological/Biological Products (November 1995)
• Q5B Quality of Biotechnological Products: Analysis of the Expression Construct in Cells Used for Production of r-DNA Derived Protein Products (February 1996)
• Q5D: Derivation and Characterisation of Cell Substrates Used for Production of Biotechnological/Biological Products (July 1997)
• Q5A Viral Safety Evaluation of Biotechnology Products Derived From Cell Lines of Human or Animal Origin (September 1998)
• Q6B: Specifications: Test Procedures and Acceptance Criteria for Biotechnological/Biological Products (August 1999)
• Q5E: Comparability of Biotechnological/Biological Products Subject to Changes in Their Manufacturing Process (June 2005)
• Q4B Annex 14: Bacterial Endotoxins Test General Chapter (July 2010)
• S6(R1) Preclinical Safety Evaluation of Biotechnology-Derived Pharmaceuticals (May 2012)
FDA Points to Consider and Other Applicable CMC Guidance Documents
• Points to Consider in the Production and Testing of New Drugs and Biologicals Produced by Recombinant DNA Technology (April 1985)
• Guideline on Validation of the Limulus Amebocyte Lysate Test as an End-Product Endotoxin Test For Human and Animal Parenteral Drugs, Biological Products, and Medical Devices (December 1987)
• Points to Consider in the Collection, Processing, and Testing of Ex-Vivo Activated Mononuclear Leukocytes for Administering to Humans (August 1989)
• Guidance for Industry: Content and Format of Investigational New Drug Applications (INDs) for Phase 1 Studies of Drugs, Including Well-Characterized, Therapeutic, Biotechnology-Derived Products (November 1995).
• Guidance for Industry: Content and Format of INDs for Phase 1 Studies of Drugs, Including Well-Characterized, Therapeutic, Biotechnology-Derived Products. Questions and Answers (November 1995)
• Demonstration of Comparability of Human Biological Products, Including Therapeutic Biotechnology-derived Products (April 1996).
• Guidance on Applications for Products Comprised of Living Autologous Cells Manipulated ex vivo and Intended for Structural Repair or Reconstruction (May 1996)
• Guidance for Industry for the Submission of Chemistry, Manufacturing, and Controls Information for a Therapeutic Recombinant DNA-Derived Product or a Monoclonal Antibody Product for In Vivo Use (August1996)
• Proposed Approach to Regulation of Cellular and Tissue-Based Products (February 1997)
• Points to Consider in the Manufacture and Testing of Monoclonal Antibody Products for Human Use (February 1997)
• Guidance for Industry: Changes to an Approved Application for Specified Biotechnology and Specified Synthetic Biological Products (July 1997)
• Guidance for Industry: Guidance for Human Somatic Cell Therapy and Gene Therapy (March 1998)
• Guidance for Industry: Environmental Assessment of Human Drug and Biologics Applications (July 1998)
• Guidance for Industry: Monoclonal Antibodies Used as Reagents in Drug Manufacturing (March 2001)
• Guidance for Industry: IND Meetings for Human Drugs and Biologics Chemistry, Manufacturing, and Controls Information (May 2001)
• Guidance for Industry: Container Closure Systems for Packaging Human Drugs and Biologics – Questions and Answers (May 2002)
• Draft Guidance for Industry: Drugs, Biologics, and Medical Devices Derived from Bioengineered Plants for Use in Humans and Animals (September 2002)
• Draft Guidance for Industry: Comparability Protocols - Protein Drug Products and Biological Products - Chemistry, Manufacturing, and Controls Information (September 2003)
• Draft Guidance for Industry: Labeling for Human Prescription Drug and Biological Products - Implementing the New Content and Format Requirements (January 2006)
• Draft Guidance for Industry: Characterization and Qualification of Cell Substrates and Other Biological Starting Materials Used in the Production of Viral Vaccines for the Prevention and Treatment of Infectious Diseases (September 2006)
• Draft Guidance for Industry: Validation of Growth-Based Rapid Microbiological Methods for Sterility Testing of Cellular and Gene Therapy Products (February 2008)
• Guidance for Food and Drug Administration Reviewers and Sponsors: Content and Review of Chemistry, Manufacturing, and Control (CMC) Information for Human Somatic Cell Therapy Investigational New Drug Applications (INDs) (April 2008)

• Guidance for Food and Drug Administration Reviewers and Sponsors: Content and Review of Chemistry, Manufacturing, and Control (CMC) Information for Human Gene Therapy Investigational New Drug Applications (INDs) (April 2008)
• Guidance for Industry: CGMP for Phase 1 Investigational Drugs (July 2008)
• Draft Guidance for Industry: Potency Tests for Cellular and Gene Therapy Products (October 2008)
• Guidance for Industry: Labeling for Human Prescription Drug and Biological Products — Determining Established Pharmacologic Class for Use in the Highlights of Prescribing Information (October 2009)
• Draft Guidance for Industry: Assay Development for Immunogenicity Testing of Therapeutic Proteins (December 2009)
• Draft Guidance for Industry: CMC Post approval Manufacturing Changes Reportable in Annual Reports (June 2010)
• Draft Guidance for Industry: Early Clinical Trials with Live Biotherapeutic Products: Chemistry, Manufacturing, and Control Information (December 2010)
• Guidance for Industry: Process Validation: General Principles and Practices (January 2011)
• Draft Guidance for Industry: Guidance for Industry on Biosimilars: Q & As Regarding Implementation of the BPCI Act of 2009 (February 2012)
• Draft Guidance for Industry: Scientific Considerations in Demonstrating Biosimilarity to a Reference Product (February 2012)
• Draft Guidance for Industry: Quality Considerations in Demonstrating Biosimilarity to a Reference Protein Product February 2012)
• Guidance for Industry: Limiting the Use of Certain Phthalates as Excipients in CDER-Regulated Products(December 2012)
• Draft Guidance for Industry: Immunogenicity Assessment for Therapeutic Protein Products ((February 2013)

meaningful review. An RTF may apply if the application contains uncorrected deficiencies (e.g., manufacturing or product specifications) that were clearly communicated to the applicant before application submission or, for electronic submissions, contains technical deficiencies sufficient to require resolution before a meaningful review can occur. An RTF is not a final determination concerning potential approvability; it can be an early opportunity for the applicant to develop a complete application, but will delay a full review of the application.

Applicants may receive additional information requests as a result of ongoing reviews and are encouraged to respond promptly and completely to such requests. During the first cycle, the FDA division ordinarily reviews all amendments solicited by the agency during the review and any amendments to the application previously agreed upon during the pre-NDA/BLA meeting. Substantial amendments submitted late in the review cycle may be reviewed in a subsequent cycle, depending on other identified application deficiencies.

Following FDA's review of a license application, the applicant and FDA may present their findings to FDA's Related Biological Products Advisory Committee. The non-FDA expert committee (scientists, physicians, biostatisticians and a consumer representative) provides advice to the agency regarding the safety and efficacy of the product for the proposed indication. Based on the discussions at the Advisory Committee meeting and committee recommendations, FDA may ask an applicant to submit additional data or analyses for review.

A CR Letter after a complete review can be issued based on critical omissions of data or analyses as well as an adverse judgment about the data, conclusions, rationale, etc., presented in the application. For example, a CR Letter could be issued if CBER concludes that effectiveness has not been demonstrated; an analysis was incorrectly carried out; clinical trials were poorly designed or conducted; safety has not been adequately demonstrated; and/or outstanding compliance issues remain. These judgments would not serve as the basis for an RTF unless the deficiencies were so severe as to render the application incomplete.

Other action letters include the IR Letter and the Discipline Review (DR) Letter. An IR Letter requests further information or clarification that is necessary to complete the discipline review. A DR Letter is sent to convey early thoughts on possible deficiencies found by a discipline review team at the conclusion of its review. A single DR letter may contain comments from multiple discipline reviews.

A PAI will be conducted for the proposed manufacturing facilities during the late stage of the application review.

Approval to market a biologic is granted by issuance of a biologics license (including US license number) as part of the approval letter. Issuance of a license is a determination that the product, the manufacturing process and the manufacturing facilities meet applicable requirements to ensure the product's continued safety, purity and potency. Among other things, safety and purity assessments must consider the storage and testing of cell substrates that are often used to manufacture biologics. A potency assay is required due to the complexity and heterogeneity of biologics.

The product approval also requires the provision of product labeling adequate to allow healthcare providers to understand the product's proper use, including its potential benefits and risks, to communicate with patients and parents, and to safely deliver the product to the public.

On 9 July 2012, the *Food and Drug Administration Safety and Innovation Act* (*FDASIA*) of 2012 was signed into law. This new law includes the reauthorization of the *Prescription Drug User Fee Act* (*PDUFA*) that provides FDA with the necessary resources to maintain a predictable and efficient review process for human drug and biologic products. Under *PDUFA V*, FDA promotes innovation through enhanced communication between FDA and sponsors during drug development. As part of its commitments in *PDUFA V*, FDA has established a new review program to promote greater transparency and increased communication between the FDA review team and the applicant on the most innovative products reviewed by the agency. The program applies to all New Medical Entity (NME) NDAs and original BLAs that are received from 1 October 2012, through 30 September 2017.

PDUFA V increases the review timeline from six to eight months for priority reviews and 10 to 12 months for standard reviews. The increase in the duration of reviews is supposed to increase the likelihood of an on-time approval (first-cycle approval).

Under the *PDUFA* provisions, submission of a major amendment during the last three months of a review may trigger a three-month extension of the review clock. *PDUFA V* modifies this, as a major amendment can extend the review clock by three months at any time during the review.

The key time points for FDA communication defined by *PDUFA V* are:
- Day 60 Filing Letter—application accepted for filing.
- Day 74 Letter (74 days after FDA receives the application)—the letter will identify substantive review issues identified during the first 14 days of the review. The letter will include the FDA's preliminary plans on whether to hold an Advisory Committee meeting.
- Mid-cycle Communication—for a priority review, this is three months after the filing date, i.e., five months after FDA receipt of the application for priority review, or nine months for standard review. The letter may include any significant issues identified to date and an update on the status of the review.
- Late-cycle Meeting—for priority applications, it is two months and 12 days prior to the approval date. The meeting will discuss the status of the review and issues that will be raised at the Advisory Committee.

Biologics Advertising and Promotional Labeling and Proprietary Name

CBER reviews draft and final professional and direct-to-consumer (DTC) advertising and promotional labeling materials submitted for licensed biological products. CBER also reviews promotional materials to ensure information about the product's risks and benefits is communicated in a truthful, non-misleading and balanced manner, and the materials are in compliance with pertinent federal laws and regulations. Final advertising and promotional labeling materials may be submitted in paper or electronic format by applicants. Submissions must contain:
- Form FDA-2253: Transmittal of Advertisements and Promotional Labeling for Drugs and Biologics for Human Use
- Two copies of final advertisements and promotional labeling materials
- Two copies of the product's current professional labeling (e.g., approved Package Labeling (PI), Patient Package Insert (PPI), medication guide and Instructions for Use)

Draft DTC television advertising and promotional labeling materials also may be submitted in paper or electronic format. For products approved under accelerated approval, all advertising and promotional materials intended for dissemination or publication within 120 days following marketing approval must be submitted to the agency for review during the preapproval review period with Form FDA 2253. Furthermore, after 120 days following marketing approval, all advertising and promotional materials must be submitted at least 30 days prior to the intended time of initial dissemination or publication.

CBER's Advertising and Promotional Labeling Branch (APLB) reviews and evaluates proposed proprietary names for biological products in accordance with SOPP 8001.4: *Review of Proprietary Names for CBER Regulated Products*. Proposed proprietary names are evaluated to avoid potential medication errors related to look-alike and sound-alike proprietary names and to avoid names that are fanciful or misleading.

APLB also evaluates other factors that could contribute to medication errors, such as unclear label abbreviations, acronyms, dose designations and error-prone label and packaging design.

Postapproval Changes

Under 21 CFR 601.12, a change in the approved product, labeling, production process, quality control, equipment or facility must be reported to FDA. The change can be reported in: a supplement requiring approval prior to distribution; a supplement submitted at least 30 days prior to distribution of the product made using the change; a supplement submitted prior to distribution of the product made using the change; or an annual report, depending on its potential to have an adverse effect on the "identity, strength, quality, purity, or potency" of the biological product as it may relate to the product's safety or effectiveness. Before distributing a licensed product manufactured using a change, the manufacturer is required to demonstrate, through appropriate validation and/or clinical or

Table 22-3. Timetable for BLA Review

	Activity	Responsibility
Day 0		Central Document Room (CDER) or Document Control Center (CBER)
Day 1-14		
By Day 14	Acknowledge application receipt in writing	Review Discipline Team Leaders (CDER) Review Division Management (CBER)
Day 0-45	Conduct filing review/convey potential RTF issues to applicant	Review team
By Day 45	Make filing decision/plan and schedule for filing meeting	Review Division Director Office Director (consulted for RTFs)/ Review Team
By Day 60		RPM/Review Division Director
By Day 74	Communicate filing review issues to applicant	RPM
By the end of Month 5	Mid-cycle Meeting	Review team
Variable	Issue Discipline Review Letters	Review team
2 months and 12 days prior to the approval date	Late-cycle Meeting	Review team
By end of Month 8 (per PDUFA IV, additional 2 months per PDUFA V)	Complete primary review/conduct Advisory Committee Meeting	Review team
4 weeks before approval action	Initiate compliance check request (BLAs)	RPM
3 weeks before approval	Labeling discussions (for Approval and Approvable Actions)	Review Team/ODS/DDMAC Labeling Team
By PDUFA goal date	Send official copy to applicant	RPM
After PDUFA goal date		Review Team

nonclinical laboratory studies, the lack of adverse effect of the change on the product's safety or effectiveness. The three reporting categories for changes to an approved application are defined in 21 CFR 601.12:

1. Prior Approval Supplement (PAS)—changes that have a substantial potential to have an adverse effect on the safety or effectiveness of the product, that require submission of a supplement and approval by FDA prior to distribution of the product made using the change (major changes)
2. Changes Being Effected (CBE) 30 or CBE—changes that have a moderate potential to have an adverse effect on the safety or effectiveness of the product, that require submission of a supplement to FDA at least 30 days prior to distribution of the product made using the change or, for some changes, the 30 days may be waived (moderate changes)
3. Annual Report—changes that have minimal potential to have an adverse effect on the safety or effectiveness of the product reported by the applicant in an Annual Report (minor changes)

Due to the sometimes limited ability to identify clinically active component(s) of complex biological products, such products are often defined by their manufacturing processes. In 1996, FDA provided recommendations in its *FDA Guidance Concerning Demonstration of Comparability of Human Biological Products, Including Therapeutic Biotechnology Products*, which explains how an applicant may demonstrate—through a combination of analytical testing, functional assay, assessment of PK, pharmacodynamics (PD) and toxicity in animals, and clinical studies—that a manufacturing change does not adversely affect identity, purity or potency of its FDA-approved product. Since 1996, FDA has approved many manufacturing process changes for licensed biological products, based on a demonstration of product comparability before and after the process change, as supported by quality criteria and analytical testing without the need for additional nonclinical data and clinical safety and/or efficacy studies. In cases where the effects of the change are uncertain, additional data may be required, including nonclinical and/or clinical studies, to demonstrate product comparability. In July 1997, CBER issued *Guidance for Industry: Changes to an Approved Application* for *Specified Biotechnology and Specified Synthetic Biological Products* to assist applicants in determining which reporting mechanism is appropriate for a change to an approved license application. These concepts were further developed by ICH and resulted in *Comparability of Biotechnological/Biological Products subject to Changes in their Manufacturing Process Q6E* (June 2005).

Advisory Committee Meetings

The *Federal Advisory Committee Act* became law in 1972 and is the legal foundation defining how these committees operate. The law places special emphasis on open meetings, chartering, public involvement and reporting. Advisory Committees are groups of experts from outside the agency that FDA sometimes turns to for advice on complex scientific, technical and policy issues. Advisory Committees provide independent, professional expertise related to the development and evaluation of FDA-regulated products, such as allergenic products; blood products; cellular, tissue and gene therapies; transmissible spongiform encephalopathies; and vaccines and related biological products. In general, Advisory Committees include a chairman, several members, plus representatives of consumer groups, industry and sometimes patients. Additional experts with special knowledge may be added for individual meetings as needed. Although the committees provide advice to the agency, FDA makes the final decisions. In some cases, FDA is required by law to refer an issue to an Advisory Committee. In others, it has discretion to consider whether to refer a matter to an Advisory Committee. For all first-of-a-kind or first-in-class products for human use, FDA either refers the product to an Advisory Committee or summarizes the reasons it does not do so before approval in the action letter.

Once the review has progressed within the reviewing division, CBER will notify the sponsor 55 days in advance if it has determined that an Advisory Committee meeting is required. The sponsor prepares materials for Advisory Committee review and designates which materials are publically releasable under the *Freedom of Information Act (FOIA)* and which are to be treated as proprietary, nonpublic materials. FDA may disagree with the sponsor's designations and request that additional information be made public. In general, product information that is not in the labeling, such as manufacturing processes, formulation information and quality control testing, as well as the raw data from preclinical and clinical studies, can be considered exempt from *FOIA*. Advisory Committee members will receive both public and proprietary materials. During the meeting, sponsors may be permitted to make presentations, but they are not allowed to approach committee members without the consent of a federal officer. The function of Advisory Committees is to provide advice to FDA, but the agency is not obligated to adopt the committee's recommendation(s).

Market Exclusivity

Biologics are allowed a 12-year market exclusivity instead of the five years allowed for NDA drugs (seven years for orphan products). With the passing of the *BPCI Act*, the additional six months of market exclusivity for pediatric indications now applies to biologics as well.

Biosimilars

The *BPCI Act*, signed into law in March 2010, amended the *PHS Act* and created an abbreviated licensure pathway in Section 351(k) of the *PHS Act* for biological products shown to be biosimilar to, or interchangeable with, an FDA-licensed biological reference. The goal of the *BPCI Act* is similar in concept to that of *Hatch-Waxman Act* since the *BPCI Act* aligns with FDA's policy of permitting appropriate reliance on what is already known about a drug, thereby saving time and resources and avoiding unnecessary duplication of human or animal testing.

Under the *BPCI Act*, a sponsor may seek approval of a "biosimilar" product under the new Section 351(k) of the *PHS Act*. A biological product may be demonstrated to be "biosimilar" if data show that it is "highly similar" to the reference product, notwithstanding minor differences in clinically inactive components, and there are no clinically meaningful differences between the biological product and the reference product in terms of safety, purity and potency. In order to meet the higher standard of interchangeability, a sponsor must demonstrate that the biosimilar product can be expected to produce the same clinical result as the reference product in any given patient and, for a biological product that is administered more than once, that the risk of alternating or switching from the reference product to the biosimilar product is not greater than the risk of maintaining the patient on the reference product. Interchangeable products may be substituted for the reference product by a pharmacist without the intervention of the prescribing healthcare provider. To be approved as a biosimilar, the following criteria must be met:

- The biological product and reference product utilize the same mechanism or mechanisms of action for the condition or conditions of use prescribed, recommended or suggested in the proposed labeling.
- The condition(s) of use prescribed, recommended or suggested in the labeling proposed for the biological product has been previously approved for the reference product.
- The route of administration, dosage form and strength of the biological product are the same as those of the reference product.
- The facility in which the biological product is manufactured, processed, packed or held meets standards designed to ensure that the product continues to be safe, pure and potent.

At this time, FDA is continuing to consider the type of information sufficient to enable the agency to determine that a biological product is interchangeable with the reference product. FDA developed three guidances in February 2012 to implement the *BPCI Act*. The guidances address a broad range of issues, including:

- *Draft Guidance for Industry: Scientific Considerations in Demonstrating Biosimilarity to a Reference Product*—This guidance discusses important scientific considerations in demonstrating biosimilarity, including: a stepwise approach to demonstrating biosimilarity, which can include a comparison of the proposed product and the reference product with respect to structure, function, animal toxicity, human PK and PD, clinical immunogenicity, and clinical safety and effectiveness; the "totality-of-the-evidence" approach FDA will use to review applications for biosimilar products; general scientific principles in conducting comparative structural and functional 66 analysis, animal testing, human PK and PD studies, clinical immunogenicity assessment, and clinical safety and effectiveness studies. Additional factors to be considered include the complexities of the therapeutic protein; use of data derived from studies comparing a proposed product with a non-US-licensed product and postmarketing safety monitoring considerations.
- *Draft Guidance for Industry: Biosimilars: Questions and Answers Regarding Implementation of the Biologics Price Competition and Innovation Act of 2009*—This guidance provides answers to common questions from sponsors interested in developing proposed biosimilar products, including: biosimilarity or interchangeability; provisions related to requirement to submit a BLA for a "biological product;" and exclusivity. The guidance recommends that sponsors of proposed biosimilar products request an initial meeting with FDA as soon as the sponsor can provide a proposed plan for its biosimilar development program, manufacturing process information and preliminary comparative analytical data with the reference product. Comparative analytical data provide the foundation for a biosimilar development program and can influence decisions about the type and amount of animal and clinical data needed.
- *Draft Guidance for Industry: Quality Considerations in Demonstrating Biosimilarity to a Reference Protein Product*—This guidance focuses on analytical studies that may be relevant to assessing whether the proposed biosimilar product and a reference product are highly similar, which is an important part of the biosimilarity assessment.

The approval of a biosimilar application under Subsection 351(k) of the *PHS Act* may not occur until 12 years after the date on which the reference product was first licensed. In addition, an application under Subsection 351(k) may not be accepted for review until four years after the date on which the reference product was first licensed.

Commercial Biologics Manufacturing and Supply

Lot Release

After a license application is approved for a biological product, some products may be subject to official lot release. As part of the manufacturing process, the manufacturer is required to perform certain tests on each lot of the product before it is released for distribution. If the product is subject to official release by CBER, the manufacturer submits samples of each lot of product to CBER together with a release protocol showing a summary of the history of manufacture of the lot and the results of all of the manufacturer's tests performed on the lot. CBER may also perform certain confirmatory tests on lots of some products, such as viral vaccines, before releasing the lots for distribution by the manufacturer.

Monitor the Safety and Stability of Approved Biological Products

Manufacturers must report certain problems to FDA's Biological Product Deviation Reporting System. Manufacturers also must report and correct product problems within established timeframes. If a significant problem is detected, a manufacturer may need to recall a product or even stop manufacturing it.

GMP Inspection

CBER inspects manufacturing facilities on a regular basis. The purpose of these inspections is to assess whether biological products are made in compliance with appropriate laws and regulations and to assist in identifying any changes needed to help ensure product quality.

Biologics Establishment Registration and Listing

Manufacturers of biological drug products are required to update the registration and listing information to CDER or CBER in the proper electronic format. FDA has adopted Structured Product Labeling (SPL) as the electronic means for submission of registration and listing information to the agency. As of 1 June 2009, FDA no longer accepts paper registration and listing submissions, unless a waiver is granted. Under Section 510 of the *FD&C Act* and the regulations in 21 CFR Part 207, manufacturers of biological drug products must:

- register their establishments annually on or before 31 December of each year
- list all of their products in commercial distribution at the time of initial registration, with bi-annual updates to their listings in June and December, as necessary

Short Supply

When a licensed biologic is in short supply, the manufacturer may obtain an initial or partially manufactured version of the product from an unlicensed, but registered facility, when the product is shipped solely to the licensee and when the licensee can ensure the product made at the unlicensed facility will be manufactured in full compliance with applicable regulations. The license holder must update its license with FDA to explain this arrangement. This provision is most commonly used to obtain source materials, such as those used in producing allergenic extracts; specific types of human plasma containing rare antibodies; venoms used in producing antitoxins and antivenins; and recovered plasma.

Divided Manufacturing

Divided manufacturing is an arrangement in which two or more manufacturers, each registered with FDA and licensed to manufacture a specific biological product in its entirety, participate jointly in the manufacture of that product by only performing part of the approved process. BLAs should be updated to describe the role of each manufacturer and may need to demonstrate equivalency and stability of the intermediate products during shipment. The intermediate should also be labeled "for further manufacturing use" as part of the proper name. Each licensed manufacturer must notify the other licensee(s) and the appropriate FDA center regarding proposed changes in the manufacture, testing or specifications of its product, in accordance with 21 CFR 601.12.

Shared Manufacturing

Shared manufacturing is an arrangement in which two or more manufacturers are registered and licensed for specific aspects of a product's manufacture but neither is licensed for the product's total manufacturing process. A common shared manufacturing arrangement makes one manufacturer responsible for an intermediate product and another for the final product. All license applications or supplements under a shared manufacturing arrangement should be submitted concurrently to FDA for BLA review. Lack of one or more related applications may result in an RTF action.

Contract Manufacturing

When the sponsor holds the BLA license, sponsors must establish, maintain and follow procedures for receiving information from the contract manufacturing facility on all deviations, complaints and adverse events that may affect product quality. Specific identification of the contractor in the product labeling is not required since it does not hold the license.

Summary

- Biologics are drug products derived from living sources, e.g., humans, animals and microorganisms, which are approved for licensure (using a BLA) under the *PHS Act*, unlike small-molecule drugs, which are approved under the *FD&C Act*. CBER is the primary reviewing center for biologics and is organized into three offices for the review of blood products, vaccines and cell, tissue and gene therapy products.
- The review of "well-characterized" biological products was moved from CBER to CDER in 2003. This category is comprised of biotechnology products and naturally- and synthetically-derived proteins and includes products such as monoclonal antibodies, cytokines, growth factors, enzymes, immunomodulators and thrombolytics.
- The IND process for biologics is much the same as for drugs; however, there are a number of preclinical, clinical and manufacturing guidance documents to assist sponsors with the issues unique to the development of biological products.
- The BLA format and general review process is also similar to that for NDAs, including the utilization of the eCTD format for submissions.
- It is now possible for a sponsor to seek approval of a "biosimilar" product under new Section 351(k) of the *PHS Act*. The sponsor must show that the product is highly similar to the reference product and that there are no clinically meaningful differences between the biological product and the reference product in terms of safety, purity and potency. However, to meet the higher standard of interchangeability, a sponsor must demonstrate that the risk of alternating or switching between use of the biosimilar product and the reference product is not greater than the risk of maintaining the patient on the reference product.

Chapter 23

Biologics Compliance

Updated by Usha Srinivasan, MS, RAC

OBJECTIVES

- Understand general biologics licensing standards

- Understand the organization, roles and responsibilities of the Office of Compliance and Biologics Quality at the Center for Biologics Evaluation and Review (CBER)

- Learn general regulatory compliance principles for biologics preapproval, including chemistry, manufacturing and controls (CMC); change control; investigational new drug (IND) safety reports; role of Bioresearch Monitoring; product naming; and pre-license inspections

- Learn general regulatory postapproval compliance principles for biologics, including inspections, postapproval commitments, change control, biologic deviations reporting and import/export

- Understand risk management plans for biologics, including setting up Risk Evaluation and Mitigation Strategies (REMS)

- Understand US Food and Drug Administration (FDA) enforcement activities for biologics

LAWS, REGULATIONS AND GUIDANCE DOCUMENTS COVERED IN THIS CHAPTER

- *Public Health Service Act* of 1946, Sections 351 and 361

- *Federal Food, Drug, and Cosmetic Act* of 1938

- The *Food and Drug Administration Amendments Act* of 2007 (*FDAAA*)

- 21 CFR 600 Biologics General

- 21 CFR 601 Biologics Licensing

- 21 CFR 610 General Biological Products Standards

- Compliance Program Guidance Manual—Inspection of Biological Drug Products—7345.848

- *Regulatory Procedures Manual*, Chapter 9, Subchapter 9.3, "Importation of Biological Products," Office of Regulatory Affairs, US Food and Drug Administration

- *Guidance for Industry: Comparability Protocols—Chemistry, Manufacturing, and Controls Information* (February 2003)

- *Guidance for Industry: Comparability Protocols—Protein Drug Products and Biological Products—Chemistry, Manufacturing, and Controls Information* (September 2003)

- ICH, *Comparability of Biotechnological/Biological Products Subject to Changes in Their Manufacturing Process Q5E* (June 2005)

Chapter 23

- *Guidance For Industry: Changes to an Approved Application for Specified Biotechnology and Specified Synthetic Biological Products (July 1997)*
- *SOPP 8410: Determining When Prelicense/Preapproval Inspections are Necessary (December 2001)*
- *SOPP 8001.4: Review of CBER Regulated Product Proprietary Names (November 2008)*
- *Draft Guidance for Industry: Contents of a Complete Submission for the Evaluation of Proprietary Names (November 2008)*
- *Guidance for Industry: Regulation of Human Cells, Tissues, and Cellular and Tissue-Based Products (HCT/Ps)—Small Entity Compliance Guide (August 2007)*
- *Exports Under the FDA Export Reform and Enhancement Act of 1996 (July 2007)*
- *Draft Guidance for Industry: Postmarketing Safety Reporting for Human Drug and Biological Products Including Vaccines (March 2001)*
- *Guidance for Industry: Biological Product Deviation Reporting for Licensed Manufacturers of Biological Products Other than Blood and Blood Components (October 2006)*
- *SOPP 8404: Refusal to File Procedures for Biologics License Applications (August 2007)*
- *Guidance for Industry: Good Pharmacovigilance Practices and Pharmacoepidemiologic Assessment (March 2005)*
- *Guidance for Industry: Premarketing Risk Assessment (March 2005)*
- *Guidance for Industry: Changes to an Approved Application: Biological Products (July 1997)*
- *Guidance for Industry: Format and Content of Proposed Risk Evaluation and Mitigation Strategies (REMS), REMS Assessments, and Proposed REMS Modifications (September 2009)*
- *Draft Guidance for Industry: Safety Reporting requirements for INDs and BA/BE Studies (September 2010)*
- *Guidance for Industry: Postmarketing Studies and Clinical Trials—Implementation of Section 505(o)(3) of the Federal Food, Drug, and Cosmetic Act (April 2011)*
- *Medications Guides - Distribution Requirements and Inclusion in Risk Evaluation and Mitigation Strategies (REMS) (February 2011)*
- *Guidance for Industry and Investigators: Safety Reporting Requirements for INDs and BA/BE Studies (December 2012)*

Introduction

Biologics licensing standards, per the *Public Health Service Act* of 1946 (*PHS Act*) and Title 21 of the *Code of Federal Regulations* (CFR) 600.3, provide that biologics must be "safe, pure, and potent." Under 21 CFR 601.20, there must be a demonstration upon inspection that the production facility assures that the product meets these standards and complies with the applicable regulations. Therefore, processes and methods to ensure these attributes are in place for licensure must be developed during the Investigational New Drug (IND) application stage. These attributes are defined as follows:

- Safety—relative freedom from harmful effect to persons affected, directly or indirectly, by a product when it is prudently administered, taking into consideration the product's character in relation to the recipient's condition at the time
- Purity—relative freedom from extraneous matter in the finished product, whether or not harmful to the recipient or deleterious to the product; purity includes, but is not limited to, relative freedom from residual moisture or other volatile and pyrogenic substances
- Potency—specific ability or capacity of the product, as indicated by appropriate laboratory tests or by adequately controlled clinical data obtained through the administration of the product in the manner intended, to effect a given result

Additional information related to chemistry, manufacturing and controls (CMC) product development and biologics submissions can be found in Chapter 22 Biologics Submissions.

Upon approval of a Biologics License Application (BLA), a manufacturer receives a license to market its product in interstate commerce. The compliance and surveillance activities related to biologics licenses during the lifecycle of biological products are overseen by the Office of Compliance and Biologics Quality (OCBQ) within the US Food and Drug Administration's (FDA) Center for

Biologics Evaluation and Research (CBER). OCBQ comprises four divisions and their associated branches:
- Division of Biological Standards and Quality Control (CBER-OCBQ-DBSQC)
  o Laboratory of Analytical Chemistry and Blood Related Products
  o Quality Assurance
  o Laboratory of Microbiology, In-Vivo Testing and Standards
- Division of Case Management
  o Advertising and Promotional Labeling Branch
  o Biological Drug and Device Compliance Branch
  o Blood and Tissue Compliance Branch (see Chapter 27 Blood and Blood Products and Chapter 28 Human Cell and Tissue Products)
- Division of Inspections and Surveillance
  o Bioresearch Monitoring Branch
  o Program Surveillance Branch
  o Program Inspection Branch
- Division of Manufacturing and Product Quality (DMPQ)
  o Product Release Branch
  o Manufacturing Review Branch I
  o Manufacturing Review Branch II

These divisions carry out a wide range of activities, including:
- developing product testing programs in a secured and controlled environment using appropriately qualified and validated methods for generating data that support center regulatory activities
- maintaining product testing programs in a manner that meets internationally recognized standards
- conducting pre-license and preapproval inspections of manufacturing facilities and products under clinical study
- monitoring the safety, purity and potency of biological products through review of:
  o Biological Product Deviation Reports (BPDRs) and Human Cell, Tissue, and Cellular and Tissue-Based Products (HCT/P) Deviation Reports
  o investigations into transfusion- and donation-related fatalities and other adverse events
  o product recalls
- monitoring research (bioresearch monitoring (BIMO)) conducted on biological products and assessing the protection of human research subjects' rights, safety and welfare and research data quality and integrity
- monitoring import and export activities
- reviewing product advertising and promotional labeling (see Chapter 24 Biologics, Labeling, Advertising and Promotion)
- monitoring reports of biological product shortages and helping to prevent or alleviate shortages of biological products, working with all parties involved to ensure medically necessary products are available within the US
- initiating regulatory action to address noncompliance with FDA regulations

These activities include both pre- and postapproval compliance surveillance activities, described in more detail below.

Preapproval Compliance

CMC Change Control

During the IND stage, CMC change control includes providing information amendments to the IND that provide data substantiating the comparability or improvements related to manufacturing changes, prior to making the change. During product development, it is likely there will be multiple changes in the manufacturing process that could impact drug product quality, safety and efficacy. Comparability studies generally are performed to demonstrate that nonclinical and clinical data generated with pre-change product are applicable to post-change product, to facilitate further development and, ultimately, to support the marketing authorization. Comparability studies conducted for products in development are influenced by factors such as the product development stage, the availability of validated analytical procedures and the extent of product and process knowledge, which can vary based on the manufacturer's experience with the process. Due to the limitations of analytical tools in early clinical development, physicochemical and biological tests alone might not be adequate to determine comparability, and it may become necessary to bridge nonclinical and/or clinical studies.

When process changes are introduced in later stages of development and no additional clinical studies are planned to support the marketing authorization, the comparability study should be as comprehensive as one conducted for an approved product. However, some comparability study outcomes on quality attributes may still require additional nonclinical or clinical studies.

IND Safety Reporting

Premarketing expedited safety reports are required for serious and unexpected adverse experiences associated with the use of the biologic, as is the case for drugs (21 CFR 312.32). These requirements were amended recently to update the definitions used for safety reporting and to clarify when to submit expedited safety reports. In summary, expedited safety reporting applies to suspected adverse reactions that are both serious and unexpected, and where there is a reasonable possibility of a causal relationship between the drug and the adverse event. For other adverse events, the sponsor should collect the information and develop a process for ongoing evaluation of accumulating safety data. The new ICH Development Safety Update Report, not yet adopted in the US, is consistent with this safety reporting framework.

FDA has issued final regulations addressing the safety reporting requirements for Investigational New Drug applications (INDs) found in 21 CFR Part 312. *Guidance for Industry and Investigators: Safety Reporting Requirements for INDs and BA/BE Studies* (December 2012) is aimed at improving the quality of safety reports submitted to FDA, thereby enhancing patient safety in clinical trials. The guidance lays out clear definitions and standards to ensure the accurate and rapid reporting of critical safety information about investigational new drugs to the agency, minimizing uninformative reports and enhancing reporting of meaningful, interpretable information.

Additional safety reporting guidance is available for specific biological products, such as those used in gene therapy clinical trials. In gene therapy trials, where there is heightened concern about the potential for delayed adverse events as a consequence of persistent biological activity of the transferred genetic material, long-term follow-up studies for safety are recommended. Adverse events associated with gene therapy trials also may need to be reported to the National Institutes of Health (NIH) if the trial includes NIH-funded sites.

Bioresearch Monitoring (BIMO)

BIMO refers to FDA's compliance program for Good Clinical Practice (GCP) and Good Laboratory Practice (GLP) inspections during development. BIMO covers clinical investigators, Institutional Review Boards (IRBs), sponsors, contract research organization (CRO) monitors, *in vivo* bioequivalence laboratories and facilities and GLP facilities. The emphasis in clinical inspections is on how sponsors ensure the validity of the data clinical investigators submit to FDA, and the adherence of sponsors, CROs and monitors to applicable regulations, such as adverse event reporting and testing the article's integrity from the time of manufacture until receipt by the investigator. To carry out these responsibilities, BIMO staff conduct preapproval data audit inspections, investigate complaints, answer questions about GCP and help evaluate data integrity concerns.

Biological Product Naming

The nonproprietary/proper name for a new biological product, as for drugs, is determined by submitting an application and fee to the United States Adopted Names Council (USANC), which is part of the American Medical Association (see www.ama-assn.org/). Sponsors should provide several selections and the naming rationale to USANC. When submitting suggested names, consideration should be given to the naming conventions used by USANC to assess submissions (i.e., use of common stems and/or syllables for existing products or product classes). For biologics, CBER has developed naming conventions for certain product categories, e.g., cellular therapies, which must be followed to the extent possible. Thus, sponsors may want to discuss nonproprietary name selection with CBER prior to submission to USANC, to assist in the naming process. For well-characterized proteins, certain suffixes are standard and must be included in the nonproprietary name, e.g., monoclonal antibodies use -mab as the final syllable.

The proprietary name for a new biological is approved by CBER and reviewed by OCBQ's Advertising and Promotional Labeling Branch (APLB). Two names may be submitted, with a clear indication of the sponsor's preference. The rationale for the choice, with summaries from marketing research studies, should be included. These studies should be designed to assess similar sounding names and to assess how names may be interpreted, including foreign language translations. Also included in the application are full descriptions of the product, therapeutic category and/or indication and the setting for use (e.g., doctor's office, hospital or home). Proprietary name submissions can be made any time after Phase 2, but a recommendation made prior to product approval will be reevaluated within 90 days of approval to ensure that no new products have entered the marketplace that could give rise to confusion because of similarity in spelling or pronunciation.

Pre-license Inspection

A pre-license inspection is an inspection of an establishment that has not yet been licensed or approved by CBER for the product under review, and may include all facilities involved in manufacturing the biologic, regardless of the manufacturing arrangement (e.g., contract, divided, shared). The inspection can also include establishments that already have one or more biologics license(s) or approvals for other products. *PHS Act* Section 351 and Section 704 of the *Federal Food, Drug and Cosmetic Act* of 1938 (*FD&C Act*) provide the regulatory authority to conduct inspections at any establishment where biological products are manufactured.

CBER's policy is that a pre-license or preapproval inspection generally will be necessary for a BLA or supplement if any of the following criteria are met:

1. The manufacturer does not hold an active US license or, in the case of a contract manufacturer, the facility is not approved for use in manufacturing a licensed product.
2. FDA has not inspected the establishment in the last two years.
3. The previous inspection revealed significant Good Manufacturing Practice (GMP) deficiencies in areas related to the processes in the submission (similar

processes) or systemic problems, such as quality control (QC)/quality assurance (QA) oversight.

4. The establishment is performing significant manufacturing step(s) in new (unlicensed) areas using different equipment (representing a process change). This would include currently dedicated areas that have not been approved as multiproduct facilities, buildings or areas.
5. The manufacturing process is sufficiently different (new production methods, specialized equipment or facilities) from that of other approved products produced by the establishment. Points to be considered:
   - Do differences in the process (e.g., different types of columns) or particulars (e.g., different production cell lines) require an on-site determination of GMP compliance?
   - Are the analytical methods accurate or sensitive enough to detect problems?
   - Are different processes or equipment being used?

In some cases, CBER relies on inspections to obtain validation and facility information that previously may have been submitted in the BLA; thus, greater coordination and efficiency are required in planning and conducting inspections. However, some BLAs and supplements include manufacturing establishments that use production areas common to other licensed products, so conducting a pre-license or preapproval inspection prior to approval of every BLA or supplement may not be necessary. In such cases, both the director of the division with product responsibility and the director of DMPQ within OCBQ must concur in the decision to waive an inspection, or the inspection should be scheduled according to established procedures.

Inspections for biologics are much the same as those for other drugs. Systems-based inspections include review of:
- production and process controls
- failure investigations
- buildings and facilities
- equipment cleaning and maintenance
- laboratory controls
- quality unit/systems

In addition, the CMC section of the BLA will be compared to manufacturing site documents during the inspection to establish the BLA submission's accuracy and integrity. Because of the complexity of the process involved in the manufacture of biologics, the investigator is likely to spend considerably more time observing the process than is typical for small-molecule inspections. The investigator usually works with the manufacturer to schedule an appropriate time to conduct the inspection so the entire manufacturing process can be observed; any delay by the sponsor in this activity may delay the BLA review. Another difference is that the CMC product specialist for the BLA review generally will participate in a biologics inspection.

Postlicensing Compliance Activities

Annual Progress Reports of Postmarketing Studies

Routine Annual Reports, such as those required under New Drug Application (NDA) or Abbreviated New Drug Application (ANDA) regulations, are not mandatory for licensed biological products. However, the regulations do require Annual Reports for products marketed under a BLA for certain situations, such as: making changes to the application (21 CFR 601.12(d)); providing information related to pediatric studies (21 CFR 601.28); and providing status reports on postmarket study requirements related to clinical safety, clinical efficacy, clinical pharmacology or nonclinical toxicology (21 CFR 601.70).

The *Food and Drug Administration Amendments Act* of 2007 (*FDAAA*), which does apply to both drugs and biologics, gave FDA authority to require additional postmarketing studies related to assessing known safety risks, including both signals of serious risk and potential serious risks associated with use of the drug. *FDAAA* also gave FDA authority to require labeling changes based on the results of such studies. Section 505(o)(3)(E)(ii), enacted under *FDAAA*, stipulates that the following information be provided in the Annual Report for required postmarketing studies: a timetable for the completion of each study; periodic reports on the status of required studies, including whether enrollment has begun, the number of participants enrolled and whether any difficulties in completing the study have been encountered; and registration information with respect to clinical trial certification. In addition, *FDAAA* requires that applicants report on each study "otherwise undertaken by the applicant to investigate a safety issue." The status of other types of postmarketing commitments (e.g., those concerning chemistry, manufacturing, production controls and studies conducted on an applicant's own initiative) are not required to be reported under Sections 314.81(b)(2)(vii) and 601.70.

Once a required postmarketing study commitment has been made, an Annual Report is due each year within 60 days after the anniversary date of application approval and must be accompanied by a completed transmittal Form FDA 2252. Sponsors must continue to report on the progress of the commitment until the postmarketing study is completed or terminated, unless the postmarketing study commitment is either no longer feasible or would no longer provide useful information (as agreed with FDA). Failure to comply with the timetable, the periodic reporting submissions or other requirements of section 505(o)(3)(E)(ii) will be considered a violation unless the applicant demonstrates good cause for the noncompliance (only as agreed with FDA). Violations could result in civil penalties of up to $250,000 per violation, and the penalties can be increased (i.e., doubled) if the violation continues for more than 30 days, and can continue to double for subsequent 30-day periods.

Inspections

After licensure, two other types of inspections may take place: the routine, periodic inspection that should occur every two years (biennial) and a directed (for cause) inspection. CBER and the Office of Regulatory Affairs (ORA) have built a partnership to focus resources on inspectional and compliance issues in the biologics area. To accomplish this, a group of specialized investigators, called Team Biologics, has been formed to inspect licensed biological drug and device product facilities regulated by CBER. The goal of Team Biologics is to assure the quality and safety of biological products and to quickly resolve inconsistencies.

Import/Export

CBER oversees the import and export of biologics to determine whether imported biological products, drugs and devices regulated by the center comply with the requirements of the *FD&C Act*, the *PHS Act* and the regulations promulgated under these statutes. Imported products regulated by FDA are subject to inspection at the time of entry by the US Customs and Border Protection (CBP) (see www.cbp.gov/). Shipments found not to comply with the law are subject to detention. For imports, FDA works with CBP to verify licensure; FDA may perform random sampling, and will issue import alerts for products that do not comply. A foreign manufacturer must have a US license to import a biological product into the US. Per FDA's *Regulatory Procedures Manual*, Chapter 9, Subchapter 9.3, "Importation of Biological Products," licensed biologics that have been lot-released (or are exempt) by CBER may be imported into the US and may proceed through Customs without FDA examination. Entry documents for IND biologics must declare a valid, active IND number. Products in short supply also may be imported under 21 CFR 601.22; however, these products must be registered with CBER, and this will be verified by CBP. Under 7 CFR Chapter III, and overseen by the US Department of Agriculture (USDA), biological products also may require an Animal and Plant Health Inspection Service (APHIS) permit to enter the country if the product contains certain microbial, plant- or animal-derived materials or is otherwise a regulated product, such as a genetically engineered organism.

A licensed biologic may be exported without FDA authorization (*Guidance for Industry: FDA Export Certificates* (August 2002)) and in accordance with Section 801(e) Exports or 802 Export of Certain Unapproved Products of the *FD&C Act* or Section 351(h) of the *PHS Act*, which states that a biologic is not adulterated or misbranded if it:
- accords to the specifications of the foreign purchaser
- is not in conflict with the laws of the country to which it is intended for export
- is labeled on the outside of the shipping package that it is intended for export
- is not sold or offered for sale in domestic commerce

FDA supplies a Certificate to Foreign Government, if requested, for the export of products that can be legally marketed in the US. It also supplies a Certificate of Exportability for the export of products that cannot be legally marketed in the US but meet *FD&C Act* requirements.

Import for export, per the *FDA Export Reform and Enhancement Act* of 1996, allows the importation of drug and device components for incorporation into a finished product that can then be exported in accordance with 801, 802 and *PHS Act* 351h.

Postapproval Changes

In accordance with Section 506A(b) of the *FD&C Act* (21 USC 356a), the effect of any postapproval CMC changes on a product's identity, strength, quality, purity or potency, as they may relate to the product's safety or efficacy, must be assessed. Such changes may include changes to:
- manufacturing processes
- analytical procedures
- manufacturing equipment
- manufacturing facilities
- container closure systems
- process analytical technology (PAT)

Before distributing a product made using a change, sponsors are required to demonstrate, through appropriate validation and/or other clinical or nonclinical laboratory studies, the lack of adverse effect of the change on identity, strength, quality, purity or potency as they may relate to the product's safety or effectiveness.

Sponsors should assess the change to determine the correct product reporting category:
- Prior Approval Supplement (PAS)—major changes that require supplement submission and approval prior to distribution of the product made using the change (21 CFR 601.12(b)). A PAS is used to report changes that have a substantial potential to adversely affect a product's identity, strength, quality, purity or potency as they may relate to the product's safety or effectiveness. Examples include: a change in manufacturing processes or analytical methods that result in change of specification limits; a change to larger-scale production; major construction; a change in the stability protocol or acceptance criteria; and extension of the expiration dating period.
- Changes Being Effected in 30 Days (CBE-30)—moderate changes (CBE-30) require a supplement

to FDA 30 days prior to distribution (21 CFR 601.12(c)(3)). A CBE-30 is used to report changes that have moderate potential to adversely affect a product's identity, strength, quality, purity or potency as they may relate to the product's safety or effectiveness. Examples include: addition of a duplicated process chain or unit process; change in the site of testing from one facility to another (e.g., from a contract lab to the sponsor; from an existing contract lab to a new contract lab; from the sponsor to a new contract lab).

- CBE—reports changes that have minimal potential to adversely affect a product's identity, strength, quality, purity or potency as they may relate to the product's safety or effectiveness. A CBE supplement would be received by FDA before, or concurrently with, distribution of the product made using the change. Examples include: addition of release tests and/or specifications; tightening of specifications for intermediates; and minor changes in fermentation batch size using the same equipment and resulting in no change in specifications of the bulk or final product.
- Annual Report—minor changes can be included in the Annual Report, which is submitted within 60 days of the anniversary date of product approval. These are changes that have minimal potential to adversely affect a product's identity, strength, quality, purity or potency as they may relate to the product's safety or effectiveness. Examples include: an increase in the scale of aseptic manufacturing for finished product without a change in equipment, e.g., increased number of vials filled; modifications in analytical procedures with no change in the basic test methodology or existing release specifications, provided the change is supported by validation data; and establishment of a new working cell bank derived from a previously approved master cell bank according to an SOP on file in the approved license application.

By using a comparability protocol that has been previously reviewed by FDA, the sponsor may be able to file certain CMC changes made under the protocol under a less-restrictive reporting category, e.g., a change that would normally be a CBE-30 may be allowed as a CBE if it has already been approved as a comparability protocol. While the submission of a comparability protocol is not required to make changes, in many cases, using one will facilitate the subsequent implementation and reporting requirements of CMC changes, which could result in moving a product into distribution more quickly than if a protocol were not submitted.

A comparability protocol is a well-defined, detailed, written plan for assessing the effect of specific CMC changes on a particular drug product's identity, strength, quality, purity and potency as they may relate to the product's safety and effectiveness. A comparability protocol describes the changes that it covers and specifies the tests and studies that will be performed, including establishing analytical procedures and acceptance criteria to demonstrate that specified CMC changes do not adversely affect the product. However, it is important to note that comparability protocols are not recommended for CMC changes that cannot be definitely evaluated, that require a new IND or that require efficacy, safety (clinical or nonclinical) or pharmacokinetic/pharmacodynamic data to evaluate the effect of the change (e.g., certain formulation changes or clinical or nonclinical studies to qualify new impurities).

The FDA review committee will determine whether the changes reported in the supplement require on-site review. If the review committee determines an inspection is necessary for one or more establishments included in the supplement, the inspection(s) will be performed prior to sending the action letter for the supplement. Failure to comply with the reporting requirements outlined in 21 CFR 601.12 could result in a request by FDA that all changes be submitted as a PAS. Two examples of failure to comply are the constant downgrading of changes (e.g., from a PAS to a CBE) and failing to supply sufficient information to support the changes.

Similarly, under 21 CFR 601.12(f), changes to a product package label, container label and package insert require one of the following:

- submission of a supplement with FDA approval needed prior to product distribution, in cases such as the addition of superiority claims or changes based on additional preclinical and/or postmarketing clinical studies
- submission of a supplement with product distribution allowed at the time of supplement submission (does not require a 30-day waiting period) in cases such as strengthening cautionary statements or instructions
- submission of the final printed label in an Annual Report in cases such as editorial changes and changes in how the product is supplied, provided there is no change in dosage strength or form

Additionally, under 21 CFR 601.12(f)(4), changes to advertising and promotional labeling must comply with the provisions of 21 CFR 314.81(b)(3)(i), which requires the submission to FDA of specimens of mailing pieces and any other labeling or advertising devised for promotion of a drug product at the time of initial dissemination of the labeling, and at the time of initial publication of the advertisement for a prescription drug product. Mailing pieces and labeling designed to contain samples of a drug product are required for the submission to be considered complete, with the exception of the sample of the drug product itself. (See Chapter 24 Biologics Labeling, Advertising and Promotion for more on labeling.)

Chapter 23

Postmarketing Reporting Requirements

Postmarketing expedited reporting requirements for serious and unexpected adverse experiences from all sources (domestic and foreign) related to biologics are similar to those for drugs and are stated in 21 CFR 600.80 and 600.81. Reporting requirements include: Postmarketing 15-day "Alert Reports," which include reports based on scientific literature; Postmarketing 15-day Alert Report follow-ups, which are also required to be reported within 15 days of receiving new information; and periodic adverse experience reports. The reporting format for individual case study reports is the MedWatch mandatory reporting form, Form FDA 3500A. However, adverse events related to vaccines must be reported on a separate form under the Vaccine Adverse Event Reporting System (VAERS). Foreign adverse experience may be reported using either the 3500A or, if preferred, a CIOMS I form. Sponsors may request waivers of the requirement to file Form FDA 3500A for nonserious, expected adverse experiences; however, FDA does not intend to grant waivers within one year of licensure for new biological molecular entities, blood products, plasma derivatives or vaccines. For biological combination products, reports must be filed with both relevant centers. Adverse events related to vaccines also are monitored by the Centers for Disease Control (CDC). The VAERS reporting system is not linked to the vaccine injury compensation program.

Periodic adverse experience reports include summaries of serious and unexpected adverse experiences as well as reports of nonserious expected adverse experiences. Periodic reports are made at quarterly intervals for three years from the date of issuance of the biologics license, and then annually. The licensed manufacturer is required to submit each quarterly report within 30 days of the close of the quarter (the first quarter beginning on the date of issuance of the biologics license) and each Annual Report within 60 days of the anniversary date of the issuance of the biologics license.

Distribution reports for biological products, including vaccines, also are required under 21 CFR 600.81; this requirement is unique for biologics with approved BLAs. The distribution report includes the bulk, fill and label lot numbers for the total number of dosage units of each strength or potency distributed, expiration date and distribution date. The licensed manufacturer submits this report every six months to either CBER or CDER, as applicable.

Risk Assessment

Risk assessment should occur throughout a product's lifecycle, from the early identification of a potential product and preclinical testing, through the premarketing development process, and after approval during marketing. Premarketing risk assessment represents a key step in this process, and product approval requires that a product's underlying risks and benefits have been adequately assessed. The adequacy of this risk assessment is a matter of both quantity (ensuring that enough patients are studied) and quality (the appropriateness of the assessments performed, the appropriateness and breadth of the patient populations studied and how results are analyzed). In reaching a final decision on approvability, both existing risk information and any outstanding questions regarding safety are considered in a product's risk assessment and weighed against the product's demonstrated benefits. The fewer a product's demonstrated benefits, the less acceptable may be higher levels of demonstrated risks.

For assessing risk in the postapproval setting, labeling and routine reporting requirements are sufficient to mitigate risks and preserve benefits for the majority of approved products. However, in other cases, FDA has requested additional risk minimization strategies, which were originally called Risk Minimization Action Plans, or RiskMAPs. Since the passage of *FDAAA,* these safety plans are now called Risk Evaluation and Mitigation Strategies or REMS. A REMS is a strategy to manage a serious safety risk associated with a drug or biological product while preserving its benefits. FDA also has the authority to apply the REMS retroactively and require sponsors to submit a REMS for an already approved product.

A REMS can include a Medication Guide, a Patient Package Insert, a communication plan for healthcare professionals, various Elements to Assure Safe Use (ETASU) and an implementation system. The Medication Guide is the most commonly used REMS, with more than 150 approved drugs now requiring a Medication Guide. Medication Guides are utilized when specific information is necessary to prevent serious adverse effects, when patient decision making should include knowledge about a serious side effect, or if patient adherence to directions for use is essential for the product's effectiveness. The responsibility for ensuring that the Medication Guides are available to patients lies with the sponsor, not the pharmacist.

ETASU may include one or more of the following requirements:
- Healthcare providers who prescribe the drug must have particular training or experience or be specially certified.
- Pharmacies, practitioners or healthcare settings dispensing the drug must be specially certified.
- The drug is dispensed to patients only in certain healthcare settings, such as hospitals.
- The drug is dispensed to patients with evidence or other documentation of safe use conditions, such as laboratory test results.
- Each patient using the drug is subject to certain monitoring requirements.
- Each patient using the drug is enrolled in a registry.

The REMS also must include a timetable for assessment; the minimum timeframe for assessments is at 18 months, three years and seven years after approval.

Biological Product Deviation Reporting (BPDR)

Manufacturers of licensed biological products are required to report events that represent unexpected or unforeseeable events or deviations from current Good Manufacturing Practice (CGMP), applicable regulations, applicable standards or established specifications that may affect a product's safety, purity or potency per 21 CFR 600.14. Prior to 2001, this reporting was termed "error and accident" reporting. The BPDR is reported on Form FDA 3486—Biological Product Deviation Report Form and the appropriate deviation code designating the type of event must be included. The report must not be dated more than 45 calendar days from the date when information that reasonably suggests a reportable event has occurred is discovered. Events that are reportable are those that occur at the sponsor's facility or at a facility under the sponsor's control, e.g., a contract manufacturer, and include events for products that have been distributed and are no longer under the sponsor's control. Therefore, procedures for the investigation of any unexplained discrepancy or failure of a lot to meet any of its specifications should include provisions for timely investigation; an appropriate corrective action plan to prevent recurrence; procedures to gain control of unsuitable products in a timely manner; and appropriate disposition of all affected products (in-date and expired). All BPDRs should be submitted to OCBQ, except in the case of biological products transferred to CDER in 2003.

FDA Enforcement Actions

Regulatory Action Letters

CBER may issue several types of regulatory action letters. These letters ordinarily are issued to biological product manufacturers in an effort to stop practices that are in violation of the regulations and to promote corrective action. Examples of regulatory action letters issued by CBER include:
- Warning Letters
- Notice of Initiation of Disqualification Proceedings and Opportunity to Explain (NIDPOE) Letters
- Untitled letters
- Administrative License Action Letters
- Orders of Retention, Recall, Destruction and Cessation of Manufacturing Related to Human Cell, Tissue, and Cellular and Tissue-Based Products (HCT/Ps)

Warning Letters are issued for violations considered to be of regulatory significance and are issued to achieve voluntary compliance. Significant violations are those violations that may lead to enforcement action if not promptly and adequately corrected. A Warning Letter is issued to a responsible individual or firm to establish prior notice that the agency considers one or more products, practices, processes or other activities to be in violation of the *FD&C Act*, its implementing regulations and other federal statutes. A Warning Letter is one of FDA's principal means of achieving prompt voluntary compliance with the *FD&C Act*.

A NIDPOE Letter informs the recipient clinical investigator that the agency is initiating an administrative proceeding to determine whether the clinical investigator should be disqualified from receiving investigational products pursuant to FDA regulations. Generally, the agency issues a NIDPOE letter when it believes it has evidence that the clinical investigator repeatedly or deliberately violated FDA's regulations governing the proper conduct of clinical studies involving investigational products or submitted false information to the sponsor.

An Untitled Letter is an initial correspondence with a sponsor citing violations that do not meet the threshold of regulatory significance for a Warning Letter. CBER has issued Untitled Letters, for example, after its review of a manufacturer's advertising and promotional labeling, after an inspection under CBER's Bioresearch Monitoring program or by Team Biologics and as a result of Internet website surveillance.

Administrative License Action Letters include license revocation and suspension. License revocation is the cancellation of a license and the withdrawal of the authorization to introduce biological products into interstate commerce. Examples of grounds for revocation include: FDA's inability to gain access for inspection; the manufacturer's failure to report a change as required; failure of the product or establishment to conform to standards in the license or to comply with CGMPs; or the product not being safe or effective, or being misbranded. Except in the case of license suspension or willful violations, CBER will issue a Notice of Intent to Revoke License Letter and provide an opportunity for the sponsor to demonstrate or achieve compliance before initiating revocation proceedings and issuing a license revocation letter. The licensee has 10 days to notify FDA of its commitment to, and plans for, achieving compliance, and then has 30 days to submit a comprehensive report with rigid timetables.

License Suspension is a summary action that provides for the immediate withdrawal, without prior notice or a hearing, of the authorization to introduce biological products into interstate commerce when there are reasonable grounds to believe that the product is a danger to public health (*PHS Act* Section 351). The Department of Justice does not need to concur. All product shipping and manufacturing activities must cease until the license is reactivated.

An Order of Retention, Recall, Destruction, or Cessation of Manufacturing may be issued when there are reasonable grounds to believe that an HCT/P is violative, or if the HCT/P is infected or contaminated and is a source of dangerous infection to humans; or if an establishment does not provide adequate protections against the risks of communicable disease transmission.

Recalls

Recalls are generally voluntary acts by sponsors because FDA has limited statutory authority to prescribe a recall. However, the *National Childhood Vaccine Injury Act* of 1986 amended the *PHS Act* to provide recall authority for biological products (42 U.S. 262). Therefore, FDA can order a recall if the biological product constitutes an imminent or substantial hazard to public health per *PHS Act* Section 351(a), or if it is considered a "dangerous" medical device per the *FD&C Act*. Recalls can be ordered for any reason, but if a recall is due to misbranding or adulteration, FDA should be notified to prevent further action. Companies can expect to work closely with the agency during a recall. There are four key stages in the recall process: discovery, planning, implementation and termination of the recall event. Final disposition of the recalled product should be discussed with FDA and typically involves destruction.

Judicial Enforcement

FDA's civil and criminal enforcement actions include:
- Seizure—an action taken to remove a product from commerce because it is in violation of the law. FDA initiates a seizure by filing a complaint with the US District Court where the product is located. A US Marshal is then directed by the court to take possession, i.e., seize the goods where they are found, until the matter is resolved.
- Injunction—a civil action taken against an individual or firm seeking to stop continued production or distribution of a violative product until the firm complies with FDA requirements.
- Prosecution—a criminal action taken as the result of acts prohibited in the *FD&C Act* that can be directed at the responsible persons in management, even if they are unaware of the violative conduct and even without intent.

For more information on FDA enforcement actions, see Chapter 36 FDA Inspection and Enforcement.

Summary

- The compliance and surveillance activities related to biologics licenses during the lifecycle of biological products are overseen by the Office of Compliance and Biologics Quality, CBER.
- Biologics licensing standards per the *PHS Act* and 21 CFR 600.3 provide that biologics must be "safe, pure, and potent." Compliance activities prior to approval include safety reporting, CMC change control and compliance with GMPs, GCPs and GLPs to ensure readiness for BIMO and/or pre-license inspections.
- For import and export of biological products, a US license is required for a foreign manufacturer to import and distribute a biological product in the US, whereas a licensed biologic may be exported from the US without FDA authorization.
- Postapproval compliance activities include post-marketing commitments, three categories of CMC change control (PAS, CBE and Annual Report), which can be reduced by using comparability protocols, postmarketing safety reporting and biologic product deviation reporting (BPDR).
- *FDAAA* authorized Risk Evaluation and Mitigation Strategies (REMS), which are safety plans designed to manage a serious risk associated with a drug or biological product if FDA determines that such a plan is necessary to ensure the product's benefits outweigh its risks.
- In cases where CBER identifies areas of noncompliance, it may issue any of several types of regulatory action letters, up to and including license revocation, to stop practices found to be in violation of the regulations and to promote corrective action. CBER also has options for judicial enforcement, including seizure, injunction and prosecution, if warranted.

Chapter 24

Biologics Labeling, Advertising and Promotion

Updated by Sherry Yanez-Gregor, JD, MSc

OBJECTIVES

❑ Review the general FDA regulations for labeling, promotion and advertising of biological drugs under the jurisdiction of CBER or CDER

❑ Understand the application of these regulations through the study of related FDA guidance documents and enforcement letters

LAWS, REGULATIONS AND GUIDELINES COVERED IN THIS CHAPTER

❑ *Federal Food, Drug, and Cosmetic Act* of 1938

❑ 21 CFR 99 Dissemination of information on unapproved/new uses for marketed drugs, biologics and devices

❑ 21 CFR 201 Labeling

  o 21 CFR 201.56–58 Labeling requirements

  o 21 CFR 201.80 Specific requirements on content and format of labeling for human prescription drug and biological products

  o 21 CFR 201.200 Disclosure of drug efficacy study evaluations in labeling and advertising

❑ 21 CFR 202.1 Prescription drug advertisements

❑ 21 CFR 203 Prescription drug marketing

❑ 21 CFR 208 Medication guides for prescription drug products

❑ 21 CFR 312.6–7 Labeling and promotion for investigational new drugs

❑ 21 CFR 314.70 Supplements and other changes to an approved application

❑ 21 CFR 314.81 Other post-marketing reports

❑ 21 CFR 601.2 Applications for biologics licenses; procedures for filing

❑ 21 CFR 601.12 Changes to an approved application

❑ 21 CFR 601.25 Review procedures to determine that licensed biological products are safe, effective, and not misbranded under prescribed, recommended, or suggested conditions of use

❑ 21 CFR 601.45 Promotional materials

❑ 21 CFR 610 Subpart G Labeling standards

❑ 21 CFR 606.120–122 Labeling, general requirements

❑ 21 CFR 660 Additional standards for diagnostic substances for laboratory tests

Chapter 24

- o 21 CFR 660.2(c) General requirements, labeling
- o 21 CFR 660.28 Blood grouping reagent labeling
- o 21 CFR 660.35 Reagent red blood cells labeling
- o 21 CFR 660.45 Hepatitis B surface antigen labeling
- o 21 CFR 660.55 Anti-human globulin labeling

- ❏ 21 CFR 801 Medical devices labeling
- ❏ 21 CFR 809 In vitro diagnostic products for human use
- ❏ *Final Guidance on Industry-Supported Scientific and Educational Activities* (November 1997)
- ❏ *Guidance for Industry: Changes to an Approved Application: Biological Products* (July 1997)
- ❏ *Draft Guidance for Industry: Product Name Placement, Size, and Prominence in Advertising and Promotional Labeling* (January 1999)
- ❏ *Draft Guidance for Industry: Accelerated Approval Products—Submission of Promotional Materials* (March 1999)
- ❏ *Guidance for Industry: Consumer-Directed Broadcast Advertisements* (August 1999)
- ❏ *Draft Guidance for Industry: Providing Regulatory Submissions in Electronic Format—Prescription Drug Advertising and Promotional Labeling* (January 2001)
- ❏ *Draft Guidance for Industry: Brief Summary: Disclosing Risk Information in Consumer-Directed Print Advertisements* (January 2004)
- ❏ *Draft Guidance for Industry: "Help-Seeking" and Other Disease Awareness Communications by or on Behalf of Drug and Device Firms* (January 2004)
- ❏ *Guidance for Industry: Providing Regulatory Submissions in Electronic Format—Content of Labeling* (April 2005)

- ❏ *Draft Guidance for Industry: Labeling for Human Prescription Drug and Biological Products—Implementing the New Content and Format Requirements* (January 2006)
- ❏ *Guidance for Industry: Indexing Structured Product Labeling* (June 2008)
- ❏ *Guidance for Industry: Good Reprint Practices for the Distribution of Medical Journal Articles and Medical or Scientific Reference Publications on Unapproved New Uses of Approved Drugs and Approved or Cleared Medical Devices* (January 2009)
- ❏ *Draft Guidance for Industry: Presenting Risk Information in Prescription Drug and Medical Device Promotion* (May 2009)
- ❏ *Guidance for Industry: Product Name Placement, Size, and Prominence in Advertising in Promotional Labeling* (January 2012)
- ❏ *Draft Guidance for Industry: Direct-to-Consumer Television Advertisements—FDAAA DTC Television Ad Pre-Dissemination Review Program* (March 2012)

Definitions

Label
The *Federal Food, Drug, and Cosmetic Act* of 1938 (*FD&C Act*) defines a "label" as a display of written, printed or graphic material on the immediate container of a drug.

Labeling
"Labeling" is defined by the US Food and Drug Administration (FDA) as any written, printed or graphic material on the drug, on any of its containers or wrappers, or on any material accompanying it. Therefore, it includes, but is not limited to, professional labeling (generally referred to as the package insert or prescribing information (PI)) and patient labeling (patient package insert (PPI) or a Medication Guide).

The umbrella term "labeling" for drugs and devices generally is divided by FDA into two subcategories that are regulated by FDA under the *FD&C Act*:
1. FDA-approved labeling is initially prepared for the original Biologics License Application (BLA) submission and then included with subsequent supplements. This includes the PI. This document includes the details and directions healthcare providers need to prescribe the product properly. It is also the basis for how sponsors can advertise their

products. FDA-approved labeling may also include a PPI; when the information is for an especially risky or difficult-to-use drug, the PPI is referred to as a Medication Guide. Risk Evaluation and Mitigation Strategies (REMS) (described later in this chapter) may also be a component of labeling. The FDA-approved labeling must be included in the package when a drug is dispensed.

2. Promotional labeling is, generally, any product material (other than the FDA-approved labeling as defined above) intended to promote the use of a drug. Unlike FDA-approved labeling, promotional labeling does not have to physically accompany the drug or be inserted in the package when a drug is dispensed. However, as per the regulations, promotional labeling must be disseminated with the full FDA-approved labeling.

Labeling Regulations and Requirements

Labeling Filed With Original BLA Submissions

Biologics labeling begins with filing of the first BLA for a biological drug product. The BLA is a request for permission to introduce, or deliver for introduction, a biologic product into interstate commerce (21 CFR 610.2). Labeling information is required in BLA submissions for approval to FDA (21 CFR 610.2). This labeling information represents the proposed labeling a sponsor intends to use for postapproval marketing. The content and format are regulated by 21 CFR 201.56–57 and 21 CFR 610.60–68 and further explained in various guidance documents, e.g., *Draft Guidance for Industry: Labeling for Human Prescription Drug and Biological Products—Implementing the New Content and Format Requirements* (January 2006). Typically, four types of labeling information are required to be submitted in the original BLA: 1) draft container and carton labels, 2) new PI format, 3) annotated draft labeling text and 4) structured product labeling (SPL). In addition, some biologics require the submission of a Medication Guide or REMS.

Container and Carton Labels

Container Label
Per 21 CFR 610.60, the container label should bear the following information:
1. proper name of the product
2. manufacturer name, address and license number
3. lot number or other lot identification
4. expiration date
5. recommended individual dose, for multiple dose containers
6. the statement: "Rx only" for prescription biologics
7. Medication Guide, if required

In special cases, certain information may be expanded or omitted. For example, expansion may be needed if the container is not inserted in any package, or text can be omitted if the container is too small to affix a label containing all the information listed above (see 21 CFR 610.60(b), (c) and (d)). To allow visual inspection of the contents, the label should not cover the container completely.

Package (Carton) Label
Per 21 CFR 610.61, the package label should contain:
1. proper name of the product
2. manufacturer name, address and license number
3. lot number or other lot identification
4. expiration date
5. preservatives, if any
6. number of containers, if more than one
7. amount of product in the container
8. recommended storage temperature
9. the words "shake well" or "do not freeze," as required
10. recommended individual dose, for multi-dose container
11. type and calculated amount of antibiotics added during manufacture
12. adjuvant, if present
13. product source, when it is a factor in safe administration
14. minimum potency of product or the statement: "No US standard of potency"
15. the statement: "Rx only" for prescription biologics
16. reference statement to PI inside the package for any other pertinent information

The font size, type, color, position and legibility of container and package labels should meet the requirements in 21 CFR 610.62. Divided manufacturing responsibility should also be shown on either the package or the container label. Bar code label requirements under 21 CFR 201.25 apply to all biologics except biological devices or blood and blood components intended for transfusion, which follow the requirements in 21 CFR 606.121(c)(13).

New Package Insert Format
The plain package insert format, also called the "draft package insert" or "draft labeling text," is required. It contains information about the sponsor's proposed labeling and should conform to the format required by regulations and guidance.

Annotated Labeling
The draft labeling text, once completed, needs to be annotated with relevant sections in the BLA submission (e.g., Module 5 clinical study reports) to substantiate each claim in the labeling. This is a separate file from the draft labeling

text required in the initial submission and is called "annotated labeling."

Structured Product Labeling (SPL)
SPL, another separate file containing all the draft labeling text in extensible markup language (xml) format, also is required by the Center for Drug Evaluation and Research (CDER) under 21 CFR 601.14 and must be submitted in the initial BLA filing. Instructions on preparing SPL are detailed in *Guidance for Industry: Providing Regulatory Submissions in Electronic Format—Content of Labeling* (April 2005) and *Guidance for Industry: Indexing Structured Product Labeling* (June 2008). Based on these guidance documents, the content of SPL labeling files is placed in a single folder named "SPL" in the electronic submission. This requirement applies to both small molecules and biologics under the jurisdiction of CDER. The Center for Biologics Evaluation and Research (CBER) will require SPL for BLAs under its jurisdiction soon. SPL in xml format enables healthcare professionals and other users to rapidly search and sort product information using new computer technologies.

Risk Evaluation and Mitigation Strategies (REMS)
Under the *Food and Drug Administration Amendments Act* of 2007 (*FDAAA*), a REMS is required for some drugs, including biologics.

> "Drug and biological products deemed to have in effect an approved REMS are those that on March 25, 2008 (the effective date of Title IX, subtitle A of FDAAA), had in effect "elements to assure safe use." "Elements to assure safe use" include the following: (1) Health care providers who prescribe the drug have particular training or experience, or are specially certified; (2) pharmacies, practitioners, or health care settings that dispense the drug are specially certified; (3) the drug is dispensed to patients only in certain health care settings, such as hospitals; (4) the drug is dispensed to patients with evidence or other documentation of safe use conditions, such as laboratory test results; (5) each patient using the drug is subject to certain monitoring; or (6) each patient using the drug is enrolled in a registry (see section 505-1(f)(3) of the act)."[1]

A drug will not be deemed to have a REMS if it has only a Medication Guide (see below), PPI and/or communication plan.

Because of this new regulation, a BLA sponsor needs to determine whether it is required to submit a proposed REMS in the BLA. If a REMS is required, it should be submitted to FDA prior to approval.

Medication Guide
A Medication Guide applies primarily to human prescription drug products used on an outpatient basis without direct supervision by a healthcare professional (21 CFR 208.1 (a)). It is approved by FDA and distributed to patients when FDA determines that such a guide is necessary to patients' safe and effective use of a drug product (21 CFR 208.1 (b)). The drug product is the basis for determining whether to file a Medication Guide in the original BLA. Self-injectable insulin to treat type I diabetes is an example of a product requiring a Medication Guide. Many new biologics, however, require healthcare professionals to administer the drug to patients in hospitals or special treatment centers to ensure safe use. Because these products often target severe diseases and unmet medical needs, patients need to be monitored closely by healthcare professionals after administration. In such cases, a REMS often is required instead of a Medication Guide.

Postapproval Labeling Changes
Lifecycle Management
The labeling lifecycle begins when the draft labeling is submitted to FDA. During the BLA review phase, the labeling content may be revised either by the sponsor or at the agency's request. Once the labeling is modified and approved by FDA, the sponsor can begin to commercialize the product by promoting and advertising the approved labeling information through various marketing channels, such as television, newspapers, magazines, the Internet, direct-to-consumer marketing, etc. However, changes to the initially approved labeling may be required, to add and/or delete any information or to clarify specific information to prevent misunderstanding in the marketplace.

Further, the initially approved full labeling may need to be adapted based on the type of marketing channel used for promotion and advertising, e.g., a television advertisement usually is limited to a brief summary of the full labeling due to time constraints (21 CFR 202.1 (e)) and a direct-to-consumer (DTC) promotional piece should be written in language that can be readily understood by ordinary consumers rather than healthcare professionals.

Any information disseminated initially by the sponsor to healthcare professionals and/or directly to consumers must follow FDA requirements (21 CFR 314.81(b)(3)(i) and 601.12(f)(4)) and be submitted to the agency at the time of dissemination. Each submission is required to be accompanied by Form FDA 2567, or its equivalent, and must include a copy of the product labeling. For products approved under the accelerated approval program (21 CFR 314 Subpart H or 21 CFR 312 Subpart E), promotional labeling and advertising must be submitted prior to dissemination (21 CFR 314.550 and 601.45).

All of these activities constitute lifecycle management of pre- and postapproval promotion and advertising.

Preparing Changes to Labeling

The labeling change lifecycle may be managed per *Guidance for Industry: Changes to an Approved Application—Biological Products* (July 1997). Postapproval changes to labeling information require submission to CDER or CBER in one of the following ways:

- Prior Approval Supplement (PAS)—Supplement submission and FDA approval are required before dissemination of the labeling change (e.g., changes to a Medication Guide, highlights of prescribed information) per 21 CFR 314.70(b)(2)(v).
- Changes Being Effected (CBE)—Supplement submission is required, but FDA approval is not necessary before dissemination of labeling changes (e.g., to add or strengthen a contraindication, warning, precaution or adverse reaction; to add or strengthen a statement about drug abuse, dependence, psychological effect or overdosage; to add or strengthen an instruction about dosage and administration that is intended to increase the safe use of the drug product; to delete false, misleading or unsupported indications for use or claims for effectiveness) per 21 CFR 314.70(c)(6)(iii). Subsequent FDA approval, however, is required.
- Annual Report—Information on labeling submitted in an Annual Report is described in 21 CFR 314.81(b)(2)(iii). It should include a summary of any labeling changes since the last Annual Report (e.g., a change in labeling description or how the drug is supplied without change of dosage strength or form, an editorial change in labeling) per 21 CFR 314.70(d)(2)(ix-x).

Depending on the category into which a change falls, the sponsor needs to develop a strategy, collect necessary information and submit the relevant regulatory documents to FDA.

Biologics Advertising and Promotional Labeling Requirements

Regulatory Oversight of Biologic Advertising & Promotion Labeling

FDA has primary jurisdiction over prescription advertising under the 1962 *Kefauver-Harris Drug Amendments* to the *FD&C Act*, over restricted medical devices and biologics advertising under the *Public Health Service Act* (*PHS Act*) and over veterinary medicines under the *FD&C Act*.

Biologics are approved primarily by CBER. At CBER, the Advertising and Promotional Labeling Branch (APLB) within the Office of Compliance and Biologics Quality is responsible for reviewing and monitoring biologic product promotion. Specific oversight activities include reviews of final and draft advertising and promotional labeling of licensed biological products to ensure that product communications are fairly balanced (with risks and benefits), truthful, non-misleading and in compliance with federal laws and regulations.

Regulatory oversight of promotion serves to ensure the following overarching principles of advertising and promotional labeling:

- Drug promotion must be consistent with approved product labeling or PI.
- Claims must be supported by substantial evidence.
- Promotion must not be false or misleading.
- Promotion must be fairly balanced.
- Promotion must reveal all material information.

It should be noted that the following requirements apply to any prescription product advertising and promotional labeling, regardless of the medium by which it is communicated—television, print media, Internet or other. Various guidance documents referenced here can be found on the FDA, CBER, CDER and CDER's Office of Prescription Drug Promotion (OPDP) websites.

Preparing Advertisements and Promotional Labeling for Submission

Submitting at First Use

Sponsors are required to submit all biologic advertisements and promotional labeling to APLB at the time of dissemination, also referred to as "time of first use" on Form FDA 2253 (21 CFR 314.81(b)(i)). The form requires sponsors to indicate the type of piece that is being submitted, using the specific coding provided on the form, and the initial date of dissemination. While CDER's OPDP and CBER's APLB require the same form for these submissions, each center provides slightly different directions on the form that the sponsor should be careful to note when completing it. Current information on how to submit biologic advertising and promotional labeling can be found at www.fda.gov/BiologicsBloodVaccines/DevelopmentApprovalProcess/AdvertisingLabelingPromotionalMaterials/ucm118171.htm. Failure to submit advertising and promotional labeling on Form FDA 2253 constitutes a violation of 21 CFR 314.81(b)(i).

Promotional Materials Requiring Presubmission Clearance

Accelerated Approval Products

While most products' materials can be submitted to FDA for the first time at the time of dissemination, there is an exception that requires prior submission for products approved under the Accelerated Approval program (21 CFR 601.45) and for products that may cause fatalities or serious damage about which information has not been widely publicized (as described in 21 CFR 202.1(j)(1)). In these cases, approval by FDA prior to dissemination is required:

- The sponsor of an accelerated approval product must submit to APLB, during the preapproval review period, all advertisements and promotional materials intended to be published within 120 days after approval. After 120 days postapproval, the applicant must submit materials at least 30 days in advance of publication. Once submitted, the sponsor must wait the minimum 30 days to receive advisory comments (often referred to as "pre-clearance") from APLB. If no comments are received at 30 days, the sponsor can choose to withdraw the submission and move ahead with the use of the piece. After receiving advisory comments or choosing to withdraw and move ahead with the piece, the sponsor still is required to submit the pieces on Form FDA 2253 at the time of dissemination.
- Products that are covered under 21 CFR 202.1(j)(1), such as those causing fatalities or serious damage but about which information has not been widely publicized, must obtain FDA approval in a similar manner prior to dissemination.

Direct-to-Consumer Television Advertisements

The Food and Drug Administration Amendments Act of 2007 (FDAAA) authorized FDA to "…require the submission of any television advertisement for a drug…not later than 45 days before dissemination of the television advertisement" (Section 901(d)(2), codified at 21 U.S.C. 353b. Under this provision, sponsors of human prescription drugs, including biological drug products approved under section 351 of the Public Health Service Act (PHS Act), are required to submit television advertisements for pre-dissemination review if the advertisement is subject to one of the following six categories:

- Category 1: the initial television advertisement for any prescription drug or the initial television advertisement for a new or expanded approved indication for any prescription drug
- Category 2: all television advertisements for prescription drugs subject to a REMS with Elements to Assure Safe Use (see Section 505-1(f) of the *FD&C Act*
- Category 3: all television advertisements for Schedule II controlled substances
- Category 4: the first television advertisement for a prescription drug following a safety labeling update that affects the Boxed Warning, Contraindications, or Warnings & Precautions section of its labeling
- Category 5: the first television advertisement for a prescription drug following the receipt by the sponsor of an enforcement letter (i.e., a Warning or untitled letter) for the product that either cites a television advertisement or causes a television advertisement to be discontinued because the advertisement contained violations similar to the ones cited in the enforcement letter
- Category 6: any television advertisement that is otherwise identified by FDA as subject to the pre-dissemination review provision

For more information about the DTC Television Ad Pre-Dissemination Review Program, please see: Draft Guidance for Industry: Direct-to-Consumer Television Advertisements—FDAAA DTC Television Ad Pre-Dissemination Review Program (March 2012).

Advisory Comments

While not a requirement, sponsors have the option of requesting APLB advisory comments on draft advertising and promotional materials. Advisory comments can be requested only for draft materials that have not yet been published or disseminated and are not currently in use or in the public domain. When sponsors are uncertain about some promotional campaigns or language, this can be a very valuable option. APLB strongly encourages the use of this option when launching a new product or indication. Specific directions on how to submit draft materials for advisory comments can be found on FDA's website (www.fda.gov/BiologicsBloodVaccines/DevelopmentApprovalProcess/AdvertisingLabelingPromotionalMaterials/ucm118171.htm). In addition, requests for advisory comments on prescription biological and drug promotional materials, other than promotional ads, can be submitted to OPDP (www.fda.gov/AboutFDA/CentersOffices/OfficeofMedicalProductsandTobacco/CDER/ucm090168.htm).

Note that even after submitting material for advisory comments or withdrawing a submission for advisory comments, the sponsor is still required to submit the pieces on Form FDA 2253 at time of dissemination/first use.

Misconception Regarding Submissions

A common misconception heard in industry is that if APLB does not comment on a piece when submitted at first use on Form FDA 2253, the piece is deemed to be "approved" by APLB. This misconception can wrongly encourage the continued use of inappropriate or violative materials. In general, the submission on Form FDA 2253 is for documentation purposes and does not constitute any type of "approval" by APLB.

Content and Format of Advertising and Promotional Labeling

The requirements for promotional and advertising materials for biologic products are described in detail in 21 CFR 202, as well as in relevant guidance documents such as *Guidance for Industry: Product Name Placement, Size, and Prominence in Advertising and Promotional Labeling* (January 2012) and *Draft Guidance for Industry: Presenting Risk Information in Prescription Drug and Medical Device Promotion* (May 2009).

Presentation of Product Name

As indicated in 21 CFR 202.1 and the draft guidance documents, product names in advertising and promotional labeling should be presented as follows:

- The entire proprietary (brand or trade) name, including the ingredients and dosage form if it is approved as such in the PI, should be presented together without any intervening written or graphic matter.
- The established (generic) name should be printed in letters that are at least half as large as the letters comprising the proprietary name, and the prominence of the established name must be comparable with the prominence of the proprietary name.
- The order of ingredients and respective quantities should be listed in the same manner as they are listed in the PI, and the information presented concerning the quantity of each ingredient should also correspond with the PI.

Product Claims

Must be Consistent With Approved Product Use/Indication

As indicated in 21 CFR 202.1, all advertising and promotional labeling may only "recommend or suggest" the approved use of the product as indicated in the product PI. Any suggestions or recommendations inconsistent with the specific product use or indication presented in the label could constitute off-label promotion or broadening of the indication. For example, in June 2003, APLB issued an enforcement letter to a company that promoted a product for a general condition when the drug was only approved for a "moderate-to-severe" condition. Failure to clarify the claim with the limitation of "moderate-to-severe" constituted broadening of the indication.

To determine whether a product claim is consistent with the product's approved use, FDA looks not just at the product indication, but also at the clinical trials section of the PI. The clinical trials section of the PI provides study background, patient populations included and study results. Generally, if a product is promoted for use in a patient population broader than that which was tested in the clinical trials used for product approval, this may constitute broadening of the indication and be considered a violation of the regulations.

Substantial Evidence or Substantial Clinical Evidence

In addition to maintaining consistency with the product's approved use, all claims of safety and effectiveness must be supported by either substantial evidence or substantial clinical evidence. Substantial evidence generally is accepted as evidence stemming from two adequate and well-controlled trials. Ideally, the trials would be prospective, randomized and blinded and would minimize confounding variables. In July 2009, APLB issued a letter to a company for presenting safety claims stemming from postmarketing data (adverse event rates observed in practice) in an exhibition panel; postmarketing data do not constitute substantial evidence (they are not from a well-controlled clinical trial) and, therefore, the panel was deemed to be misbranded.

Product claims that are held to this standard include not just verbal and textual communications, but also graphics. Graphics in advertising and promotional labeling must be consistent with the FDA-approved product label and be supported by substantial evidence. For instance, a patient depicted in an advertisement generally should represent the average patient in the clinical trials conducted for product approval. An example of an inconsistent advertising claim would contain a graphic of a patient climbing a mountain when the product is indicated for a seriously physically disabling disease; if the majority of patients in the clinical trial had seriously debilitating physical disabilities, this depiction could constitute overstating the product's efficacy.

Fair Balance and Presentation of Risk Information

The manner in which a product's risks are presented in advertising and promotional labeling in comparison to the efficacy information is of utmost importance to APLB. Essentially, safety and effectiveness claims in advertising and promotional labeling must be fairly balanced with risk information. In addition, the risk information must be presented with equal prominence to the promotional claims (21 CFR 202.1(e)(5)). Material facts about the product being promoted also must be communicated, including facts about consequences that may result from the use of the product as suggested in the promotional piece (21 CFR 202.1 (e)(5)(iii)).

Draft Guidance for Industry: Presenting Risk Information in Prescription Drug and Medical Device Promotion (May 2009) provides insight into FDA's thinking on appropriate risk presentation and the various factors used to evaluate adequate risk disclosure. A key aspect of the draft guidance is that when FDA evaluates risk communication in promotional pieces, it does not look only at specific risk statements, but rather at the net impression. The net impression is the message communicated by the promotional piece in its entirety; the piece as a whole should convey an accurate and non-misleading impression of the product's benefits and risks. Furthermore, even if individual claims are not misleading, if the piece as a whole provides a misleading impression (e.g., that the drug is safer than has been proven by substantial evidence), the piece may be deemed to be violative.

Provided below are some general factors that FDA will consider when reviewing risk communication:
- Consistent use of language appropriate for target audience—If a promotional piece is directed toward patients, it should be written in patient-friendly language likely to be understood by the general public.
- Use of signals—Headlines and subheads should accurately identify the risk information.
- Framing risk information—Information should be stated clearly and specifically without inaccurately emphasizing positive or negative aspects.
- Hierarchy of risk information—The ordering of risks is important and, generally, serious risks should be communicated first to ensure increased emphasis.
- Quantity—The amount of benefits conveyed generally should not exceed the amount of risks conveyed (fair balance) in number, completeness, time and space.
- Formatting—The layout, location of risk information and the contrast between text and background will be evaluated to ensure that the benefits are not highlighted more than the risk information.

Consistent with these guidelines, APLB issued an enforcement letter to a company in May 2010 for an audio news release in which efficacy claims were presented in a "slow and deliberate manner that is understandable in terms of the pacing and articulation" while the risk information was presented in a "fast and inarticulate" manner. APLB stated that the piece "fail[ed] to present information about risks of a drug with a prominence reasonably comparable with the presentation of information relating to the effectiveness." In this example, the benefits were highlighted more than the risk information and, thus, the risks associated with the product were minimized.

Misconception About Fair Balance
In previous years, there may have been a general misconception that merely providing a statement of the serious and most common risks in any piece, regardless of the amount of benefits or effectiveness claims provided would be sufficient risk disclosure. This statement of risks was often referred to as the "Fair Balance Statement." Through more recent enforcement letters and the draft guidance, it has become clear that FDA is looking not for a concise statement, but rather for a balance (as described in the section above) between benefit and risk information and disclosure of material information.

Distinctions between Advertising and Promotional Labeling

While "advertising" is technically not defined in the CFR, 21 CFR 202.1(l)1 states that advertisements subject to Section 502(n) of the *FD&C Act* include advertisements published in journals, magazines, other periodicals and newspapers; and broadcast through media such as radio, television and telephone communications systems. This is not a comprehensive list of advertising media subject to regulation. For example, FDA also regulates advertising on the Internet. To date, FDA has not issued a guidance related to online-advertising, social media platforms and mobile advertisements. Instead, one must glean Internet advertising rules from recently issued Warning Letters related to online content.

Generally, advertising and promotional labeling are treated in the same manner, except for the three following distinctions.

Broadcast Advertising

Television and radio advertising (broadcast advertising) must include a statement of the drug's most important risks; this statement is called the "Major Statement" (21 CFR 202.1(e)(1)). This presentation must be spoken, and it can also be included in the video portion of a television advertisement.

The law enables broadcast advertising to include only the most important risk information if the advertisement makes "adequate provision" and directs viewers and/or listeners on how they can obtain the full FDA-approved prescribing information. Broadcast advertisements can meet the "adequate provision" requirement by communicating the following sources for locating a drug's prescribing information:
- website address
- toll-free telephone number
- current issue of a magazine running a print advertisement
- referring to a healthcare provider (e.g., a doctor)

Brief Summary in Print Advertising

Regulations allow advertising to contain a "statement of information in brief summary relating to side effects, contraindications, and effectiveness" (21 CFR 202.1(e)) rather than requiring dissemination of the full FDA-approved labeling (PI), which must be presented directly adjacent to the advertisement. Promotional labeling must always be disseminated with the full PI.

Draft Guidance for Industry: Brief Summary: Disclosing Risk Information in Consumer-Directed Print Advertisements provides the following advice:

- Risk information in brief summaries should be presented in patient-friendly language (language that can be easily understood).
- Consumers should be directed to a toll-free number or a website for additional information.
- A statement clarifying that the brief summary does not provide a comprehensive list of risks associated with the product should be included.

FDAAA

Section 906 of *FDAAA* went into effect in March 2008 and mandates that all published direct-to-consumer advertisements for prescription drugs include the following statement printed in conspicuous text: "You are encouraged to report negative side effects of prescription drugs to the FDA. Visit www.fda.gov/medwatch, or call 1-800-FDA-1088." This requirement only applies to advertising and not to promotional labeling.

General Exception to Risk Disclosure Requirement: Reminder Labeling

"Reminder labeling" is the only type of pharmaceutical promotional labeling that is exempt from the requirement to disclose risk information (21 CFR 201.100(f)). Reminder labeling generally calls attention to the biologic product's name but does not include indications or dosage recommendations for use. Promotional labeling qualifies as a reminder if the following elements are met:

- The product proprietary name and established name of each active ingredient are disclosed.
- Certain specific descriptive information relating to quantitative ingredients statements, dosage form, quantity of package contents, price and other limited information may be included.
- The product indication or dosage recommendation is not conveyed.
- There are no claims or representations about the product.
- The product does not have a "black box" warning in its labeling.

Note that merely indicating a patient population in the material, either through text or a graphic, would be a violation of this exemption and would require the sponsor to provide risk disclosure. For instance, if along with the name, Product X, there was a graphic of a child in the background, this would provide a representation about the product in that it is appropriate for use in a pediatric population; therefore, the sponsor would have to include the appropriate risk disclosure.

Nonpromotional Communications

The following communications generally are not considered to be "promotional" in nature; however, they are still monitored by FDA to ensure that they do not cross the line into advertising and promotional labeling.

Preapproval Product Communications

FDA generally prohibits any promotional activity and claims of safety and efficacy for investigational products prior to approval. Specifically, 21 CFR 312.7(a) states: "A sponsor or investigator, or any person acting on behalf of a sponsor or investigator, shall not represent in a promotional context that an investigational new drug is safe or effective for the purposes for which it is under investigation or otherwise promote the drug."

However, companies often need to provide product information to the public prior to approval (e.g., clinical trial recruitment, press releases, etc.). In these instances, the following recommendations can help ensure that product information is not linked to promotional claims of safety and efficacy:

- When presenting efficacy information, provide an objective presentation of data; state all endpoints and provide data without bias.
- When presenting safety information, include all grades of adverse events with material percentages and/or incidences.
- Avoid characterizing data descriptions such as well-tolerated, revolutionary or robust.
- Always clarify that the product is not yet approved by using descriptions such as "investigational" or "study medication."

It is important to note that this regulation applies not only to sponsors, but also to investigators. In recent years, FDA has issued enforcement letters to investigators who, in their product communications, suggested that a product was safe or efficacious prior to approval.

Scientific Exchange

21 CFR 312.7 also states: "This provision is not intended to restrict the full exchange of scientific information concerning the drug, including dissemination of scientific findings in scientific or lay media. Rather, its intent is to restrict promotional claims of safety or effectiveness of the drug for a use under which it is under investigation and to preclude commercialization of the drug before it is approved for commercial distribution."

Scientific media include journal publications and scientific abstracts and presentations at purely scientific forums. To determine whether a communication is truly a scientific exchange, FDA generally looks at who is communicating it as well as the media by which it is communicated. If a promotional individual (e.g., pharmaceutical sales representative) provides the communication in a promotional venue (e.g., promotional presentation), this is unlikely to be considered a scientific exchange. However, if a clinical researcher from the company, in response to a request from a medical society, provides a presentation on current findings in a purely scientific forum, this may qualify as a scientific exchange.

The nuances are slight and sometimes difficult to discern; therefore, this is an area of much discussion. Consequently, in one-on-one communications, sponsors generally do not allow any proactive communication of information that may be deemed inconsistent with the label and restrict any sharing of additional information to reactive responses to unsolicited requests from medical customers. Also, many sponsors hire medical professionals to fill this communication role.

Dissemination of purely scientific information before a drug is approved is generally allowed since there is no promotional activity or commercial incentive involved, and the sponsor is not allowed to sell an IND biologic. *Final Guidance on Industry-Supported Scientific and Educational Activities* (November 1997) states that truly independent and nonpromotional industry-supported activities have not been subject to FDA regulation. Thus, the agency does not have specific regulations for such an activity.

Disease Awareness and "Help-seeking" Advertising

"Help-seeking" communications or advertisements are disease awareness communications directed at consumers or healthcare practitioners that discuss a particular disease or health condition but do not mention any specific drug or device or make any representation or suggestion concerning a particular drug or device. Because no drug is mentioned or implied, this type of communication is not considered to be a product advertisement, and therefore, it is not subject to the requirements of the *FD&C Act* or FDA regulations (see *Draft Guidance for Industry: "Help-Seeking" and Other Disease Awareness Communications by or on Behalf of Drug and Device Firms* (January 2004)).

To qualify as a disease awareness and help-seeking advertisement as outlined in the draft guidance, a piece must meet the following requirements:
- It should discuss a disease or health condition.
- If it is directed toward consumers, it should advise the consumer to "see your doctor."
- If it is directed at healthcare practitioners, it should encourage awareness of the signs of the disease or condition to assist in diagnosis.
- It should not mention or identify a particular drug.
- It should not contain any representation or suggestion relating to the drug.

The most important element here is that the piece should not mention or identify a particular drug. The guidance also provides principles on how to help ensure a help-seeking or disease awareness communication is not linked to product promotion and does not identify a product. Essentially, the guidance suggests that help-seeking and disease awareness communications should be distinct from commercial and product marketing communications. FDA will examine the following elements to determine whether they are distinct:
- Perceptual similarity—themes, presentation (branding) elements, colors, logos, graphics (Do the two presentations look alike?)
- Physical proximity (Are the advertisements running close to one another?)
- Linking by audience (Is the audience able to associate the two presentations with one another?)

Also, when a communication relates to a drug or device that is the only one in its diagnostic or therapeutic class or the only product manufactured by a company, the agency may treat the communication as labeling or advertising under the *FD&C Act*.

FDA Oversight and Enforcement

FDA can enforce violations of the FD&C Act or agency regulations through a variety of mechanisms, including: Notices of Violations (NOVs), also known as Untitled Letters; Warning Letters; and, if the violation warrants, referral for judicial action. All three mechanisms are intended to induce compliance with regulations. It should be noted that OPDP is responsible for the review and oversight of all prescription drug advertising and promotional labeling, including many therapeutic biological products. OPDP's mission is to protect public heath by assuring prescription drug information is truthful, balanced and accurately communicated. OPDP recently divided into two review divisions and is now responsible for both consumer-directed promotion and professional-directed promotion. The majority of advertising and promotion NOVs are issued by OPDP and can be found on FDA's website (www.fda.gov/Drugs/GuidanceComplianceRegulatoryInformation/EnforcementActivitiesbyFDA/WarningLettersandNoticeofViolationLetterstoPharmaceuticalCompanies/ucm339597.htm#DDMAC.)

NOVs are reserved for those violations that are generally less serious and do not greatly jeopardize public health but are still significant concerns. An NOV usually requires only that the sponsor discontinue use of the violative materials along with any other pieces that may contain a similar violation.

Warning Letters usually are reserved for more serious violations that may pose a risk to public safety. They typically contain stronger language and commonly are addressed to the company's CEO. In addition to ceasing use of the violative materials, Warning Letters also may require the company to conduct corrective actions. For example, a company may be required to run a remedial advertisement to reach the same audience as the original violative advertisement, or disseminate corrective information through a "Dear Healthcare Professional" letter as described in 21 CFR 200.5(c)(3). Generally, the corrective action is meant to be communicated in the same medium as the original violative piece. Warning Letters frequently direct the sponsor to provide FDA with information on any other promotional items that contain similar messages. All FDA Warning Letters, regardless of issuing center or office, are available at www.fda.gov/ICECI/EnforcementActions/WarningLetters/default.htm.

In determining whether a sponsor should be issued an enforcement letter and, if so, which grade, FDA often looks at the following elements:

- Do the product materials have recurrent violations?
- Is there a pattern and/or consistency of these violations through different forms of media?
- Is there a risk to public health?

If FDA is not satisfied by the sponsor's response to the Warning Letter, it may recommend such enforcement actions as injunctions, seizures and/or criminal prosecution. The Department of Justice carries out these activities. One possible outcome is the company agreeing to enter into an arrangement with the government, called a consent decree, which places severe restrictions on the company's operations to ensure it comes into compliance.

Corrective actions that can be taken by FDA on inadequate dissemination of medical and scientific information relating to an unapproved use of an approved biologics are outlined in 21 CFR 99.401–405.

Summary

- Promotion and advertising activities generally are prohibited for investigational products prior to FDA approval.
- The labeling lifecycle usually begins with the original BLA, when draft labeling information is prepared and submitted by the sponsor to FDA for review and approval. The draft labeling information should contain, at a minimum, container and carton labels, package insert, annotated labeling and SPL. The draft labeling information also may contain a REMS and a Medication Guide. Upon approval, the labeling content can be applied appropriately to promotional and advertising activities.
- The content and format of labeling information are subject to FDA regulations.
- Postapproval changes to the original labeling as well as promotional labeling and advertising content need to be reported to FDA. Depending on the nature of the change, it is reported via one of three mechanisms: Prior Approval Supplement, Changes Being Effected or Annual Report.
- Biologics labeling, whether contained in the original BLA or submitted as a postapproval change, is reviewed and approved under the jurisdiction of CDER and CBER. In CDER, OPDP reviews, approves and monitors all labeling. In CBER, APLB oversees all labeling activities.
- Advertising and promotional labeling utilize many formats, including direct-to-consumer, reminder advertisements, print advertisements and radio and television broadcasting. Each is governed by specific regulations.
- Generally, advertising and promotional labeling must be consistent with the FDA-approved product labeling, must be supported by substantial evidence, must not be false or misleading and must reveal all material information.
- Product communications intended to be "non-promotional" in nature can be subject to FDA regulations if they make product claims.
- Dissemination of scientific or medical information regarding an approved biologic must be conducted in accordance with the *FD&C Act* and should adhere to appropriate regulatory guidelines.
- Disease awareness and "help-seeking" advertising do not mention any specific drug or make any representations about a drug, and therefore, are not subject to the requirements of the *FD&C Act*.
- FDA uses a variety of enforcement tools, such as Notices of Violations, Warning Letters and other corrective actions to ensure industry compliance with the *FD&C Act* and to ensure safe and effective use of biologics in patients. Most NOVs related to prescription drug advertising, including many therapeutic biologicals, are issued by OPDP.

References

1. FDA, Identification of Drug and Biological Products Deemed to Have Risk Evaluation and Mitigation Strategies for Purposes of the Food and Drug Administration Amendments Act of 2007. Federal Register 73:16313 (27 March 2008). Federal Register website. www.federalregister.gov/articles/2008/03/27/E8-6201/identification-of-drug-and-biological-products-deemed-to-have-risk-evaluation-and-mitigation. Accessed 1 May 2013.

Chapter 25

Combination Products

Updated by Jocelyn Jennings, MS, RAC

OBJECTIVES

- Review the regulatory definition of a combination product
- Understand the overall regulatory scheme for combination products
- Explain how combination product jurisdictional determinations are made
- Discuss the premarket review process for combination products
- Describe the proposed combination product postmarket safety reporting regulation
- Describe the proposed CGMP requirements for combination products
- Discuss relevant combination product guidance documents
- Discuss how user fees are applied for combination products

LAWS, REGULATIONS AND GUIDELINES COVERED IN THIS CHAPTER

- 21 CFR 3 Product Jurisdiction
- Proposed 21 CFR 4 Regulation of Combination Products
- 21 CFR 210 Current Good Manufacturing Practice in Manufacturing, Processing, Packing, or Holding of Drugs; General
- 21 CFR 211 Current Good Manufacturing Practice for Finished Pharmaceuticals
- 21 CFR 820 Quality System Regulation
- *Federal Food, Drug, and Cosmetic Act* of 1938
- *Safe Medical Devices Act* of 1990
- *Medical Device User Fee and Modernization Act* of 2002
- *Public Health Service Act* of 1944

Introduction

Combination products raise a variety of regulatory and review challenges. Although the US regulatory frameworks for drugs, devices and biological products share many of the same basic features, each is also somewhat unique. Drugs, devices and biological products each have their own types of marketing applications, Good Manufacturing Practice (GMP) regulations and adverse event reporting requirements. When drugs and devices, drugs and biologics or devices and biologics are combined to create a new product, consideration must be given to how the combination product as a whole will be regulated.

Until 1990, there was no clear process or mandate for the US Food and Drug Administration (FDA) to determine the regulatory pathway of "borderline" products, or products comprised of more than one type of regulated article.

Chapter 25

The *Safe Medical Devices Act* of 1990 (*SMDA*) introduced the notion of a combination product in Section 503(g) of the *Federal Food, Drug, and Cosmetic Act* of 1938 (*FD&C Act*) and provided that a combination product be assigned to a lead agency center based on its "primary mode of action" (PMOA). In 1991, FDA implemented the *SMDA* provision in Title 21 of the Code of Federal Regulations (CFR) Part 3. This regulation vested jurisdictional authority for both combination and non-combination products in FDA's Product Jurisdiction Officer (originally FDA's Office of the Ombudsman, and later reassigned to FDA's newly established Office of Combination Products in 2003).

21 CFR Part 3 also established a "Request for Designation" (RFD) process to determine which FDA center would be assigned review responsibility for combination products, or for any product for which jurisdiction is unclear or in dispute. This regulation was intended to eliminate in most cases, but did not preclude, the need for separate approvals for each individual component of a combination product.

Despite the changes brought with the *SMDA*, the perception persisted that combination products were still vulnerable to "falling through the cracks" between the medical product centers. To address these issues, in the *Medical Device User Fee and Modernization Act* of 2002, Congress amended Section 503(g) of the *FD&C Act* to mandate that FDA establish an Office of Combination Products (OCP) with the following responsibilities for combination product assignment, premarket review and postmarket regulation:

- prompt assignment of the center with primary jurisdiction ("lead center") for the review and regulation of a combination product
- ensure timely and effective premarket review by overseeing the timeliness of and coordinating reviews involving more than one center
- ensure consistent and appropriate postmarket regulation
- resolve disputes regarding review timeliness
- review and/or revise agreements, guidance and practices specific to the assignment of combination products
- report to Congress on the activities and impact of OCP

While not part of its statutory mandates, OCP also works with FDA centers to develop guidance and regulations to clarify combination product regulation, and serves as a focal point for combination product issues for internal and external stakeholders. Note that OCP does not itself review combination products, but assigns the product to the lead reviewing center and oversees the intercenter consultation process.

Definition of a Combination Product

A "combination product" is defined in 21 CFR 3.2(e) as a combination of two or more different types of regulated products, i.e.:
- a drug and a device
- a device and a biological product
- a drug and a biological product
- a drug, a device and a biological product

The individual components (called "constituent parts") of a combination product can be:
- physically or chemically combined (21 CFR 3.2(e)(1))[1]
- co-packaged (21 CFR 3.2(e)(2))[2]
- separate, cross-labeled products (21 CFR 3.2(e)(3)[3] and (e)(4))[4]

Combinations of two drugs, two devices or two biological products are not combination products as defined by 21 CFR Part 3.

Examples of combination products include:
- drug-coated or drug-eluting device
- drug packaged with a syringe or injector pen
- controlled-release drug delivery device
- orthopedic implant coated or packaged with biologic growth factor
- chemotherapy drug and monoclonal antibody (biologic) conjugate
- scaffold (device) seeded with autologous cells (biologic)
- cross labeled drug/in vitro pharmacogenomic test

A list of recent FDA examples of combination approvals can be found at www.fda.gov/CombinationProducts/AboutCombinationProducts/ucm101598.htm.

Determining Combination Product Jurisdiction and Regulatory Path

FDA is required to assign a combination product to a lead center based on its PMOA. In the 25 August 2005 *Federal Register* FDA promulgated a final regulation (PMOA rule) to describe the principles for how combination products will be assigned to an agency center. The regulation defined "mode of action" and "primary mode of action" and set forth an algorithm for how FDA would assign combination products for which the PMOA cannot be determined with "reasonable certainty."

FDA defined "mode of action" as the means by which a product achieves an intended therapeutic effect or action. For purposes of this definition, "therapeutic" action or effect includes any effect or action of the combination product intended to diagnose, cure, mitigate, treat or prevent disease, or affect the structure or any function of the body. Because combination products are comprised of more than one type of regulated article (biological product, device or drug), and each constituent part contributes a biological product, device or drug mode of action, combination products typically will have more than one identifiable mode of action. The definitions of biological product, device and drug mode of actions are closely related to the statutory definitions of a biological product, device and drug, respectively:

1. A constituent part has a biological product mode of action if it acts by means of a virus, therapeutic serum, toxin, antitoxin, vaccine, blood, blood component or derivative, allergenic product or analogous product applicable to the prevention, treatment or cure of a disease or condition of human beings, as described in section 351(i) of the *Public Health Service Act*. (Note: while not currently reflected in the definition of a biological product mode of action, it should be noted that the statutory definition of a biological product was amended in 2010 to also include proteins (except any chemically synthesized polypeptide).)
2. A constituent part has a device mode of action if it meets the definition of device contained in section 201(h)(1) to (h)(3) of the *FD&C Act*, it does not have a biological product mode of action and it does not achieve its primary intended purposes through chemical action within or on the body of man or other animals and is not dependent upon being metabolized for the achievement of its primary intended purposes.
3. A constituent part has a drug mode of action if it meets the definition of drug contained in section 201(g)(1) of the *FD&C Act* and it does not have a biological product or device mode of action.

"PMOA" is defined as "the single mode of action of a combination product that provides the most important therapeutic action of the combination product." The regulation further clarifies that PMOA is the "mode of action expected to make the greatest contribution to the overall intended therapeutic effects of the combination product." For example, if the PMOA of a drug-device combination product is attributable to its device constituent part, the Center for Devices and Radiological Health (CDRH) would have primary jurisdiction for the combination product, whereas if the PMOA of a drug-device combination product is attributable to its drug constituent part, the Center for Drug Evaluation and Research (CDER) would have primary jurisdiction.

In cases where FDA is unable to determine the most important therapeutic action with reasonable certainty, 21 CFR 3.4 sets out an "assignment algorithm," describing the assignment process. First, FDA would look at historical precedents to assign the combination product to the agency component that regulates other combination products that present similar questions of safety and effectiveness with regard to the combination product as a whole. When there are no other combination products that present similar questions of safety and effectiveness with regard to the combination product as a whole, FDA would look to direct the most appropriate assignment based on the safety and effectiveness questions raised by the new combination product. FDA assigns the product to the agency component with the most expertise related to the most significant safety and effectiveness questions presented by the combination product. For example, if the most significant safety and effectiveness issues presented by a drug-device combination product in this scenario were attributable to the drug constituent part, the combination product would likely be assigned to CDER.

Understanding the regulatory pathway early in the development phase of a combination product is often essential for the sponsor to establish a realistic regulatory strategy. There are two ways in which a manufacturer can seek FDA's feedback for determining the product's jurisdiction: informal processes or formal processes. Informal processes involve seeking advice from center or OCP staff, typically by telephone, email or meeting. Informal procedures are generally appropriate where the most important therapeutic action of the combination product is clear or when FDA has previous experience with similar combination products for which jurisdiction has been previously determined. However, one of the disadvantages of the informal approach is that the advice is not binding on FDA and may be subject to change.

Formal designation of a product, whether a single entity (i.e., non-combination drug, device or biologic) or a combination product, is achieved by submitting a Request for Designation (RFD). An RFD is a written submission to OCP requesting designation of the center with primary jurisdiction for a product. An RFD submission is not necessary for every product, but it generally is indicated when the jurisdiction of a single entity or combination product is unclear or in dispute.

FDA action on an RFD is a binding jurisdictional determination with respect to center assignment and is subject to change only under conditions specified in 21 CFR 3.9 and Section 563 of the *FD&C Act*. However, while a designation is binding as to assignment of a particular product, such assignment pertains only to the product described in the RFD. For example, if the product's configuration, composition, modes of action, intended use or any other key aspect changes after the designation letter is issued, it may be necessary to submit a new RFD to determine the modified product's appropriate assignment.

An RFD is limited by regulation to 15 pages, including attachments. Under the regulation, if FDA does not provide an answer within 60 days of the RFD filing date, the sponsor's request for classification or assignment is granted.

As described in 21 CFR 3.7(c), the following information is required in an RFD submission. FDA has issued a guidance document *How to Write a Request for Designation* that further elaborates on these requirements:[5]

- sponsor's identity, including company name and address, establishment registration number, company contact person and telephone number
- product description, including:
    - classification, name of the product and all component products
    - common, generic or usual name of the product and all components
    - proprietary name
    - identification of any component of the product that already has received premarket approval, is marketed as not being subject to premarket approval or has received an investigational exemption
    - status of any discussions or agreements between the sponsors regarding the use of this product as a component of a new combination product
    - chemical, physical or biological composition
    - status and brief report of the results of developmental work, including animal testing
    - description of the manufacturing processes, including the sources of all components
    - proposed use or indications
    - description of all known modes of action, the sponsor's identification of the single mode of action that provides the most important therapeutic action of the product and the basis for that determination
    - schedule and duration of use
    - dose and route of administration of drug or biologic
    - description of related products, including their regulatory status
    - any other relevant information
- sponsor's recommendation as to which agency component should have primary jurisdiction

FDA generally reviews an RFD for completeness within five working days of receipt. An incomplete RFD is "not filed," and the applicant is notified of the information necessary to permit OCP to undertake a substantive review. If an RFD is filed, the sponsor is notified of the filing date, as well as the date by which OCP will respond. Within 60 days after the filing of the RFD, OCP issues a letter specifying the agency component with primary jurisdiction for the product's premarket review and regulation. The designation letter usually also identifies any consulting agency components and sometimes also describes the regulatory authorities (e.g., device or drug provisions of the *FD&C Act*) to which the product will be subject.

If the sponsor disagrees with the designation, it may request that OCP reconsider the decision. The Request for Reconsideration (RFR) must be submitted within 15 days of receipt of the designation letter, may not include new information, and must not exceed five pages. OCP will in turn respond in writing to the RFR within 15 days.

A variety of resources are available to help sponsors understand the jurisdiction of a combination product. The original resources were the three intercenter agreements (ICAs) between the Center for Biologics Evaluation and Research (CBER) and CDER, CDER and CDRH, and CBER and CDRH, established in 1991. The usefulness of the ICAs has decreased over time due to organizational realignments within FDA, the development of new products not envisioned in the original ICAs, new uses of existing products and laws that have been enacted since 1991. In 2006 (71 *FR* 56988[6]), the agency announced that it had reviewed these agreements and preliminarily proposed to continue using the CBER-CDRH and CDER-CDRH ICAs as they provide helpful, nonbinding guidance, with the understanding that they should not be independently relied upon as the agency's most current, complete jurisdictional statements. Due to the transfer of many therapeutic biologic products from CBER to CDER in 2003, the agency stated that the CBER-CDER ICA is out of date.

The 2006 notice also explained that while FDA does not plan to update the existing ICAs, it believes transparency in jurisdictional decision making should result in greater predictability and reduce ambiguity about FDA perspectives. A number of mechanisms have been implemented by FDA to provide this transparency. For example, the agency has used its website to disseminate information concerning product jurisdiction. Some examples of these are:

- Jurisdictional determinations—Approximately 250 capsular descriptions of selected RFD decisions have been posted on OCP's website. www.fda.gov/CombinationProducts/JurisdictionalInformation/RFDJurisdictionalDecisions/CapsularDescriptions"One-Liners"/default.htm
- Jurisdictional updates—Detailed statements on updated classification and assignment of specific product classes are available on OCP's website. www.fda.gov/CombinationProducts/JurisdictionalInformation/JurisdictionalUpdates/default.htm
- RFD decision letters—For approximately 50 products covered by an RFD that have since been approved or cleared, the OCP website includes the written jurisdictional determination respecting the RFD, redacted to remove trade secret and confidential commercial information in accordance with the *Freedom of Information Act*. www.fda.gov/

CombinationProducts/JurisdictionalInformation/
RFDJurisdictionalDecisions/
RedactedDecisionLetters/default.htm

Premarket Review

The assigned lead center has primary responsibility for the review and regulation of a combination product; however, a second center is often involved in the review process, especially to provide input regarding the "secondary" component. In some cases, secondary center involvement may be extensive, depending on the issues raised by a particular product or submission.

To make the combination product review process more efficient, FDA established a standard operating procedure (SOP), the *Intercenter Consultative and Collaborative Review Process*.[7] This SOP provides the procedures for FDA staff to follow when requesting, receiving, handling, processing and tracking formal consultative and collaborative reviews of combination products, devices, drugs and biologics. The objectives of the SOP are to improve intercenter communication on combination products as well as the timeliness and consistency of intercenter consultative and collaborative reviews.

While a combination product's PMOA dictates the lead center assignment, it does not dictate the regulatory authorities that may be applied to a combination product. In most cases, the lead center applies its usual regulatory pathway. For example, a drug-device combination product assigned to CDRH typically is reviewed under the 510(k) or Premarket Approval Application (PMA) process, while a drug-device combination product assigned to CDER will typically be reviewed under a New Drug Application (NDA). In most cases, a single marketing application is sufficient to review a combination product, but in some cases, particularly where the two components are themselves separate products, two applications (e.g., a PMA and an NDA) may be desirable or required.

FDA published the concept paper "Number of Marketing Applications for a Combination Product" for stakeholder comment.[8] The document describes FDA's thinking about when single or separate marketing applications may be appropriate for the constituent parts of a combination product. While separate marketing applications are sometimes appropriate, normally only one investigational application (Investigational New Drug (IND) or Investigational Device Exemption (IDE)) is submitted to authorize a clinical investigation of a combination product.

It is recommended that the sponsor contact the agency, ideally during early product development, to determine the nature of technical and scientific information that may be necessary for investigational and marketing applications for a combination product. In September 2006, FDA published *Guidance for Industry and Staff: Early Development Considerations for Innovative Combination Products*,[9] which provides helpful perspectives on combination product development.

Special consideration also should be given to intellectual property when more than one manufacturer is co-developing a combination product. For example, the sponsor of an IDE or PMA for a device-drug combination product may not be given access by the drug manufacturer to confidential or trade secret drug information, such as drug synthesis, formulation, purification or manufacturing processes, yet such information may be required for regulatory purposes.

Confidentiality of such information can usually be maintained while providing FDA the necessary information to support the investigational or marketing application in one of two ways. One is through a letter of authorization (LOA), which allows the applicant to cross-reference an existing application and allows FDA to consider this information in its review of the application used for the combination product. The second alternative is the use of master files. Drug Master Files (DMFs) or Device Master Files (MAFs) are voluntary submissions to FDA used to provide confidential information about a product or process (e.g., manufacturing processes or toxicology data) that one sponsor wishes to keep confidential but that is necessary for the other sponsor to support the premarket review process. It should be noted that FDA does not approve information or data in a master file, but rather accesses and reviews the information in context of the referring application. Additional information on DMFs can be found in 21 CFR 314.420 and on FDA's website.

New Regulations Proposed in 2009 for Combination Products

In late 2009, FDA published two proposed rules that would amend the combination product regulations by creating new 21 CFR 4. Subpart A would address current GMP (CGMP) requirements for combination products, while Subpart B would promulgate postmarketing safety reporting requirements for combination products. A similar legal framework underlies both proposed rules and sets forth FDA's view that drugs, devices and biological products do not lose their individual regulatory identities when they become constituent parts of a combination product. Under this framework, in general, the CGMP and postmarket safety reporting requirements specific to each constituent part of a combination product also apply to the combination product itself. However, rather than impose duplicative requirements for manufacturers to fully comply with both sets of requirements, the proposed rules set out a streamlined framework whereby a manufacturer would comply with one set of requirements, as well as specific, additional provisions to ensure that any unique requirements attributable to the "other" component are not lost if the product were to comply with only one set of requirements. The application of this general approach is further described below for both postmarket safety reporting and CGMP requirements.

Good Manufacturing Practice Requirements

In 2004, FDA published *Draft Guidance for Industry and FDA: Current Good Manufacturing Practice for Combination Products* on the applicability of GMP requirements to combination products. In the 23 September 2009, *Federal Register*,[10] FDA proposed codifying an approach similar to the one taken in the draft guidance, by establishing new 21 CFR 4, Subpart A. The proposed rule embodied the legal framework that, in FDA's view, drugs, devices and biological products do not lose their individual regulatory identities when they become constituent parts of a combination product. In other words, a drug-device combination product is both a drug and a device, and both sets of CGMP requirements (21 CFR 210 and 211 for drugs and 21 CFR 820 for devices) apply to the combination product itself. FDA published the final rule on GMP requirements for combination products 22 January 2013 in the *Federal Register*.[11] The rule will be effective 22 July 2013.

The final rule recognizes that 21 CFR 210 and 211 and 820 are similar in most respects. In this context, for single entity and co-packaged combination products, the rule provides a streamlined approach as an alternative to fully implementing and complying with both sets of CGMP requirements. Under this streamlined approach, a manufacturer could choose to operate under and comply with either 21 CFR 210 and 211 or 21 CFR 820, rather than both, provided that additional specific aspects of the other CGMP framework are also incorporated.

Specifically, under the final rule, a manufacturer choosing to operate under and comply with drug CGMP regulations under 21 CFR 210 and 211 for its single-entity or co-packaged drug-device combination product, would also be considered to have complied with all provisions of the device Quality System Regulations at 21 CFR 820, if it complies with the following specific provisions from 21 CFR 820:

1. 820.20 Management responsibility
2. 820.30 Design controls
3. 820.50 Purchasing controls
4. 820.100 Corrective and preventive action
5. 820.170 Installation
6. 820.200 Servicing

In an analogous manner, a manufacturer choosing to operate under and comply with device QSR requirements under 21 CFR 820 for its single-entity or co-packaged drug-device combination product, would also be considered to have complied with all provisions of the drug CGMP requirements in 21 CFR 210 and 211, if it complies with the following specific provisions from 21 CFR 210 and 211:

1. 211.84 Testing and approval or rejection of components, drug product containers, and closures
2. 211.103 Calculation of yield
3. 211.132 Tamper-evident packaging for over-the-counter (OTC) human drug products
4. 211.137 Expiration dating
5. 211.165 Testing and release for distribution
6. 211.166 Stability testing
7. 211.167 Special testing requirements
8. 211.170 Reserve samples

The streamlined approach may be used when two or more types of constituents are manufactured in the same facility. When manufacture of a constituent part occurs at a separate facility from all other types of constituent parts, it would require the manufacture of that part to occur under the CGMP regulations applicable to that part. For example, the manufacture of a drug constituent part at a facility separate from all other combination product constituent parts would be subject to 21 CFR 210 and 211, while the facility where that drug constituent part is manufactured with the device into a single-entity or co-packaged constituent part could implement the streamlined approach.

For a combination product that includes a biological product constituent part, in addition to demonstrating compliance with either the drug CGMPs or the device QSR, the CGMP operating system would also have to comply with additional CGMP requirements that apply to that constituent part as a biological product (see 21 CFR 600–680). Similarly, if the combination product includes a human cellular or tissue (HCT/P) constituent part, it would also have to be shown to comply with the requirements of 21 CFR 1271.

Finally, for combination products where the constituent parts are separately packaged (21 CFR 3.2(e)(3) and (e)(4)), each constituent part would remain separate for purposes of applying the CGMP regulations. For example, for a combination product comprised of a drug and a cross-labeled but separately packaged delivery device, the drug constituent part would be subject to 21 CFR 210 and 211, while the delivery device would be subject to 21 CFR 820.

Postmarket Safety Reporting for Combination Products

The 1 October 2009 proposed rule,[12] which has not been finalized as of the date of this publication, recognizes that the individual reporting requirements for drugs (21 CFR 310 and 314), devices (21 CFR 803) and biological products (21 CFR 600 and 606) share many similarities and have a common underlying purpose, i.e., to protect the public health by ensuring a product's continued safety and effectiveness. For example, each set of regulations requires reports of death and serious adverse events; each provides for periodic and follow-up reports; and each provides a method to signal certain types of safety events that warrant expedited reporting. Despite these similarities, each set of regulations

Table 25-1. Unique Proposed Postmarket Safety Reporting Provisions for Combination Products

Type of Requirement	Name of Requirement	Regulatory Citation
Device	5-Day Report	21 CFR 803.53(a)
Device	30-Day Device Malfunction Report	21 CFR 803.20(b)(3)(ii)
Drug/Biological Product	15-Day Alert Report	21 CFR 314.80(c)(1) and (e) 21 CFR 600.80(c)(1) and (e)
Drug	3-Day Field Alert Report	21 CFR 314.81(b)(1)
Biological Product	Expedited Blood Fatality Report	21 CFR 606.170

also has certain reporting standards and timeframes with unique requirements based on the characteristics of the products for which the regulations were designed. For example, the drug reporting provisions have no requirement analogous to device malfunction reporting, while the device reporting provisions have no requirement analogous to drug 3-Day Field Alert Reporting. The intent of the proposed rule is to consolidate the requirements so that a combination product is subject primarily to the reporting requirements associated with the type of marketing application under which the product is approved or cleared, while at the same time ensuring that the public health benefit of the specific unique provisions is not lost if the combination product were subject solely to the reporting requirements associated with the type of marketing application.

FDA has identified five such provisions, described in **Table 25-1**, that are unique to drugs, devices and biological products that FDA believes need to be preserved to appropriately reflect the combination nature of the product and to ensure consistent and appropriate postmarketing safety reporting for combination products.

Under the proposed rule, a drug-device combination product approved or cleared under the device provisions of the *FD&C Act* would be subject to Medical Device Reporting under 21 CFR 803, and in addition, would be subject to 15-Day Alert Reporting under 21 CFR 314.80(c)(1) and 3-Day Field Alert Reporting under 21 CFR 314.81(b)(1). A drug-device combination product approved under the drug provisions of the *FD&C Act* would be subject to the drug reporting provisions under 21 CFR 314.80 and 314.81, as well as 5-Day Reporting under 21 CFR 803.53(a) and 30-Day Malfunction Reporting under 21 CFR 803.20(b)(3)(ii). Expedited blood fatality reporting under 21 CFR 606.170 would apply to combination products with a blood constituent part.

The proposed rule also describes how reporting would work in less frequent situations, e.g., where there are separate marketing applications for the constituent parts of the combination product or where there are multiple reporters (i.e., one application holder for one constituent part of the combination product and a second application holder for another constituent part of the combination product).

In the case of multiple reporters, each reporter would be subject to the applicable requirements for that reporter's constituent report. The application holder for the device constituent part would submit in accordance with 21 CFR 803, while the application holder for the drug constituent part would submit in accordance with 21 CFR 314. In addition, to ensure each reporter is aware of and can investigate and follow-up on events the other may learn about that may impact a constituent part, the proposed rule would require each application holder to submit information learned about the "other component" to the other manufacturer for investigation or follow-up, or to FDA.

The proposed requirements are not currently in effect and may be revised to incorporate stakeholder comments, but it is expected that the final rule will be similar in overall approach.

User Fees for Combination Products

FDA published *Guidance for Industry and Staff: Application User Fees for Combination Products*[13] in April 2005 to clarify the application of user fees for combination products. The guidance explains that a combination product, as defined in 21 CFR 3.2(e), is subject to the application fee associated with the type of application submitted for the product's premarket approval or clearance. For example, a biologic-device or a drug-device combination product for which a PMA is submitted is subject to the PMA fee under the *Medical Device User Fee and Modernization Act* (*MDUFMA*). Likewise, a combination product for which an NDA is submitted is subject to the NDA fee under the *Prescription Drug User Fee Act* (*PDUFA*).

In specific situations, a sponsor may opt to submit separate marketing applications for each constituent part of the combination product, even though one application (covering the entire combination product) would suffice. Usually, this is done to pursue some type of benefit, such as new drug product exclusivity, orphan status or proprietary data protection when two firms are involved. Because the submission of two applications when one would suffice places an extra burden on FDA resources, a user fee for each application ordinarily would be required.

However, in cases where two marketing applications are required by FDA for the combination product (rather than at the discretion of the sponsor), an "innovative combination product waiver" might allow for reduction of the dual application user fees. More information on the eligibility for fee reduction provided by this waiver is available in the guidance document referenced above.

Summary

- As defined in 21 CFR 3.2(e), a "combination product" is any combination of a drug and a device; a biological product and a device; a drug and a biological product; or a drug, a device and a biological product. There are four definitions within 3.2(e) explaining these combinations.
- The *FD&C Act* gives OCP broad responsibilities covering the lifecycle of combination products. However, primary responsibility and oversight reside with the lead center (CDRH, CDER or CBER) to which the product is assigned.
- OCP is responsible for the prompt assignment of a lead center that will have primary jurisdiction for the review and regulation of a combination product based on a determination of its primary mode of action (PMOA).
- Formal designation of a single entity (i.e., drug, device or biologic) or combination product is achieved by submitting a Request for Designation (RFD).
- In 2009, FDA proposed new regulations for postmarket safety reporting and CGMP requirements for combination products. The proposed regulations are predicated on the general legal framework that a combination product is subject to the legal authorities governing its constituent parts; however, streamlined approaches are proposed that recognize the similarities while also preserving the unique differences among the respective regulations for drugs, devices and biologics.
- A marketing application for a combination product is subject to the usual fee associated with that type of application. In unique situations where two applications are required and the eligibility criteria are met, an "innovative combination product waiver" may apply.

References

1. 21 CFR 3.2(e)(1): a product comprised of two or more regulated components, i.e., drug/device, biologic/device, drug/biologic or drug/device/biologic, that are physically, chemically or otherwise combined or mixed and produced as a single entity.
2. 21 CFR 3.2(e)(2): two or more separate products packaged together in a single package or as a unit and comprised of drug and device products, device and biological products or biological and drug products.
3. 21 CFR 3.2(e)(3): a drug, device or biological product packaged separately that, according to its investigational plan or proposed labeling, is intended for use only with an approved, individually specified drug, device or biological product where both are required to achieve the intended use, indication or effect and where, upon approval of the proposed product, the labeling of the approved product would need to be changed, e.g., to reflect a change in intended use, dosage form, strength, route of administration or significant change in dose.
4. 21 CFR 3.2(e)(4): any investigational drug, device or biological product packaged separately that, according to its proposed labeling, is for use only with another individually specified investigational drug, device or biological product where both are required to achieve the intended use, indication or effect.
5. *Guidance for Industry: How to Write a Request for Designation* (April 2011). FDA website. www.fda.gov/RegulatoryInformation/Guidances/ucm126053.htm. Accessed 10 May 2013.
6. *Federal Register*, 71:56988 (September 28, 2006). "Review of Agreements, Guidances, and Practices Specific to Assignment of Combination Products in Compliance With the Medical Device User Fee and Modernization Act of 2002; Request for Comments." GPO website. http://edocket.access.gpo.gov/2006/pdf/E6-15967.pdf. Accessed 10 May 2013.
7. *Manual of Standard Operating Procedures and Policies, General Information—Review, Intercenter Consultative/Collaborative Review Processes, Version 4* (June 18, 2004). FDA website. www.fda.gov/downloads/RegulatoryInformation/Guidances/UCM126016.pdf. Accessed 10 May 2013.
8. Concepts for Comment Purposes Only—Not for Implementation; Number of Marketing Applications for a Combination Product. FDA website. www.fda.gov/downloads/CombinationProducts/RequestsforComment/UCM108197.pdf. Accessed 10 May 2013.
9. *Guidance for Industry and FDA Staff: Early Development Considerations for Innovative Combination Products* (September 2006). FDA website. www.fda.gov/downloads/RegulatoryInformation/Guidances/ucm126054.pdf. Accessed 10 May 2013.
10. *Federal Register* 74:48423 (September 23, 2009). "Current Good Manufacturing Practice Requirements for Combination Products " Proposed Rule GPO website. http://edocket.access.gpo.gov/2009/pdf/E9-22850.pdf. Accessed 10 May 2013.
11. *Federal Register* 78:4307 (January 22, 2013) "Current Good Manufacturing Practice Requirements for Combination Products" Final Rule. FDA website. http://www.fda.gov/downloads/CombinationProducts/UCM336194.pdf. Accessed 22 May 2013.
12. *Federal Register* 74:50744 (October 1, 2009). "21 CFR Part 4, Postmarketing Safety Reporting for Combination Products." GPO website. http://edocket.access.gpo.gov/2009/pdf/E9-23519.pdf. Accessed 10 May 2013.
13. *Guidance for Industry and FDA Staff: Application User Fees for Combination Products* (April 2005). FDA website. www.fda.gov/downloads/RegulatoryInformation/Guidances/UCM147118.pdf. Accessed 10 May 2013.

Recommended Reading

- Product Jurisdiction, 21 CFR 3 www.accessdata.fda.gov/scripts/cdrh/cfdocs/cfCFR/CFRSearch.cfm?CFRPart=3&showFR=1

Chapter 26

Products for Small Patient Populations

Updated by Min Chen, PhD, RAC

OBJECTIVES

- Review regulations for small patient populations

- Recognize that orphan products include not only drugs but also devices and medical foods

- Learn about US orphan drug regulatory history and process, HUD and the HDE process

- Understand differences between patent protection and exclusivity provisions

- Recognize that many countries or regions have their own orphan product regulations or policies

- Learn about the joint orphan application between the US and the EU

LAWS, REGULATIONS AND GUIDELINES COVERED IN THIS CHAPTER

- *Orphan Drug Act* of 1983, Public Law 97-414, 1983 with amendments in 1985 and 1988

- 21 U.S. Code 360bb(a)(2) Designation of drugs for rare diseases or conditions

- 21 CFR 316.3(b)(13) Definition of same drug

- 21 CFR 814.20(b)(10) Proposed labeling and 21 CFR 814.102 Designation of HUD status

- 21 CFR 814, Subpart H Humanitarian Use Devices

- 21 CFR 814.104 Original applications

Introduction

Orphan Drug Act

The *Orphan Drug Act* of 1982 (*ODA*) was signed into law (Public Law 97-414)[1] on 4 January 1983 to provide tax incentives and exclusive licensing that would encourage manufacturers to develop and market drugs or biologics for diseases affecting relatively few people (fewer than 200,000 in the US). *ODA* defines an "orphan drug" as one developed for a disease or condition that occurs so infrequently in the US that there is no reasonable expectation that the costs of research, development and marketing would be recovered from sales revenues.[2]

FDA's Office of Orphan Product Development (OOPD) administers *ODA*'s major provisions as well as the Orphan Products Grants Program, which provides funding for clinical research on rare diseases. OOPD also works on rare disease issues with the medical and research communities, professional organizations, academia, governmental agencies, industry and rare disease patient groups.

Prior to this legislation, private industry had little incentive to invest in the development of treatments for small patient populations when the drugs were expected to be unprofitable. The law provides several incentives, including seven-year marketing exclusivity for approved orphan products; a tax credit of 50% of clinical trial costs; and the Orphan Products Grants Program. Marketing exclusivity prevents competition by preventing other companies from marketing the same drug for the same orphan indication.

The original *ODA* required a sponsor to establish a lack of commercial viability. *ODA* expanded the definition of "orphan drugs" to include biological products, antibiotics, medical devices and medical foods.[3] It also was amended to clarify the term "rare disease or condition" as any disease or condition in the US that affected:

- fewer than 200,000 people (for vaccines and blood products, the figure of 200,000 or fewer applies to patients receiving the product annually)
- more than 200,000 people and offering no reasonable expectation that the costs of development and distribution of the drug will be recovered from sales[4]

As amended, the standard for orphan designation changed from profitability to prevalence. The requirement to show lack of economic viability applies only when prevalence exceeds 200,000. Only one drug has been approved for orphan status under the second criteria. Manufacturers rarely attempt to prove compliance with the second set of criteria because regulation requires FDA to verify unprofitability and examine all relevant financial and sales records.[5]

ODA further states that an orphan medical device is one treating "any disease or condition that occurs so infrequently in the US that there is no reasonable expectation that a medical device for such disease or condition will be developed without the assistance" of grants and contracts from OOPD. A similar statement regarding medical foods and biologics is included.

ODA also created an Orphan Products Board within the Department of Health and Human Services (DHHS) to determine policy on orphan product development and to coordinate federal efforts and private sector activities.

The impact of *ODA* has been far-reaching. In the 30 years following *ODA* enactment in 1983, FDA has approved 425 drugs for rare diseases that otherwise would not have been incentivized to be developed and marketed. Prior to that, fewer than 10 products were approved between 1973 and 1983. In addition, the Orphan Products Grants Program helped bring more than 45 products to markets. The Humanitarian Use Device (HUD) program helped approve more than 50 Humanitarian Device Exemptions (HDE). It is important to note, though, when approving orphan product marketing applications, FDA holds products to the same standards as non-orphan products.

Conditions for Orphan Status

To be eligible for orphan status, a product must:
- have a sponsor (i.e., a company, individual, scientific institution or government agency)
- not have been approved previously under a New Drug Application (NDA), Biologic License Application (BLA) or Premarket Approval (PMA) application for the disease or condition for which orphan status is requested
- not be the subject of a marketing application submitted prior to the filing of an orphan designation request

Orphan Drug Designation Application Process

To receive orphan drug designation, the sponsor must first submit an orphan drug designation request to OOPD for the product proposed for a specific rare disease or condition. The request should include:
- description of the rare disease or condition and proposed indication
- description of the product and the scientific rationale (including data available) supporting its use in the disease or condition
- documentation supporting the assertion that potential users number fewer than 200,000 in the US

As of 15 March 2013, approximately 2773 drugs had been granted orphan drug designation. Of these, 425 drugs had received marketing approval. A sponsor may request orphan drug designation at any time during drug development prior to submitting a marketing application. An orphan drug also can have more than one orphan drug designation. Such multiple designations can include:
- same drug with different indications sponsored by the same company
- identical or different drugs with same indications sponsored by different companies

For example, Interferon has six designations for cancer or viral infections, and Interferon Alfa-2b has 10 designations. Similarly, there may be multiple designations for the same orphan indication.

Until recently, FDA decided on a case-by-case basis whether two drugs were different for the purposes of determining marketing exclusivity. A case involving a human growth hormone and a slight variation of the same product resulted in regulations promulgated in 1992 to use structural similarity to create a presumption of "sameness" between two drugs.[7]

Typically, the orphan designation is granted to the active ingredient only. However, if superiority is expected or demonstrated, uniqueness is presumed. For example, if a product with an active ingredient has been approved for an orphan indication, another orphan designation with the same active ingredient but with different formulation can still be requested only when the different formulation is believed to be "clinically superior" to the approved product either in greater effectiveness, greater safety or providing a major contribution to patient care. Therefore, to break orphan exclusivity before expiration of the first orphan drug's marketing exclusivity, the subsequent entry needs to demonstrate "clinical superiority" if the two products are to be considered the same.

Orphan Drug Designation Annual Reports (21 CFR 316.30)

Within 14 months after the date on which a drug was designated as an orphan product and annually thereafter until marketing approval, the sponsor of a designated drug shall submit a brief progress report (21 CFR 316.30) to OOPD that includes:

- short account of the drug development progress, including a review of preclinical and clinical studies initiated, ongoing and completed, and a short summary of the status or results of such studies
- description of the coming year's investigational plan, as well as any anticipated difficulties in development, testing and marketing
- brief discussion of any changes that may affect the product's orphan drug status (For example, sponsors of products nearing the end of the approval process should discuss any disparity between the probable marketing indication and the designated indication as related to the need for an amendment to the orphan drug designation pursuant to 21 CFR 316.26.)

Regulatory and Financial Incentives for Orphan Drugs

The sponsor may be eligible for the following incentives for a product with US orphan drug designation:

- FDA protocol assistance
- 50% federal tax credit for qualified clinical testing expenses (Under the tax-credit provision, no credit is allowed for clinical testing conducted outside the US, unless there is an insufficient patient population available for testing within the US.)
- *Pediatric Research Equity Act* (*PREA*) requirements exemption
- *Prescription Drug User Fee Act* (*PDUFA*) fee waiver for marketing application
- Research grants from OOPD to support clinical studies to develop orphan drugs

FDA Protocol Assistance

ODA Section 525 provides for formal protocol assistance when requested by orphan drug sponsors. The formal review of such a request is the direct responsibility of the Center for Drug Evaluation and Research (CDER) or the Center for Biologics Evaluation and Research (CBER), whichever has jurisdiction for review of the product. OOPD is responsible for ensuring that the request qualifies for consideration under Section 525 of the *Federal Food, Drug, and Cosmetic Act* (*FD&C Act*). FDA utilizes these meetings to guide the sponsor to ensure that studies are properly designed to meet regulatory requirements.

The Orphan Products Grants Program

FDA, through OOPD, funds the development of qualifying orphan products through its clinical study grants program, whose fund availability is announced in the *Federal Register*. Eligibility for grant funding is extended to drugs, medical devices and medical foods for which there is no reasonable expectation of development without such assistance. An orphan designation for a drug does not guarantee a research grant will be awarded. Grant applications, submitted in response to a Request for Application (RFA), are reviewed by panels of outside experts and funded by priority score. The grant program is very competitive, and only about 30% of the applicants receive awards each year. Any organization, whether domestic or foreign, public or private, or profit or nonprofit, is eligible to apply for the grants. Small businesses are encouraged to apply as well. Although rare, large pharmaceutical companies have qualified for some grants.

Applications are first reviewed by the OOPD program staff for relevance and responsiveness to the RFA. Responsive applications are reviewed and evaluated for scientific and technical merit by an ad hoc panel of experts. A national advisory council conducts a second review for concurrence with the recommendations made by the initial review group. Rank-ordered priority scores determine the final awards.

OOPD plans to further facilitate orphan drugs by:[6]

- developing a simplified application based entirely on the prevalence requirement and rationale of the proposed product (Is there reason to believe this is a promising drug that can be expected to be effective against the proposed rare disease or condition?) and working to revise current regulations and ways of dividing patients with a specific disease or disorder into credible subsets acceptable to OOPD (What is the acceptable medical rationale for a particular disease?)
- addressing study design for small clinical trials, which are appropriate for small patient populations
- informing policymakers of the grant program's success ($14 million awarded per year); greater awareness might lead to an increase in the grant budget, which has not changed in recent years

Common Mistakes in Requesting Orphan Drug Designation

Depending on the type of rare condition or disease, applicants requesting orphan designation tend to make the following common mistakes in attempting to meet the requirements for orphan designation:

- dividing a subset of patients with a common disease condition, which is not medically plausible

- orphan requests with words such as severe, refractory, metastatic, late-stage, acute or chronic, which may raise questions on subset issues
- erroneously using incidence instead of prevalence for a disease or condition when incidence does not apply
- inadequate scientific rationale to support the use of the product for the proposed indication

Increase in Population and Its Impact on Orphan Drug Status

In general, if orphan drug status was granted for the treatment of a disease or condition estimated to affect fewer than 200,000 people in the US, the status of the drug designation holds. This can be illustrated by multiple sclerosis (MS). Although MS is no longer considered a rare disease because its prevalence is now known to exceed 250,000 in the US, orphan drug regulations regarding marketing exclusivity still apply to the beta-interferons, since they were granted orphan drug status for the treatment of MS at a time when the disease was estimated to affect fewer than 200,000 in the US.

Public Knowledge of Orphan Drug Designations

Once a drug or biologic receives orphan designation, the following information is available from the OOPD website (www.accessdata.fda.gov/scripts/opdlisting/oopd/index.cfm), including the drug's chemical name, trade name, date of designation and proposed indication, sponsor name, address and contact information, and, if applicable, the approved indication and marketing exclusivity date (typically the date of NDA or BLA approval). None of the scientific rationale used to define a medically plausible subset of patients is revealed.

After the designated orphan product receives marketing approval from FDA, however, additional information regarding the product and the application, including a copy of the written review conducted by the FDA OOPD officer, can be requested through the *Freedom of Information Act* (*FOIA*).

Pharmacogenomics, Disease Stratification and Potential Orphan Status

The use of genetic profiling techniques could benefit drug development and clinical testing, as this would allow subjects to be included in or excluded from certain clinical trials. Screening subjects with pharmacogenomic approaches could potentially indicate whether the drug is effective, ineffective or unsuitable for an individual. This methodology also opens the door to include subjects selectively in a clinical trial, provided they are screened for a known genetic diversity or genetic composition. This process is called patient stratification and could make clinical trials smaller, faster and more cost-effective. When a pharmacogenomic approach is effective, it has the potential to reduce overall drug development costs. The consequences of disease stratification could create a much smaller market for an individual drug that may reach "orphan" levels. As the field expands and the understanding of disease stratification deepens, it may be possible to stratify the patient population for a certain disease into a smaller subset reaching orphan levels, based on genetic variants.

ODA has been very successful, resulting in new drugs for more than 200 rare diseases, and FDA is actively encouraging drug companies to pursue pharmacogenomic approaches to more of the 7,000 remaining rare diseases identified by NIH.[7] However, from a regulatory perspective, pharmacogenomics could drastically change disease classification schemes and basic assumptions about what constitutes a rare disease.[8,9] It is possible that diverse rare diseases may turn out to share molecular genetic disease processes that are amenable to the same drug. Additional indications for the drug that are driven by a common set of genes likely will be found. At some point, understanding these mechanisms could lead to a redefinition of rare disease.[10]

Exclusivity and Patents

Another amendment to the act changed the exclusivity provision and made orphan status available to both patentable and unpatentable drugs.[11] The 1985 amendment extended exclusivity to orphan drugs having either of two characteristics:

1. no use or product patent issued
2. no use patent issued and an expired product patent

The biotechnology industry, where some products have been known to take as long as four to six years to receive patent approval, while the approval of others are delayed by legal challenges, has benefited from the exclusivity provision. Biotech drugs with orphan status may use the seven-year exclusivity provision as a surrogate patent. The *Food and Drug Administration Modernization Act* of 1997 (*FDAMA*)[12] extended exclusivity to an additional six months for orphan drugs for a pediatric indication.

There are, however, important differences between patent protection and *ODA*'s seven-year exclusivity provision. The seven years of marketing exclusivity for patented products run concurrently with any outstanding patent. Further, the protected use is only for the rare disease approved. Patent protection is broader; a product patent covers an active ingredient and all its uses. A second company cannot receive approval for any use of the active ingredient until the patent has expired. Use patents and process patents similarly provide broad protection. Exclusivity differs from patent protection, which gives the patent holder exclusive rights, regardless of whether patent rights are exercised. Under the exclusivity provisions, during the seven-year period that begins with the product's approval, a second company can receive approval to market the product for a common disease or some other rare one (provided the patent has expired).[13] The sponsor may grant other manufacturers or distributors the privilege of marketing the orphan product; however, a written request for the privilege must be submitted to FDA. A firm can lose its research and development investment while studying an orphan product because a second firm attains market approval first. To minimize these risks, companies may file cross-licensing agreements or shared exclusivity for the same or different indications. If a sponsor fails to make adequate quantities of the orphan product available, it may lose exclusivity. The sponsor also may relinquish orphan drug status, as with the AIDS drug didanosine (DDI).

Under the new biosimilar legislation *Biologics Price Competition and Innovation Act* of 2009[14] enacted on 23 March 2010, biologic orphan drugs now are granted protection for 12 years of data exclusivity or seven years of market exclusivity.

Postmarketing Approval Conditions

Once an orphan product is on the market, there are no constraints against a physician prescribing it to treat other diseases. It is possible for an orphan drug to achieve "blockbuster" status despite being an orphan drug. The drug may have a market much broader than that of the approved orphan indication, although the sponsor must only advertise the product in compliance with the approved rare indication(s).[15] Also, the seven-year market exclusivity immunizes the sponsor from market competition and provides no price controls. Finally, a company can divide a projected market of more than 200,000 patients into several subsets and attempt to achieve orphan approvals for each indication. FDA does scrutinize orphan drug applications for evidence of "arbitrary subsets" (medically implausible) and can impose penalties, including revocation of orphan drug status. Although many legislative attempts have tried to close *ODA* loopholes (e.g., by capping profits), none has become law.

In recent years, orphan drug development has become not only a focus of organizations such as the National Organization of Rare Disorders (NORD),[16] the Pharmaceutical Research and Manufacturers of America's (PhRMA) Commission on Drugs for Rare Diseases, and the rare disease patient advocacy groups, but also a hot area that an increasing number of pharmaceutical companies are entering due to the incentives provided and decreasing productivity in other traditional therapeutic areas.

Orphan Drugs Globally

The impact of the *Orphan Drug Act* on the international stage has been significant. Japan adopted an orphan drug regulation in 1993 (offering 10 years of data exclusivity), followed by Australia in 1997 with an orphan drug policy (offering 5 years of marketing exclusivity, similar to other drugs), and the EU in 2000. Even some emerging markets, such as Brazil, Mexico, Russia, Singapore, South Korea and Taiwan, have partial orphan drug policies.

European Union (EU)

In 2000, the EU passed its first legislation specifically for orphan drugs, Regulation (EC) 141/2000 of the European Parliament and the Council on orphan medicinal products.[17,18]

Under the EU *Orphan Medicinal Product Regulation*, a rare disease is defined as affecting no more than five in 10,000 people in the community. The legislation offers protocol assistance, 10 years of market exclusivity and financial incentives (fee reduction or exemptions).[19,20]

The legislation is overseen by the European Medicines Agency (EMA), which has the authority to award orphan status and also approves drugs for marketing. However, each Member State has responsibility for making the drug available and dealing with reimbursement issues.

The EMA's Committee for Orphan Medicinal Products examines all applications for orphan designation and advises the European Commission on the establishment and development of policies on orphan medicinal products in the EU, as well as drawing up detailed guidelines and working internationally on matters relating to orphan medicinal products.

Joint US-EU Orphan Drug Designation Application and Orphan Annual Report

In recent years Regulatory agencies have significantly increased their collaborative efforts in achieving global harmonization, one example being the introduction of a joint US-EU orphan drug designation application. When a sponsor wishes to submit orphan drug designation applications for the same product for the same indication in both the US and the EU, the sponsor may use the "Common EMA/FDA Application Form for Orphan Medicinal Product Designation" in conjunction with other supporting documents.

Subsequently, on 26 February 2010, FDA and EMA announced in the International Collaboration Announcement[21] that both agencies now allow for a single orphan annual report for products designated in both the US and the EU. The orphan annual reports can be submitted either on World Rare Disease Day (last day of February) or the normal US or EU annual reporting date.

Chapter 26

Humanitarian Device Exemptions

History

Although the *Orphan Drug Act* does not specifically mention medical devices, the *Safe Medical Devices Act* of 1990 (*SMDA*) does include orphan medical devices. In 1996, FDA promulgated a final rule describing the orphan devices process that subsequently was codified in 21 CFR 814, Subpart H.13.22. OOPD is responsible for granting orphan designation to devices known as humanitarian use devices (HUDs), which must meet the following criteria:
- device treats or diagnoses a disease in fewer than 4,000 patients per year in the US
- no comparable FDA-approved therapy exists for the proposed indication
- evidence is provided that the applicant could not otherwise bring the device to market

Incentives to manufacturers for developing HUDs are identical to those for developing orphan drugs.

Process

The Humanitarian Device Exemption (HDE) process[22, 23] involves two steps:
1. The applicant must request and obtain HUD designation from OOPD. The application's required contents are outlined in 21 CFR 814.102. Among other requirements, the application must precisely define the proposed indication for use. If the applicant proposes using the device for a limited subset of a larger group of patients suffering from a more common disease or condition, the application must contain evidence that the subset is medically plausible and justify the proposed limitation. The application also must document, with appended authoritative references, that the rare disease affects fewer than 4,000 individuals per year in the US. Upon receipt of the application, OOPD has 75 days to approve or deny the HUD request under 21 CFR 814.114. A 30-day filing period is included in this 75 days. After the initial review to determine the completeness of the package, if OOPD asks the applicant to provide more information, the clock stops and resets upon receiving the requested information.
2. Once the applicant receives HUD designation, it must submit an HDE application to the Office of Device Evaluation (ODE) at the Center for Devices and Radiological Health (CDRH). Contents of the HDE application are set forth in 21 CFR 814.104. The purpose of the application is to assist ODE reviewers in understanding why the device deserves the HDE. One major difference between a Premarket Approval Application (PMA) and one for an HDE is that the HDE is exempt from the PMA effectiveness requirements, unless specifically requested by FDA. Otherwise, effectiveness would be required under Sections 514 and 515 of the *FD&C Act*. However, the application must contain an explanation of probable device benefits and demonstrate that those probable benefits outweigh the risk of injury or illness from use. If the intended price of the device is more than $250, the HDE application must include verification that the amount charged does not exceed the costs of research, development, fabrication and distribution per either of two statements:
- report by a certified public accountant
- attestation by a responsible individual of the applicant organization

FDA makes a threshold determination as to whether the HDE application is sufficiently complete to permit substantive review. The agency can refuse to file for any of four reasons:
1. application is incomplete
2. comparable device already is available to treat or diagnose the disease or condition
3. application contains an untrue statement or omits material information
4. HDE lacks a statement of certification or disclosure, or both, as required by 21 CFR 54

ODE has 75 days to review the application and send the applicant an approval order, an approvable letter, a nonapprovable letter or an order denying approval.

Labeling

HDE labeling requirements match those for PMA-approved devices in 21 CFR 814.20(b)(10). In addition, the labeling of an approved HDE device must bear the following statement: "Humanitarian Device. Authorized by Federal law for use in the treatment [or diagnosis] of [specify disease or condition]. The effectiveness of this device for this use has not been demonstrated."

Distribution

The HDE holder is responsible for ensuring that an HUD is administered only at hospitals or institutions that have an Institutional Review Board (IRB) constituted and acting in accordance with 21 CFR 56. The initial use of the HUD must be approved by the IRB, and the IRB must provide continuing oversight of the use of the HUD. The IRB does not have to review and approve each individual use of the HUD. Instead, the IRB may approve the use of the device in general for groups of patients meeting certain criteria or for devices under a treatment protocol. The IRB may specify limitations on the use of the device based on any criterion it deems appropriate. Unless the data are intended for use in a clinical investigation, informed consent is not required because an HDE provides temporary marketing approval and does not constitute research or an investigation.

Additional Indication(s)

Once an HUD is approved, the applicant may seek different indications for use by requesting and obtaining HUD designation and filing a new, original HDE for the new indication. The new, original HDE may incorporate by reference any information or data submitted to the agency under the previous HDE.

Quality System

An approved HDE is subject to the same Quality System Regulation (QSR) in 21 CFR 820 and postapproval requirements as a PMA-approved product. The latter may include the following:

- restriction of the device's sale, use and distribution (prescription only)
- Phase 4 studies to evaluate the device's safety, effectiveness and reliability for its intended use; in the HDE-approval order, FDA states the study conditions, which include:
  o a reason or purpose
  o number of patients to be evaluated
  o reports required
- prominent display in the labeling (and advertising/promotional materials) of warnings, hazards or precautions important for safe and effective device use, including any patient information
- inclusion of identification codes on the device or its labeling
- records pertaining to patient tracing if such information is necessary to protect public health
- maintenance of records for specified periods of time and records organization and indexing into identifiable files to enable FDA to determine whether there is reasonable assurance of the device's safety or effectiveness
- periodic reports in accordance with the HDE approval order, the contents of which are described in 21 CFR 814.126(b)(1)
- batch testing of the device
- Medical Device Reports (MDRs) submitted to FDA in compliance with 21 CFR 803 (also should be submitted to the IRB of record)
- records of the facility names and addresses to which the HUD has been shipped and all correspondence with reviewing IRBs

Revocation

Once FDA approves a PMA or clears a 510(k) for treating (or diagnosing) the same disease or condition, the HDE can be revoked.

Misbranding

The HDE holder cannot promote the device for any patient population other than the target population for the indicated HDE use. Promotion to groups other than the target population constitutes misbranding. In addition, an HDE holder cannot imply that its device is effective for the indicated use because there is no requirement to submit clinical effectiveness data in the HDE. Through 11 March 2013, 57 devices had been approved under the HDE program.

Summary

- Worldwide regulatory agencies attempt to incentivize orphan drug and humanitarian device development.
- Patients with rare diseases are benefiting from having access to orphan drugs or humanitarian devices.

References

1. *Orphan Drug Act*, Public Law 97-414, 4 January 1983. FDA website. www.fda.gov/regulatoryinformation/legislation/federalfooddrugandcosmeticactfdcact/significantamendmentstothefdcact/orphandrugact/default.htm. Accessed 10 May 2013.
2. Ibid.
3. *Orphan Drug Amendments* of 1988, Public Law 100-290, 18 April 1988. GPO ebsite. www.gpo.gov/fdsys/pkg/STATUTE-102/pdf/STATUTE-102-Pg90.pdf. Accessed 10 May 2013.
4. *Health Promotion and Disease Prevention Amendments* of 1984, Public Law No. 98–551, 30 October 1984). NIH website. http://history.nih.gov/research/downloads/PL98-551.pdf. Accessed 10 May 2013.
5. Op cit 1.
6. Tankosic T. "Orphan Drug Development: commercial strategies flourish." *SCRIP* "Drug Market Developments," 2008; 19(5)
7. The Office of Rare Diseases at the NIH maintains a list of rare diseases and conditions on its website. http://rarediseases.info.nih.gov/. Accessed 10 May 2013.
8. Maher PD and Haffner M. "Orphan Drug Designation and Pharmacogenomics: Options and Opportunities." *BioDrugs*, 20, no. 2 (2006): pp. 71–79.
9. Shah J. "Economic and regulatory considerations in pharmacogenomics for drug licensing and healthcare." *Nature Biotechnology*, 21, no. 7 (July 2003): pp. 747–753.
10. Tucker L. "Pharmacogenomics: A Primer for Policymakers" National Health Policy Forum, Background Paper, 28 January 2008.
11. *Orphan Drug Amendments* of 1985, Public Law 99-91, 99, 15 August 1985. NIH website. http://history.nih.gov/research/downloads/PL99-91.pdf. Accessed 10 May 2013.
12. *Food and Drug Administration Modernization Act* of 1997. FDA website. www.fda.gov/RegulatoryInformation/Legislation/FederalFoodDrugandCosmeticActFDCAct/SignificantAmendmentstotheFDCAct/FDAMA/. Accessed 10 May 2013.
13. Op cit 11.
14. *Biologics Price Competition and Innovation Act of* 2009. FDA website. www.fda.gov/downloads/drugs/guidancecomplianceregulatoryinformation/ucm216146.pdf. Accessed 10 May 2013.
15. 21 CFR 312.2.

16. Myers AS. "Orphan Drugs: The Current Situation in the United States, Europe and Asia." *Drug Information Journal* 31 (1997): 101–104.
17. Regulation (EC) 141/2000 of the European Parliament and of the Council of 16 December 1999 on orphan medicinal products. EUR-Lex website. http://eur-lex.europa.eu/LexUriServ/LexUriServ.do?uri=OJ:L:2000:018:0001:0005:en:PDF. Accessed 10 May 2013.
18. Commission Regulation (EC) 847/2000 of 27 April 2000 laying down the provisions for implementation of the criteria for designation of a medicinal product as an orphan medicinal product and definitions of the concepts "similar medicinal product' and 'clinical superiority." EC website. http://ec.europa.eu/health/files/eudralex/vol-1/reg_2000_847/reg_2000_847_en.pdf. Accessed 10 May 2013.
19. *SCRIP* "Drug Market Developments," 2008; 19(5).
20. 21 CFR 814, Subpart H Humanitarian Use Devices. FDA website. www.accessdata.fda.gov/scripts/cdrh/cfdocs/cfcfr/CFRSearch.cfm?CFRPart=814&showFR=1&subpartNode=21:8.0.1.1.11.7. Accessed 10 May 2013.
21. FDA news release: "International Collaboration: FDA and European Medicines Agency Agree to Accept a Single Orphan Drug Designation Annual Report," 26 February 2010. FDA website. www.fda.gov/NewsEvents/Newsroom/PressAnnouncements/ucm202300.htm. Accessed 10 May 2013.
22. FDA. "Final Rule: Medical Devices; Humanitarian Use of Devices," *Federal Register* 61:33232. (1996).
23. FDA. "Final Rule: Medical Devices; Humanitarian Use of Devices," *Federal Register* 63:59222 (1998).

Recommended Reading
- Carter MJ and Bennett AR. "Developments in Orphan Drugs." *Food, Drug, Cosmetic Law Journal* 44 (1989): 627–632.
- Clissold DB. "Prescription for the Orphan Drug Act: The Impact of the FDA's 1992 Regulations and the Latest Congressional Proposals for Reform," *Food and Drug Law Journal* 50 (1995): 125–147.
- Finke MJ. "Orphan Products and the Pharmaceutical Industry."*Clinical Research Practices and Drug Regulatory Affairs* (1983): 19–25.
- Grossman DB. "The Orphan Drug Act: Adoption or Foster Care." *Food, Drug, Cosmetic Law Journal* 39 (1984): 128–132.
- Henkel J. "Orphan Products: New Hope for People With Rare Disorders," *FDA Consumer* (18 June 1994): 17–20.
- Levitt JA and Kelsey JV. "The Orphan Drug Regulations and Related Issues," *Food and Drug Law Journal* 48 (1993): 526–530.
- Shah J. "Economic and regulatory considerations in pharmacogenomics for drug licensing and healthcare". 2003 Nature Publishing Group, http://www.nature.com/naturebiotechnology
- Shulman SR et. al. "Implementation of the Orphan Drug Act: 1983–1991," *Food and Drug Law Journal* 47 (1992): 363–401.
- Tucker L. "Pharmacogenomics: A Primer for Policymakers." National Health Policy Forum, Background Paper, 28 January 2008.

Chapter 27

Blood and Blood Products

Updated by Joseph C. Fratantoni, MD

OBJECTIVES

- Understand FDA strategies to protect the blood supply
- Understand the regulatory authority used by FDA for blood and blood products
- Understand the advisory apparatus employed by FDA for blood and blood products
- Learn about licensing requirements for a new type of blood product

LAWS, REGULATIONS AND GUIDELINES COVERED IN THIS CHAPTER

- *Public Health Service Act* of 1944, Section 351
- *Federal Food, Drug, and Cosmetic Act* of 1938
- 21 CFR 201.25 Bar Code Label Requirements
- 21 CFR 211.100 Written Procedures; Deviations
- 21 CFR 601 Licensing Requirements
- 21 CFR 606 Current Good Manufacturing Practice for Blood and Blood Components
- 21 CFR 607 Establishment Registration and Product Listing For Manufacturers of Human Blood and Blood Products
- 21 CFR 610 General Biologics Products Standards
- 21 CFR 640 Additional Standards for Human Blood and Blood Products
- 21 CFR 820 Quality System Regulation
- *Guidance for Industry: Blood Establishment Computer System Validation in the User's Facility,* (April 2013)
- *Guidance for Industry: Minimally Manipulated, Unrelated Allogeneic Placental/Umbilical Cord Blood Intended for Hematopoietic Reconstitution for Specified Indications* (October 2009)

Introduction

The US Food and Drug Administration (FDA) is responsible for ensuring the safety of the US blood supply. This responsibility includes regulation of the collection of both blood and blood components, such as clotting factors used for transfusion or manufacture of drugs. FDA's authority for the review and approval of blood products resides in Section 351 of the *Public Health Service Act* of 1944 (*PHS Act*), and the regulation of these products resides under the *Federal Food, Drug, and Cosmetic Act* of 1938 (*FD&C Act*). The Center for Biologics Evaluation and Research (CBER) is the center within FDA responsible for the regulation of blood and blood products. CBER develops and enforces quality standards, performs inspections of blood establishments and monitors reports of deviations and adverse events.

Advisory Committees

There are three Advisory Committees related to blood and blood products. CBER manages the Blood Products Advisory Committee and Transmissible Spongiform Encephalopathies Advisory Committee. The Blood Products Advisory Committee advises the commissioner in discharging his or her responsibilities as they relate to helping ensure safe and effective biological products and related medical devices, and, as required, any other product for which FDA has regulatory responsibility.[1] The Transmissible Spongiform Encephalopathies Advisory Committee[2] advises the commissioner in discharging responsibilities as they relate to helping to ensure safe and effective products. This committee specifically focuses on the safety of products that may be at risk for transmission of spongiform encephalopathies having an impact on the public health. The third committee, the Advisory Committee on Blood Safety and Availability, is overseen by the Department of Health and Human Services (DHHS). This committee provides advice to the secretary and assistant secretary for health regarding research initiatives on diseases involving blood and blood products and for issuing and enforcing regulations concerning the collection, preparation and distribution of these products and regulations related to the transmission of communicable diseases.[3] The meetings of these Advisory Committees can be viewed online (see http://www.fdalive.com/webcast.cfm for additional details).

FDA Strategies for the Safety of Blood and Blood Products

HIV infection resulting from blood transfusion has been documented repeatedly since the first case report in late 1982. In the US, almost all cases are due to blood transfused before March 1985, when HIV antibody testing became available to screen donated blood.[4] Since that time, FDA has focused on ensuring the safety of blood and blood products by advocating the use of new technologies, standards, guidelines and strategies to minimize the risk of consumer exposure to unsafe products. Blood donors are required to answer risk-based questions geared to eliminate the potential for individuals from donating unsafe blood. These questions identify behaviors, transmittable disease states or exposure to certain geographic areas for periods of time that may indicate the donor is unsuitable. By regulation, unsuitable donors may be excluded from blood donations permanently or for a specified period. Further, all donated blood is tested for seven infectious diseases to help prevent unsuitable blood from being administered to patients.

In 1995, the Institute of Medicine released its report, "HIV and the Blood Supply," an analysis of decisions and actions on blood related to the AIDS crisis.[5] FDA responded to the criticisms contained in the report and, in 1997, initiated the Blood Action Plan.[6] The plan was approved by DHHS in 1998 and ensures coordination between CBER and FDA's Office of Regulatory Affairs (ORA), Office of Chief Counsel and Office of Policy, and the Centers for Disease Control (CDC), the National Institutes of Health (NIH) and the Centers for Medicare and Medicaid (CMS). The intent is to leverage scientific and regulatory information and actions to further elevate the safety of blood and blood products. The program focuses on improvement in seven areas:

1. updating blood regulations
2. reinventing blood regulations
3. emerging infectious diseases
4. ensuring compliance of plasma fractionation establishments
5. notification and lookback
6. FDA response to emergencies and Class I recalls affecting blood safety
7. monitoring and increasing the blood supply

Through this collaborative program, new or revised standards, guidance documents and compliance programs are put into place. These documents can be found electronically at www.fda.gov/BiologicsBloodVaccines/GuidanceComplianceRegulatoryInformation/Guidances/Blood/default.htm.

FDA's "Five Layer Approach"

The efforts of FDA to improve and promote the safety of blood and blood products through the Blood Action Plan, leveraging technology and science, has resulted in a key systematic program. This program has a "five layer" approach to ensure the safety of the blood supply and products derived from blood or blood components. These five layers create a seamless safety system from the initial collection of blood at the donor center all the way though to distribution and use of a blood product.

1. Donor Screening

The first layer is donor screening. Potential donors must answer questions about their health and risk factors. Transmission of HIV and other blood-borne viruses can occur during transfusion of blood components (e.g., whole blood, packed red cells, fresh-frozen plasma, cryoprecipitate and platelets) derived from the blood of an infected individual. Depending on the production process used, blood products derived from pooled plasma can also transmit HIV and other viruses, but recombinant clotting factors cannot. Donor screening establishes a donor's eligibility to donate blood and blood components by documenting that the individual is free of any diseases transmissible by blood transfusion. This process must be done on the day of the donation (21 CFR 640.3(a) and 640.63(a)).

After completing the questionnaire at the donation site, the potential donor is interviewed by a trained healthcare professional about his medical history and given a physical examination. Donors may be temporarily deferred from donating blood for what may seem to be minor illnesses, such as a fever, cold, cough or sore throat, or if they are taking certain drugs. These precautions are necessary to prevent any unintentional transmission of a disease. Once the donor has recovered and has no symptoms of the minor illness, he may donate. Permanent exclusion from donating is covered by a specific guidance citing risk factors such as human immunodeficiency virus (HIV) infection, male homosexual activity since 1977, or a history of intravenous drug use or viral hepatitis. Individuals who respond "yes" to any questions about such risk factors are not allowed to donate blood for injectable use. In certain circumstances, to avoid being singled out as a transmission risk in the volunteer setting, a volunteer donor may be allowed to donate blood; however, the technician should indicate with a bar code that the unit not be used.

2. Donor Testing

The second layer ensuring blood supply safety is testing of each unit of blood collected. Each unit or bag of donor blood must be tested for hepatitis B, hepatitis C, syphilis, HIV 1 and 2, or human T-lymphotropic virus (HTLV) Types I and II. Any donor who is positive for one of the seven diagnostic tests above will be placed on a deferred donor list and the unit collected will be destroyed. In some situations, such as donation of platelets, testing for CMV (cytomegalovirus) may be performed; however, this test is not routine for all blood collections.

3. Donor Lists

The third layer of control is the requirement that all blood donation establishments keep a current list of deferred donors and check donor names against that list each time a person offers to donate blood. Any person whose name appears on the list may not donate. These lists are shared among blood donation establishments to ensure that an individual who has been identified as a risk for transmission of infectious disease cannot avoid detection by going to another establishment.

4. Quarantine of Untested Blood

Blood products collected must be appropriately stored and are not released for use until all testing has been completed and the information has been checked for accuracy. Whenever a donor has repeatedly reactive screening tests for HBsAg, anti-HBc, anti-HCV or anti-HTLV-I, blood establishments should promptly, within 72 hours if possible, identify and quarantine within-date blood and blood components in inventory from prior collections, extending back five years. For a test that is repeatedly reactive, and there is a record available of the donor's last negative test results from a licensed screening test, quarantine of prior collections should only extend back to 12 months before such a test. In addition, blood establishments should promptly request consignees of such products to immediately quarantine all previously distributed products extending back five years or 12 months before the donor's last negative test results from licensed serological tests. Quarantined units should be destroyed or appropriately labeled either as 1) "biohazard" and "Not for use for transfusion or further manufacturing into injectable products," in the case of products originating from donors who subsequently test repeatedly reactive for HBsAg or anti-HCV, or 2) "biohazard" and "Not for use for transfusion," in the case of products originating from donors who subsequently test repeatedly reactive for anti-HBc or anti-HTLV-I.

5. Deviations and Nonconformances

Lastly, blood establishments must investigate any deviations where the safeguards cited in items 1–4 were ineffective and must correct the system deficiencies that allowed the failure to occur. Licensed establishments must report to FDA any manufacturing problems, errors or accidents that may affect the safety, purity or potency of their distributed finished products using a Biological Product Deviation Report (BPDR). On 7 November 2000, FDA published a final rule to amend the requirements for reporting errors and accidents during the manufacture of products. The rule amended the regulation at 21 CFR 600.14 for licensed biological products and added a requirement at 21 CFR 606.171 applicable to all manufacturers of blood and blood components. The amended regulation at 21 CFR 600.14 and the new regulation at 21 CFR 606.171 require the reporting of any event associated with manufacturing to include testing, processing, packing, labeling or storage, or with the holding or distribution of a licensed biological product or a blood or a blood component, in which the safety, purity, or potency of a distributed product may be affected. A manufacturer is required to report to CBER's Office of Compliance and Biologics Quality (OCBQ) as soon as possible, but not to exceed 45 calendar days from the date of discovery of information reasonably suggesting a reportable event has occurred. To facilitate reporting, FDA has developed a standardized reporting format that may be used for electronic or hard copy submissions. Directions for completing and mailing the forms are provided by CBER and can be accessed at www.fda.gov/downloads/AboutFDA/ReportsManualsForms/Forms/UCM061463.pdf.

CBER's Direct Recall Classification (DRC) program provides blood and plasma establishments the opportunity to electronically report recall-related information directly to CBER. The standardized reporting established for the submission of electronic Biological Product Deviation Reports (eBPDRs) has been expanded to include the collection of Additional Information (AI) necessary for recall classification purposes. Electronically submitted eBPDRs that represent a potential recall situation and contain 18 or fewer components are candidates for DRC. Currently, for recall classification purposes, eBPDRs that contain more than 18 components require collection of recall documentation through the local district office. Healthcare professionals and consumers may report adverse events voluntarily through the FDA MedWatch program or through the FDA Consumer Complaint Coordinator in their geographic area.

"Lookback" Procedures

"Practices for Blood and Blood Components; Notification of Consignees Receiving Blood and Blood Components at Increased Risk for Transmitting HIV Infection," published in the *Federal Register* of 30 June 1993 (58 FR 34962) establishes the requirement for "lookback" procedures for all blood and blood products within a 90-day implementation timeframe. The short implementation phase emphasizes the importance of being able to address post-donation information and donors whose status may change over time. Analogous procedures related to donor screening for HIV antigen and to post-donation information on increased risk of Creutzfeldt-Jacob Disease (CJD) were recommended in three memoranda issued on 8 August 1995, entitled "Recommendations for Donor Screening with a Licensed Test for HIV-1 Antigen," "Disposition of Products Derived from Donors Diagnosed with, or at Known High Risk for, Creutzfeldt-Jakob Disease" and "Precautionary Measures to Further Reduce the Possible Risk of Transmission of Creutzfeldt-Jakob Disease by Blood and Blood Products." As a result, all licensed and registered blood establishments must implement lookback procedures and are audited by FDA to ensure that they are functional at each inspection. Under a lookback procedure, blood establishments retrieve and quarantine units previously collected from a donor who originally tested negative for HIV or another infectious disease, but subsequently tested positive at a later donation. As part of the investigation, the blood establishment will conduct additional testing on a current sample of the donor's blood to confirm the positive result. If the results are confirmed, previously donated units from that individual cannot be used in transfusions or the manufacture of injectable products, and anyone receiving such units must be notified. Further guidance for lookback procedures may be found on the CBER website: *Guidance for Industry: "Lookback" for Hepatitis C Virus (HCV): Product Quarantine, Consignee Notification, Further Testing, Product Disposition, and Notification of Transfusion Recipients Based on Donor Test Results Indicating Infection with HCV* and Memorandum to All Registered Blood and Plasma Establishments: "Recommendations for the Quarantine and Disposition of Units from Prior Collections from Donors with Repeatedly Reactive Screening Tests for Hepatitis B Virus (HBV), Hepatitis C Virus (HCV) and Human T-Lymphotropic Virus Type I (HTLV-I)," 19 July 1996.

Notification Process for Transfusion Related Fatalities and Donation Related Deaths

21 CFR 606.170(b) requires that facilities notify CBER's OCBQ as soon as possible after confirming a complication of blood collection or transfusion to be fatal. The collecting facility is to report donor fatalities, and the compatibility testing facility is to report recipient fatalities. The regulation also requires the reporting facility to submit a report of the investigation within seven days after the fatality. In addition, 21 CFR 640.73 requires notification by telephone as soon as possible if a source plasma donor has a fatal reaction which, in any way, may be associated with plasmapheresis.

Computers and Software Used to Control the Collection Process in Blood Banks

A Blood Establishment Computer System includes: computer hardware, computer software, peripheral devices, personnel and documentation. The computer software used in a Blood Establishment Computer System includes Blood Establishment Computer Software, which is a medical device. FDA considers a Blood Establishment Computer System to be equipment under 21 CFR 606.60, and automated or electronic equipment under 21 CFR 211.68.

Blood Establishment Computer Software is software, designed to be used in a blood establishment, which is intended for use in the diagnosis of disease or other conditions in donors, or in the prevention of disease in humans by the release of unsuitable blood and blood components. CBER recently issued updated guidance to assist blood establishments in their use of computer systems, *Guidance for Industry: Blood Establishment Computer System Validation in the User's Facility* (April 2013).

Blood Establishment Registration (BER)

All owners or operators of establishments that manufacture blood products are required to register with FDA, pursuant to Section 510 of the *FD&C Act*, unless they are exempt under 21 CFR 607.65. A list of every blood product manufactured, prepared or processed for commercial distribution must be submitted with the registration documentation. Products must be registered and listed within five days of beginning operation, and annually between 15 November and 31 December. Blood product listings must be updated in June and December each year. Form FDA 2830, Blood Establishment Registration and Product Listing, is used to submit registration and product listing information to the agency.

Section 351(a) of the *PHS Act*, as amended 21 November 1997 (the *Food and Drug Administration Modernization Act*

(*FDAMA*)); Public Law 105-115), mandates in part that no person shall introduce or deliver for introduction into interstate commerce any biological product unless a biologics license is in effect for that product. In the past, both an establishment license (one per legal entity) and product license (one for each approved product) have been issued. However, as of 19 February 1998 (effective date of *FDAMA*), biologics license certificates will be issued for all new biological products and when existing licenses are reissued.

Barcode Labeling for Blood and Blood Products

The requirement for barcodes on certain products is another step in ensuring blood safety by preventing mistakes in the handling of blood products. The intent of FDA's barcode rule is to reduce medication errors, including transfusion errors in the hospital setting. The regulation requiring barcode labeling that is machine-readable for blood and blood components intended for transfusion is 21 CFR 606.121(c)(13). This requirement applies to all blood establishments that manufacture, process, repack or relabel blood and blood components, including hospital transfusion services that pool or aliquot blood components. FDA also requires that specific human drug and biological product labels contain a barcode consisting of, at a minimum, the National Drug Code (NDC) number. This regulation can be found in 21 CFR 201.25.

Inspection of Blood Establishments

FDA began conducting inspections of establishments that manufacture blood or blood products for human use in 1972 under Section 351 of the *PHS Act*. The purpose of the inspections is to "ensure that blood establishments manufacture biological products that are safe, pure, potent and have the quality they represent and the establishment manufactures them according to Current Good Manufacturing Practice (CGMP) for Blood and Blood Component regulations and applicable standards."

In 1997, FDA established Team Biologics, a group of specialized investigators who conduct routine and CGMP follow-up inspections of manufacturers of biologic products regulated by CBER. The Team Biologics Operations Group, made up of senior managers from ORA and CBER, provides guidance and support for Team Biologics and supplies a forum for setting policy and discussing regulatory issues.

The inspection strategy takes a system-based approach, identifying five elements in blood establishment operations required to achieve the five layers of protection for the blood supply:
- quality assurance system—various planned activities providing confidence that all procedures/processes that influence product manufacture and overall quality are monitored to ensure they are working as expected (21 CFR 211.100 and 606.100)
- donor (suitability) eligibility system—the system that protects donor safety, determines a donor's suitability for blood collection (including donor deferral from history screening and/or testing), notifies donors of unsuitability for donation and, where acceptable to FDA, permits donor re-entry (21 CFR610.40, 610.41, 640.63,640.65)
- product testing system—the system(s) that tests for communicable diseases, blood grouping and typing, and cross-matches blood for transfusion by direct testing or electronically (21 CFR 606.40)
- quarantine/inventory management system—the system(s) pertaining to product storage, distribution and retrieval, quarantine and distribution (release for use or destruction) (21 CFR 606.60)
- production and processing system—process controls in the manufacture of specific blood and blood components and equipment quality control, calibration and maintenance (21 CFR 606.160)

The inspection of each element should review:
- the accuracy, availability and appropriateness of procedures
- the adequacy of qualifications, training and number of personnel for the operations
- the appropriateness of the facility for operations and the adequacy of its maintenance
- equipment maintenance to ensure it will perform as intended
- record maintenance to ensure traceability of steps and that a complete history of work performed is provided

Routine inspections are required by statute and generally occur biennially. They may be conducted at two levels:
- Level 1—a comprehensive review of all elements employed at the establishment
- Level 2—a review of the quality assurance system plus two others; eligibility is based on favorable inspectional history, recent Level 1 inspection and no evidence of unfavorable trends in monitoring data (recalls, deviation reports, fatality reports, etc.)

CBER Announces Acceptance of License Applications for Cord Blood

Cells derived from placentas or umbilical cords include populations with the properties and functions of hematopoietic stem cells. Research has demonstrated that these cells can be used for reconstitution of bone marrow in patients whose marrow reserve has been depleted by disease or chemotherapy. Such stem cell therapy has been accomplished by bone marrow transplantation and by use of stem cells derived from cytapheresis procedures. The cord blood approach has some logistic advantages, and FDA has chosen to accept license applications for cord blood.

The guidance issued addresses submission of a BLA (21 CFR 601) for placental/umbilical cord blood products that are: 1) minimally manipulated and 2) intended for hematopoietic reconstitution in patients with hematologic malignancies, certain genetic disorders, primary immunodeficiency diseases, bone marrow failure and beta thalassemia. It is noted that manufacturing processes that involve other than minimal manipulation or indications other than those cited may lead to the requirement for an IND and premarket application appropriated for the product. Acceptance of license applications for cord blood constitutes the first approval for marketing of a stem cell product by FDA. *Guidance for Industry: Minimally Manipulated, Unrelated Allogeneic Placental/Umbilical Cord blood Intended for Hematopoietic Reconstitution for Specified Indications* describes the regulatory history of these products and explains the processes followed to reach this point.

Summary

- FDA is responsible for ensuring the safety of the US blood supply and regulates the collection of blood and blood components, such as clotting factors used for transfusion or manufacture of drugs.
- FDA's authority for the review and approval of blood products resides in Section 351 of the *PHS Act,* and the regulation of these products resides under the *FD&C Act.*
- All owners or operators of establishments that manufacture blood products are required to register with FDA, pursuant to section 510 of the *FD&C Act*, unless they are exempt under 21 CFR 607.65.
- FDA has a "five layer" approach to ensure the safety of the blood supply and products derived from blood or blood components. These five layers overlap from the initial collection of blood at the donor center all the way though to the distributor of a blood product.
- All licensed and registered blood establishments must implement lookback procedures.
- FDA regulates blood establishment computer software as medical devices.

References

1. Blood Products Advisory Committee Charter. FDA website. www.fda.gov/AdvisoryCommittees/CommitteesMeetingMaterials/BloodVaccinesandOtherBiologics/BloodProductsAdvisoryCommittee/ucm121602.htm. Accessed 18 April 2013.
2. Transmissible Spongiform Encephalopathies Advisory Committee Charter. FDA website. www.fda.gov/AdvisoryCommittees/CommitteesMeetingMaterials/BloodVaccinesandOtherBiologics/TransmissibleSpongiformEncephalopathiesAdvisoryCommittee/ucm129558.htm. Accessed 18 April 2013.
3. Amended Charter, Advisory Committee on Blood and Tissue Safety and Availability. DHHS website. www.hhs.gov/ash/bloodsafety/advisorycommittee/charter/charter_acbsa.pdf. Accessed 18 April 2013.
4. Peterman TA, Jaffe HW, Feorino PM, Getchell JP, Warfield DT, Haverkos HW, Stoneburner RL, Curran JW. "Transfusion-associated acquired immunodeficiency syndrome in the United States." *JAMA*. 1985 Nov 22–29;254(20):2913–7.
5. *HIV and the Blood Supply: An analysis of crisis decisionmaking*. Leveton LB, Sox HC and Stoto MA, eds. Institute of Medicine, National Academy Press, Washington, DC, 1995.
6. FDA's Role in Regulating and Protecting the Nation's Blood Supply. Testimony of Lead Deputy Commissioner Michael A. Friedman before the Subcommittee on Human Resources and Intergovernmental Affairs of the House Committee on Government Reform and Oversight. 5 June 1997. FDA website. www.fda.gov/newsevents/testimony/ucm114940.htm. Accessed 9 May 2013.

Recommended Reading

- 21 CFR 600–680. FDA website. www.accessdata.fda.gov/scripts/cdrh/cfdocs/cfcfr/cfrsearch.cfm?cfrpart=600. Accessed 18 April 2013.
- *Guideline for Quality Assurance in Blood Establishments* (July 1995). FDA website. www.fda.gov/downloads/BiologicsBloodVaccines/GuidanceComplianceRegulatoryInformation/Guidances/Blood/ucm164981.pdf. Accessed 18 April 2013.
- Compliance Program Manual 7342.001 "Inspection of Licensed and Unlicensed Blood Banks, Brokers, Reference Laboratories, and Contractors" & 7342.002 "Inspection of Source Plasma Establishments." FDA website. www.fda.gov/biologicsbloodvaccines/guidancecomplianceregulatoryinformation/complianceactivities/enforcement/complianceprograms/ucm095226.htm. Accessed 18 April 2013.
- *Guidance for Industry: Implementation of Acceptable Full-Length Donor History Questionnaire and Accompanying Materials for Use in Screening Donors of Blood and Blood Components* (October 2006). FDA website. www.fda.gov/biologicsbloodvaccines/guidancecomplianceregulatoryinformation/guidances/blood/ucm073445.htm. Accessed 18 April 2013.
- FDA memorandum, "Revised Recommendations for the Prevention of Human Immunodeficiency Virus (HIV) Transmission by Blood and Blood Products" (23 April 1992). FDA website. www.fda.gov/downloads/BiologicsBloodVaccines/GuidanceComplianceRegulatoryInformation/OtherRecommendationsforManufacturers/MemorandumtoBloodEstablishments/UCM062834.pdf. Accessed 18 April 2013.
- FDA memorandum, "Revised Guideline for the Collection of Platelets, Pheresis" (7 October 1988). FDA website. www.fda.gov/downloads/BiologicsBloodVaccines/GuidanceComplianceRegulatoryInformation/OtherRecommendationsforManufacturers/MemorandumtoBloodEstablishments/UCM063003.pdf. Accessed 18 April 2013.
- *Guidance for Industry: Changes to an Approved Application: Biological Products: Human Blood and Blood Components Intended for Transfusion or for Further Manufacture* (July 2001). FDA website. www.fda.gov/BiologicsBloodVaccines/GuidanceComplianceRegulatoryInformation/Guidances/Blood/ucm076729.htm. Accessed 18 April 2013.
- FDA Correspondence, Letter to Blood Establishment Computer Software Manufacturers (31 March 1994). FDA website. www.fda.gov/downloads/BiologicsBloodVaccines/GuidanceComplianceRegulatoryInformation/OtherRecommendationsforManufacturers/

MemorandumtoBloodEstablishments/UCM062804.pdf. Accessed 18 April 2013.
- FDA, *General Principles of Software Validation; Final Guidance for Industry and FDA Staff* (January 2002). FDA website. www.fda.gov/MedicalDevices/DeviceRegulationandGuidance/GuidanceDocuments/ucm085281.htm. Accessed 18 April 2013.
- *Guidance for Industry and FDA Staff: Guidance for the Content of Premarket Submissions for Software Contained in Medical Devices* (11 May 2005). FDA website. www.fda.gov/MedicalDevices/DeviceRegulationandGuidance/GuidanceDocuments/ucm089543.htm. Accessed 18 April 2013.
- *Reviewer Guidance for a Premarket Notification Submission for Blood Establishment Computer Software* (13 January 1997). FDA website. www.fda.gov/downloads/BiologicsBloodVaccines/GuidanceComplianceRegulatoryInformation/OtherRecommendationsforManufacturers/MemorandumtoBloodEstablishments/UCM062208.pdf. Accessed 18 April 2013.
- Memorandum to All Registered Blood Establishments—Requirements for Computerization of Blood Establishments (8 September 1989). FDA website. www.fda.gov/downloads/BiologicsBloodVaccines/GuidanceComplianceRegulatoryInformation/OtherRecommendationsforManufacturers/MemorandumtoBloodEstablishments/UCM062883.pdf. Accessed 18 April 2013.
- Memorandum to All Registered Blood Establishments - Recommendations for Implementation of Computerization in Blood Establishments (6 April 1988). FDA website. www.fda.gov/downloads/BiologicsBloodVaccines/GuidanceComplianceRegulatoryInformation/OtherRecommendationsforManufacturers/MemorandumtoBloodEstablishments/UCM063007.pdf. Accessed 18 April 2013.
- *Guidance for Industry—Process Validation: General Principles and Practices* (January 2011). FDA website. www.fda.gov/downloads/Drugs/GuidanceComplianceRegulatoryInformation/Guidances/UCM070336.pdf. Accessed 18 April 2013.
- *Inspection Guide: Computerized Systems in Drug Establishments* (February 1983). FDA website. www.fda.gov/ICECI/Inspections/InspectionGuides/ucm074869.htm. Accessed 18 April 2013.

Chapter 28

Human Cell and Tissue Products

Updated by Rafael Cassata, MS, RAC (US, EU)

OBJECTIVES

❑ Review the history of human tissue regulations

❑ Explain the legal basis and authority for human tissue regulation under the *Public Health Service Act*

❑ Identify the differences between 21 CFR Part 1270 and 21 CFR Part 1271

❑ Differentiate between cell and tissue-related products that are regulated by FDA and those that are not

❑ Identify the criteria that allow regulation of a cell or tissue without premarket approval

❑ Understand the key concepts of the cell and tissue product regulations

❑ Identify new policies for streamlined licensure of cord blood products regulated as biological products

LAWS, REGULATIONS AND GUIDELINES COVERED IN THIS CHAPTER

❑ *Public Health Service Act*, 42 USC 264

❑ *Federal Food, Drug, and Cosmetic Act* of 1938

❑ 21 CFR Part 1270 Human Tissue Intended for Transplantation

❑ 21 CFR Part 1271 Human Cells, Tissues, and Cellular and Tissue-Based Products

❑ *Guidance for Industry: Regulation of Human Cells, Tissues, and Cellular and Tissue-Based Products (HCT/Ps)—Small Entity Compliance Guide* (August 2007)

❑ *Guidance for Industry: Eligibility Determination for Donors of Human Cells, Tissues, and Cellular and Tissue-Based Products (HCT/Ps)* (August 2007)

❑ *Guidance for Industry: Current Good Tissue Practice (CGTP) and Additional Requirements for Manufacturers of Human Cells, Tissues, and Cellular and Tissue-Based Products (HCT/Ps)* (December 2011)

❑ *Final Guidance for Industry: Minimally Manipulated, Unrelated Allogeneic Placental/Umbilical Cord Blood Intended for Hematopoietic Reconstitution for Specified Indications* (October 2009)

History and Background of Human Cell and Tissue Regulation

In the early 1990s, the US Centers for Disease Control and Prevention (CDC) reported that human immunodeficiency virus (HIV) had been transmitted through transplantation of human tissue. Information reported also suggested that potentially unsafe tissue was being imported into the US for transplantation into humans. Prompted by reports that potentially unsafe bone was being imported, the commissioner of food and drugs ordered an investigation, the results

Table 28-1. 21 CFR 1271 at a Glance

Final Rule	21 CFR 1271 Subpart(s)	Effective Date (Published Date)	Issues Addressed
Establishment Registration and Listing	A, B	4 April 2001, 21 January 2003 (19 January 2001)	Applicability: types and uses of products that will be regulated by these rules; requirements for registering and listing HCT/Ps
Donor Eligibility	C	25 May 2005 (25 May 2004)	Requirements for donor screening and testing for relevant communicable disease agents and diseases
Current Good Tissue Practices (CGTP)	D, E, F	25 May 2005 (24 November 2004)	Manufacturing to ensure that HCT/Ps do not contain communicable disease agents; reporting; labeling and compliance/inspections

of which identified an immediate need to protect the public health from the transmission of HIV and Hepatitis B and C through transplantation of unsuitable tissue. Concerns that disease transmission could occur, coupled with information derived from these investigations, prompted the US Food and Drug Administration (FDA) to publish an interim final rule in December 1993 that specifically required testing for certain communicable diseases and screening of donors, and recordkeeping for certain human tissues intended for transplantation. This regulation, in Title 21 of the Code of Federal Regulations (CFR) Part 1270,[1] only applied to musculoskeletal, ocular and skin products from non-living human donors. A final rule was issued in July 1997.

21 CFR 1270

The regulations concerning human tissues intended for transplantation are listed in 21 CFR 1270. FDA regulates tissues under the legal authority of Section 361 of the *Public Health Service Act* (*PHS Act*).[2] This section authorizes the surgeon general, with the approval of the secretary of the Department of Health and Human Services, to make and enforce such regulations as are judged necessary to prevent the introduction, transmission or spread of communicable diseases from foreign countries into the US or from state to state. Tissues and cells regulated only under the authority of Section 361 do not require premarket approval. Applicable regulations apply to these products regardless of intra- or interstate distribution. The regulations in 21 CFR 1270 are divided into four subparts:
- Subpart A: General provisions
- Subpart B: Donor screening and testing
- Subpart C: Procedures and records
- Subpart D: Inspection of tissue establishments

21 CFR 1271

In 1997, FDA announced its plans for a comprehensive, tiered, risk-based approach for regulation of cellular and tissue-based products.[3] The goals of FDA's new regulatory framework for cells and tissues were to prevent the unwitting use of contaminated tissues with the potential for transmitting infectious disease, prevent improper handling or processing that might contaminate or damage tissues and ensure that clinical safety and effectiveness are demonstrated for cells and tissues that are highly processed (used for purposes other than replacement or combined with non-tissue components, or that have systemic effects). Since that time, the agency has proposed and finalized three rules to implement this proposed approach. These requirements were promulgated under Section 361 of the *PHS Act* and are codified as 21 CFR 1271.[4] These rules became wholly effective for cells and tissues recovered on or after 25 May 2005. Summaries of the three rules are listed in **Table 28-1**.[5]

FDA defines human cells, tissues and cellular and tissue-based products (HCT/Ps) as articles containing or consisting of human cells or tissues that are intended for implantation, transplantation, infusion or transfer into a human recipient. Some examples of HCT/Ps are listed in **Table 28-2**. Some examples of products that are not considered HCT/Ps along with their respective regulation also are provided in **Table 28-2**. FDA's Center for Biologics Evaluation and Research (CBER) regulates HCT/Ps under 21 CFR 1270 and 1271. The Health Resources Services Administration (HRSA), a separate agency within DHHS, is responsible for the oversight of vascularized human organs such as kidney, liver, heart, lung or pancreas; CBER does not regulate vascularized human organ transplants.

General Provisions (21 CFR 1271, Subpart A)

The criteria that form the foundation of FDA's tiered, risk-based approach to regulating HCT/Ps are found in 21 CFR 1271.10(a). If an HCT/P meets all of these criteria, it is regulated under Section 361 of the *PHS Act* and subject to the regulations in Part 1271. The four criteria are:
- minimal manipulation
- intended for homologous use
- not combined with another article
- no systemic effect and not dependent on metabolic activity of living cells, or has a systemic effect and is dependent on metabolic activity of living cells,

but is for autologous use, use in a first-degree or second-degree blood relative, or for reproductive use

For HCT/Ps that meet all of the criteria listed in 21 CFR 1271.10(a), no premarket approval is required and compliance is determined at FDA inspection. HCT/Ps that do not meet all four of these criteria are regulated as drugs, devices and/or biological products under Section 351 of the *PHS Act* and the *Federal Food, Drug, and Cosmetic Act*. In addition to applicable sections of 21 CFR 1271, these HCT/Ps would be subject to the regulations specific to drugs, biological products or medical devices. In other words, the 21 CFR 1271 requirements supplement the current Good Manufacturing Practice (CGMP) requirements for HCT/Ps regulated as biological products and the Quality Systems (QS) regulations for HCT/Ps regulated as medical devices. Examples of HCT/Ps regulated under Section 351 of the *PHS Act* include, but are not limited to, the following:

- autologous chondrocytes expanded *in vitro* for repair of cartilage defects
- allogeneic hematopoietic stem/progenitor cells, cord blood
- genetically modified cell therapy

In determining whether an HCT/P is regulated under Section 351 or 361 of the PHS Act, it is important to understand the following definitions:

- "autologous use"—use in the individual from whom the cells or tissue were recovered
- "allogeneic use"—use in a first- or second-degree blood relative, including parents, children, siblings, aunts, uncles, nieces, nephews, first cousins, grandparents and grandchildren (important for hematopoietic stem cell therapies)
- "minimal manipulation"—for structural tissue, processing that does not alter the original relevant characteristics of the tissue relating to the tissue's utility for reconstruction, repair or replacement; for cells or nonstructural tissues, processing that does not alter the relevant biological characteristics of the cells or tissues
- "homologous use"—repair, reconstruction, replacement or supplementation of a recipient's cells or tissues with an HCT/P that performs the same basic function or functions in the recipient as in the donor

Registration and Listing (21 CFR 1271, Subpart B)

FDA requires any establishment that manufactures HCT/Ps to register and submit a list of every HCT/P it manufactures within five days of beginning operation, and to re-register annually in December. In the context of the HCT/P regulations, "manufacture" is defined as any or all steps in the recovery, processing, storage, labeling or distribution of any human cell or tissue, and the screening or testing of the cell or tissue donor. Furthermore, changes in an establishment's HCT/P listing must be updated within six months of the change. If an establishment's ownership or location is changed, an amendment to the establishment registration also must be reported within five days. Furthermore, all foreign establishments exporting HCT/Ps to the US are also subject to the HCT/P registration and listing requirements. Under 21 CFR 1271.15, some establishments may not be required to complete the aforementioned registration and listing requirements. Establishments engaged in the following activities are not required to register and list:

- use HCT/Ps solely for nonclinical scientific or educational purposes
- remove and implant autologous HCT/Ps in the same surgical procedure
- accept, receive, carry or deliver HCT/Ps in the usual course of business as a carrier
- receive or store HCT/Ps solely for implantation, transplantation, infusion or transfer within the same

Table 28-2. Examples of Cell and Tissue-Based Products

Regulated Solely HCT/Ps	Non-HCT/Ps
• bone (including demineralized bone) • ligaments • tendons • fascia • cartilage • ocular tissue (corneas and sclera) • skin • arteries and veins • pericardium • amniotic membrane • dura mater • heart valves • hematopoietic stem/progenitor cells derived from peripheral and cord blood • semen, oocytes and embryos	• vascularized human organs for transplantation • whole blood or blood components or blood derivative products • secreted or extracted human products such as milk, collagen and cell factors • minimally manipulated bone marrow for homologous use and not combined with another article • products used in the manufacture of an HCT/P, cells, tissues and organs derived from animals other than humans (xenotransplantation) • in vitro diagnostic products • blood vessels recovered with organs for use in organ transplantation • products recovered and transplanted in the same surgical procedure

Figure 28-1. Form FDA 3356

See Instructions for OMB Statement. FORM APPROVED: OMB No. 0910-0543. Expiration Date: 8/31/10

DEPARTMENT OF HEALTH AND HUMAN SERVICES FOOD AND DRUG ADMINISTRATION **ESTABLISHMENT REGISTRATION AND LISTING FOR HUMAN CELLS, TISSUES, AND CELLULAR AND TISSUE-BASED PRODUCTS (HCT/Ps)** *(See reverse side for instructions)*	**1. REGISTRATION NUMBER** (Field Establishment Identifier) FEI	**2. REASON FOR SUBMISSION** a. ☐ INITIAL REGISTRATION/LISTING b. ☐ ANNUAL REGISTRATION/LISTING c. ☐ CHANGE IN INFORMATION d. ☐ INACTIVE	**VALIDATION – FOR FDA USE ONLY**

PART I – ESTABLISHMENT INFORMATION

3. OTHER FDA REGISTRATIONS

a. BLOOD FDA 2830   NO. _____

b. DEVICE FDA 2891   NO. _____

c. DRUG FDA 2656   NO. _____

4. PHYSICAL LOCATION *(Include legal name, number and street, city, state, country, and post office code.)*

a. PHONE:

b. ☐ SATELLITE RECOVERY ESTABLISHMENT
(MANUFACTURING ESTABLISHMENT FEI NO. _____)

c. ☐ TESTING FOR MICRO-ORGANISMS ONLY

5. ENTER CORRECTIONS TO ITEM 4

6. MAILING ADDRESS OF REPORTING OFFICIAL *(Include institution name if applicable, number and street, city, state, country, and post office code.)*

a. PHONE:

7. ENTER CORRECTIONS TO ITEM 6

8. U.S. AGENT

a. E-MAIL ADDRESS:

b. PHONE:

9. REPORTING OFFICIAL'S SIGNATURE

a. TYPED NAME:

b. E-MAIL ADDRESS:

c. TITLE: d. DATE:

PART II – HCT / P INFORMATION

10. ESTABLISHMENT FUNCTIONS AND TYPES OF HCT / Ps

Types of HCT / Ps	Recover	Screen	Test	Package	Process	Store	Label	Distribute	11. HCT / Ps DESCRIBED IN 21 CFR 1271.10	12. HCT / Ps REGULATED AS MEDICAL DEVICES	13. HCT / Ps REGULATED AS DRUGS OR BIOLOGICAL DRUGS	14. PROPRIETARY NAMES
a. Bone												
b. Cartilage												
c. Cornea												
d. Dura Mater												
e. Embryo ☐ SIP ☐ Directed ☐ Anonymous												
f. Fascia												
g. Heart Valve												
h. Ligament												
i. Oocyte ☐ SIP ☐ Directed ☐ Anonymous												
j. Pericardium												
k. Peripheral Blood Stem Cells ☐ Autologous ☐ Family Related ☐ Allogeneic												
l. Sclera												
m. Semen ☐ SIP ☐ Directed ☐ Anonymous												
n. Skin												
o. Somatic Cell Therapy Products ☐ Autologous ☐ Family Related ☐ Allogeneic												
p. Tendon												
q. Umbilical Cord Blood Stem Cells ☐ Autologous ☐ Family Related ☐ Allogeneic												
r. Vascular Graft												
s.												
t.												
u.												
v.												

FORM FDA 3356 (4/08)   PSC Graphics (301) 443-1090   EF   **Page 1 of 2**

INSTRUCTIONS FOR COMPLETING FORM 3356: ESTABLISHMENT REGISTRATION AND LISTING FOR HUMAN CELLS, TISSUES, AND CELLULAR AND TISSUE-BASED PRODUCTS (HCT/Ps)

Completion of Form FDA 3356 is required under 21 CFR Part 1271, 207.20 and 807.20 for all establishments engaged in the recovery, processing, storage, labeling, packaging, or distribution of any HCT/P, or the screening or testing of a cell or tissue donor. After we receive your form, we will update our records and send a validated form to the reporting official.

PART I. ESTABLISHMENT INFORMATION

NOTE: You are required to register and list your HCT/Ps by submitting this form if you recover, process, store, label, package, or distribute any HCT/P, or screen or test the HCT/P donor unless one of the following exceptions applies. You are not required to submit this form if:

a. You use HCT/Ps solely for nonclinical scientific or educational purposes,
b. You remove and then implant HCT/Ps solely for autologous use during the same surgical procedure,
c. You are a carrier who accepts, receives, carries, or delivers HCT/Ps in the usual course of business as a carrier,
d. You only receive or store HCT/Ps solely for implantation, transplantation, infusion, or transfer within your facility,
e. You only recover reproductive cells or tissue and immediately transfer them into a sexually intimate partner of the cell or tissue donor, or
f. You are an individual person who works under contract, agreement, or other arrangement with or for a registered establishment and only recover and send HCT/Ps to the registered establishment.

Item 3. OTHER FDA REGISTRATIONS – Provide the registration number if your establishment is already registered with FDA as a Blood, Medical Device or Drug establishment. Your establishment will not be given a new registration number and you are not required to fill in items 4 to 8 of Part I. Item 9 must be filled out and signed on all forms. If you choose not to complete, Items 4 to 8 of Part I, you still must complete and sign Item 9. Then proceed to Part II and provide product information.

Item 4. PHYSICAL LOCATION – Provide the legal name, street address including the postal code of the actual location and
a. Telephone number.
b. Indicate (with an X) if you are a satellite recovery establishment that supports recovery personnel in the field by providing temporary storage for recovered HCT/Ps for shipment to your parent manufacturing establishment, but do not perform any other activities or manufacturing steps. Provide the FEI NO. of your parent manufacturing establishment.
c. Indicate (with an X) if you are an establishment that performs testing of HCT/Ps for micro-organisms if that is the only HCT/P processing function that you perform.

Item 6. MAILING ADDRESS OF THE REPORTING OFFICIAL – Provide the reporting official's mailing address including the postal code if it is different from the actual location of the establishment.

Items 8. U.S. AGENT – Non-U.S. establishments only. Provide your U.S. agent name, institution name if applicable, street address, e-mail address, and telephone number. United States agent means a person residing or maintaining a place of business in the United States whom a foreign establishment designates as its agent.

Item 9. REPORTING OFFICIAL'S SIGNATURE – The reporting official as listed in item 6 is the person appointed by the owner or operator to register the firm and answer all the correspondence and inquiries relative thereto. The dated signature by the reporting official affirms that all information contained on the form is true and accurate, to the best of his or her knowledge.

PART II. HCT/P INFORMATION (If item 2.c is checked, only indicate the information being changed.)

Item 10. ESTABLISHMENT FUNCTIONS AND TYPES OF HCT/Ps – Indicate (with an X) the activity (ies) performed by the registered establishment in conjunction with the type of HCT/P that the registered establishment manufactures. Test and screen refer to the donor, not the HCT/P. For reproductive HCT/Ps, indicate whether the HCT/Ps are from sexually intimate partners (SIP), directed, or anonymous. For hematopoietic stem/progenitor cells and somatic cells, indicate whether the HCT/Ps are autologous, family related, or allogeneic. Family related means allogeneic use in a first degree or second degree relative.

Item 11. LISTING FOR HCT/Ps DESCRIBED IN 21 CFR 1271.10 – To list HCT/Ps that are described in 21 CFR 1271.10 (a) indicate (with an X) each HCT/P that fulfills all of the following criteria:

a. The HCT/P is minimally manipulated,
b. The HCT/P is intended for homologous use only, as reflected by the labeling, advertising, or other indications of the manufacturer's objective intent,
c. The manufacture of the HCT/P does not involve the combination of the cell or tissue component with a drug or a device, except for a sterilizing, preserving, or storage agent, if the addition of the agent does not raise new clinical safety concerns with respect to the HCT/P, and either
d. The HCT/P does not have a systemic effect and is not dependent upon the metabolic activity of living cells for its primary function; or the HCT/P has a systemic effect or is dependent upon the metabolic activity of living cells for its primary function, and (i) is for autologous use, (ii) is for allogeneic use in a first-degree or second-degree blood relative, or (iii) is for reproductive use.

If your HCT/P type is not preprinted on the form, list it on lines s-v.

Item 12. HCT/P LISTING FOR MEDICAL DEVICES – Indicate (with an X) each HCT/P that is regulated as a medical device under the Federal Food, Drug, and Cosmetic Act.

Item 13. HCT/P LISTING FOR DRUGS OR BIOLOGICAL DRUGS – Indicate (with an X) each HCT/P that is regulated as a drug or biological drug under the Federal Food, Drug, and Cosmetic Act and/or section 351 of the Public Health Service Act.

NOTE: For items 11, 12, and 13 indicate changes to HCT/P listing such as discontinuance (indicate with a D), or resumption (indicate with an R) of a HCT/P into commercial distribution in June and December or at the time the change occurs as directed under 21 CFR Part 1271.21. Dates of HCT/P discontinuance / resumption should be provided on an additional page.

Item 14. PROPRIETARY NAMES – Indicate any applicable proprietary names used for the HCT/Ps listed, such as a trademark.

NOTE: If necessary add an additional page to complete items 11, 12, 13, or 14.

After completion, return the form to:
Food and Drug Administration
Center for Biologics Evaluation and Research (HFM-775)
1401 Rockville Pike, Rockville, MD 20852-1448
ATTENTION: Tissue Establishment Registration Coordinator
FAX No. (301) 827-2844

FORM FDA 3356 (4/08)

Public reporting burden for this collection of information is estimated to average .75 hour per response, including the time for reviewing instructions, searching existing data sources, gathering and maintaining the data needed, and completing and reviewing the collection of information. Send comments regarding this burden estimate or any other aspect of this collection of information, including suggestions for reducing this burden to:
Department of Health and Human Services
Food and Drug Administration
Office of Chief Information Officer (HFA-250)
5600 Fishers Lane
Rockville, MD 20857

An agency may not conduct or sponsor, and a person is not required to respond to, a collection of information unless it displays a currently valid OMB control number.

Table 28-3. Overview of the Core CGTP Requirements (21 CFR 1271, Subpart D)

Core CGTP	Brief Description
Facilities	• Facilities must be of suitable size, construction, and location to prevent contamination of HCT/Ps with communicable disease agents and maintained in a good state of repair—kept in a clean, sanitary, and orderly manner. They should be divided into separate or defined areas of adequate size for each operation that takes place in the facility, or establish and maintain other control systems to prevent improper labeling, mix-ups, contamination, cross-contamination, and accidental exposure of HCT/Ps to communicable disease agents. • Establish and maintain procedures for facility cleaning and sanitation. • Document, and maintain records of (and retain for three years after their creation) all cleaning and sanitation activities performed to prevent contamination of HCT/Ps.

Environmental control	• Where appropriate, provide for the following control activities or systems:
	  o temperature and humidity controls
	  o ventilation and air filtration
	  o cleaning and disinfecting of rooms and equipment to ensure aseptic processing operations
	  o maintenance of equipment used to control conditions necessary for aseptic processing operations
	• Each environmental control system should be periodically inspected and records should be maintained.

Equipment	• The equipment used in the manufacture of HCT/Ps must be of appropriate design for its use and must be suitably located and installed to facilitate operations, including cleaning and maintenance. • Any automated, mechanical, electronic, or other equipment used for inspection, measuring or testing in accordance with this part must be capable of producing valid results. • The procedures and schedules, calibration of equipment, inspections, and records are also addressed.
Supplies and reagents	• Only supplies and reagents verified to meet specifications shall be used. Verification may be accomplished by the establishment that uses the supply or reagent, or by the vendor of the supply or reagent. • Reagents used in processing and preservation of HCT/Ps must be sterile, where appropriate. • The production of in-house reagents must be validated and records pertaining to supplies and reagents must be maintained.
Recovery	• The recovery of each HCT/P should be performed in a way that does not cause contamination or cross-contamination during recovery, or otherwise increase the risk of the introduction, transmission or spread of communicable disease.
Processing and process controls	• Human cells or tissues from two or more donors must not be pooled (placed in physical contact or mixed in a single receptacle) during manufacturing. • The in-process control and testing requirements must be met and controlled until the required inspection and tests or other verification activities have been completed, or necessary approvals are received and documented. Sampling of in-process HCT/Ps must be representative of the material to be evaluated. • With respect to dura mater, when there is a published validated process that reduces the risk of transmissible spongiform encephalopathy, such a process should be used (or an equivalent process that has been validated), unless following this process adversely affects the clinical utility of the dura mater.
Labeling controls	• Procedures to control the labeling of HCT/Ps should be established and maintained. They must be designed to ensure proper HCT/P identification and to prevent mix-ups. Procedures must include verification of label accuracy, legibility, and integrity. • Procedures must also be in place to ensure that each HCT/P is labeled in accordance with all applicable labeling requirements, including those in 1271.55, 1271.60, 1271.65, 1271.90, 1271.290 and 1271.370, and that each HCT/P made available for distribution is accompanied by documentation of the donor eligibility determination as required under 1271.55.
Storage	• Storage areas and stock rooms are to be controlled to prevent mix-ups, contamination and cross-contamination of HCT/Ps, supplies and reagents. These areas also should be designed to prevent an HCT/P from being improperly made available for distribution. • Temperature, expiration date, corrective action and acceptable temperature limits also are addressed.
Receipt, predistribution shipment and distribution	• Upon receipt, each incoming HCT/P must be tested for the presence and significance of microorganisms and inspected for damage and contamination. • A determination of whether to accept, reject or place in quarantine each incoming HCT/P, based on pre-established criteria designed to prevent communicable disease transmission, should be established. • Pre-distribution shipment, availability for distribution, packaging and shipping, procedures and returns to inventories also are covered.
Donor eligibility determination, donor screening and donor testing	• See "Donor Eligibility (21 CFR 1271, Subpart C)" section.

facility (and do not recover, screen, test, process, label, package or distribute)
- recover reproductive cells or tissue and immediately transfer them into a sexually intimate partner of the cell or tissue donor
- solely recover cells or tissues and send them to a registered establishment under contract, agreement or other arrangement with a registered establishment

To facilitate the registration and listing process, FDA developed Form FDA 3356 (see **Figure 28-1**), which can be submitted electronically, in paper form or by fax. Establishment registration does not imply that an establishment is in compliance with all requirements; compliance is determined at inspection. By the end of 2012, more than 4,100 establishments were registered with FDA and approximately 1,400 establishments are inactive.

Donor Eligibility (21 CFR 1271, Subpart C)

Donor eligibility determination is based on donor screening and testing for relevant communicable disease agents and disease (RCDADs). It is required for all donors of HCT/Ps, with some exceptions such as autologous donors and sexually intimate donors of reproductive cells and tissues. HCT/Ps must not be administered until the donor has been determined to be eligible, with some exceptions.

Donors must be screened by reviewing relevant medical records for risk factors for and clinical evidence of the RCDADs and for communicable disease risks associated with xenotransplantation (live cells, tissue or organs from a nonhuman animal source) and human transmissible spongiform encephalopathy including Creutzfeldt-Jakob Disease. Prospective HCT/P donors also must be screened for other RCDADs such as West Nile Virus, sepsis and vaccinia (recent smallpox vaccination). Relevant medical records are a collection of documents that includes a current donor medical history interview; a current report of the physical assessment of a cadaveric donor or the physical examination of a living donor and other available records.

All HCT/P donors must be tested for the following RCDADs:
- HIV, types 1 and 2
- Hepatitis B virus
- Hepatitis C virus
- Treponema pallidum

Donors of leukocyte-rich HCT/Ps such as hematopoietic stem/progenitor cells and semen also must be tested for the following RCDADS:
- Cytomegalovirus
- Human T-lymphotropic virus, types I and II

In addition, donors of reproductive HCT/Ps must be tested for the sexually transmitted agents:
- Chlamydia trachomatis
- Neisseria gonorrhea

Donor testing must be performed using the appropriate FDA-licensed, approved or cleared donor screening tests, in accordance with the manufacturer's instructions, to adequately and appropriately reduce the risk of transmission of RCDADS. Required donor testing must be performed by a laboratory that either is certified to perform such testing on human specimens under the *Clinical Laboratory Improvement Amendments* of 1988 (42 U.S.C. 263a) and 42 CFR Part 493, or has met equivalent requirements as determined by the Centers for Medicare and Medicaid Services. A donor must be determined to be ineligible if any of the criteria in 21 CFR 1271.80(d) are met. FDA has provided detailed guidance concerning its current thinking regarding donor screening and testing, which also recognizes new RCDADS not previously listed in 21 CFR 1271.[6]

Current Good Tissue Practices (21 CFR 1271, Subpart D)

The current Good Tissue Practices (CGTPs) requirements address the methods, facilities and controls used for manufacturing HCT/Ps to prevent the introduction, transmission and spread of communicable disease. Communicable diseases include, but are not limited to, those transmitted by viruses, bacteria, fungi, parasites and transmissible spongiform encephalopathy agents. The core CGTP requirements along with brief descriptions are listed in **Table 28-3**. They address all aspects of manufacture from recovery to distribution, with a specific focus on establishing a comprehensive quality program to oversee such manufacture. The quality program must be designed to prevent, detect and correct deficiencies that may lead to an increased risk of introduction, transmission or spread of communicable diseases.

The donor eligibility requirements discussed above are also considered to be CGTPs. These requirements are applicable to the manufacture of HCT/Ps regulated under Section 361 of the *PHS Act* and, to some extent, to HCT/Ps regulated as drugs, biological products and medical devices (i.e., under Section 351 of the *PHS Act*). FDA has published a guidance document with recommendations for complying with the CGTP regulations in 21 CFR 1271 Subparts D and E.[7]

Reporting and Labeling (21 CFR 1271, Subpart E)

The 21 CFR 1271 requirements for reporting and labeling currently apply only to nonreproductive HCT/Ps regulated under Section 361 of the *PHS Act*. The labeling requirements focus on information that must appear on the HCT/P label, including a distinct identification code and

Chapter 28

Figure 28-2.

DEPARTMENT OF HEALTH AND HUMAN SERVICES
FOOD AND DRUG ADMINISTRATION

BIOLOGICAL PRODUCT DEVIATION REPORT

FDA USE ONLY
Date Received:
Date Reviewed:
BPD ID:
BPD No.

* Indicates required information

A. FACILITY INFORMATION

1. Reporting Establishment Information

* Reporting Establishment Name
* Street Address Line 1
  Street Address Line 2
* City
* State
  Country
* Zip Code
* Point of Contact
* Telephone #
  E-mail

2. * Reporting Establishment Identification Number

FDA Registration #
CLIA #

3. If the BPD occurred somewhere other than the above facility, please complete this Section and Section A4; otherwise, continue on to Section B1.

* Establishment Name
  Street Address Line 1
  Street Address Line 2
* City
* State
* Country
  Zip Code

4. Establishment Identification Number

FDA Registration #
CLIA #

B. BIOLOGICAL PRODUCT DEVIATION (BPD) INFORMATION

1. Establishment Tracking #
2. Date BPD Occurred
3. * Date BPD Discovered
4. * Date BPD Reported
5. * Description of BPD *(use Page 2 for additional space)*
6. * Description of Contributing Factors or Root Cause *(use Page 3 for additional space)*
7. * Follow-Up *(use Page 4 for additional space)*
8. * Please Enter the 6 Character BPD Code

C. UNIT / PRODUCT INFORMATION

Please check the type of product:
- Blood ☐ (Continued on Page 5)
- Non-Blood ☐ (Continued on Page 6)

FORM FDA 3486 (10/12)
Form Approved:
OMB No. 0910-0458
Expires: 1/31/2014

See PRA Statement on Page 8.

Page 1 of 8

Biological Product Deviation Report

B5. DESCRIPTION OF BPD *(continued)*

FORM FDA 3486 (10/12)   Page 2 of 8

Biological Product Deviation Report

B6. DESCRIPTION OF CONTRIBUTING FACTORS OR ROOT CAUSE *(continued)*

FORM FDA 3486 (10/12)

Biological Product Deviation Report

B7. FOLLOW-UP *(continued)*

Biological Product Deviation Report

C1. BLOOD PRODUCTS / COMPONENTS

TOTAL NUMBER OF UNITS: _____

Unit #	Collection Date (MM/DD/YYYY)	Expiration Date (MM/DD/YYYY)	Product Code	Disposition	Notification (Y,N,RN)
1.)					
2.)					
3.)					
4.)					
5.)					
6.)					
7.)					
8.)					
9.)					
10.)					
11.)					
12.)					
13.)					
14.)					
15.)					
16.)					
17.)					
18.)					

FORM FDA 3486 (10/12)

Human Cell and Tissue Products

Biological Product Deviation Report

C2. NON-BLOOD PRODUCTS

TOTAL NUMBER OF LOTS: _____

Lot #	Expiration Date (MM/DD/YYYY)	Product Type	Product Code	Disposition	Notification (Y,N)
1.)					
2.)					
3.)					
4.)					
5.)					
6.)					
7.)					
8.)					
9.)					
10.)					
11.)					
12.)					
13.)					
14.)					
15.)					
16.)					
17.)					
18.)					

FORM FDA 3486 (10/12)

Biological Product Deviation Report

D. ADDITIONAL COMMENTS

FORM FDA 3486 (10/12)   Page 7 of 8

Biological product deviation reports required by 21 CFR 600.14, 21 CFR 606.171, or 21 CFR 1271.350(b), involving products regulated by the Center for Biologics Evaluation and Research (CBER), mail to:

Director, Office of Compliance and Biologics Quality (HFM-600)
Center for Biologics Evaluation and Research
Food and Drug Administration
1401 Rockville Pike, Suite 200N
Rockville, MD 20852-1448

Biological product deviation reports required by 21 CFR 600.14, involving licensed biological products regulated by the Center for Drug Evaluation and Research (CDER), mail to:

Division of Compliance Risk Management and Surveillance
Office of Compliance
Center for Drug Evaluation and Research
Food and Drug Administration
10903 New Hampshire Ave.
Silver Spring, MD 20993-0002

This section applies only to requirements of the Paperwork Reduction Act of 1995.

DO NOT SEND YOUR COMPLETED FORM TO THE PRA STAFF ADDRESS BELOW.

The burden time for this collection of information is estimated to average 2 hours per response, including the time to review instructions, search existing data sources, gather and maintain the data needed and complete and review the collection of information. Send comments regarding this burden estimate or any other aspect of this information collection, including suggestions for reducing this burden, to:

Department of Health and Human Services
Food and Drug Administration
Office of Chief Information Officer
Paperwork Reduction Act (PRA) Staff
1350 Piccard Drive, Room 400
Rockville, MD 20850

"An agency may not conduct or sponsor, and a person is not required to respond to, a collection of information unless it displays a currently valid OMB control number."

FORM FDA 3486 (10/12)

Table 28-4. FDA Regulation of Minimally Manipulated Cord Blood Products

Origin and Use of Cord Blood	Applicable FDA Requirements	Premarket Application Required
Autologous	21 CFR 1271 (exempt from donor eligibility requirements)	No, if 1271.10 criteria met
Allogeneic: first or second degree blood relative	21 CFR 1271 (donor eligibility required)	No, if 1271.10 criteria met
Allogeneic: unrelated	Parts of 1271, 201, 211, 600, 610	Yes, IND and/or BLA

a description of the type of HCT/P. Other requirements address information that may accompany the HCT/P or appear on the label, such as the name and address of the establishment that determined release criteria and made the HCT/P available for distribution. HCT/Ps regulated under Section 351 of the *PHS Act* must comply with the applicable drug, biological product or medical device labeling requirements.

Adverse reactions involving a communicable disease must be reported to FDA if they are fatal, life-threatening, result in permanent impairment or damage or necessitate medical or surgical intervention, including hospitalization. As required for other FDA adverse event reports, HCT/P adverse reaction reports are submitted to FDA's MedWatch system.[8,9]

All deviations related to a distributed HCT/P for which an establishment performed a manufacturing step must be investigated. If the deviation occurred at the facility or in a contracted facility during manufacture, it must be reported as related to core CGTP requirements. The deviation report should include a description of the HCT/P deviation, information relevant to the event and manufacture of the HCT/P, and information on all follow-up actions that have happened or will be taken. FDA has developed a standardized format (Form FDA 3486—see **Figure 28-2**) for reporting HCT/P deviations.[10,11,12] Deviation reporting is not required for reproductive HCT/Ps and HCT/Ps regulated as drugs, biological products and medical devices.

Inspection and Enforcement (21 CFR 1271, Subpart F)

The general inspectional provisions are described for notification, frequency and copying of records. This subpart applies only to HCT/Ps regulated solely under Section 361 of the *PHS Act*. What distinguishes these Part 1271 provisions from the inspection and enforcement requirements for other FDA-regulated products is that compliance actions are focused on providing protection against risks of communicable disease transmission. FDA has provided its investigators with detailed descriptions of how to conduct HCT/P inspections and address HCT/P importation.[13,14,15]

Regulation of Hematopoietic Progenitor Cells from Umbilical and Cord Blood Products

FDA has developed a streamlined approach to licensure of hematopoietic progenitor cells derived from cord blood (HPC-C) for allogeneic use. Though some cord blood products for autologous and family-related use are regulated only under the new requirements in 21 CFR 1271 and Section 361 of the *PHS Act*, those intended for allogeneic unrelated recipients are considered biological products (**Table 28-4**). Effective 20 October 2011, HPC-C for unrelated allogeneic use requires the submission of Biological License Applications (BLAs) and/or must be distributed under an Investigational New Drug Applications (INDs). FDA published two guidances (one for BLAs and one for INDs) on 20 October 2009 to assist sponsors with preparing BLAs and INDs.[16,17] The BLAs required for the specified indications listed in the BLA guidance will be streamlined in that they will not require each establishment to demonstrate clinical efficacy, but can rely on clinical data that were submitted to FDA for review in a public docket. In addition, FDA has updated a *Compliance Program Guidance for Biological Products*[18] to include HPC-C compliance issues to assist investigators with both pre-licensure and annual investigations.

FDA has not yet completed its policy for another HCT/P, hematopoietic progenitor cells derived from peripheral blood. Because these are also life-saving therapies where access to the best human leukocyte antigen (HLA) match for a patient is crucial, FDA is being very careful to develop guidance that will ensure product safety and efficacy but will not impede patient care.

Summary

- FDA has developed and implemented comprehensive, tiered, risk-based regulations that apply to a wide range of HCT/Ps which ensure:
  - the level and type of regulation is commensurate with the risk posed by the product characteristic
  - like products are treated alike
  - FDA exercises regulatory oversight only to the degree appropriate to protect the public health

- These requirements are broad and focus on ensuring that HCT/Ps are neither contaminated nor capable of transmitting communicable diseases.
- Unlike many other FDA-regulated products, most HCT/Ps are not required to undergo premarket review and approval before distribution.
- For certain HCT/Ps (regulated under Section 361 of the *PHS Act*), the new regulations comprise the sole regulatory requirements.
- FDA has completed policy development for streamlined licensure for allogeneic cord blood and is still developing policy for peripheral blood stem cell products.
- For HCT/Ps regulated as drugs, devices and/or biological products, the new tissue regulations supplement other requirements (CGMP/QS).
- All establishments that perform a manufacturing function must register and list with FDA.

References

1. 21 CFR 1270. Human tissue intended for transplantation. FDA website. www.accessdata.fda.gov/scripts/cdrh/cfdocs/cfcfr/CFRSearch.cfm?CFRPart=1270. Accessed 2 May 2013.
2. *Public Health Service Act*. FDA website. www.fda.gov/RegulatoryInformation/Legislation/ucm148717.htm. Accessed 2 May 2013.
3. "A Proposed Approach to the Regulation of Cellular and Tissue-Based Products." 62 *FR* 9721 (4 March 1997). Federal Register website. http://www.gpo.gov/fdsys/pkg/FR-1997-03-04/pdf/97-5240.pdf. Accessed 2 May 2013.
4. 21 CFR 1271 Human cells, tisssues, and cellular and tissue-based products. FDA website. www.accessdata.fda.gov/scripts/cdrh/cfdocs/cfcfr/CFRSearch.cfm?CFRPart=1271. Accessed 2 May 2013.
5. *Guidance for Industry: Regulation of Human Cells, Tissue, and Cellular and Tissue-Based Products (HCT/Ps) Small Entity Compliance Guide* (August 2007). FDA website. www.fda.gov/BiologicsBloodVaccines/GuidanceComplianceRegulatoryInformation/Guidances/Tissue/ucm073366.htm. Accessed 2 May 2013.
6. *Guidance for Industry: Eligibility Determination for Donors of Human Cells, Tissue, and Cellular and Tissue-Based Products (HCT/Ps)* (August 2007). FDA website. www.fda.gov/BiologicsBloodVaccines/GuidanceComplianceRegulatoryInformation/Guidances/CellularandGeneTherapy/ucm072929.htm. Accessed 2 May 2013.
7. *Guidance for Industry: Current Good Tissue Practice (CGTP) and Additional Requirements for Manufacturers of Human Cells, Tissues, and Cellular and Tissue-Based Products (HCT/Ps)* (December 2011). FDA website. www.fda.gov/downloads/BiologicsBloodVaccines/GuidanceComplianceRegulatoryInformation/Guidances/Tissue/UCM285223.pdf. Accessed 2 May 2013.
8. *Guidance for Industry: MedWatch Form FDA 3500A: Mandatory Reporting of Adverse Reactions Related to Human Cells, Tissue, and Cellular and Tissue-Based Products (HCT/Ps)* (November 2005). FDA website. www.fda.gov/BiologicsBloodVaccines/GuidanceComplianceRegulatoryInformation/Guidances/Tissue/ucm074000.htm. Accessed 2 May 2013.
9. SOPP 8508—*Procedures for Handling Adverse Reaction Reports Related to "361" Human Cells, Tissues, and Cellular and Tissue Based Products* (March 2008). FDA website. www.fda.gov/BiologicsBloodVaccines/GuidanceComplianceRegulatoryInformation/ProceduresSOPPs/ucm073048.htm. Accessed 2 May 2013.
10. Form FDA 3486: Biological Product Deviation Report. FDA website. www.fda.gov/downloads/AboutFDA/ReportsManualsForms/Forms/UCM061463.pdf. Accessed 2 May 2013.
11. "Compliance Program 7341.002: Inspection of Human Cells, Tissues, and Cellular and Tissue-Based Products (HCT/Ps)." Covers human tissue recovered after 25 May 2005. FDA website. www.fda.gov/biologicsbloodvaccines/guidancecomplianceregulatoryinformation/complianceactivities/enforcement/complianceprograms/ucm095207.htm. Accessed 2 May 2013.
12. "Compliance Program 7341.002A: Inspection of Tissue Establishments." Covers human tissue recovered before 25 May 2005. FDA website. www.fda.gov/BiologicsBloodVaccines/GuidanceComplianceRegulatoryInformation/ComplianceActivities/Enforcement/CompliancePrograms/ucm095218.htm. Accessed 2 May 2013.
13. "Compliance Program 7342.007 Addendum: Imported Human Cells, Tissues, and Cellular and Tissue-based Products (HCT/Ps)." FDA website. www.fda.gov/downloads/BiologicsBloodVaccines/GuidanceComplianceRegulatoryInformation/ComplianceActivities/Enforcement/CompliancePrograms/ucm095253.pdf. Accessed 2 May 2013.
14. Op cit 11.
15. Op cit 12.
16. *Final Guidance for Industry: Minimally Manipulated, Unrelated Allogeneic Placental/Umbilical Cord Blood Intended for Hematopoietic Reconstitution for Specified Indications* (October 2009). FDA website. www.fda.gov/downloads/BiologicsBloodVaccines/GuidanceComplianceRegulatoryInformation/Guidances/Blood/UCM187144.pdf. Accessed 2 May 2013.
17. *Draft Guidance for Industry and FDA Staff: IND Applications for Minimally Manipulated, Unrelated Allogeneic Placental/Umbilical Cord Blood Intended for Hematopoietic Reconstitution for Specified Indications* (October 2009). FDA website. www.fda.gov/downloads/BiologicsBloodVaccines/GuidanceComplianceRegulatoryInformation/Guidances/Blood/UCM187146.pdf. Accessed 2 May 2013.
18. *Compliance Program Guidance Manual 7345.848: Inspection of Biological Drug Products* (October 2010). FDA website. www.fda.gov/BiologicsBloodVaccines/GuidanceComplianceRegulatoryInformation/ComplianceActivities/Enforcement/CompliancePrograms/ucm095393.htm. Accessed 2 May 2013.

Reading List

- FDA CBER Tissue website. www.fda.gov/BiologicsBloodVaccines/TissueTissueProducts/default.htm. Accessed 2 May 2013.
- "Keeping Human Tissue Transplants Safe," *FDA Consumer Magazine*, May-June 2005. GPO website. http://permanent.access.gpo.gov/lps1609/www.fda.gov/fdac/features/2005/305_tissue.html. Accessed 2 May 2013.
- Consumer Frequently Asked Questions, 2007 FDA, CBER website. www.fda.gov/BiologicsBloodVaccines/TissueTissueProducts/QuestionsaboutTissues/ucm101559.htm. Accessed 2 May 2013.
- Frequently asked Questions about Tissue Transplants from the Centers for Disease Control and Prevention Website. AATB website. www.aatb.org/files/2006bulletin16.pdf. Accessed 2 May 2013.
- Office of Cellular, Tissue and Gene Therapies (OCTGT) Learn: Educational Webinars Regarding OCTGT and Products Regulated in the Office www.fda.gov/BiologicsBloodVaccines/NewsEvents/ucm232821.htm. Accessed 2 May 2013.
- Prebula R. "Current Good Tissue Practices: The Core Requirements when Donating Human Tissue," *FDLI Update*, November/December 2007.
- Shapiro JK and Wesoloski BJ. "FDA's Regulatory Scheme for Human Tissue, A Brief Overview," *FDLI Update*, November/December 2007.
- Weber DJ. "Understanding and Implementing Good Tissue Practices (GTPs)," *Regulatory Focus*, July 2008, 13(7):18–28.

- Weber DJ. "Navigating FDA Regulations for Human Cells and Tissue," *BioProcessing International*, 2(8): 22-26, 2004.
- Wells MA. "Overview of FDA Regulation of Human Cellular and Tissue-Based Products," *Food and Drug Law Journal*, 52, 401-408, 1997.
- Wells MA and Lazarus EF. "FDA Streamlines Licensure approach for Certain Cord Blood Products," *Regulatory Focus*, April 2010, 15(4):36–39.

Acknowledgements
We acknowledge and thank the contribution of Martha Wells, MPH, RAC, whose prior version of this chapter formed the core for this current iteration.

Chapter 29

Regulations Pertaining to Pediatrics

Updated by Min Chen, PhD, RAC

OBJECTIVES

❑ Familiarize readers with US regulations pertaining to pediatric products

❑ Review the requirements of the *Pediatric Research Equity Act (PREA)* and the changes mandated in the *Food and Drug Administration Admendments Act of 2007 (FDAAA)* and the *Food and Drug Administration Safety and Innovation Act of 2012 (FDASIA)*

❑ Review the requirements of the *Best Pharmaceuticals for Children Act (BPCA)* and the changes mandated in *FDAAA* and *FDASIA*

❑ Review the requirements of the *Pediatric Medical Safety and Improvement Act* mandated in *FDAAA*

❑ Understand the difference between *PREA* and *BPCA*

❑ Understand the pediatric written request process in the US

❑ Familiarize readers with international collaboration on pediatric product development between FDA and other regulatory agencies

LAWS, REGULATIONS AND GUIDELINES COVERED IN THIS CHAPTER

❑ *Guidance for Industry: General Considerations for the Clinical Evaluation of Drugs in Infants and Children* (1977)

❑ American Academy of Pediatrics *Guidelines for the Ethical Study of Drugs in Infants and Children* (1977)

❑ *Orphan Drug Act of 1983*

❑ American Academy of Pediatrics *Guidelines for the Ethical Conduct of Studies to Evaluate Drugs in Pediatric Populations* (1995)

❑ *Guidance for Industry: The Content and Format of Pediatric Use Section* (May 1996)

❑ *Food and Drug Administration Modernization Act of 1997*

❑ *Best Pharmaceuticals for Children Act of 2002*

❑ *Pediatric Research Equity Act of 2003*

❑ *Food and Drug Administration Amendments Act of 2007*

❑ *Pediatric Medical Device Safety and Improvement Act of 2007*

❑ *Food and Drug Administration Safety and Innovation Act of 2012*

Introduction

Children are not small adults. When taking drugs, children do not necessarily respond as might be expected by simply adjusting the dose for a smaller person. There have been instances where children have died or suffered serious injury as a result of taking drugs shown to be safe in adults but never specifically tested in children. With regard to the use of medical devices, medical devices that function properly in adults may be inappropriate to use in children if differences in growth, metabolism and activity levels between the two have not been taken into consideration.

As such, significant medical needs must be considered for drugs and devices to be used in pediatric populations. In the past, a number of steps have been taken to provide additional information on pediatric treatments (see below "History of Pediatric Initiatives"). Of note, in the mid-1990s, two major advancements took place.

"Up to 1994 most drugs (75–80%) were not labeled as either safe or effective for infants and children and off label use was the norm for these therapeutic orphans. There was little awareness among practitioners that prescribing for children was not evidence-based."[1] The Eunice Kennedy Shriver National Institute of Child Health and Human Development (NICHD) established the Pediatric Pharmacology Research Unit (PPRU) Network in 1994. This organization was formed to respond to the need for appropriate drug therapy studies in pediatric patients.

Reasons for possible gaps in the pediatric knowledge base include:
- ethical concerns in enrolling pediatric patients in studies
- limited populations for certain diseases
- technical difficulties in conducting pediatric trials
- belief that dosing could be determined by weight-based calculations
- lack of accepted endpoints and validated pediatric assessment tools
- limited marketing potential compared to adults

Since the inception of the PPRU Network, researchers have conducted a variety of drug studies, including pharmacokinetic studies, pharmacodynamic studies and studies of trial design.

In 1997, a major change occurred when the US Food and Drug Administration (FDA) issued new regulatory approaches that expanded and created systems to encourage development of medical and surgical devices for pediatric patients; to ensure that drugs that are or will be prescribed for children are tested for safety and effectiveness in children; and to review study designs to ensure that pediatric patients are protected and that these studies result in data that are medically and ethically appropriate for pediatric therapeutics.

History of Pediatric Initiatives

- 1972—Former FDA Commissioner Charles Edwards stated at the annual meeting of the American Academy of Pediatrics (AAP) that most prescription products used in children are given based on empirical evidence.
- 1973—The National Academy of Sciences issued a report calling for innovative investigative programs to provide information on the use of pharmacologic agents in the pediatric population.
- 1974—AAP issued a report commissioned by FDA on the evaluation of drugs to be used in the treatment of pregnant women, infants and children.
- 1975—Professor John Wilson of the Department of Pediatrics at LSU Medical Center published a survey of prescription drug package inserts noting that 78% of package inserts state the that the product either had not been studied in infants and children or had no pediatric statement.[2]
- 1977—Publication of three documents related to pediatric research:
  o FDA published *Guidance for Industry: General Considerations for the Clinical Evaluation of Drugs in Infants and Children.*
  o National Commission on Pediatric Research issued *General Considerations for the Clinical Evaluation of Drugs in Infants and Children.*
  o AAP issued *Guidelines for the Ethical Study of Drugs in Infants and Children.*
- 1979—FDA published a regulation adding a pediatric use subsection to the precautions section of the approved product package insert.
- 1983—The *Orphan Drug Act* established the precedent of incentives, provided by the federal government, to develop new therapeutics for underserved populations.
- 1994—FDA revised the pediatric use regulation to allow extrapolation of adult efficacy data if the disease course in adults and children is similar.
- 1994—NICHD established the first national network for pediatric pharmacology.
- 1995—AAP revised *Guidelines for the Ethical Conduct of Studies to Evaluate Drugs in Pediatric Populations.*
- 1996—FDA issued *Guidance for Industry: The Content and Format of Pediatric Use Section.*
- 1996—The National Institutes of Health (NIH) initiated a policy of requiring NIH-funded clinical research to address applicability to pediatric populations.
- 1997—The *Food and Drug Administration Modernization Act* (*FDAMA*) established an incentive program for pediatric studies for medicinal products. Incentives, such as additional six months'

exclusivity or patent extension, may be permitted after FDA issues a Written Request for relevant pediatric studies to the sponsor. The incentive is granted after a review confirms the study has been conducted in accordance with the FDA agreement. The program is limited to chemical moieties and excludes biological products and some antibiotics.
- 1998—FDA published a regulation ("Pediatric Rule") mandating pediatric studies when the disease or condition is similar in adults and children, and if either widespread use is anticipated or the product is a therapeutic advance.
- 2002—The Federal Court in the District of Columbia invalidated the 1998 Pediatric Rule, holding that FDA overstepped its authority in requiring pediatric testing unless the manufacturer can show it is highly unlikely the drug will be used in pediatric populations.
- 2002—The *Best Pharmaceuticals for Children Act* (*BPCA*) renewed the pediatric incentive program and established a program for the study of off-patent products through the NICHD.
- 2003—The *Pediatric Research Equity Act* (*PREA*) established the mandates of the 1998 Pediatric Rule as law for drugs and biological products, excluding products with Orphan Drug designation. (See the section on *PREA* below for details.)
- 2006—FDA, under the incentive programs defined in the *BPCA*, revised product package inserts for 118 products with new pediatric information.
- 2007—As of the end of the first quarter of the calendar year, FDA:
  o had issued 340 Written Requests for pediatric studies since the incentive program began
  o had granted an incentive for pediatric studies to 136 products for 129 active chemical moieties of 149 determinations (91% favorable determination rate)
  o had revised product package inserts for 55 products under *PREA*
- 2007—The *Food and Drug Administration Amendments Act* (*FDAAA*)[3] became law and renewed, with modification, *PREA* and *BPCA* and introduced the *Pediatric Medical Device Safety and Improvement Act*. In general, the pediatric population includes patients' age "birth to 16 years, including age groups often called neonates, infants, children and adolescents."[4] Each of these is reviewed below in detail.
- 2012 – The *Food and Drug Administration Safety and Innovation Act (FDASIA)*[5] was signed into law, renewed and strengthened three essential laws on pediatric research (*PREA, BPCA,* and the *Pediatric Medical Device Safety and Improvement Act)* and made *PREA* and *BPCA* permanent. The changes made in *FDASIA* are outlined below.

Changes to Pediatric Provisions Under FDASIA

FDASIA made both *PREA* and *BPCA* permanent, so they no longer require periodic reauthorization.

Under *PREA*, FDA is given new authority to help to ensure *PREA* requirements are addressed in a more-timely manner and sponsors subject to *PREA* now are required to submit pediatric study plans earlier.

In addressing neonatal needs, FDA's Office of Pediatric Therapeutics (OPT) is required to have a staff member with expertise in a pediatric subpopulation that is less likely to be studied under *BPCA* or *PREA*, and have a staff member with expertise in neonatology within five years after *FDASIA* enactment. Further, an FDA employee with neonatology expertise should sit on the Pediatric Review Committee. Under *BPCA*, a rationale for not including neonatal studies in the *BPCA* requests must be included if none are requested.

For products that received pediatric exclusivity and a pediatric labeling change under *BPCA* 2002, FDA is required to post not just the medical and clinical pharmacology summaries on its website, but also the medical, statistical and clinical pharmacology reviews and corresponding written requests in the same manner as currently posted materials.

For product development related to pediatric orphan diseases, FDA is required to hold a public meeting and to issue a report on the efforts taken to accelerate such matter.

Pediatric Research Equity Act (PREA)

PREA originally became law on 3 December 2003. It requires pediatric studies of certain drugs and biologicals whose indications are under development unless waived or deferred. The designated orphan indications are exempted from *PREA* requirements. The "Pediatric Mandate" is included in the *PREA* law. *FDASIA* in 2012 made *PREA* permanent.

A pediatric assessment is required for applications with new ingredients, new indications, new dosage forms, new dosing regimens or new routes of administration. The assessment must contain sufficient data to adequately assess the drug or biological product's safety and effectiveness and to support dosing and administration for each relevant pediatric subpopulation.

Pediatric studies should either have minimal risk, or have the prospect of direct benefit with greater than minimal risk, or have no prospect of direct benefit but with a minor increase over minimal risk, and they should likely yield generalized knowledge about the subject's disorder or condition. The types of data submitted under *PREA* will depend on the nature of the application, what is known about the product in pediatric populations and the underlying disease or condition being treated. *PREA* does not require applicants to conduct separate safety and effectiveness studies in pediatric patients in every case.

For a course of disease or effect similar to adults, effectiveness can be extrapolated from adequate and well-controlled studies in adults, when supplemented with other information (e.g., safety, pharmacokinetics and pharmacodynamics). Extrapolation from one age group to another is permitted, where appropriate.

FDA may grant a deferral when the drug or biologic is ready for approval in adults or when additional safety and effectiveness data are determined to be necessary. The deferral is tracked as a Phase 4 or postmarketing commitment.

A full waiver is granted when the condition does not occur in the pediatric population or the required studies are impossible or highly impractical. A waiver also may be granted when strong evidence suggests that the drug or biologic would be ineffective or unsafe in children. If the drug or biologic does not represent a meaningful therapeutic benefit over existing therapies and is not likely to be used in a substantial number of pediatric patients, a full waiver may also be granted. FDA has used 50,000 patients as representing a "substantial number."

A partial waiver may be granted for an age subset of the pediatric population using the same conditions and criteria that apply for a full waiver. A partial waiver also may be granted if reasonable attempts to produce a pediatric formulation for a particular subset of the pediatric population have failed. An update in *PREA* 2007 requires the sponsor to submit documentation to FDA explaining why a pediatric formulation cannot be developed. Labeling should include information that states that a full or partial waiver has been granted because there is evidence the drug or biologic would be ineffective or unsafe.

If a waiver is granted, FDA will make the application for the waiver publically available.

For marketed drugs and biological products, FDA can require study data after providing notice to the sponsor of the approved application and providing an opportunity for a written response and a meeting. This situation may occur if the drug or biologic is used for a substantial number of pediatric patients for the labeled indication and in the absence of adequate labeling that could pose significant risks to a pediatric population. Additional studies also may be required if there is a reason to believe the drug or biologic would represent a meaningful therapeutic benefit over existing therapies and the absence of adequate studies could pose significant risks to pediatric patients. Waiver and deferral criteria are the same as those for new drugs and biologics.

A pediatric plan is a statement of intent that outlines the applicant's planned pediatric studies. It also should indicate whether the applicant plans to request a waiver or deferral and the basis for the request. FDA encourages applicants to discuss pediatric plan at pre-Investigational New Drug (pre-IND) application meetings, especially for products intended for life-threatening or severely debilitating diseases. For products that are not intended for treating life-threatening or severely debilitating diseases, applicants may submit and discuss the pediatric plan no later than the End-of-Phase 2 meeting.

PREA 2007 requires the sponsor's annual review to document study status, reasons for lack of progress and plans for completing studies in a timely fashion. Such information will become publically available on FDA's website.

FDAAA contains the *PREA* provisions in Title IV, which includes a number of changes to the original *PREA*. The updates include:

- requires an annual review from an applicant that has received a deferral
- makes annual deferral reviews public
- requires manufacturers that have tried but have been unsuccessful in producing a pediatric formulation to submit to FDA the reasons why the formulation cannot be developed
- changes the criteria for applying *PREA* to already marketed drugs; new language allows FDA to use a "benefit" standard as opposed to a "risk" standard
- shortens the "request and response" period for the holder to an expedited 30-day review of private funding before referral to *PREA*
- requires an FDA internal committee to review study plans and assessments as well as deferrals and waivers
- requires FDA to track the number and type of studies completed, as well as labeling changes and other data resulting from *PREA*
- modifies the *BPCA* dispute resolution process and applies it to *PREA*; the modified language reduces the overall time period for resolving disputes over labeling and removes the provision requiring labeling to be the only remaining open issue before referral for resolution
- requires FDA to make medical, statistical and clinical pharmacology reviews publically available
- requires sponsors to provide physicians and other healthcare providers with new pediatric labeling information
- requires reporting of adverse events for drugs studied under *PREA* and provides for review by the Pediatric Advisory Committee
- requests the Institute of Medicine to review past study requests issued by FDA and make recommendations to the agency for future requests
- continues linkage of *PREA* to the expiration of *BPCA* on 1 October 2012
- establishes a coordinated internal review committee to *BPCA* and *PREA*

- requires the Government Accountability Office to produce a report on the results of *BPCA* and *PREA* with recommendations for improving the programs

FDASIA in 2012 made *PREA* permanent and contains the *PREA* provisions in Title V, where it requires sponsors to submit pediatric study plans earlier and gives FDA new authority to ensure *PREA* requirements are addressed in a more timely manner.

Best Pharmaceuticals for Children Act (BPCA)

The *Best Pharmaceuticals for Children Act* of 2002 (*BPCA*) followed the 1998 Pediatric Rule, which was invalidated in 2002 by the District of Columbia federal court. *FDAAA* increased the authority and effectiveness of *BPCA*, and *FDASIA* made *BPCA* permanent. It is important to note that the pediatric studies under *BPCA* cover drugs and biologics with a broad range of indications and formulations including orphan drugs, which are voluntary, in contrast to those required under *PREA*. *BPCA* provides the incentive of a six-month extension of marketing exclusivity or patent protections by fulfilling the terms of an agreed FDA issued Written Request.

To initiate the process defined in *BPCA*, FDA issues a Written Request to holders of approved applications. The sponsor also may submit a proposed pediatric study request, which may generate a formal Written Request by FDA. The Written Request is a legal document requesting the sponsor to conduct studies in the pediatric population. The Written Request specifies the indication, population, type of studies, safety parameters, longer-term follow-up and timeframe for completion and response.

The criteria for issuing a Written Request include:
- serious or life-threatening condition
- frequency of disease or condition
- whether other therapeutic options are available
- how often the drug is used or expected to be used in the pediatric population
- whether adequate safety data are available to move into the pediatric population (based on animal studies and adult experience)
- whether there is an appropriate and acceptable benefit compared to the risks

There are defined processes for both on- and off-patent drugs.
- On-patent process—The sponsor has 180 days to respond to FDA's Written Request for an on-patent drug. The manufacturer can agree to conduct studies or decline the request. If it agrees, the potential incentive is six months of exclusivity added to and covering the same scope as any exclusivity currently covering the product. There is a specific time when this exclusivity can be requested and a formal procedure for granting it, which is discussed below. If the sponsor declines, FDA may publicize the fact that the sponsor has declined the Written Request. If the drug is not developed by the current supplier, referral is made to the Foundation for the NIH for possible funding of studies by grant mechanism.
- The formal mechanism to allow the additional six months of exclusivity is a three-step process. It starts with the Written Request by FDA to the sponsor. After completing the studies or otherwise complying with the Written Request, the sponsor replies with a report that addresses the information requested and makes a claim for the six months' exclusivity. FDA then takes action based on an evaluation of the report. The study results do not need to be positive or lead to a change in the label in order for the exclusivity to be granted.
- Off-patent process—NIH, in consultation with FDA, develops a list of pediatric therapeutic needs. FDA issues Written Requests based on a priority list to all current suppliers. The suppliers have 30 days to respond to the Written Request. This is a right of first refusal. If all current suppliers decline, NIH will issue a request for proposals to perform studies under contract using a special fund. Study reports are submitted to FDA for evaluation and inclusion in product labeling.

Dissemination of Information

FDA can publicize the fact that the innovator of a drug with exclusivity has declined a Written Request. Study reports in response to Written Requests are published in the FDA dockets, as are the reviews of the study reports and recommended label changes. Summaries of clinical and pharmacology submissions are published in the dockets and in the *Federal Register*.

BCPA Dispute Resolution

If FDA recommends changes to the label and the supplier does not accept the recommendations, the issue is referred to the Pediatric Subcommittee for advice. If the Pediatric Subcommittee recommends label changes and the supplier declines, FDA may declare the product misbranded.

Major Provisions of BPCA

BPCA renewed the pediatric incentive program and established a program for the study of off-patent products through NICHD.

Provisions included in the 2007 update established procedures to ensure proper pediatric labeling and adverse event reporting and tracking, and required a pediatric plan for investigational drugs or INDs. Reports are required to be submitted by the Institute of Medicine on pediatric study practices; by the General Accounting Office on the enrollment of minority children and pediatric exclusivity; and by FDA on patient access to new cancer therapeutics.

FDAAA contains the provisions for *BPCA* in Title V. The updates include:
- allows FDA to request preclinical studies as part of a Written Request
- requires pediatric studies under *BPCA* to be submitted and exclusivity awarded nine months before the expiration of the patent
- allows FDA to issue one study request for more than one use of a drug, and to issue one study request to capture both on- and off-label uses
- requires a manufacturer that declines a Written Request, on the basis that it was unable to produce a pediatric formulation, to submit to FDA the reasons why the formulation cannot be developed
- requires manufacturers to submit all postmarket adverse events as part of the exclusivity application or supplement
- lengthens the time FDA has to review submitted studies from 90 to 180 days
- shortens the "request and response" period for the patent holder to an expedited 30-day review of private funding before referral to *PREA*
- requires FDA to make study requests public after the drug has been granted the additional exclusivity
- requires prominent public disclosure when a manufacturer creates a pediatric formulation and fails to market it
- requires an internal FDA committee to review Written Requests prior to issuance
- provides authority for internal committee review of studies submitted in response to Written Requests
- requires FDA to track the number and type of studies completed, as well as labeling changes and other data resulting from *BPCA*
- applies dispute resolution to all drugs that are issued study requests, not just those granted exclusivity; sets a time for referral to the Pediatric Advisory Committee if the sponsor does not make the requested label change
- grants FDA explicit authority to indicate on a label when a product has been studied in children
- requires FDA to make the actual medical, statistical and clinical pharmacology review (not summaries) publicly available
- requires sponsors that have been granted exclusivity to provide physicians and other healthcare providers with any new pediatric labeling information

- provides for Pediatric Advisory Committee review of all adverse events for one year following the awarding of exclusivity
- requires FDA to determine whether a drug should be studied under *PREA* if a study is declined by a manufacturer; if applicable, FDA will report why it did not use *PREA*
- allows only 30 days to determine whether private donations are available to completely fund all studies in a declined Written Request before referral to *PREA*
- provides for review by the Institute of Medicine of past Written Requests issued by FDA to make recommendations to FDA for future requests and to make recommendations of incentives to encourage the study of biologics in children
- grants NIH expanded authority to examine needs in pediatric therapeutics, including drugs

The *Patient Protection and Affordable Care Act* of 2010 expanded *BPCA* to include biologics.[6]

FDASIA in 2012 made *BPCA* permanent and contains the *BPCA* provisions in Title V, where under *BPCA*, a rationale for not including neonatal studies shall be included if none are requested in the pediatric studies. Also, for products that received pediatric exclusivity and a pediatric labeling change under *BPCA* 2002, FDA is required to post on its website the medical, statistical and clinical pharmacology reviews and corresponding written requests in the same manner as currently posted materials.

Pediatric Medical Device Safety and Improvement Act

The *Pediatric Medical Device Safety and Improvement Act* is in Title III of *FDAAA*.

Section 302—Tracking Pediatric Device Approvals

This section specifies that device protocols and applications must include an evaluation that describes any pediatric subpopulations suffering from the disease or condition the device is intended to treat, diagnose or cure, and the number of affected pediatric patients, if readily available. If the course of the disease or condition and the effects of the device are sufficiently similar in adult and pediatric patients, FDA has the specific authority to conclude that adult data may be used to support a determination of a reasonable assurance of effectiveness in pediatric populations, as appropriate. A study may not be needed in each pediatric subpopulation if data from one subpopulation can be extrapolated to another subpopulation. This section requires that FDA provide an annual report to Congress containing information pertaining specifically to pediatric usage of devices, allowing tracking of the number and types of devices approved specifically for children or for conditions that occur in children, as well as the timelines for completing premarket approvals and humanitarian device exemptions.

Section 303—Modification to Humanitarian Device Exemption

This section modified the *Food, Drug, and Cosmetic Act* of 1938 (*FD&C Act*), Section 520, to allow exemptions from the requirements for demonstrating effectiveness for treatment or diagnosis of diseases or conditions that affect fewer than 4,000 individuals. It also allows sponsors to make a profit on devices approved under the Humanitarian Device Exemption (HDE) that are specifically designed to meet a pediatric need. This exemption from the usual HDE requirements is conditional, based on appropriate labeling for use in the pediatric population and approval of the HDE after passage of *FDAAA*, and sets a limit on the number of devices that can be distributed annually (i.e., the annual distribution number (ADN)). The device distributor is obligated to notify FDA if the number of devices distributed during any calendar year exceeds the ADN. Adverse event reports are to be reviewed and evaluated by the FDA Pediatric Advisory Committee and reported to Congress. This section also defines pediatric populations as under the age of 21; subpopulations are defined in **Table 29-1**. Additional subpopulations also may be defined.

Section 304—Encouraging Pediatric Medical Device Research

This section requires the NIH director to designate an office to serve as a point of contact to identify and access funding for pediatric medical device research. It directs NIH, FDA and the Agency for Healthcare Research and Quality (AHRQ) to submit a plan to expand pediatric medical device research. The plan must include a survey of pediatric healthcare providers to assess unmet pediatric medical device needs and provide a research agenda for improving pediatric medical device development and FDA clearance or approval of pediatric medical devices, and for evaluating the short- and long-term safety and effectiveness of those devices.

Section 305—Demonstration Grants for Improving Pediatric Device Availability

Demonstration grants for nonprofit consortia were established by this section to facilitate the development, production, approval and distribution of pediatric devices. This section requires the consortia to coordinate with NIH to identify research issues that require further study and with FDA to facilitate pediatric medical device approval. These funds aim to encourage innovation and connect qualified individuals with potential manufacturers; mentor

Table 29-1. Definition of Pediatric Subpopulations

Pediatric Subpopulation	Approximate Age Range
newborn	birth to 1 month of age
infant	1 month to 2 years of age
child	2 to 12 years of age
adolescent	12-21 years of age

and manage pediatric device projects from concept through development and marketing; assess the scientific and medical merit of medical device projects; and provide other assistance and advice consistent with the purposes of this section.

Section 306—Amendments to Office of Pediatric Therapeutics and Pediatric

Advisory Committee

FDA's Pediatric Advisory Committee has the authority to monitor medical devices and make recommendations for improving their availability and safety.

Section 307—Postmarket Surveillance

For Class II or Class III devices that are expected to have significant pediatric usage, FDA may require a manufacturer to conduct postmarket surveillance. FDA may require a prospective surveillance period of more than 36 months for these devices as a condition of approval. Dispute resolution may be requested by a manufacturer.

Premarket Assessment of Pediatric Medical Devices

FDA assesses device safety and effectiveness in the pediatric population using the same regulatory basis, scientific approaches and processes as those for adult medical devices. However, special consideration is given to devices meant for use in pediatric patients.

The agency does not believe that clinical data are always necessary to demonstrate safety and effectiveness for all devices intended for pediatric populations. A number of factors will be used to determine the need for clinical data, including the nature of the device, the device's adult use history, whether known factors can be extrapolated to the pediatric population and the underlying disease or condition being treated. Well-designed bench and animal testing may be considered sufficient in some cases.

If a device is modified to meet the needs of a pediatric population, the manufacturer must conduct a risk analysis of the changes and develop methods to adequately address or mitigate the identified risks.

FDA may require clinical testing in the following circumstances:

- Supporting information from sources such as preclinical bench or animal testing, literature or adult clinical trials is inadequate to establish safety and effectiveness for the pediatric indication.
- Adult data are inadequate to predict pediatric risks and adverse events.
- Pediatric data are needed for validation of device design modifications.
- Pediatric data are needed to develop an age-appropriate treatment regimen.

When minors are involved in research, the regulations require the assent of the child and the permission of the parent(s) rather than the consent of the subject.

Indications for use should be supported by appropriate data for the targeted populations and subpopulations.

Contraindications, warnings and precautions for devices intended for pediatric use should clearly address the risks associated with the pediatric subject's age, size and maturity, and alert the user to specific hazards associated with the use of the device in the target population.

The manufacturer should make a concerted effort to obtain and report the frequency of device-related adverse events according to the various subgroups in which the device will be used.

Any instructions for use provided specifically for the pediatric patient should be age appropriate with respect to written language and other visual and auditory tools. The labeling must be satisfactory for all pediatric subgroups.

International Collaboration on Pediatric Product Development[7]

- Since August 2007, FDA and the European Medicines Agency (EMA) established monthly teleconferences to discuss product-specific pediatric development and topics related to product classes under the terms of a Confidentiality Agreement.
- Between August 2007 and January 2013, FDA and EMA have exchanged information on a total of 294 products and held 52 discussions on general topics (not product-specific).
- In November 2009 and September 2010, respectively, Japan's Pharmaceuticals and Medical Devices Agency (PMDA) and Health Canada joined the FDA/EMA teleconferences as observers and now are active participants.
- In 2011, FDA's OPT expanded the collaboration to include regulatory agencies in Latin America.

Summary

Legal, regulatory and policy actions have been taken to expand the participation of children in clinical research, recognizing both the need for pediatric research and protection of welfare and rights of children as research projects. New programs and incentives have been developed to expedite the development of pediatric therapies. Since 1998, FDA has issued 362 Written Requests for pediatric studies,[8] and there have been 467 revised product inserts (425 with new pediatric studies).[9]

The vision of global pediatric drug development is that children shall receive therapeutics that have been evaluated in an appropriate, timely and ethical manner, and dosing, efficacy and safety information shall be available for all appropriate pediatric age groups.

References

1. National Institutes of Health. Pediatric Pharmacology and Therapeutics Research Consortium. NIH website. http://nih.gov/grants/guide/rfa-files/RFA-HD-08-021.html. Accessed 13 May 2013.
2. Curry JI, Lander TD and Stringer MD. Review article: "Erythromycin as a prokinetic agent in infants and children." *Aliment Pharmacol Ther* 2001:15:595-603.
3. *Food and Drug Administration Amendments Act* of 2007. FDA website. www.fda.gov/Regulatoryinformation/legislation/federalfooddrugandcosmeticactfdcact/significantamendmentstothefdcact/foodanddrugadministrationamendmentsactof2007/fulltextoffdaaalaw/default.htm. Accessed 13 May 2013.
4. 21 CFR 201.57(f)(9) Specific requirements on content and format of labeling for human prescription drug and biological products described in 201.56(b)(1). FDA website. www.accessdata.fda.gov/scripts/cdrh/cfdocs/cfCFR/CFRSearch.cfm?fr=201.57. Accessed 13 May 2013.
5. *Food and Drug Administration Safety and Innovation Act* of 2012. FDA website. www.fda.gov/RegulatoryInformation/Legislation/FederalFoodDrugandCosmeticActFDCAct/SignificantAmendmentstotheFDCAct/FDASIA/. Accessed 13 May 2013.
6. *Patient Protection and Affordable Care Act* of 2010. HealthCare.gov website. http://www.healthcare.gov/law/full/. Accessed 13 May 2013.
7. International Collaborations. FDA website. www.fda.gov/ScienceResearch/SpecialTopics/PediatricTherapeuticsResearch/ucm106621.htm. Accessed 13 May 2013.
8. Written Requests Issued. FDA website. www.fda.gov/Drugs/DevelopmentApprovalProcess/DevelopmentResources/ucm050002.htm. Accessed 13 May 2013.
9. New Pediatric Labeling Information Database through 26 February 2013. FDA website. www.accessdata.fda.gov/scripts/sda/sdNavigation.cfm?sd=labelingdatabase. Accessed 13 May 2013.

Recommended Reading

- US Food and Drug Administration Pediatric Drug Development webpage. www.fda.gov/Drugs/DevelopmentApprovalProcess/DevelopmentResources/UCM049867.htm. Accessed 13 May 2013.
- US Food and Drug Administration Pediatric Therapeutics webpage. www.fda.gov/ScienceResearch/SpecialTopics/PediatricTherapeuticsResearch/default.htm. Accessed 13 May 2013.
- FDA. Developing Products for Rare Diseases & Conditions. www.fda.gov/ForIndustry/DevelopingProductsforRareDiseasesConditions/default.htm. Accessed 13 May 2013.
- FDA. Pediatric Written Request Template (updated January 2013). www.fda.gov/downloads/Drugs/DevelopmentApprovalProcess/DevelopmentResources/UCM207644.pdf. Accessed 13 May 2013.

- FDA. *Guidance for Industry: Qualifying for Pediatric Exclusivity Under Section 505A of the Federal Food, Drug, and Cosmetic Act* (Revised, September 1999).
- www.fda.gov/downloads/Drugs/DevelopmentApprovalProcess/DevelopmentResources/UCM049924.pdf. Accessed 13 May 2013.
- FDA. *Draft Guidance for Industry: How to Comply with the Pediatric Research Equity Act* (September 2005). www.fda.gov/downloads/Drugs/GuidanceComplianceRegulatoryInformation/Guidances/ucm079756.pdf. Accessed 13 May 2013.
- FDA. *Guidance for Industry and FDA Staff: Premarket Assessment of Pediatric Medical Devices* (May 2004). www.fda.gov/downloads/MedicalDevices/DeviceRegulationsandGuidance/GuidanceDocuments/UCM089742.htm. Accessed 13 May 2013.
- FDA. *Guidance for HDE Holders, Institutional Review Boards (IRBs), Clinical Investigators, and FDA Staff: Humanitarian Device Exemption (HDE) Regulation: Questions and Answers* (July 2010). www.fda.gov/MedicalDevices/DeviceRegulationandGuidance/GuidanceDocuments/ucm110194.htm. Accessed 13 May 2013.
- Grylack L. "Pediatric Drug Development: Focus on US Regulatory Issues." *Regulatory Focus*, Vol. 13, No. 3, March 2008, pp 26–31.
- Klimek J. "US Pediatric Developments." *Regulatory Focus*, Vol. 13, No. 3, March 2008, pp 32–35.

Chapter 30

Dietary Supplements and Homeopathic Products

Updated by Matthew T. Rycyk, MS, RAC

OBJECTIVES

❏ Develop a broad understanding of the regulation of dietary supplements

❏ Understand claims permitted for dietary supplements

❏ Understand basic current Good Manufacturing Practice regulations (CGMPs) for dietary supplements

❏ Understand the basic regulatory requirements for adverse event reporting

❏ Develop a broad understanding of the regulation of homeopathic drug products

---

LAWS, REGULATIONS AND GUIDELINES COVERED IN THIS CHAPTER

❏ *Dietary Supplement Health Education Act of 1994 (DSHEA)*

❏ 21 CFR 101.36 Nutrition labeling of dietary supplements

❏ 21 CFR 101.93 Structure/function claims

❏ 21 CFR 111 Current Good Manufacturing Practice in manufacturing, packaging, labeling, or holding operations for dietary supplements

❏ 21 CFR 190.6 Requirement for premarket notification of new dietary ingredients

❏ *Public Health Security and Bioterrorism Preparedness and Response Act* of 2002 (Public Law 107-188). 107th Congress

❏ 21 CFR 110.310: Prior notice of imported food under the Public Health Security and Bioterrorism Preparedness and Response Act of 2002

❏ *Guidance for Industry: A Dietary Supplement Labeling Guide* (April 2005)

❏ 21 CFR 190.6 New Dietary Ingredient Notifications

❏ *Draft Guidance for Industry: Questions and Answers Regarding Adverse Event Reporting and Recordkeeping for Dietary Supplements as Required by the Dietary Supplement and Nonprescription Drug Consumer Protection Act* (October 2007)

❏ *Guidance for Industry: Substantiation for Dietary Supplement Claims Made Under Section 403(r) (6) of the Federal Food, Drug, and Cosmetic Act* (January 2009)

❏ "Claims That Can Be Made for Conventional Foods and Dietary Supplements" (September 2003)

Chapter 30

- FTC, *Dietary Supplements: An Advertising Guide for Industry*

- *Guidance for Industry: Evidence-Based Review System for the Scientific Evaluation of Health Claims* (January 2009)

- *Guidance for Industry: Iron-Containing Supplements and Drugs: Label Warning Statements Small Entity Compliance Guide* (October 2003)

- *Guidance for Industry: Notification of a Health Claim or Nutrient Content Claim Based on an Authoritative Statement of a Scientific Body* (June 2998)

- *Guidance for Industry: Evidence-Based Review System for the Scientific Evaluation of Health Claims* (January 2009)

- *Guidance for Industry: Food Labeling; Nutrient Content Claims; Definition for "High Potency" and Definition for "Antioxidant" for Use in Nutrient Content Claims for Dietary Supplements and Conventional Foods; Small Entity Compliance Guide* (July 2008)

- *Guidance for Industry: Statement of Identity, Nutrition Labeling, and Ingredient Labeling of Dietary Supplements; Small Entity Compliance Guide* (January 1999)

- *Guidance for Industry: Structure/Function Claims, Small Entity Compliance Guide* (January 2002)

- *Guidance for Industry: Evidence-Based Ranking System for Scientific Data* (January 2009)

- *Guidance for Industry: Interim Procedures for Qualified Health Claims in the Labeling of Conventional Human Food and Human Dietary Supplements* (July 2003)

- *Guidance for Industry: Prior Notice of Imported Food Questions and Answers* (Edition 2) (May 2004)

- *Guidance for Industry: Questions and Answers Regarding Establishment and Maintenance of Records (Edition 4); Final Guidance* (September 2006)

- *Draft Guidance for Industry: Questions and Answers Regarding Adverse Event Reporting and Recordkeeping for Dietary Supplements as Required by the Dietary Supplement and Nonprescription Drug Consumer Protection Act* (October 2007)

- *Draft Guidance for Industry: Questions and Answers Regarding the Labeling of Dietary Supplements as Required by the Dietary Supplement and Nonprescription Drug Consumer Protection Act* (Revision 1) (December 2008)

- *Guidance for Industry: Questions and Answers Regarding Food Allergens, Including the Food Allergen Labeling and Consumer Protection Act of 2004* (Edition 4) (October 2006)

- *Guidance for Industry: FDA Export Certificates* (July 2004)

- *Compliance Policy Guide, Guidance for FDA and CBP Staff. Sec. 110.310 Prior Notice of Imported Food Under the Public Health Security and Bioterrorism Preparedness and Response Act of 2002* (May 2009)

- *Guidance for Industry: Questions and Answers Regarding Registration of Food Facilities* (Edition 4) (August 2004)

- "Criteria Needed With Request For Certificate Of Free Sale For Dietary Supplement(s), Infant Formula(s), & Medical Food(s)" December 2006)

- *Guidance for Industry: FDA Export Certificates* (July 2004)

- Compliance Policy Guide 7132.15, Section 400.400 "Conditions Under Which Homeopathic Drugs May Be Marketed" (Revised March 1995)

- 21 CFR 207 Registration of producers of drugs and listing of drugs in commercial distribution

- 21 CFR 211 Current Good Manufacturing Practice for finished pharmaceuticals

- *Current Good Manufacturing Practice in Manufacturing, Packaging, Labeling, or Holding*

Operations for Dietary Supplements; Small Entity Compliance Guide (December 2010)

❑ 21 CFR 201 Labeling

❑ The Homeopathic Pharmacopoeia of the United States, Guidelines For Homeopathic Drugs

Introduction

Controversies over the regulation of vitamin and mineral dietary supplement product dosages and health claims arose in the 1960s and 1970s.[1] Between 1941 and 1979, the US Food and Drug Administration (FDA) attempted to limit the dosages of dietary supplements that could be sold without a prescription, limit the claims that could be made and require a disclaimer on supplement products stating that there was no scientific basis for the routine use of vitamins and minerals.[2,3] Litigation and eventually legislation limited FDA's ability to regulate supplements, with the end result that final rules were never enacted, and proposed rules were withdrawn.[4]

In November 1989, FDA first issued a warning against the use of L-tryptophan products and subsequently recalled them. There was growing evidence that linked L-tryptophan, an amino acid promoted to relieve occasional sleeplessness, among other things, to a serious but rare blood disorder, eosinophilia. In 1990, sufficient evidence had been developed to link the disorder to a product from a Tokyo firm, Showa Denko KK, which had introduced a new production method in early 1989. Unfortunately, by that time, 1,478 cases and 21 deaths due to eosinophila linked to L-tryptophan use had been reported.[5]

Concurrently, the *Nutrition Labeling Education Act* (*NLEA*) was passed in 1990, requiring FDA to regulate food labeling and include references to dietary supplements. In the early 1990s, several bills were introduced in both the House and Senate that would have impacted the dietary supplement industry. One such bill introduced in the House was the *Nutrition Advertising Coordination Act* of 1991 (HR 1662 SC2). This bill was thought to threaten the future availability of vitamins and other supplements because it defined misbranding in part as a claim that "characterizes the relationship of any nutrient … to a health-related condition."[6] Another bill, the *Dietary Supplement Consumer Protection Act* of 1993 (HR 2923 IH), also introduced in the House, stated that a dietary supplement would be deemed unsafe unless the ingredient was "generally recognized, among experts qualified by adequate training and experience to evaluate its safety, as having been adequately shown through scientific procedures to be safe under the conditions of its intended use."[7] This provision was retroactive to products that were on the market. The legislation further stated that FDA would establish regulations stipulating the uses as well as "the maximum quantity which may be used or permitted in the dietary supplement."[8] The interpretation of this proposed legislation was that dietary supplements, which had previously been regulated as foods, would be moved into a regulatory status very similar to drugs.

While neither of these bills passed, in response to the proposed legislation, the supplement and health foods industries promoted a public letter-writing campaign that declared FDA was seeking to regulate some dietary supplements as drugs, and in fact they were. In early 1991 David Kessler, MD, the commissioner of FDA at the time, created the Dietary Supplements FDA Task Force.[9] This task force was given the job by Kessler of taking a new look at how FDA could possibly regulate dietary supplements and creating a proposal that would best serve the public health of the US. The Dietary Supplement Task Force was headed by chairman, Gary Dykstra. The final report finished in May of 1992 became forever known in the dietary supplement industry at the "Dykstra Report."[10]

The Dykstra Report stated several generalized conclusions proposed by the Dietary Supplements Task force with safety as FDA's overriding concern in the regulation of dietary supplements. In addition, it recommended that the industry assume the burden of ensuring the safety of these products. The task force divided supplements into three main categories: 1) vitamins and minerals, 2) amino acid products and 3) all other types of dietary supplements. The primary recommendation for vitamins and minerals was to establish safe daily intake levels through rulemaking. These daily intake levels would provide a benchmark for some essential nutrients that are toxic when consumed in excess to avoid hazards associated with them. The recommendation for amino acids was that each individual amino acid be analyzed on a case-by-case basis, but overall the products would be regulated as drugs if any non-NLEA claims were associated with them. The final category, all other types of dietary supplements, was recommended to be regulated under the food additives provisions of the statute, unless drug claims were made for the product. The task force also recommended the establishment of Good Manufacturing Practices (GMPs), purity and identity standards and disintegration and dissolution standards to ensure bioavailability.

Although the Dykstra Report was completed in May 1992, it was not released by Kessler for many months afterward. The dietary supplement industry had been working on its own proposal, the *Dietary Supplement Health Education Act* (*DSHEA*), with the help of Senator Orin Hatch, Representative Bill Richardson and Senator Tom Harkin.[11] The public write-in campaign resulted in an estimated two million[12] letters to Congress, prompting passage of *DSHEA*.[13] The first paragraph of the executive summary in the Report of the Commission on Dietary Supplement Labels, states:

"The *Dietary Supplement Health and Education Act* (*DSHEA* or the Act) of 1994 was enacted by Congress following public debate concerning the importance of dietary supplements in leading a healthy life, the need for consumers to have current and accurate information about supplements, and controversy over the Food and Drug Administration (FDA) regulatory approach to dietary supplements. President Clinton, in signing the legislation into law on October 25, 1994, said: After several years of intense efforts, manufacturers, experts in nutrition, and legislators, acting in a conscientious alliance with consumers at the grassroots level, have moved successfully to bring common sense to the treatment of dietary supplements under regulation and law."

In *DSHEA*, Congress defined dietary supplements and dietary ingredients; required ingredient and nutrition labeling; provided for claims and nutritional support statements that can be used for dietary supplements; outlined guidelines for information that can be provided on supplement products; and gave FDA the authority to establish GMP regulations for dietary supplements. In addition, *DSHEA* allowed the continued sale of dietary ingredients on the market as of 15 October 1994. The law also established a framework for assuring the safety of new dietary ingredients (NDIs).

Prior to 1994, vitamins, minerals and other dietary supplements were regulated as foods;[14] however, with the passage of *DSHEA*, a new class of FDA-regulated products was created. In addition, the law allowed statements of nutritional support to be made regarding dietary supplement products. The resulting dietary supplement regulations promulgated by FDA are very similar to food regulations. Like foods, dietary supplements are not subject to agency approval prior to marketing. Dietary supplement product labels must include a supplement facts box that is similar, but not identical to the nutrition facts boxes used on food products. Dietary ingredients that were not on the market as of 15 October 1994 must be the subject of NDI petitions that are similar in content to "generally regarded as safe" (GRAS) notifications used for new food additives. Additionally, most nutrient content claims, which were established in *NLEA*, also may be used on dietary supplement products.

Definition of Dietary Ingredients and Dietary Supplements

Dietary ingredients traditionally were viewed as essential vitamins, minerals and other nutrients, such as fats, carbohydrates and proteins. In 1990, *NLEA* added "herbs, or similar nutritional substances"[15] to the definition of dietary supplement. In *DSHEA*, this definition was expanded further as Congress defined dietary supplements as

"products (other than tobacco) intended to supplement the diet that bear or contain one or more of the following dietary ingredients:

A vitamin;
A mineral;
An herb or other botanical;
An amino acid;
A dietary substance for use by man to supplement the diet by increasing the total dietary intake; or
A concentrate, metabolite, constituent, extract, or a combination of any ingredient mentioned above.
Further, dietary supplements are products intended for ingestion, are not represented for use as a conventional food or as a sole item of a meal or the diet, and are labeled as dietary supplements."[16]

The prohibition on representing dietary supplements as conventional foods was underscored by the agency's 2009 publication of a guidance document regarding liquid dietary supplements.[17] FDA noted that this guidance was issued to address the trend of marketing beverages as dietary supplements and of including ingredients in beverages and conventional foods that are not GRAS. The guidance states in part, "Liquid products that suggest through their serving size, packaging, or recommended daily intake that they are intended to be consumed in amounts that provide all or a significant part of the entire daily drinking fluid intake of an average person in the U.S., are represented as beverages. In addition, the name of a product can represent the product as a conventional food. Product or brand names that use conventional food terms such as "beverage," "drink," "water," 'juice" or similar terms represent the product as a conventional food."

NDI Notifications

Dietary supplement ingredients and products are not subject to premarket approval; however, FDA must be notified prior to introducing any dietary ingredients onto the marketplace that were not marketed in the US prior to 15 October 1994.[18] Notification must be given to the Office of Nutritional Products, Labeling and Dietary Supplements (ONPLDS) at least 75 days before introducing the NDI into interstate commerce. The notification must include:

- name and address of the manufacturer or distributor of the NDI or supplement product that contains the NDI
- NDI name, including the Latin binomial name of any herb or other botanical
- description of the products that contain the NDI along with the level of the NDI in the product; conditions of ordinary or recommended uses of the supplement
- history of use or other evidence establishing the safety of the dietary ingredient under the conditions of use, including any citation to and reprint, copy or English translation of published articles or other evidence that is the basis upon which the

distributor or manufacturer has concluded that the NDI or product containing the NDI will reasonably be expected to be safe
- signature of the person designated by the manufacturer or distributor of the NDI or dietary supplement that contains the NDI

FDA will acknowledge and provide the date of receipt of the NDI notification. The date FDA provides is the filing date for the notification, and the NDI may not be introduced into interstate commerce for 75 days after the filing date. FDA will put the NDI notification, with the exception of any trade secret or confidential information, "on public display" 90 days after receipt of the submission. Although the NDI may be introduced into the marketplace 75 days after filing, this does not guarantee that FDA agrees there is sufficient information to presume reasonable safety. As stated in 21 CFR 190.6 (f), "Failure of the agency to respond to a notification does not constitute a finding by the agency that the NDI or the dietary supplement that contains the NDI is safe or is not adulterated under section 402 of the act." A list of NDIs submitted between 1995 and early 2000, along with their status and links to the notifications, can be found at www.fda.gov/Food/DietarySupplements/ucm109764.htm.

Labels and Labeling

As for all other classes of FDA-regulated products, "labels" are "any display of written, printed, or graphic matter on the immediate container of any article, or any such matter affixed to any consumer commodity or affixed to or appearing upon a package containing any consumer commodity,"[19] and "labeling" "includes all written, printed, or graphic matter accompanying an article at any time while such article is in interstate commerce or held for sale after shipment or delivery in interstate commerce."[20] Labeling regulations for dietary supplement products are found in 21 CFR 101.36.[21] This section frequently references 21 CFR 101.9,[22] which covers food labeling. Both food and dietary supplement labels must include a statement of identity; a net quantity of contents statement; an ingredient list; the address of the manufacturer, packer or distributor; and a facts box that declares the nutrients present in the product.

Dietary supplement facts boxes are very similar to the nutrition facts boxes used on food labels. While both must list key nutrients when present at threshold levels defined by regulation, the order in which some of the nutrients must appear differs between foods and dietary supplements. Another key difference is that nutrition facts boxes must list certain nutrients such as fats even when they are not present in the product; for dietary supplements, so called "zero-value" nutrients must not be listed in the facts box unless claims are being made about them. Supplement facts boxes also may list the quantities of dietary ingredients such as herbs, amino acids, concentrates or metabolites (see **Figure 30-1**).

The *Food Allergen Labeling and Consumer Protection Act of 2004* (*FALCPA*) requires that foods and dietary supplements alert consumers to the presence of the any of the "major" allergens.[23] Congress defined "major allergens" as the eight foods responsible for 90% of food allergies. The so-called "big 8" allergens are: milk, eggs, fish, crustacean shellfish, tree nuts, peanuts, wheat and soybeans. Allergens must be declared by their common or usual name (i.e., milk, peanuts, wheat, etc.) and may be declared in either the ingredient list or in a separate statement. The species must be listed when fish, crustacean shellfish or tree nut allergens are declared.

Claims Permitted on Dietary Supplement Products

NLEA permitted nutrient content claims such as "high in fiber" or "rich source of vitamin C" on foods and dietary supplements. The guidelines for determining whether a product is eligible to bear such claims are found in the following sections of the CFR:
- 21 CFR 101.13 Nutrient content claims—general principles.
- 21 CFR 101.54 Nutrient content claims for "good source," "high," "more," and "high potency"
- 21 CFR 101.56 Nutrient content claims for "light" or "lite"
- 21 CFR 101.60 Nutrient content claims for the calorie content of foods
- 21 CFR 101.61 Nutrient content claims for the sodium content of foods
- 21 CFR 101.62 Nutrient content claims for fat, fatty acid and cholesterol content of foods
- 21 CFR 101.65 Implied nutrient content claims and related label statements
- 21 CFR 101.67 Use of nutrient content claims for butter
- 21 CFR 101.69 Petitions for nutrient content claims

In addition, *NLEA* provided for the establishment of allowable health claims. Petitions for such claims may be made for foods, supplements or related ingredients when the benefits of the ingredients have been documented in publicly available scientific literature. As a result, FDA has approved allowable health claims based on significant scientific agreement of data supporting the claims. Examples of claims include:
- Calcium—Regular exercise and a healthy diet with enough calcium help teen and young adult white and Asian women maintain good bone health and may reduce their high risk of osteoporosis later in life.
- Soluble Fiber—Soluble fiber from foods such as oats, as part of a diet low in saturated fat and cholesterol,

Chapter 30

Figure 30-1. Sample Supplement Facts Boxes

Supplement Facts
Serving Size: 1 capsule
Servings per container: 30

	Amount per serving	% Daily Value*
Vitamin A	2,500 IU	50%
Vitamin C	2.3 mg	4%
Vitamin D	165 IU	41%
Vitamin E	1.6 IU	5%
Thiamin	4.8 mg	320%
Riboflavin	2.2 mg	130%
Niacin	26 mg	130%
Vitamin B6	4.2 mg	210%
Vitamin B12	2.4 mcg	40%
Pantothenic acid	8.8 mg	88%
Calcium	11 mg	1%
Iron	1.6 mg	9%
Magnesium	0.2 mg	<1%
Zinc	0.2 mg	1%
Selenium	15 mcg	21%
Copper	0.04 mg	2%
Manganese	0.03 mg	2%
Molybdenum	20 mcg	27%
Potassium	0.4 mg	<1%
Cobalt	10 mcg	†
Lecithin (from soybean)	14 mg	†
Rutin (from Dimorphandra mollis) (pods)	5 mg	†

*Percent Daily Values are based on a 2,000 calorie diet.
†Daily value not established.

INGREDIENTS: THIAMIN HYDROCHLORIDE, PYRIDOXINE HYDROCHLORIDE, CYANOCOBALMIN, SODIUM SELENITE, ASCORBIC ACID, NIACINAMIDE, RIBOFLAVIN, CALCIUM PANTOTHENATE, DICALCIUM PHOSPHATE, FERROUS FUMARATE, MAGNESIUM SULFATE, COPPER SULFATE, MANGANESE SULFATE, POTASSIUM SULFATE, COBALT SULFATE, SODIUM MOLYBDENATE, RUTIN, ZINC OXIDE, RETINYL PALMITATE, CHOLECALCIFEROL, DL-ALPHA TOCOPHEROL ACETATE, SOYBEAN OIL, GELATIN, BEESWAX, TITANIUM DIOXIDE, FD&C YELLOW # 5, FD&C BLUE #1, FD&C RED # 40.
ALLERGENS: CONTAINS SOY

Supplement Facts
Serving Size 1 Capsule

	Amount Per Capsule	% Daily Value
Calories	20	
Calories from Fat	20	
Total Fat	2 g	3%*
Saturated Fat	0.5 g	3%*
Polyunsaturated Fat	1 g	†
Monounsaturated Fat	0.5 g	†
Vitamin A	4250 IU	85%
Vitamin D	425 IU	106%
Omega-3 fatty acids	0.5 g	†

* Percent Daily Values are based on a 2,000 calorie diet.
† Daily Value not established.

Ingredients: Cod liver oil, gelatin, water, and glycerin.

may reduce the risk of heart disease. A serving of oats supplies x grams of the 3 grams of soluble fiber from oats necessary per day to have this effect.

Specific information about allowable health claims can be found in the following regulations:
- 21 CFR 101.70 Petitions for health claims
- 21 CFR 101.71 Health claims: claims not authorized
- 21 CFR 101.72 Health claims: calcium and osteoporosis
- 21 CFR 101.73 Health claims: dietary lipids and cancer
- 21 CFR 101.74 Health claims: sodium and hypertension
- 21 CFR 101.75 Health claims: dietary saturated fat and cholesterol and risk of coronary heart disease
- 21 CFR 101.76 Health claims: fiber-containing grain products, fruits and vegetables and cancer
- 21 CFR 101.77 Health claims: fruits, vegetables and grain products that contain fiber, particularly soluble fiber, and risk of coronary heart disease
- 21 CFR 101.78 Health claims: fruits and vegetables and cancer
- 21 CFR 101.79 Health claims: Folate and neural tube defects
- 21 CFR 101.80 Health claims: dietary noncariogenic carbohydrate sweeteners and dental caries
- 21 CFR 101.81 Health claims: Soluble fiber from certain foods and risk of coronary heart disease (CHD)
- 21 CFR 101.82 Health claims: Soy protein and risk of coronary heart disease (CHD)
- 21 CFR 101.83 Health claims: plant sterol/stanol esters and risk of coronary heart disease (CHD)

Provisions in the *Food and Drug Administration Modernization Act* of 1997 (*FDAMA*)[24] allow the use of claims based on current, published authoritative statements from "a scientific body of the United States with official responsibility for public health protection or research directly related to human nutrition." The law specifically notes that some such authoritative scientific bodies include the National Academy of Sciences (NAS) or any of its subdivisions, the National Institutes of Health (NIH) and the Centers for Disease Control and Prevention (CDC). *FDAMA* further stated that such claims could be made 120 days after submission of a notification of the claim. *FDAMA* claim notifications must include: the exact wording of the claim; a concise description of the basis for determining that the requirements for an authoritative statement have been satisfied; a copy of the referenced authoritative statement; and, for a health claim, "a balanced representation of the scientific literature relating to the relationship between a nutrient and a disease or health-related condition to which the claim refers," or, for a nutrient content claim, "a

balanced representation of the scientific literature relating to the nutrient level to which the claim refers." FDA has issued guidance[25] but has not published specific regulations on *FDAMA* claims. Current authorized *FDAMA* claims cover:
- choline nutrient content claims
- fluoride and the risk of dental caries
- potassium and the risk of high blood pressure and stroke
- saturated fat, cholesterol and trans fat, and the risk of heart disease
- substitution of saturated fat with unsaturated fatty acids and risk of heart disease
- whole grain foods and the risk of heart disease and certain cancers

Yet another class of claims, "qualified health claims," has been created as a result of the court decision in *Pearson v. Shalala*. In this suit, FDA's general health claims regulations for dietary supplements and the agency's decision not to authorize health claims for four specific substance/disease relationships were challenged. A district court first ruled for FDA (14 F. Supp. 2d 10 (D.D.C. 1998)). However, on appeal, the US Court of Appeals for the DC Circuit reversed the lower court's decision (164 F.3d 650 (D.C. Cir. 1999)). The appeals court ruled that the First Amendment does not permit FDA to reject health claims that are deemed potentially misleading unless the agency also determines that no disclaimer would eliminate the potential deception. The disclaimers mentioned in the decision are what "qualify" the health claim. In general, qualified health claims are not supported by data that meet the standard of significant scientific agreement[26] required for health claims and are qualified by inclusion of a statement regarding the strength of the data. Examples of qualified health claims include:
- Omega-3 Fatty Acids—Supportive but not conclusive research shows that consumption of EPA and DHA omega-3 fatty acids may reduce the risk of coronary heart disease. One serving of [Name of the food] provides [ ] gram of EPA and DHA omega-3 fatty acids. [See nutrition information for total fat, saturated fat, and cholesterol content.]
- B Vitamins—As part of a well-balanced diet that is low in saturated fat and cholesterol, Folic Acid, Vitamin B6 and Vitamin B12 may reduce the risk of vascular disease. FDA evaluated the above claim and found that, while it is known that diets low in saturated fat and cholesterol reduce the risk of heart disease and other vascular diseases, the evidence in support of the above claim is inconclusive.

Other qualified health claims cover the relationships between:
- selenium and cancer
- antioxidant vitamins and cancer
- phosphatidylserine and cognitive dysfunction and dementia
- nuts and heart disease
- walnuts and heart disease
- monounsaturated fatty acids from olive oil and coronary heart disease
- green tea and cancer
- chromium picolinate and diabetes
- calcium and colon/rectal cancer and calcium and recurrent colon/rectal polyps
- calcium and hypertension, pregnancy-induced hypertension and preeclampsia
- tomatoes and/or tomato sauce and prostate, ovarian, gastric and pancreatic cancers
- unsaturated fatty acids from canola oil and reduced risk of coronary heart disease
- corn oil and corn oil-containing products and a reduced risk of heart disease
- folic acid and neural tube birth defects[27]

DSHEA allowed statements of nutritional support to be made for dietary supplements. Statements of nutritional support may discuss: the benefit of the supplement in relation to a classical nutrient deficiency disease; the role of a nutrient or dietary ingredient in affecting the structure or function of the human body or its systems; the documented mechanism by which a nutrient or dietary ingredient acts to maintain the structure or function of the body; or general well-being supported from consumption of a nutrient or dietary ingredient. All such claims must be truthful, not misleading, supported by scientific data and accompanied by the following disclaimer: "This statement has not been evaluated by the Food and Drug Administration. This product is not intended to diagnose, treat, cure, or prevent any disease."[28]

If claims are made regarding nutrient deficiency diseases, such as scurvy from lack of vitamin C, the prevalence of the disease in the US must be disclosed. Since such nutrient deficiency diseases are rare, most claims made about dietary supplement products discuss the manner and/or mechanism by which a dietary ingredient affects or maintains human structure or function. Since dietary supplements may not be marketed to "diagnose, treat, cure, or prevent any disease," these so-called structure/function claims may only describe how the supplement affects or maintains the normal, healthy structure or normal, healthy function of the human body and its systems.

To assist industry in crafting acceptable structure/function claims, FDA has published regulations[29] and guidance[30] that define disease and provide criteria for evaluating whether dietary supplement claims are disease claims. The definition of "disease" is listed in 21 CFR 101.93(g)(1) as "damage to an organ, part, structure, or system of the body such that it does not function properly (e.g., cardiovascular disease), or a state of health leading to such dysfunctioning (e.g., hypertension); except that diseases resulting from essential nutrient deficiencies (e.g., scurvy, pellagra) are not included in this definition." Section 101.93(g)(2) lists 10 criteria for identifying statements that are prohibited disease claims, which state explicitly or imply that a dietary supplement product:

1. has an effect on a specific disease or class of diseases
2. has an effect on the characteristic signs or symptoms of a specific disease or class of diseases, using scientific or lay terminology
3. has an effect on an abnormal condition associated with a natural state or process, if the abnormal condition is uncommon or can cause significant or permanent harm
4. has an effect on a disease or diseases through: a) the name of the product; b) a statement that the product contains an ingredient that is not listed in the definition of dietary ingredients and that has been regulated by FDA as a drug and is well known to consumers for its use or claimed use in preventing or treating a disease; c) citation of a publication or reference, if the citation refers to a disease use; d) use of the term "disease" or "diseased," except in general statements about disease prevention that do not refer explicitly or implicitly to a specific disease or class of diseases or to a specific product or ingredient; or e) use of pictures, vignettes, symbols or other means
5. belongs to a class of products that is intended to diagnose, mitigate, treat, cure or prevent a disease
6. is a substitute for a product that is a therapy for a disease
7. augments a particular therapy or drug action that is intended to diagnose, mitigate, treat, cure or prevent a disease or class of diseases
8. has a role in the body's response to a disease or to a vector of disease
9. treats, prevents or mitigates adverse events associated with a therapy for a disease, if the adverse events constitute diseases
10. otherwise suggests an effect on a disease or diseases

Dietary supplements may be marketed to affect certain conditions that are considered part of typical, everyday living due to their mild nature and infrequent occurrence. Such conditions that are not considered diseases typically resolve without requiring medical attention. They include occasional irregularity and mild stress due to everyday living and occasional sleeplessness. It is clear that these same symptoms can indicate disease if they are not mild or occasional.

In order to legally make structure/function or any other type of claim about dietary supplement products, the manufacturer must have data to substantiate the claim. FDA has published a draft guidance on dietary supplement claim substantiation.[31] The guidance refers to the FTC standard of competent and reliable scientific evidence, defined in FTC case law as "tests, analyses, research, studies, or other evidence based on the expertise of professionals in the relevant area, that has been conducted and evaluated in an objective manner by persons qualified to do so, using procedures generally accepted in the profession to yield accurate and reliable results."[32] The level of substantiating evidence sufficient for a particular claim is affected by the language and meaning of the claim, the quality of the studies and the relevance of the studies to the actual product, as well as the total body of evidence relating to the claim. The data substantiating product claims are not submitted to FDA but should be available if needed to answer any questions that may arise regarding the claim.

Third-Party Literature

Although dietary supplements may not be marketed to "diagnose, treat, cure or prevent any disease," many dietary ingredients—particularly herbs, botanicals and glandular extracts—have been used historically in traditional and folk medicine of various cultures. This body of information is difficult to use in dietary supplement promotional materials without violating regulations on allowable claims for dietary supplement products. Section 403B of *DSHEA* makes provision for the use of "third-party literature" by stating that "a publication, including an article, a chapter in a book, or an official abstract of a peer-reviewed scientific publication that appears in an article and was prepared by the author or the editors of the publication, which is reprinted in its entirety, shall not be defined as labeling when used in connection with the sale of a dietary supplement to consumers."[33]

The provision for the use of third-party literature goes on to list criteria to which the information must conform. Any articles, books or other literature used in the sale of dietary supplements must:

- be truthful and not misleading
- not promote a particular manufacturer or brand of a dietary supplement
- be displayed or presented with other such items on the same subject matter, so as to present a balanced view of the available scientific information on a dietary supplement
- be displayed physically separated from the dietary supplements
- not have appended to it any information by sticker or any other method

The act also states that these criteria "shall not apply to or restrict a retailer or wholesaler of dietary supplements in any way whatsoever in the sale of books or other publications as a part of the business of such retailer or wholesaler."[34]

Claim Submission

Dietary supplement manufacturers must notify ONPLDS of any claims or statements of nutritional support they wish to make about their products. The claims must be submitted no later than 30 days after first using the claims in the marketplace. Claims submitted to ONPLDS are reviewed but not approved; however, FDA may send a letter objecting to the claims in response to the submission.

Supplement Advertising and the FTC

FTC is dually charged with ensuring that US consumers are protected from fraud, deception and unfair business practices and that a fair and competitive marketplace exists for businesses. The agency has investigative, enforcement and litigation authority over many areas that impact businesses and consumers daily. FTC's Division of Advertising Practices is the nation's enforcer of federal truth-in-advertising laws. Among other things, this division's law enforcement activities focus on claims for products promising health benefits including foods, drugs, medical devices and dietary supplements.

FDA works closely with FTC under a 1971 memorandum of understanding[35] governing the division of responsibilities between the two agencies. FDA has primary responsibility for claims appearing on product labeling, including packaging, inserts and other promotional materials distributed at the point of sale. FTC has primary responsibility for claims made in advertising, including print and broadcast advertisements, infomercials, websites, catalogs and similar direct marketing materials.

The most basic requirement of FTC regulations is that all advertisements must be truthful, not misleading and appropriately substantiated. FTC's advertising guide for the supplement industry[36] provides detailed examples of claims, how to identify claims and ways to determine adequate levels of substantiation.

Other Regulations

The *Public Health Security and Bioterrorism Preparedness and Response Act* of 2002[37] (*Bioterrorism Act*) amended the *FD&C Act* to require facilities that manufacture, process, hold or package food to register with FDA. FDA has stated that, according to the *FD&C Act*, dietary supplements and dietary ingredients are "food" and therefore, facilities that manufacture these products must register.[38] Registration may be submitted electronically[39] or by mail or facsimile. As detailed in 21 CFR 1.232, the following information must be included to register a dietary supplement facility:

- facility name, full address and telephone number
- parent company name, address and telephone number, if the facility is a subsidiary
- owner, operator and agent in charge names, addresses and telephone numbers; foreign facilities must also provide the name, address and telephone number of their US agent
- emergency contact telephone number; foreign facilities must also provide an emergency contact phone number for their US agent
- all trade names the facility uses
- applicable food product categories as identified in 21 CFR 170.3
- a statement in which the owner, operator or agent in charge certifies that the information submitted is true and accurate; the person submitting the registration must also provide a statement certifying that the information submitted is true and accurate if he or she is someone other than the owner, operator or agent in charge

Facility registrations must be updated within 60 days of any changes in the information submitted. In 2012, FDA completed an update of its Food Facility Registration Module (FFRM) (www.fda.gov/Food/GuidanceRegulation/FoodFacilityRegistration/default.htm).[40] Food facilities are now able to register biannually and update information via FDA's website instead of using Form FDA 3537.

The *FDA Food Safety Modernization Act* (*FSMA*),[41] enacted on 4 January 2011, amended Section 415 of the *FD&C Act* to require that facilities engaged in manufacturing, processing, packing or holding food for consumption in the US submit additional registration information to FDA, including an assurance that FDA will be permitted to inspect the facility at the times and in the manner permitted by the *FD&C Act*. Section 415 of the *FD&C Act*, as amended by *FSMA*, also requires food facilities required to register with FDA to renew such registrations every other year and provides FDA with authority to suspend the registration of a food facility in certain circumstances. Specifically, if FDA determines that food manufactured, processed, packed, received or held by a registered food facility has a reasonable probability of causing serious adverse health consequences or death to humans or animals, the agency may suspend the registration of a facility that:

- created, caused or was otherwise responsible for such reasonable probability

or

- knew of, or had reason to know of, such reasonable probability; and packed, received or held such food

Dietary Supplement GMPs

More than a decade after receiving authorization from Congress to establish CGMPs for dietary supplements, and four years after FDA published its proposed rule,[42] the agency released its final rule,[43] 21 CFR 111 Current Good Manufacturing Practice in manufacturing, packaging, labeling, or holding operations for dietary supplements ("dietary supplement CGMP rule"). Previously, dietary supplement manufacturing and distribution were regulated under "umbrella" CGMPs established for food generally and were not subject to individualized CGMPs. Although the general food CGMPs in 21 CFR 110 apply to a variety of food products, including dietary supplements, they do not address the unique characteristics of dietary supplements.

The dietary supplement CGMP rule in 21 CFR 111 establishes the minimum CGMPs necessary for activities related to manufacturing, packaging, labeling or holding dietary supplements to ensure product quality.

The dietary supplement CGMP rule went into effect 24 August 2007. However, FDA established the following compliance dates, which are associated with the size of the dietary supplement company in terms of full-time equivalent employees. The compliance date was 25 June 2008 for companies with more than 500 employees; June 2009 for companies with fewer than 500 employees; and June 2010 for companies with fewer than 20 employees.

The dietary supplement CGMP rule applies to all domestic and foreign establishments that manufacture, package, label or hold dietary supplements, including those involved with testing, quality control, packaging and labeling and distribution in the US. The dietary supplement CGMP rule does not apply to retail establishments holding dietary supplements only for purposes of direct retail sale to individual consumers, although this exception does not include a retailer's warehouse or other storage facility or a warehouse or other storage facility that sells directly to individual consumers. The dietary supplement CGMP rules do not apply to dietary ingredient suppliers.

The dietary supplement CGMP rule requires:
- written procedures for personnel (Subpart B)
- cleaning the physical plant, including pest control (Subpart C)
- calibrating instruments and controls (Subpart D)
- calibrating, inspecting and checking automated, mechanical or electronic equipment (Subpart D)
- maintaining, cleaning and sanitizing equipment and utensils (Subpart D)
- quality control operations, including conducting a material review and making a disposition decision (Subpart F)
- components, packaging, labels and labeling (Subpart G)
- laboratory operations (Subpart J)
- manufacturing operations (Subpart K)
- packaging and labeling operations (Subpart L)
- holding and distributing operations (Subpart M)
- returned dietary supplements (Subpart N)
- product complaints (Subpart O)

The dietary supplement CGMP rule is divided into 16 user-friendly question and answer subparts (Subparts A–P) and was published in *Federal Register* Volume 72, No. 121 on 25 June 2007. Each subpart is presented according to its specific operations to make it easier to find the relevant production and process control requirements.

Following is the general outline of GMP concepts. The outline is not intended to be complete or all-inclusive, but does provide some key points:

- Establish minimum requirements for personnel, including rules to prevent microbial contamination from sick personnel, employee and supervisor qualifications and record retention (21 CFR 111.10, 21 CFR 111.12, 21 CFR 111.13 and 21 CFR 111.14).
- Establish minimum requirements for physical plant and grounds, equipment and utensils, design and construction, including requirements for written procedures, the use of automated, mechanical or electronic equipment, and record development, retention and maintenance (21 CFR 111.15, 21 CFR 111.16, 21 CFR 111.20, 21 CFR 111.23, 21 CFR 111.25, 21 CFR 111.27, 21 CFR 111.30, 21 CFR 111.35).
- Establish specifications in the production and process control system that will ensure dietary supplements meet the identity, purity, strength and composition established in specifications and are properly packaged and labeled as specified in the master manufacturing record (21 CFR 111.55, 21 CFR 111.60, 21 CFR 111.70, 21 CFR 111.75, 21 CFR 111.77).
- Permit the use of a "certificate of analysis" from a component supplier for specifications other than the identity of a dietary ingredient in lieu of having manufacturers conduct tests or examinations on all components received (21 CFR 111.75).
- Establish minimum requirements for representative samples and reserve samples (21 CFR 111.80, 21 CFR 111.83).
- Establish minimum requirements for quality control and require implementation of quality control operations to ensure the quality of a dietary supplement (21 CFR 111.105, 21 CFR 111.110, 21 CFR 111.113, 21 CFR 111.117, 21 CFR 111.120).
- Require the preparation and use of a written master manufacturing record for each unique formulation of manufactured dietary supplement and for each batch size to ensure manufacturing process is performed consistently and to ensure uniformity in the finished product from batch to batch (21 CFR 111.205, 21 CFR 111.210, 21, CFR 111.123)
- Require design and conduct of all manufacturing operations of dietary supplements in accordance with adequate sanitation principles to prevent contamination of components or dietary supplements (21 CFR 111.355, 21 CFR 111.360, 21 CFR 111.365).

- Require testing of a subset of finished product batches, basing the testing system on either a sound statistical sampling plan or testing of all finished batches (21 CFR 111.75).
- Establish minimum requirements for the batch production record (21 CFR 111.255, 21 CFR 111.260).
- Require the establishment and use of laboratory control processes related to establishing specifications and to the selection and use of testing and examination methods (21 CFR 111.303, 21 CFR 111.310, 21 CFR 111.315, 21 CFR 111.320, 21 CFR 111.325).
- Establish minimum requirements for packaging and labeling operations to assure the quality of the dietary supplement and that the dietary supplement is packaged and labeled as specified in the master manufacturing record (21 CFR 111.160, 21 CFR 111.415).
- Require reserve samples of dietary supplements to be held in a manner that protects against contamination and deterioration (21 CFR 111.465).
- Require holding of components and dietary supplements under appropriate conditions of temperature, humidity and light so that the identity, purity, strength and composition of the components and dietary supplements are not affected and are protected against mix-up, contamination or deterioration (21 CFR 111.455).
- Establish minimum quality control operations required for returned dietary supplements and require identification and quarantine of returned dietary supplements until quality control personnel conduct a material review and make a disposition decision (21 CFR 111.130, 21 CFR 111.503, 21 CFR 111.510, 21 CFR 111.515, 21 CFR 111.525, 21 CFR 111.530, 21 CFR 111.535).
- Require a qualified person to investigate any "product complaint" that involves a possible failure of a dietary supplement to meet any CGMP requirement, with oversight by quality control personnel (21 CFR 111.553, 21 CFR 111.560).
- Establish minimum requirements for records and recordkeeping (21 CFR 111.605, 21 CFR 111.610).
- Require records associated with the manufacture, packaging, labeling or holding of a dietary supplement to be kept for one year beyond the shelf life dating or, if shelf life dating is not used, for two years beyond the date of distribution of the last batch of dietary supplements associated with those records (21 CFR 111.605).

FDA examined the economic implications of the dietary supplement CGMP rule as required by the *Regulatory Flexibility Act* (5 U.S.C. 601–612) and determined that the rule would have a significant economic impact on a substantial number of small entities. In compliance with Section 212 of the *Small Business Regulatory Enforcement Fairness Act* (Public Law 104–121), FDA has released a Small Entity Compliance Guide[44] (SECG), stating in plain language the requirements of the 21 CFR 111 regulations. FDA issued this SECG as Level 2 guidance consistent with the agency's good guidance practices regulation (21 CFR 10.115(c)(2)). This SECG restates, in simplified format and language, FDA's requirements for Current Good Manufacturing Practice in Manufacturing, Packaging, Labeling, or Holding Operations for Dietary Supplements, including the requirements for a Petition to Request an Exemption from 100 Percent Identity Testing of Dietary Ingredients. In addition, the SECG includes several recommendations made by FDA in the dietary supplement CGMP rule so the guidance in those recommendations will be readily accessible to small businesses.

On 15 December 2010, FDA took new steps aimed at keeping consumers safe from harmful products that are marketed as dietary supplements and that contain undeclared or deceptively labeled ingredients.

The new steps include:
- a letter from the FDA commissioner to the dietary supplement industry emphasizing its legal obligation and responsibilities to prevent tainted products from reaching the US market[45]
- a new rapid public notification system (RSS Feed) on its website to more quickly warn consumers about these products[46]

Companies that make or distribute tainted products may receive Warning Letters and/or face enforcement actions, such as product seizures, injunctions and criminal prosecution. Responsible individuals also may face criminal prosecution.

Adverse Event Reporting

On 22 December 2006, President George W. Bush signed into law the *Dietary Supplement and Nonprescription Drug Consumer Protection Act* (Pub. L. 109-462, 120 Stat. 3469). This law amends the *FD&C Act* with respect to adverse event reporting and recordkeeping for dietary supplements and nonprescription drugs marketed without an approved application.

The manufacturer, packer or distributor whose name (pursuant to Section 403(e)(1) of the *FD&C Act*) appears on the label of a dietary supplement marketed in the US is required to submit to FDA all serious adverse event reports associated with use of the dietary supplement in the US. The effective date for compliance with the requirements of this law was 22 December 2007.

An "adverse event" is "any health-related event associated with the use of a dietary supplement that is adverse."

A "serious adverse event" is an adverse event that results in:
- death
- a life-threatening experience
- inpatient hospitalization
- a persistent or significant disability
- incapacity
- a congenital anomaly or birth defect
- a medical or surgical intervention, based on reasonable medical judgment, to prevent an outcome described above

The *Dietary Supplement and Nonprescription Drug Consumer Protection Act* usually refers to the entity (manufacturer, packer or distributor) that is required to submit a serious adverse event report to FDA as the "responsible person." Serious adverse event reports, as well as all follow-up reports of new medical information received within one year after the initial report, must be submitted to FDA on MedWatch Form 3500A along with a copy of the dietary supplement label and any other attachments no later than 15 business days after the report is received by the responsible person. However, voluntary reports of adverse events associated with a dietary supplement may be submitted on MedWatch Form 3500, the voluntary reporting form.

FDA requires that mandatory reports using MedWatch Form 3500A for serious adverse events associated with the use of dietary supplements be submitted in hard copy by mail only. FDA does not currently accept dietary supplement serious adverse event reports electronically or by facsimile.

The following five data elements,[47] at a minimum, are necessary for FDA to avoid duplication in its adverse event reports database and to interpret the significance of adverse events, facilitate follow-up and detect fraud:
- an identifiable injured person
- an identifiable initial reporter
- responsible person's identity and contact information (i.e., the manufacturer, packer or distributor submitting the serious adverse event report to FDA)
- a suspect dietary supplement
- a serious adverse event or fatal outcome

If a serious adverse event involves multiple dietary supplements that are manufactured, packaged or distributed by the same responsible person, the responsible person should submit only one serious adverse event report to FDA on Form 3500A. If a serious adverse event involves multiple suspect dietary supplements that were manufactured, packaged or distributed by more than one responsible person (e.g., manufacturers A and B), and if the event is reported to one of the responsible persons (manufacturer A), that responsible person (manufacturer A) should submit a serious adverse event report to FDA, identifying both its own product(s) and manufacturer B's product(s) in the Suspect Product section (Section C) of Form 3500A. In such a case, manufacturer A should send manufacturer B a copy of the submitted Form 3500A, including manufacturer A's report number. Manufacturer B need not submit a separate report to FDA for the serious adverse event unless manufacturer B has information about the serious adverse event that was not provided to FDA in manufacturer A's report. If manufacturer B does have such information, it must be reported to FDA as a follow-up report of new medical information, accompanied by a copy of manufacturer A's serious adverse event report. It is not necessary for manufacturer B to submit its own separate serious adverse event report on Form 3500A.

If the serious adverse event involves a nonprescription drug product marketed without an approved application and a dietary supplement that is also manufactured, packaged or distributed by the same responsible person, and the initial reporter views each product as suspect, the responsible person should submit one report about the serious adverse event to both the Center for Drug Evaluation and Research (CDER) and the Center for Food Safety and Applied Nutrition (CFSAN). The report should include information about both suspect products in Section C of the form and should use one manufacturer report number.

There is no requirement to provide a sample of the dietary supplement to FDA with the adverse event report, and the agency does not recommend that a sample be submitted unless requested.

Instructions for completing MedWatch Form 3500A to report a serious adverse event associated with a dietary supplement can be found on FDA's website (www.fda.gov/Safety/MedWatch/HowToReport/DownloadForms/ucm149238.htm).

The responsible person must maintain records related to each report of a serious adverse event for six years. These records should include, at a minimum, copies of the following:
- the responsible person's serious adverse event report to FDA on MedWatch Form 3500A, with attachments
- any new medical information about the serious adverse event received by the responsible person
- any reports to FDA of new medical information related to the serious adverse event
- communications between the responsible person and
    - the initial reporter
- any other person(s) who provided information related to the adverse event

Any new medical information received within one year of the initial report must be submitted to FDA within 15 business days of receipt.

Dietary supplements labeled on or after 22 December 2007 need to include a domestic address or domestic phone number at which the responsible person can receive reports of adverse events.[48] Products that do not include such information (such as those imported from foreign manufacturers) will be deemed "misbranded" and subject to regulatory action by FDA.

Import and Export Regulations

The *Bioterrorism Act* of 2002, Section 307, added Section 801(m) to the *FD&C Act*, requiring that FDA receive prior notice for food imported or offered for import into the US. Prior notice is notification to FDA that an article of food, including animal feed or pet food, is being imported or offered for import into the US in advance of the arrival of the article of food at the US border. Section 801(m) also provides that if an article of food arrives at the port of arrival with inadequate prior notice (e.g., no prior notice, inaccurate prior notice or untimely prior notice), the food is subject to refusal of admission under Section 801(m)(1) of the act and may not be delivered to the importer, owner or consignee.

The prior notice must be submitted to FDA electronically via either the US Customs and Border Protection (Customs) Automated Broker Interface (ABI) of the Automated Commercial System (ACS) or FDA's Prior Notice System Interface (FDA PNSI).

Prior notice must be received and confirmed electronically by FDA no more than five days before arrival and, as specified by the mode of transportation below, no less than:
1. two hours before arrival by land by road
2. four hours before arrival by air or by rail
3. eight hours before arrival by water
4. the time consistent with the timeframe established for the mode of transportation for an article of food carried by or otherwise accompanying an individual if it is subject to prior notice

Instructions for submitting prior notice and information on prior notice of imported foods can be found on the FDA website (cwww.fda.gov/Food/GuidanceRegulation/ImportsExports/Importing/ucm2006836.htm). Additional information on Customs' procedures for prior notice can be found at www.cbp.gov.

Failure to submit prior notice by a person who imports or offers for import an article of food is a prohibited act under Section 301(ee) of the act (21 U.S.C. 331(ee)) and could result in the US bringing civil, criminal and debarment actions against him or her. When it is consistent with the agency's public protection responsibilities, and depending on the nature of the violation, FDA gives individuals and firms an opportunity to take voluntary and prompt corrective action before initiating regulatory actions.[49] Accordingly, FDA may elect to refuse prior notices or send compliance letters to give the responsible parties warning before pursuing other regulatory actions, e.g., injunction, prosecution, etc.

The regulatory actions for violations include:
- refusal under Section 801(m) of the act for no prior notice, inaccurate prior notice or untimely prior notice
- hold under Section 801(l) of the act for importing or offering for import food from a foreign facility that is not registered under section 415 of the act
- injunction under Section 302 of the act
- prosecution under Sections 301 and 303 of the act
- debarment under Section 306 of the act
- Customs seizure and assessment of civil monetary penalties for violation of any laws enforced by Customs and Border Protection, including 19 U.S.C. 1595a(b), against any person who directs, assists financially or otherwise, or is in any way concerned in the importation of any merchandise contrary to law

The *Bioterrorism Act* requires domestic and foreign facilities that manufacture, process, pack or hold food for consumption in the US to register with FDA. In addition, the act amended Chapter VIII of the *FD&C Act* by adding Section 801(l), which requires any food for human and animal consumption from an unregistered foreign facility that is imported or offered for import to be held at the port of entry until the foreign facility has been registered.

In addition, the *Bioterrorism Act*, Section 305, added Section 415 to the *FD&C Act* to require domestic and foreign facilities that manufacture, process, pack or hold food for human or animal consumption in the US to register with FDA. Dietary supplements and dietary ingredients are regulated as foods by FDA. The *Bioterrorism Act* makes failure to register a prohibited act under Section 301 of the *FD&C Act*.

Owners, operators or agents in charge of domestic or foreign facilities that manufacture/process, pack or hold foods for human or animal consumption in the US are required to register the facility with FDA. Domestic facilities are required to register whether or not food from the facility enters interstate commerce.

Foreign facilities that manufacture, process, pack or hold food also are required to register unless food from that facility undergoes further processing (including packaging) by another foreign facility before the food is exported to the US. However, if the subsequent foreign facility performs only a minimal activity, such as putting on a label, both facilities are required to register. Foreign facilities are required to designate a US agent for purposes of the registration regulation. The US agent acts as a communications link between FDA and the foreign facility. FDA will treat representations by the US agent as those of the foreign facility and will consider information or documents provided to the US agent equivalent to providing the information or documents to the foreign facility.

Registrants must register using Form FDA 3537. Registrations can be submitted in hard copy format by mail, electronically via the Internet, on CD-ROM or by fax. Instructions for completing Form FDA 3537 and additional information on registration of food facilities can be found on FDA's website (www.fda.gov/Food/GuidanceRegulation/FSMA/ucm314178.htm).

Section 801(e)(1) of the *FD&C Act* states that a food intended for export must not be deemed to be adulterated or misbranded under the act if it: (A) accords to the specifications of the foreign purchaser; (B) is not in conflict with the laws of the country to which it is intended for export; (C) is labeled on the outside of the shipping package that it is intended for export; and (D) is not sold or offered for sale in domestic commerce.[50] Dietary ingredients and dietary supplements for export are subject to Section 801(e)(1) of the act and would be subject to the notification and recordkeeping requirements of 21 CFR 1.101.[51]

Currently, FDA issues the "certificate of free sale" as an export certificate for food, including dietary supplements that are legally marketed in the US.[52] The criteria needed to request a certificate of free sale for dietary supplements can be found at www.food-drug.com/fda_expoert_certificate.htm. A certificate of free sale is only issued for products manufactured in the US.

The requirements for prior notice do not apply to dietary supplements that are imported and then exported without leaving the port of arrival until export.

Homeopathic Products

The term "homeopathy" is derived from the Greek words *homeo* (similar) and *pathos* (suffering or disease). Homeopathy is the practice of treating the syndromes and conditions constituting disease with remedies that have produced similar syndromes and conditions in healthy subjects.[53]

History of Homeopathy in Food and Drug Law

As both the chief sponsor of the *FD&C Act* and a homeopathic physician, Senator Royal Copeland of New York amended the *Food and Drugs Act* of 1906 by defining "drug" to include those homeopathic drugs listed in the *Homeopathic Pharmacopoeia of the United States* (*HPUS*).

For five decades (from 1938–88), homeopathic drugs were sold in a regulatory vacuum. FDA action was based on institutional understanding and informal agreements between agency officials and industry members. From 1982–88, the industry, professional and consumer members of the community through the American Homeopathic Pharmacists Association worked with FDA in the development of a regulatory framework called a Compliance Policy Guide, CPG 7132.15 "Conditions under which homeopathic drugs may be marketed." CPG 7132.15 provides guidance on the regulation of over-the-counter (OTC) and prescription homeopathic drugs, and delineates those conditions under which homeopathic drugs may ordinarily be marketed in the US.

FDA does not regulate homeopathic drugs in precisely the same way as conventional or allopathic drugs; in fact, the agency treats homeopathic drugs, both prescription and OTC, quite differently. Unlike conventional drugs, homeopathic drugs are not subject to premarket approval, which involves filing a new drug application (NDA) in order to market the drug. Furthermore, unlike other OTC drugs, which are either required to be submitted for OTC review or to file an NDA, OTC homeopathic drugs are not subject to the FDA review process. Like some drug OTC products, homeopathic drugs need to comply with a monograph.

The FDA Compliance Policy Guide, CPG 7132.15 and *HPUS* form the basis for the regulation of homeopathic drugs in the US.[54]

Definition of Homeopathic Drugs

A homeopathic drug is any drug labeled as being homeopathic that is listed in *HPUS*, an addendum to it or its supplements. The potencies of homeopathic drugs are specified in terms of dilution, i.e., 1x (1/10 dilution), 2x (1/100 dilution), etc. Homeopathic drug products must contain diluents commonly used in homeopathic pharmaceuticals. Drug products containing homeopathic ingredients in combination with nonhomeopathic active ingredients are not homeopathic drug products.

Homeopathic drugs generally must meet the standards for strength, quality and purity set forth in *HPUS*. *HPUS* is declared a legal source of information on homeopathic drug products in Section 201(g)(1) of the *FD&C Act*. *HPUS* is a compilation of standards for source, composition and preparation of homeopathic drugs, which the *FD&C Act* also recognized as an official compendium. Section 201(j) of the act (21 U.S.C. §321) defines the term "official compendium" as the "official *United States Pharmacopoeia*, official *Homeopathic Pharmacopoeia of the United States*, official *National Formulary* or any supplement to them."

Introduction to the Homeopathic Pharmacopoeia Convention of the United States (HPCUS)

The Homeopathic Pharmacopoeia Convention of the United States (HPCUS) is a nongovernmental, nonprofit, scientific organization composed of experts who have appropriate training and experience and have demonstrated additional knowledge and interest in the principles of homeopathy. HPCUS is an autonomous body that works closely with FDA and homeopathic organizations. The HPCUS board appoints a Monograph Review Committee (MRC), a Pharmacopoeia Revision Committee (PRC) and a Council on Pharmacy to assist in its ongoing responsibilities.

HPCUS is responsible for the production and constant updating of *HPUS*. *HPUS* is published as the *Homeopathic Pharmacopoeia of the United States Revision Service*. *HPUS* is "written" by a group of pharmacists, physicians and lay people who meet three to six times a year to review monographs and pharmacy procedures. The *HPUS Revision Service*, also known as the subscription service, began in December 1988. One or two revisions are published each year. Annual subscription updates are required to keep the *HPUS Revision Service* current and official.

HPUS is divided into two sections, General Pharmacy and Drug Monographs. General Pharmacy contains all official manufacturing procedures for all official homeopathic dosage forms as well as labeling guidelines and administrative information. In addition, criteria and procedures for inclusion in *HPUS* are published. *HPUS* contains approximately 1,300 individual monographs of official drug substances. Each monograph lists complete identifying data for the drug as well as specific manufacturing standards.

The *HPUS* online database is a powerful tool that provides quick access to all *HPUS* publications. The database includes the most current monograph and quality control specifications, along with real-time updates. To access the *HPUS* online database, visit www.hpus.com.

HPUS Approval Process

To be included in *HPUS*, a drug must have sufficient clinical data or "drug proving" to show efficacy. In a homeopathic drug proving, a homeopathically prepared substance is administered to healthy volunteers in order to produce the symptoms specific to that substance and thereby reveal its inherent curative powers. During a homeopathic drug proving, the goal is to provoke temporary symptoms associated with the homeopathic medication. These symptoms are then arranged to form a symptom pattern or "remedy picture" that is specific to that particular homeopathic substance and provides the basis for a better understanding of its possible effects in patients.

To be eligible for inclusion in *HPUS*, the drug must meet the first three criteria and at least one of the latter four (4, 5, 6 or 7):

1. HPCUS has determined that the drug is safe and effective.
2. The drug must be prepared according to the specifications of the General Pharmacy and relevant sections of *HPUS*.
3. The submitted documentation must be in an approved format as set forth in the relevant sections of *HPUS*.
4. The therapeutic use of a new and nonofficial homeopathic drug is established by a homeopathic drug proving and clinical verification acceptable to HPCUS.
5. The therapeutic use of the drug is established through published documentation that the substance was in use prior to 1962. This documentation must include the symptom picture, including subjective and any available objective symptoms.
6. The therapeutic use of the drug is established by at least two adequately controlled, double-blind clinical studies using the drug as the single intervention; and the study is to be accompanied by adequate statistical analysis and adequate description of the symptom picture acceptable to HPCUS, including the subjective symptoms and, where appropriate, the objective symptomatology.
7. The drug's therapeutic use is established by: data gathered from clinical experience encompassing the symptom picture and pre- and post-treatment, including subjective and any available objective symptoms; or data documented in the medical literature (all sources of medical literature may be considered on a case-by-case basis) subjected to further verification (statistical and/or other forms of verification).

Homeopathic drug provings on healthy volunteers are carried out according to Hahnemann's classical directions and also adhere to the current regulations for conventional clinical trials

Clinical verification of all or part of the symptom picture established in a homeopathic drug proving is designed to further demonstrate a homeopathic medication's potential clinical applicability. Clinical verification may also use a variety of methodologies in a prospective or retrospective fashion. The design and sample size will vary on a case-by-case basis, depending on what is being verified (symptom picture, keynotes or a specific clinical indication). The responsibility for a scientifically sound clinical verification protocol lies with the sponsor. The study design for the clinical verification of the symptoms gathered in a drug proving should be submitted to the MRC and the PRC for review prior to beginning clinical verification. For additional information, refer to the HPCUS Guidelines for Homeopathic Drug Provings, HPCUS Outline for Protocols for Homeopathic Drug Provings and HPCUS Guidelines for Clinical Verification on the HPUS website.

To be considered for inclusion in *HPUS*, a monograph must adhere to the specified format and must be accompanied by documentation verifying that it meets the eligibility criteria for inclusion in *HPUS*.

A sponsor desiring to have monographs considered for inclusion in *HPUS* must submit them to the editor. If the monographs are acceptable, the editor will forward them, with any comments and accompanying documentation, to the chairman of the MRC. The MRC will perform a comprehensive review of each monograph and recommend its categorization under one of three headings: approved for publication in *HPUS*; deferred for presentation of additional data; or not approved for publication in *HPUS*.

The editor will publish a list of the monographs that the MRC has recommended for the approved category and those in the not-approved category, and the reasons for the actions taken, in an appropriate medium such as the *Journal of the American Institute of Homeopathy, Homeopathy Today* or *American Homeopathy*. The editor also will forward the annotated monographs, the monograph list and any accompanying documentation to the chairman of the PRC. A minimum of 90 days, beginning on the 15th day of the month of publication of the monograph list, is permitted for receipt of comments from the general public. At the end of the 90-day period, any public comments received by the editor will be forwarded to the PRC chairman. The PRC will perform a comprehensive review of each monograph and recommend categorization under one of three headings: approved for publication in *HPUS*; deferred for presentation of additional data; or not approved for publication in *HPUS*. MRC and PRC recommendations are reviewed and acted upon by the board of directors. If acceptable, the monograph is granted final approval for inclusion in *HPUS*, and the secretary notifies the sponsor of the board's decision.

Labeling and Advertising

All homeopathic products are drugs within the meaning of the *FD&C Act* and, therefore, are subject to applicable FDA regulations for labeling, advertising and promotion. Homeopathic drug product labeling must comply with the provisions of Sections 502 and 503 of the *FD&C Act* and 21 CFR 201. The label shall contain, in prominent type, the word "HOMEOPATHIC" or "Homeopathic."

The Statement of Ingredients must appear in accordance with Section 502(e) of the *FD&C Act* and 21 CFR 201.10. Labeling must bear a statement of the quantity and amount of ingredient(s) in the product in conformance with Section 502(b) of the act, as well as 21 CFR 201.10, expressed in homeopathic terms, e.g., 1x, 2x. On each label and package, the letters "HPUS" should be appended to the name of each official drug or drugs present in the product, e.g., "Arnica Montana 3X HPUS." In addition, the following statement must appear at the end of the formula section of each label when all product(s) contained therein are official: "The letters 'HPUS' indicate that the component(s) in this product is (are) officially monographed in the *Homeopathic Pharmacopoeia of the United States*. The designation 'HPUS' is restricted (or may be appended only) to those substances (or Homeopathic Drug Products) whose monographs have been reviewed by the Convention and have been approved for publication in the current Pharmacopoeia by the Board of Directors."

Other general labeling requirements include the manufacturer, packer or distributor's name and place of business, in conformance with Section 502(b) and 21 CFR 201.1, adequate directions for use (Section 502(f) and 21 CFR 201.5) and Established Name (Section 502(e)(3) of the *FD&C Act* and 21 CFR 201.10). The label and labeling must be in the English language as described and provided for under 21 CFR 201.15(c)(1), although it is permissible for industry to include the labeling in both English and Latin.

The label of prescription homeopathic drug products shall bear a statement of identity (21 CFR 201.50), declaration of net quantity of contents (21 CFR 201.51), a statement of the recommended or usual dosage (21 CFR 201.55) and information described under 21 CFR 201.56 and 21 CFR 201.57. An exemption from adequate directions for use under Section 503 is applicable only to prescription drugs. All prescription homeopathic drug products must bear the prescription legend, "Caution: Federal law prohibits dispensing without prescription" (Section 503(b)(1)), and a package insert bearing complete labeling information for the homeopathic practitioner must accompany the product.

The label of OTC homeopathic drug products must comply with the principal display panel provision (21 CFR 201.62); a statement of identity (21 CFR 201.61) shall conform to the provisions for declaring net quantity of contents under 21 CFR 201.62. OTC homeopathic drugs intended for systemic absorption, unless specifically exempted, must bear a warning statement in conformance with 21 CFR 201.63(a). Other warnings, such as those for indications conforming to those in OTC drug final regulations, are required as appropriate.

Homeopathic products intended solely for self-limiting disease conditions amenable to self-diagnosis (of symptoms) and treatment may be marketed OTC. Homeopathic products offered for conditions not amenable to OTC use must be marketed as prescription products. The criteria specified in Section 503(b) of the *FD&C Act* apply to the determination of prescription status for all drug products, including homeopathic drug products. If *HPUS* specifies a distinction between nonprescription and prescription status of products that is based on strength and is more restrictive than Section 503(b) of the act, the more stringent criteria will apply.

Any drug included in *HPUS* is considered "official," and those not included in *HPUS* are "nonofficial." According to the understanding, any official drug can be sold without any further documentation being generated by the manufacturer. Nonofficial drugs require the manufacturer to produce a proving or sufficient clinical data for FDA to make a determination as to whether the drug was, in fact, homeopathic.

If any homeopathic drug is promoted significantly beyond the recognized or customary practice of homeopathy, the priorities and procedures concerning FDA's policy on health fraud will apply (CPG 7150.10 "Health Fraud-Factors in Considering Regulatory Action" 5 June 1987).

Good Manufacturing Practices

All firms that manufacture, prepare, propagate, compound or otherwise process homeopathic drugs must register as drug establishments in conformance with Section 510 of the *FD&C Act* and 21 CFR 207.[55]

Homeopathic drug products must be manufactured in conformance with current Good Manufacturing Practice, Section 501(a)(2)(B) of the *FD&C Act* and 21 CFR 211. However, due to the unique nature of these drug products, there are two exemptions to this requirement. First, homeopathic drugs need not have expiration dating (21 CFR 211.137). Second, FDA proposed an amendment that exempted homeopathic drug products from the requirement for laboratory determination of identity and strength of each active ingredient prior to the release and distribution of the drug on the market (21 CFR 211.165). Until there is a final ruling on this proposed testing requirement amendment, FDA has a policy of not enforcing this regulation against homeopathic drugs.

Summary

- Dietary supplements are regulated as a class of food products and may be marketed to support the normal, healthy structure or function of the human body and its systems.
- Dietary supplements are subject to GMP regulations and adverse event reporting requirements, and facilities must be registered with FDA; however, product listing and premarket approval are not required.
- Homeopathic products are a class of drug products regulated through a Compliance Policy Guide.
- Homeopathic drug products are not subject to the NDA process. They are subject to approval by the Homeopathic Pharmacopoeia Convention of the United States (HPCUS) or must conform to monographs published in the *Homeopathic Pharmacopoeia of the United States* (HPUS).
- Homeopathic drug products must comply with labeling regulations found in 21 CFR 201.

References

1. Pray WS. *A History of Nonprescription Product Regulation*, Pharmaceutical Products Press, New York (2003).
2. "Chapter II: Background on dietary supplements." Commission on Dietary Supplement Labels. Office of Disease Prevention and Health Promotion website. http://www.health.gov/dietsupp/ch2.htm. Accessed 3 May 2013.
3. "Vitamin and Mineral Drug Products for Over-the-Counter Human Use." *Federal Register*, Vol 44, No. 53, p. 16126 (16 March 1979).
4. Pray WS. "The FDA, Vitamins, and the Dietary Supplement Industry." *US Pharm*. 2008;33(10):10–15.
5. Op cit 1.
6. *Nutrition Advertising Coordination Act* of 1991 (HR 1662 SC2).
7. *Dietary Supplement Consumer Protection Act* of 1993 (HR 2923 IH).
8. Op cit 3.
9. *The Dietary Supplements Task Force Final Report*, Dept. of Health and Human Services, Public Health Service, Food and Drug Administration, 1992.
10. Interview Mr. Loren Isrealsen, JD, Executive Director UNPA, 1 October 2009.
11. Ibid.
12. Soller RW. "Regulation in the Herb Market: The Myth of the 'Unregulated Industry.'" *HerbalGram*. 2000;49:64 American Botanical Council.
13. *Dietary Supplement Health and Education Act* of 1994 (Public Law 103-417, 103rd Congress).
14. FDA information on *Dietary Supplement Health and Education Act* of 1994, 1 December 1995. FDA website. www.fda.gov/Food/DietarySupplements/default.htm. Accessed 3 May 2013.
15. *Nutrition Labeling Education Act* of 1990 (Public Law 101-535, 101st Congress).
16. Op cit 6.
17. *Draft Guidance for Industry: Factors that Distinguish Liquid Dietary Supplements from Beverages*, Considerations Regarding Novel Ingredients, and Labeling for Beverages and Other Conventional Foods (December 2009). FDA website. www.fda.gov/Food/GuidanceRegulation/GuidanceDocumentsRegulatoryInformation/DietarySupplements/ucm196903.htm. Accessed 3 May 2013.
18. 21 CFR 190.6 Requirement for premarket notification. GPO website. www.gpo.gov/fdsys/pkg/CFR-2011-title21-vol3/pdf/CFR-2011-title21-vol3-part190-subpartB.pdf. Accessed 13 May 2013.
19. 21 CFR 1.3(b). Defintions; Label. FDA website. www.accessdata.fda.gov/scripts/cdrh/cfdocs/cfcfr/CFRSearch.cfm?fr=1.3. Accessed 13 May 2013.
20. 21 CFR 1.3(a). Definitions, Labeling. FDA website. www.accessdata.fda.gov/scripts/cdrh/cfdocs/cfcfr/CFRSearch.cfm?fr=1.3. Accessed 13 May 2013.
21. 21 CFR 101.36 Nutrition labeling of dietary supplements. FDA website. www.accessdata.fda.gov/scripts/cdrh/cfdocs/cfcfr/CFRSearch.cfm?fr=101.36. Accessed 13 May 2013.
22. 21 CFR 101.9 Nutrition labeling of food. FDA website. www.accessdata.fda.gov/scripts/cdrh/cfdocs/cfcfr/cfrsearch.cfm?fr=101.9. Accessed 13 May 2013.
23. *Food Allergen Labeling Consumer Protection Act* of 2004 (Public law 108-282).
24. *Food and Drug Administration Modernization Act* of 1997 (*FDAMA*) (Public Law 105-115).
25. "*FDA Modernization Act of 1997 (FDAMA)* Claims." FDA website. www.fda.gov/Food/IngredientsPackagingLabeling/LabelingNutrition/LabelClaims/FDAModernizationActFDAMAClaims/default.htm. Accessed 3 May 2013.
26. 21 CFR 101.14(c). Health claims: general requirements; Validity claims. FDA website. www.accessdata.fda.gov/scripts/cdrh/cfdocs/cfcfr/CFRSearch.cfm?fr=101.14. Accessed 13 May 2013.
27. "Qualified Health Claims." FDA website. www.fda.gov/Food/IngredientsPackagingLabeling/LabelingNutrition/LabelClaims/QualifiedHealthClaims/default.htm. Accessed 3 May 2013.
28. Op cit 6.
29. 21 CFR 101.93 Certain types of statements for dietary supplements. FDA website. www.accessdata.fda.gov/scripts/cdrh/cfdocs/cfcfr/CFRsearch.cfm?fr=101.93. Accessed 13 May 2013.
30. *Guidance for Industry: Structure/Function Claims Small Entity Compliance Guide* (January 2002). FDA website. www.fda.gov/Food/

GuidanceRegulation/GuidanceDocumentsRegulatoryInformation/DietarySupplements/ucm103340.htm Accessed 3 May 2013.
31. *Guidance for Industry: Substantiation for Dietary Supplement Claims Made Under Section 403(r)(6) of the Federal Food, Drug, and Cosmetic Act* (December 2008). FDA website. www.fda.gov/Food/GuidanceRegulation/GuidanceDocumentsRegulatoryInformation/DietarySupplements/ucm073200.htm. Accessed 3 May 2013.
32. *Draft Guidance for Industry: Substantiation for Dietary Supplement Claims Made Under Section 403(r)(6) of the Federal Food, Drug, and Cosmetic Act.*
33. "Section 5 Dietary Supplement Claims, Dietary Supplement Labeling Exemptions," *Dietary Supplement Health and Education Act* of 1994 (Public Law 103-417, 103rd Congress).
34. Op cit 6.
35. Memorandum of Understanding Between Federal Trade Commission and the Food and Drug Administration, Federal Register, Vol 36, No. 180, 16 September 1971.
36. Federal Trade Commission, *Dietary Supplements: An Advertising Guide for Industry*. FTC website. http://business.ftc.gov/documents/bus09-dietary-supplements-advertising-guide-industry. Accessed 3 May 2013.
37. *Public Health Security and Bioterrorism Preparedness and Response Act* of 2002 (Public law 107-188).
38. *Guidance for Industry: Questions and Answers Regarding Registration of Food Facilities* (Edition 5) (December 2012). FDA website. www.fda.gov/Food/GuidanceRegulation/GuidanceDocumentsRegulatoryInformation/FoodDefense/ucm331959.htm. Accessed 3 May 2013.
39. "Registration of Food Facilities." FDA website.. www.fda.gov/Food/GuidanceRegulation/FoodFacilityRegistration/default.htm. Accessed 3 May 2013.
40. Food, Registration. FDA website. www.fda.gov/Food/GuidanceRegulation/FSMA/ucm314178.htm. Accessed 3 May 2013.
41. *The FDA Food Safety Modernization Act of 2011* (Public Law 111-353)
42. 68 Fed. Reg. 12158 (13 March 2003). Current Good Manufacturing Practice in Manufacturing, Packing, or Holding Dietary Ingredients and Dietary Supplements. GPO website. www.gpo.gov/fdsys/pkg/FR-2003-03-13/pdf/03-5401.pdf. Accessed 3 May 2013.
43. 21 CFR Part 111 Current Good Manufacturing Practice in manufacturing, packaging, labeling, or holding operations for dietary supplements; final rule. FDA website. www.accessdata.fda.gov/scripts/cdrh/cfdocs/cfcfr/cfrsearch.cfm?cfrpart=111 . Accessed 3 May 2013.
44. *Current Good Manufacturing Practice in Manufacturing, Packaging, Labeling, or Holding Operations for Dietary Supplements; Small Entity Compliance Guide* (December 2010). FDA website. www.fda.gov/Food/GuidanceRegulation/GuidanceDocumentsRegulatoryInformation/DietarySupplements/ucm238182.htm. Accessed 3 May 2013.
45. FDA News Release: Tainted products marketed as dietary supplements potentially dangerous (15 December 2010). FDA website. www.fda.gov/NewsEvents/Newsroom/PressAnnouncements/ucm236967.htm. Accessed 3 May 2013.
46. Tainted Products That are Marketed as Dietary Supplements RSS Feed. FDA website. www.fda.gov/AboutFDA/ContactFDA/StayInformed/RSSFeeds/TDS/rss.xml. Accessed 3 May 2013.
47. *Guidance for Industry: Questions and Answers Regarding Adverse Event Reporting and Recordkeeping for Dietary Supplements as Required by the Dietary Supplement and Nonprescription Drug Consumer Protection Act* (October 2007; Revised June 2009). FDA website. www.fda.gov/Food/GuidanceRegulation/GuidanceDocumentsRegulatoryInformation/DietarySupplements/ucm171383.htm. Accessed 3 May 2013.
48. *Draft Guidance for Industry: Questions and Answers Regarding the Labeling of Dietary Supplements as Required by the Dietary Supplement and Nonprescription Drug Consumer Protection Act* (December 2007; Revised December 2008 and September 2009). FDA website. http://www.fda.gov/Food/GuidanceRegulation/GuidanceDocumentsRegulatoryInformation/DietarySupplements/ucm179018.htm. Accessed 3 May 2013.
49. Compliance Policy Guide, *Guidance for Industry and CBP Staff: Sec. 110.310 Prior Notice of Imported Food Under the Public Health Security and Bioterrorism Preparedness and Response Act* of 2002 (May 2009). FDA website. www.fda.gov/Food/GuidanceRegulation/GuidanceDocumentsRegulatoryInformation/FoodDefense/ucm153055.htm. Accessed 3 May 2013.
50. *FD&C Act*, Section 801 (21 USC 381) Imports and exports. GPO website. http://www.gpo.gov/fdsys/pkg/USCODE-2010-title21/html/USCODE-2010-title21-chap9-subchapVIII-sec381.htm. Accessed 3 May 2013.
51. 21 CFR 1.101 Notification and recordkeeping. FDA website. www.accessdata.fda.gov/scripts/cdrh/cfdocs/cfcfr/CFRSearch.cfm?fr=1.101. Accessed 3 May 2013.
52. FDA Export Certificates to Foreign Governments FAQs. FDA website. www.fda.gov/downloads/Drugs/GuidanceComplianceRegulatoryInformation/ImportsandExportsCompliance/UCM318409.pdf Accessed 3 May 2013.
53. Compliance Policy Guide 7132.15, Sec. 400.400, "Conditions Under Which Homeopathic Drugs May Be Marketed." FDA website. www.fda.gov/ICECI/ComplianceManuals/CompliancePolicyGuidanceManual/ucm074360.htm. Accessed 3 May 2013.
54. *Homeopathic Pharmacopoeia of the United States*, "The Regulation of Homepathic Medicines." HPUS website. www.hpus.com/regulations.php. Accessed 3 May 2013.
55. "Drug Registration and Listing System (DRLS & eDRLS)." FDA website. www.fda.gov/Drugs/GuidanceComplianceRegulatoryInformation/DrugRegistrationandListing/default.htm. Accessed 3 May 2013.

Recommended Reading
- 21 CFR Part 1 Subpart I: Prior Notice of Imported Food Under the Public Health Security and Bioterrorism Preparedness and Response Act of 2002.. FDA website. www.accessdata.fda.gov/scripts/cdrh/cfdocs/cfcfr/CFRSearch.cfm?CFRPart=1&showFR=1&subpartNode=21:1.0.1.1.1.7. Accessed 3 May 2013.
- 21 CFR 101.93 Certain types of statements for dietary supplements. FDA website. www.accessdata.fda.gov/scripts/cdrh/cfdocs/cfcfr/CFRsearch.cfm?fr=101.93. Accessed 3 May 2013.
- *Public Health Security and Bioterrorism Preparedness and Response Act* of 2002 (Public Law 107-188, 107th Congress). FDA website. www.fda.gov/regulatoryinformation/legislation/ucm148797.htm. Accessed 3 May 2013.
- New Dietary Ingredient in Dietary Supplements. FDA website. www.fda.gov/Food/DietarySupplements/ucm109764.htm. Accessed 3 May 2013.
- *Guidance for Industry: Substantiation for Dietary Supplement Claims Made Under Section 403(r) (6) of the Federal Food, Drug, and Cosmetic Act* (December 2008). FDA website. www.fda.gov/Food/GuidanceRegulation/GuidanceDocumentsRegulatoryInformation/DietarySupplements/ucm073200.htm. Accessed 3 May 2013.
- "Claims That Can Be Made for Conventional Foods and Dietary Supplements" (September 2003). FDA website. www.fda.gov/Food/IngredientsPackagingLabeling/LabelingNutrition/ucm111447.htm. Accessed 3 May 2013.
- *Guidance for Industry: Evidence-Based Review System for the Scientific Evaluation of Health Claims* (January 2009). FDA website. www.fda.gov/Food/GuidanceRegulation/GuidanceDocumentsRegulatoryInformation/LabelingNutrition/ucm073332.htm. Accessed 3 May 2013.
- *Guidance for Industry: Iron-Containing Supplements and Drugs: Label Warning Statements Small Entity Compliance Guide* (October 2003). FDA website. www.fda.gov/Food/GuidanceRegulation/GuidanceDocumentsRegulatoryInformation/DietarySupplements/ucm073014.htm. Accessed 3 May 2013.
- *Guidance for Industry: Notification of a Health Claim or Nutrient Content Claim Based on an Authoritative Statement of a Scientific Body* (June 1998). FDA

- website. www.fda.gov/Food/GuidanceRegulation/GuidanceDocumentsRegulatoryInformation/LabelingNutrition/ucm056975.htm. Accessed 3 May 2013
- *Guidance for Industry: Food Labeling; Nutrient Content Claims; Definition for "High Potency" and Definition for "Antioxidant" for Use in Nutrient Content Claims for Dietary Supplements and Conventional Foods Small Entity Compliance Guide* (July 2008). FDA website. www.fda.gov/Food/GuidanceRegulation/GuidanceDocumentsRegulatoryInformation/LabelingNutrition/ucm063064.htm. Accessed 3 May 2013.
- *Guidance for Industry: Statement of Identity, Nutrition Labeling, and Ingredient Labeling of Dietary Supplements Small Entity Compliance Guide* (January 1999). FDA website. www.fda.gov/Food/GuidanceRegulation/GuidanceDocumentsRegulatoryInformation/DietarySupplements/ucm073168.htm. Accessed 3 May 2013.
- *Guidance for Industry: Structure/Function Claims Small Entity Compliance Guide* (January 2002). FDA website. www.fda.gov/Food/GuidanceRegulation/GuidanceDocumentsRegulatoryInformation/DietarySupplements/ucm103340.htm. Accessed 3 May 2013.
- *Guidance for Industry: Interim Procedures for Qualified Health Claims in the Labeling of Conventional Human Food and Human Dietary Supplements* (July 2003). FDA website. www.fda.gov/Food/GuidanceRegulation/GuidanceDocumentsRegulatoryInformation/LabelingNutrition/ucm053832.htm. Accessed 3 May 2013.
- *Guidance for Industry: Prior Notice of Imported Food Questions and Answers (Edition 2)* (May 2004). FDA website. www.fda.gov/Food/GuidanceRegulation/GuidanceDocumentsRegulatoryInformation/FoodDefense/ucm078911.htm. Accessed 3 May 2013.
- *Guidance for Industry: Questions and Answers Regarding Establishment and Maintenance of Records by Persons Who Manufacture, Process, Pack, Transport, Distribute, Receive, Hold or Import Food (Edition 5)* (February 2012). FDA website. www.fda.gov/Food/GuidanceRegulation/GuidanceDocumentsRegulatoryInformation/FoodDefense/ucm292746.htm. Accessed 3 May 2013.
- *Guidance for Industry: Questions and Answers Regarding Adverse Event Reporting and Recordkeeping for Dietary Supplements as Required by the Dietary Supplement and Nonprescription Drug Consumer Protection Act* (October 2007; Revised June 2009). FDA website. www.fda.gov/Food/GuidanceRegulation/GuidanceDocumentsRegulatoryInformation/DietarySupplements/ucm171415.htm. Accessed 3 May 2013.
- *Draft Guidance for Industry: Questions and Answers Regarding the Labeling of Dietary Supplements as Required by the Dietary Supplement and Nonprescription Drug Consumer Protection Act* (December 2007; Revised December 2008; Revised September 2009). FDA website. www.fda.gov/Food/GuidanceRegulation/GuidanceDocumentsRegulatoryInformation/DietarySupplements/ucm179018.htm. Accessed 3 May 2013.
- *Guidance for Industry: Questions and Answers Regarding Food Allergens, including the Food Allergen Labeling and Consumer Protection Act of 2004* (Edition 4); Final Guidance (October 2006). FDA website. www.fda.gov/Food/GuidanceRegulation/GuidanceDocumentsRegulatoryInformation/Allergens/ucm059116.htm. Accessed 3 May 2013.
- Clarke JH. *A Dictionary of Practical Materia Medica.* (3 vol.). London (U.K.): The Homeopathic Publishing Co.; 1902.

Chapter 31

Cosmetics

By Evelyn D. Cadman

OBJECTIVES

❏ Understand the classification of cosmetics and related products

❏ Understand the basic regulations covering cosmetic product sales in the US

REGULATIONS AND GUIDELINES FOR THE COSMETIC INDUSTRY

❏ 21 CFR 1 General enforcement regulations

❏ 21 CFR 250 Section 250.250 Requirements for drugs and cosmetics—hexachlorophene

❏ 21 CFR 700 Subpart A (Section 700.3) Cosmetics—General provisions

❏ 21 CFR 700 Subpart B (Sections 700.11–700.35) Requirements for specific cosmetic products

❏ Amendment to Section 700.27 (71 *FR* 59653) 11 October 2006

❏ 21 CFR 701 Subpart A (Sections 701.1–701.9) Cosmetic labeling—General provisions

❏ 21 CFR 701 Subpart B (Sections 701.10–701.19) Package form

❏ 21 CFR 701 Subpart C (Sections 701.20–701.30) Labeling of specific ingredients

❏ 21 CFR 710 Voluntary registration of cosmetic product establishments

❏ 21 CFR 720 Voluntary filing of cosmetic product ingredient and cosmetic raw material composition statements

❏ 21 CFR 740 Cosmetic product warning statements

❏ Cosmetics Good Manufacturing Practice Guidelines

❏ Cosmetics Labeling Manual

❏ "Intercenter Agreement Between the Center for Drug Evaluation and Research and the Center for Food Safety and Applied Nutrition to Assist FDA in Implementing the Drug and Cosmetic Provisions of the Federal Food, Drug and Cosmetic Act for Products that Purport to be Cosmetics but Meet the Statutory Definition of a Drug"

❏ FDA Recall Policy for Cosmetics

Introduction

In spite of the fact that skin is the body's largest organ, the regulation of cosmetic products used on the skin is not tightly regulated by the US Food and Drug Administration (FDA). The agency was given responsibility for cosmetics as a result of the *Federal Food, Drug, and Cosmetic Act* of 1938 (*FD&C Act*), which defined cosmetic adulteration and misbranding and made provisions for FDA to write regulations defining exemptions to compliance. The act further affected cosmetics by requiring that FDA certify color additives. No other premarket approval is required for cosmetic products or their ingredients. It is the manufacturer's responsibility to ensure that its cosmetic products and ingredients are safe and properly labeled in full compliance with the law. FDA's Center for Food Safety and Applied Nutrition (CFSAN) regulates cosmetics only after they have been introduced onto the marketplace. Cosmetic manufacturers may voluntarily register their facilities and product lists, but there is no regulatory requirement for registration. Good Manufacturing Practices (GMPs) are encouraged but are not required by regulation.

In recent years, bills to increase cosmetic safety and regulation have been introduced in the US Congress but have not been enacted.[1-4] These bills seek to amend the *FD&C Act* to require cosmetic manufacturers to register cosmetic products and cosmetic manufacturing facilities; follow GMPs; establish a file containing scientific evidence substantiating the product's safety; report information received on any serious adverse events; and maintain records of the manufacturing, safety and adverse events associated with their products. The proposed legislation also would provide for mandatory recalls of adulterated products. Some versions of the bills would require FDA to review cosmetic ingredients and establish a list of those deemed to be safe for use.[5-7] To date, all such proposed legislation has died in committee, leaving the cosmetic industry to voluntarily register and follow GMPs.

The *FD&C Act* defines "cosmetics" as "(1) articles intended to be rubbed, poured, sprinkled, or sprayed on, introduced into, or otherwise applied to the human body or any part thereof for cleansing, beautifying, promoting attractiveness, or altering the appearance, and (2) articles intended for use as a component of any such articles; except that such term shall not include soap."[8] Interestingly, soaps are defined by regulation as articles made primarily of alkali salts of fatty acids whose detergent properties are due to the alkali-fatty acid compounds and that are labeled and sold only as soap and without cosmetic claims such as 'moisturizing' or 'deodorant.'[9]

These definitions and, in particular, the stipulation that soaps may only be labeled and sold as soap allude to the principle that the intended use of the product determines how it is regulated. If a product to be applied to the body in some fashion is intended to do anything other than cleanse or beautify, that product is not a simple cosmetic. As such, shampoos with ingredients for treating dandruff are regulated both as cosmetics and as over-the-counter (OTC) drugs. Similarly, toothpaste with fluoride to prevent cavities is both a cosmetic and an OTC drug.

The following 13 categories of cosmetic products are listed in 21 CFR 720.4(c):

- baby products
- bath preparations
- eye makeup preparations
- fragrance preparations
- hair preparations (non-coloring)
- hair coloring preparations
- makeup preparations (not eye)
- manicuring preparations
- oral hygiene products
- personal cleanliness products
- shaving preparations
- skin care preparations (creams, lotions, powder and sprays)
- suntan preparations

Safety and Adulteration

As noted previously, FDA does not approve cosmetics or cosmetic ingredients, other than colors, prior to their introduction into the marketplace. Only after market introduction do cosmetic products come under FDA's authority. Nevertheless, Section 601 of the *FD&C Act* prohibits the introduction into interstate commerce of cosmetics that are adulterated.[10] Cosmetic products may be considered adulterated if they:

- may be injurious to users under conditions of customary use (except for hair dyes)
- are composed of a potentially harmful substance
- contain filthy, putrid or decomposed substances
- contain a non-permitted or non-certified color additive
- are manufactured or held under unsanitary conditions that may have caused them to become injurious to users or contaminated with filth
- are packaged in containers composed of harmful substances

While injurious products other than hair dyes[11] are not permitted, cosmetic manufacturers are not required to conduct product testing to substantiate product performance or safety. However, if safety testing has not been conducted, the regulations require that the following warning be included on the product label: "WARNING: The safety of this product has not been determined." As noted in the regulation, this warning statement "does not constitute an exemption to the adulteration provisions of the Act or to any other requirement in the Act or this chapter."[12] Since cosmetic ingredients do not require prior FDA approval or certification of safety and since safety testing is not required, FDA must prove that an ingredient is harmful or unsafe under conditions of use prior to removing unsafe, adulterated products from the market.

Although FDA does not certify or approve cosmetic ingredients other than colors, the use of a few ingredients is prohibited or restricted by regulation due to safety concerns. The prohibited ingredients, listed in 21 CFR 700, are:

- bithionol

- mercury compounds
- vinyl chloride
- halogenated salicylanilides
- zirconium complexes in aerosol cosmetics
- chloroform
- methylene chloride
- chlorofluorocarbon propellants
- hexachlorophene
- methyl methacrylate monomer in nail products

Additionally, FDA restricts the use of certain materials from cattle due to concerns regarding Bovine Spongiform Encephalopathy.[13] FDA also promotes the use of safe ingredients in cosmetics by participating in the Cosmetic Ingredient Review (CIR). CIR is an industry-sponsored organization that reviews cosmetic ingredient safety and publishes its results in open, peer-reviewed literature. FDA participates in CIR in a non-voting capacity.

Cosmetic Labeling and Misbranding

The *FD&C Act* gives FDA regulatory authority over cosmetic product labeling. Federal Trade Commission (FTC) regulations authorized by the *Fair Packaging and Labeling Act* (*FPLA*) also apply to cosmetic products. The labeling regulations promulgated by FDA are found in 21 CFR 701 and 740, while those promulgated by FTC are found in 16 CFR 500.

The definition of "label" differs between the *FD&C Act* and *FPLA*. The *FD&C Act* definition is "a display of written, printed or graphic matter upon the immediate container," while *FPLA* defines the term as "written, printed or graphic matter affixed to any consumer commodity or affixed to or appearing upon a package containing any consumer commodity." However, any disparity in the definition is overcome by the *FD&C Act* requirement that any information required on the label of the immediate container shall also appear on any outer container.[14]

Taken together, the acts and regulations listed above require five basic elements on cosmetic product labels:
- statement of identity
- net quantity of contents
- ingredient list
- signature line declaring the product manufacturer or distributor's name and location
- certain warning statements

Some of these required elements must appear on the principal display panel (PDP) of the label. The PDP is the portion of the label most likely to be displayed under customary conditions of retail sale. Typically, the PDP is the front panel of the package; however, any other panel that includes the product name is considered an alternate PDP and must include any label elements required by regulation to appear on the PDP. Some cosmetics are marketed in very small or highly stylized or decorative containers. The regulation under 21 CFR 710.13 states that the PDP of cosmetics in "'boudoir-type' container[s] including decorative cosmetic containers of the 'cartridge,' 'pill box,' 'compact,' or 'pencil' variety, and those with a capacity of one-fourth ounce or less" may be affixed to the container via a tag.

Statement of Identity

A statement of identity must appear on cosmetic label PDPs. According to 21 CFR 701.11, the statement of identity shall be the common or usual name of the cosmetic; a descriptive name; a fanciful name commonly understood to identity such a cosmetic; or an illustration or vignette depicting the intended cosmetic use of the product. The categories and subcategories of cosmetic products listed in 21 CFR 720.4 may serve as appropriate statements of identity.

The statement of identity may appear anywhere on the PDP but must be generally parallel to the container. The statement must be in bold type of "a size reasonably related to the most prominent printed matter on such panel."[15]

Net Quantity of Contents Statement

The regulations stipulating the format, placement and size of the net quantity of contents (net contents) statements are found in 21 CFR 701.13. The net contents statement must accurately declare the quantity of cosmetic in the container whether in terms of weight, volume, measure, numerical count or a combination thereof. The net contents statement on aerosol products must declare the net quantity of contents expelled.

Generally, if the cosmetic is a liquid, the net contents statement must be expressed as a fluid measure such as the US fluid ounce, pint, quart, etc. Fluid measures must declare the volume at 68°F (20°C). Cosmetics that are solid, semi-solid, viscous or a mixture of solid and liquid must be declared in avoirdupois pounds and ounces. Net contents declarations for aerosol products are made in terms of weight. Net contents may additionally be stated in metric units. The term "net weight" or "net wt." must be used in conjunction with a weight statement; terms such as "net contents" or "net" may be used in a liquid statement of contents.

The net contents statement must appear on the PDP and any alternate PDPs in the lower 30% of the panel, generally parallel to the base of the package as displayed. The statement must be distinct and conspicuous, printed in boldface type that is in distinct contrast to other matter on the package. The statement must be at least one-sixteenth inch in height for PDPs smaller than five square inches and one-eighth inch for PDPs of 5 to 25 square inches.

The net contents statement must be separated from other text above or below it by a space at least equal to the height of the lettering used in the statement itself. Separation of the statement from other label items on either side must be by a space at least twice the width of the letter "N" of the text used in the contents statement.

Ingredient List

Cosmetic product ingredients must be listed on the immediate container as well as any outer container in descending order of prominence, unless the ingredients are flavors, fragrances or trade secret[16] elements. The ingredient list must be in a type size not less than one-sixteenth of an inch in height as measured on the lower-case "o" for most packages. If the total area available to bear labeling is less than 12 square inches, the ingredient list may be in type of one-thirty-second of an inch in height. The ingredient list may appear on any information panel. If there is no information panel, the ingredient list must appear on the PDP.

Ingredient Naming Conventions

Cosmetic ingredients must be identified by established names specified in 21 CFR 701.30. If no name for an ingredient has been specified by FDA, regulations stipulate that the names used in the following references are to be used in the order listed.

- CTFA (Cosmetic, Toiletry and Fragrance Association, Inc.) *Cosmetic Ingredient Dictionary*, Second Ed., 1977
- *United States Pharmacopeia*, 19th Ed., 1975, and Second Supplement to the USP XIX and NF XIV, 1976
- *National Formulary*, 14th Ed., 1975, and Second Supplement to the USP XIX and NF XIV, 1976.)
- *Food Chemicals Codex*, 2d Ed., 1972; First Supplement, 1974, and Second Supplement, 1975
- United States Adopted Name (USAN) and the USP dictionary of drug names, USAN 1975, 1961–1975 cumulative list

If the ingredient is not listed in any of the above sources, it should be designated by a common name generally recognizable to consumers. If the ingredient does not have a common name, it should be listed by its chemical name.

It has become common to see cosmetic ingredients listed using International Nomenclature Cosmetic Ingredient (INCI) names. This nomenclature system, used by the EU, was originally adopted from CTFA's *Cosmetic Ingredient Dictionary*.[17] While CTFA has petitioned FDA repeatedly since the mid-1990s,[18] and although FDA participates in the International Cooperation on Cosmetic Regulation (ICCR),[19] FDA has yet to fully embrace INCI naming conventions, which include the use of genus and species names for botanical ingredients. Consequently, it is common to see both the INCI name followed by a US common name in parentheses in cosmetic ingredient lists.

Name and Place of Business

Cosmetic labels also are required to conspicuously declare the manufacturer, packer or distributor's name and place of business. If the name listed is not that of the manufacturer, it must be preceded by an appropriate statement such as "distributed by" or "packed by." The corporate name must be used, and the business address must include the street, city, state and zip code. The street address is not required if the corporation is listed in a current city directory or telephone directory.

Warning Statements

As noted previously, labels on cosmetics whose safety has not been substantiated must include a warning noting that fact. Specific warning statements are also required on:
- cosmetics in self-pressurized containers (21 CFR 740.11)
- feminine deodorant sprays (21 CFR 740.12)
- foaming detergent bath products (21 CFR 740.17)
- coal tar hair dyes posing a risk of cancer (21 CFR 740.18)
- sun tanning preparations (21 CFR 740.19)

In addition, the label of any product that may pose a health hazard must include a warning statement, as appropriate, regarding the associated hazard. Any required warning statements must be prominent and conspicuous using bold type no less than one-sixteenth inch in height on a contrasting background.

Incomplete or improper labeling may render a cosmetic misbranded. Section 602 of the *FD&C Act* prohibits the introduction into interstate commerce of cosmetics that are misbranded.[20] Cosmetic products are considered misbranded if:
- labeling is false or misleading
- label fails to state prominently and conspicuously any required information
- container presentation or fill is misleading

Claims

By definition, cosmetics are intended to cleanse, beautify, promote attractiveness or alter appearance. Accordingly, claims about cosmetic products are restricted to stating how the product changes appearance, beautifies or cleanses and may not discuss changes to the structure or any function of the human body. As noted previously, the intended use of a product determines how it is regulated. Intended use can be established in part by claims on the product label, labeling, advertising or promotional material, including websites. Cosmetic products marketed to change the body's structure or function or to diagnose, treat, cure or prevent disease are drugs or medical devices. A product that "improves the appearance of fine lines or wrinkles" is a cosmetic, but products that remove or physically alter wrinkles, such as injected collagen or Botox, are medical devices and drugs, respectively.

FDA has begun to issue Warning Letters regarding anti-aging and wrinkle repair claims.[21–25] In recent letters to Avon[26] and Lancome,[27] FDA cited claims for wrinkle reduction that included detailed descriptions of the products' mechanisms of action that were clearly to alter the structure or function of the skin. While claims such as 'reduces the appearance of fine lines and wrinkles' would be an acceptable cosmetic claim, FDA considered the following to be drug claims:

- "Rebuild collagen to help plump out lines and wrinkles."
- "Stimulate elastin to help improve elasticity and resilience."
- "Regenerate hydroproteins to help visibly minimize creasing."
- "Improve fine & deep wrinkles up to 50%."
- "Immediately plumps out wrinkles and fine lines."
- "See significant deep wrinkle reduction in UV damaged skin, clinically proven."
- "Immediate lifting, lasting repositioning. Inspired by eye-lifting surgical techniques . . . helps recreate a younger, lifted look in the delicate eye area."

It is common today to see products that are labeled as "cruelty free" or "not tested on animals." These terms have no legal meaning, and their use has not been restricted by FDA. Consequently, it is unclear what meaning is intended by the companies using these claims. No matter the intended meaning, these and any other claims on cosmetics and all other consumer products must meet the basic standard of the FTC that they be truthful and not misleading. FDA and FTC published a memorandum of understanding in 1971 stating that the agencies would work in tandem on cases of improper claims and advertising.[28]

GMPs

GMPs are not included in cosmetic regulations; however, compliance with GMPs can minimize the risk that products will be adulterated or misbranded. Consequently, the agency has published guidelines for the industry based upon FDA's Inspection Operations Manual.[29]

Section 301 of the *FD&C Act* authorizes FDA to enter and inspect cosmetic company facilities to prevent introduction of adulterated or misbranded cosmetics into interstate commerce. Companies complying with these guidelines are less likely to encounter regulatory problems.

These guidelines are basic to all GMP procedures and cover the building, equipment, personnel, raw materials, production procedures, laboratory controls, recordkeeping, labeling and customer complaint files. In brief, the building construction and design should be adequate to permit orderly, sanitary manufacturing operations. Production, storage and handling equipment and utensils should be appropriate for the application and easy to clean and maintain. Personnel are to be properly trained, and all materials used in the manufacture of the cosmetics should be stored and handled so as to prevent contamination and ensure certain identification and regulatory status. Manufacturing control procedures should be in place to ensure that the product will be properly made and match specifications and labeling. The guidelines outline procedures for examining or testing incoming raw materials to ensure identification and purity as well as retention of manufactured lots for compliance checks. Additionally, the maintenance of records is covered in the GMP guidelines. Records should be kept of all materials; batch manufacturing, processing, handling, transferring, holding and filling; and labeling and distribution of all finished products. Records of any consumer complaints also should be kept.

While it is not clear how Vienna Beauty Products came to the attention of FDA and was subsequently inspected, the Warning Letter cited many violations that would have been less likely if a GMP program were in place and being followed. Vienna Beauty Products, which at the time was supplying cosmetics to several large drug store chains, received a Warning Letter in May 2012 after inspections in October, November and December of 2011. The Warning Letter cited the following conditions that led to microbial contamination of the finished goods:

"Specifically, there was apparent filth and dust build up on manufacturing equipment in the production area. A layer of sediment and encrusted material was observed on the exterior and tops of production kettles in use. Information obtained during the inspection indicates that the production room floor is cleaned and sanitized once per year; the last cleaning was performed November 2010 during a shutdown period. Based on other information obtained during the inspection, the 250 and 500 gallon kettles were last cleaned 15 years ago. The last cleaning of the 400 gallon shower gel kettle could not be determined. Additionally, the finished product storage tank and storage totes were said to have last been cleaned over 20 years ago."[30]

Cosmetics That are Also Drugs or Medical Devices

According to the definition above, shampoo used for cleansing the hair is a cosmetic. However, shampoo that includes ingredients to control dandruff, and toothpaste containing fluoride for prevention of cavities are also OTC drugs and must conform to regulations for both drugs and cosmetics.[31] Similarly, contact lenses used to alter the appearance of eye color are regulated as medical devices, as are breast implants.[32]

When a cosmetic product is also an OTC drug, the label must have a "Drug Facts" box to declare the active drug ingredients, indications, uses, etc., as required by regulation (See Chapter 15 Over-the-Counter Drug Products). The cosmetic ingredients in cosmetic/OTC combination products must be declared in the inactive ingredient portion of the drug facts box. Cosmetics that are also medical devices must be the subject of Premarket Approval Application or 510(k) submissions, as appropriate, and must conform to all applicable medical device regulations.

Related Products

Some companies market products as "cosmeceuticals," a term that has no recognized regulatory status.[33] Such products may be promoted only to cleanse or beautify. However, if their labeling includes claims that they affect the structure or function of the body, these products would be regulated as drugs or devices. Aromatherapy products pose interesting regulatory questions: perfumes are regulated as cosmetics by FDA, while room deodorizers are regulated by the Consumer Product Safety Commission. If a scented product is marketed to treat or prevent a disease or otherwise affect the body's structure or function, it is regulated as a drug.[34]

Permanent and temporary tattoos as well as permanent make-up are regulated as cosmetics.[35] The pigments used in these products are regulated as color additives and are subject to premarket approval. It is difficult to determine the contents of permanent tattoo pigments since products for professional use are exempt from labeling regulations. The resurgence in the popularity of tattoos has prompted FDA to update communications regarding the safety of tattooing.[36] It is interesting to note that even though henna is approved only for use in hair dye and not for direct application to skin, products containing henna are on the market for use in *mehndi*, the South Asian practice of skin decoration that is popular among some groups in the US. FDA has issued an import alert requiring that henna products intended for use on the skin be detained.[37]

Products that are used to cleanse or beautify animals are classified as grooming aids and are not regulated by FDA. In recent years, some grooming aids designed for animals have become popular with people.[38] Bag Balm, originally intended for use on cows' udders, became a popular hand cream, and products formulated to keep horses' hooves healthy have been used by people to strengthen fingernails. If a manufacturer markets grooming aids to humans, labeling must comply with cosmetic regulations.

Facility and Product Registration

Cosmetic companies are not subject to mandatory establishment registration or ingredient reporting, but they may voluntarily register their establishments and their product compositions through FDA's Voluntary Cosmetic Registration Program (VCRP).[39,40] Data provided through the VCRP help CIR prioritize its safety testing program. Unless noted as proprietary, information provided through VCRP may be obtained through the *Freedom of Information Act*.

Registration also enables FDA to notify cosmetic companies about potential problems with the ingredients in their products and helps the agency with inspections that may be necessary. The VCRP is not an approval program, and registrants are prohibited from using participation in the VCRP as a promotional tool.[41] Close to two thousand companies have registered voluntarily over 36,000 cosmetic formulations since the online registration system was launched in December 2005.[42]

Importing and Exporting Cosmetic Products

Cosmetic products imported into the US must comply with the same regulations as those produced domestically. While registration is not required, foreign cosmetic companies are encouraged to participate in the VCRP. Any companies or individuals wishing to import cosmetics or any other FDA-regulated product into the US must file an entry notice and entry bond with the US Customs Service. The Customs Service notifies FDA of the import, and FDA makes a determination regarding the product's admissibility. FDA may admit the product into the US, refuse entry or examine the product for compliance, including performing laboratory testing of the ingredients.

Cosmetic products for export from the US do not have to comply with US regulations, but only with those of the importing country.[43] Some countries require certificates for imported products. FDA does issue certificates for cosmetic products intended for export; however, since cosmetics are not approved by FDA these certificates simply list the product names provided by the exporter and do not indicate agency review or approval of the product. Form FDA 3613d is used for requesting cosmetics certificates.

Compliance and Enforcement

FDA carries out enforcement activities against cosmetics companies despite the fact that cosmetic manufacturing facilities are not required to register with FDA or comply with GMP regulations, and that cosmetic products are not subject to premarket review or approval. The discussion of the findings noted above during an inspection of Vienna Beauty Products is an example.[44] Many FDA enforcement actions are carried out to ensure that cosmetic products are not adulterated or misbranded. Recently, FDA took enforcement action against GIB LLC doing business as Brazilian Blowout. The Warning Letter sent to the company noted that the product was adulterated due to the presence of methylene glycol, which was described as 'the liquid form of formaldehyde' and as 'releas[ing] formaldehyde when hair treated with the product is heated with a blow dryer'.[45]

As noted previously, FDA works with FTC to enforce cosmetics labeling regulations. In addition, CFSAN, which has regulatory responsibility for cosmetics, works with the Center for Drug Evaluation and Research (CDER) through an intercenter agreement when reviewing cosmetic products with labeling that includes drug claims.[46] Under this agreement, a product promoted as a cosmetic to enhance eyelashes was the subject of Warning Letters and finally product seizure due to the presence of a glaucoma drug.[47] Similarly, Warning Letters were issued regarding various skin care products marketed with drug claims.[48] While FDA does not have authority to recall cosmetic products, the agency can request that a company recall its products.[49] On 5 January 2009, FDA announced recall of a make-up remover due to contamination with *Pseudomonas aeruginosa*.[50]

FDA also has undertaken enforcement actions against devices marketed for cosmetic use to beautify the skin and hair. Gaunitz Hair Sciences LLC was marketing a laser for hair growth,[51] while Sunetics International Corporation was marketing laser skin and hair brushes,[52] and Rejuvenu International Ltd. was marketing a hair removal system.[53] None of these devices had premarket clearance and most were being promoted to change the structure or function of the body and were, therefore, unapproved medical devices. All of these companies received letters notifying them that their products were adulterated and misbranded.

Summary

- Cosmetics are products that are applied or introduced to the body for cleansing, beautifying, promoting attractiveness or altering the appearance.
- Cosmetics are not subject to premarket approval or GMP regulations; facility registration and product listing are voluntary.
- Regulations require that cosmetic products be safe but do not require safety testing.
- Regulations prohibit the marketing of cosmetic products that are adulterated or misbranded.
- Five basic elements must appear on cosmetic product labels:
- statement of identity
- net quantity of contents statement
- ingredient list
- signature line
- certain warning statements
- Products that alter both appearance and the structure or function of the body are regulated as cosmetic-drug combination products or cosmetic-medical device combination products.

References

1. H.R. 5786 (111th): *Safe Cosmetics Act* of 2010. GovTrack.us website. www.govtrack.us/congress/bills/111/hr5786. Accessed 6 April 2013.
2. H.R. 2359 (112th): *Safe Cosmetics Act of 2011*. GovTrack.us website. www.govtrack.us/congress/bills/112/hr2359. Accessed 6 April 2013.
3. H.R. 4262 (112th): Cosmetics Safety Enhancement Act of 2012, GovTrack.us website. www.govtrack.us/congress/bills/112/hr4262#overview. Accessed 8 April 2013.
4. H.R. 4395 (112th): Cosmetic Safety Amendments Act of 2012, GovTrack.us website. www.govtrack.us/congress/bills/112/hr4395/text. Accessed 6 April 2013.
5. Op cit 1.
6. Op cit 2.
7. Op cit 4.
8. *Federal Food, Drug, and Cosmetic Act* of 1938 (*FD&C Act*), Chapter II. FDA website. www.fda.gov/opacom/laws/fdcact/fdcact1.htm. Accessed 6 April 2013.
9. 21 CFR Part 701.20. www.accessdata.fda.gov/scripts/cdrh/cfdocs/cfcfr/CFRSearch.cfm?fr=701.20. Accessed 6 April 2013.
10. *FD&C Act*, Chapter VI. FDA website. www.fda.gov/RegulatoryInformation/Legislation/FederalFoodDrugandCosmeticActFDCAct/FDCActChapterVICosmetics/. Accessed 6 April 2013.
11. Hair Dye Products. FDA website. www.fda.gov/Cosmetics/ProductandIngredientSafety/ProductInformation/ucm143066.htm. Accessed 6 April 2013.
12. 21 CFR Sec. 740.10(c). FDA website. www.accessdata.fda.gov/scripts/cdrh/cfdocs/cfcfr/CFRSearch.cfm?fr=740.10. Accessed 6 April 2013.
13. Bovine Spongiform Encephalopathy (BSE). FDA website. www.fda.gov/Cosmetics/ProductandIngredientSafety/PotentialContaminants/ucm136786.htm. Accessed 6 April 2013.
14. *FD&C Act*, Section 201(k). GPO website. www.gpo.gov/fdsys/pkg/USCODE-2010-title21/pdf/USCODE-2010-title21-chap9-subchapII-sec321.pdf. Accessed 8 April 2013.
15. 21 CFR 710.11. FDA website. www.accessdata.fda.gov/scripts/cdrh/cfdocs/cfcfr/CFRSearch.cfm?fr=701.11. Accessed 8 April 2013.
16. 21 CFR 720.8. FDA website. www.accessdata.fda.gov/scripts/cdrh/cfdocs/cfcfr/CFRSearch.cfm?fr=720.8&SearchTerm=identity%20labeling. Accessed 8 April 2013.
17. FDA Response to CTFA Requests Regarding Harmonization of Ingredient Names (Color Additives, Denatured Alcohol, and Plant Extracts). FDA website. www.fda.gov/Cosmetics/CosmeticLabelingLabelClaims/IndustryRequestsFDAResponses/ucm075032.htm. Accessed 8 April 2013.
18. International Harmonization of Nomenclature: Industry Requests and FDA Responses. FDA website. www.fda.gov/Cosmetics/InternationalActivities/InternationalHarmonizationofNomenclature/default.htm. Accessed 8 April 2013.
19. International Programs: International Cooperation on Cosmetic Regulation ICCR-2. FDA website. www.fda.gov/InternationalPrograms/HarmonizationInitiatives/ucm114520.htm. Accessed 8 April 2013.
20. Op cit 3.
21. Warning Letter Hydroderm 25-Sep-05. FDA website. www.fda.gov/ICECI/EnforcementActions/WarningLetters/2005/ucm075572.htm. Accessed 8 April 2013.
22. Warning Letter Avon Products, Inc. (U.S. Headquarters) 10/5/12. FDA website. www.fda.gov/ICECI/EnforcementActions/WarningLetters/2012/ucm323738.htm. Accessed 8 April 2013.
23. Warning Letter Bioque Technology 10/5/12. FDA website. www.fda.gov/ICECI/EnforcementActions/WarningLetters/2012/ucm323767.htm. Accessed 8 April 2013.
24. Warning Letter Janson-Beckett 9/21/12. FDA website. www.fda.gov/ICECI/EnforcementActions/WarningLetters/2012/ucm321111.htm. Accessed 8 April 2013.
25. Warning Letter Lancome 9/7/12. FDA website. www.fda.gov/ICECI/EnforcementActions/WarningLetters/2012/ucm318809.htm. Accessed 8 April 2013.
26. Op cit 22.
27. Op cit 25.

28. "Memorandum of Understanding Between Federal Trade Commission and the Food and Drug Administration," *Federal Register*, Vol 36, No. 180, 16 September 1971.
29. Cosmetic Good Manufacturing Practice Guidelines/Inspection Checklist, 12 February 1997; Updated 24 April 2008. FDA website. www.fda.gov/Cosmetics/GuidanceComplianceRegulatoryInformation/GoodManufacturingPracticeGMPGuidelinesInspectionChecklist/default.htm Accessed 8 April 2013.
30. Warning Letter Vienna Beauty Products 5/17/12. FDA website. www.fda.gov/ICECI/EnforcementActions/WarningLetters/2012/ucm313452.htm. Accessed 8 April 2013.
31. "Is It a Cosmetic, a Drug, or Both? (Or Is It Soap?)." FDA website. www.fda.gov/Cosmetics/GuidanceComplianceRegulatoryInformation/ucm074201.htm. Accessed 8 April 2013.
32. *Guidance for Industry, FDA Staff, Eye Care Professionals, and Consumers: Decorative, Non-corrective Contact Lenses* (November 2006). FDA website. www.fda.gov/MedicalDevices/DeviceRegulationandGuidance/GuidanceDocuments/ucm071572.htm. Accessed 8 April 2013.
33. "Cosmeceuctical" (24 February 2000). FDA website. http://www.fda.gov/Cosmetics/ProductandIngredientSafety/ProductInformation/ucm127064.htm. Accessed 8 April 2013.
34. Aromatherapy (13 March 2000). FDA website. www.fda.gov/Cosmetics/ProductandIngredientSafety/ProductInformation/ucm127054.htm. Accessed 8 April 2013.
35. Tattoos & Permanent Makeup (Updated 23 June 2008). FDA website. www.fda.gov/Cosmetics/ProductandIngredientSafety/ProductInformation/ucm108530.htm. Accessed 8 April 2013.
36. Ibid.
37. Import Alert. Detention Without Physical Examination of Henna Based Skin Color. FDA website. www.accessdata.fda.gov/cms_ia/importalert_138.html. Accessed 8 April 2013.
38. Willman M. "Using Pet Products on People." *Los Angeles Times* (22 October 1999).
39. 21 CFR 710. FDA website. www.accessdata.fda.gov/scripts/cdrh/cfdocs/cfcfr/CFRSearch.cfm?CFRPart=710. Accessed 8 April 2013.
40. 21 CFR 720. FDA website. www.accessdata.fda.gov/scripts/cdrh/cfdocs/cfcfr/CFRSearch.cfm?CFRPart=720. Accessed 8 April 2013.
41. Voluntary Cosmetic Registration Program (VCRP). FDA website. www.fda.gov/Cosmetics/GuidanceComplianceRegulatoryInformation/VoluntaryCosmeticsRegistrationProgramVCRP/default.htm. Accessed 8 April 2013.
42. Voluntary Cosmetic Registration Program (VCRP) Monthly Status Reports. FDA website. www.fda.gov/Cosmetics/GuidanceComplianceRegulatoryInformation/VoluntaryCosmeticsRegistrationProgramVCRP/ucm280194.htm. Accessed 8 April 2013.
43. Cosmetics Exports. FDA website. www.fda.gov/Cosmetics/InternationalActivities/ImportsExports/CosmeticExports/default.htm. Accessed 8 april 2013.
44. Op cit 30.
45. Warning Letter GIB LLC dba Brazilian Blowout 8/22/11. FDA website. www.fda.gov/ICECI/EnforcementActions/WarningLetters/2011/ucm270809.htm. Accessed 8 April 2013.
46. "Intercenter Agreement Between the Center for Drug Evaluation and Research and the Center for Food Safety and Applied Nutrition to Assist FDA in Implementing the Drug and Cosmetic Provisions of the Federal Food, Drug and Cosmetic Act for Products that Purport to be Cosmetics but Meet the Statutory Definition of a Drug" (1 June 2006). FDA website. www.fda.gov/Cosmetics/GuidanceComplianceRegulatoryInformation/ComplianceEnforcement/ucm2005170.htm. Accessed 8 April 2013.
47. Approximately $2 Million of Potentially Harmful "Cosmetic" Eye Product Seized. News release 16 November 2007. FDA website. www.fda.gov/NewsEvents/Newsroom/PressAnnouncements/2007/ucm109028.htm. Accessed 8 April 2013.
48. Freedom Plus Corporation Warning Letter (29 March 2007). FDA website. www.fda.gov/ICECI/EnforcementActions/WarningLetters/2007/ucm076343.htm. Accessed 8 April 2013.
49. Cosmetics Recall and Alerts policy (29 July 2002). FDA website. www.fda.gov/Cosmetics/ProductandIngredientSafety/RecallsAlerts/default.htm. Accessed 8 April 2013.
50. Recall—Firm Press Release. Celeste Industries Corporation Recalls All Lots of simplySmart Remove Make Up Remover (5 January 2009). FDA website. www.fda.gov/Safety/Recalls/ArchiveRecalls/2009/ucm128452.htm. Accessed 8 April 2013.
51. Gaunitz Hair Sciences LLC Warning Letter (7 August 2008). FDA website. www.fda.gov/ICECI/EnforcementActions/WarningLetters/2008/ucm1048189.htm. Accessed 8 April 2013.
52. Sunetics International Corporation Warning Letter (7 August 2008). FDA website. www.fda.gov/ICECI/EnforcementActions/WarningLetters/2008/ucm1048188.htm. Accessed 8 April 2013.
53. Rejuvenu International Ltd. Warning Letter (16 August 2004). FDA website. www.fda.gov/ICECI/EnforcementActions/WarningLetters/2004/ucm146892.htm. Accessed 8 April 2013.

Chapter 32

Veterinary Products

Updated by Jeffrey Zinza, RAC

OBJECTIVES

❑ Identify the regulations and agencies governing veterinary products

❑ Develop a broad understanding of the regulation of veterinary drugs, feeds, devices and biologics

---

LAWS, REGULATIONS AND GUIDELINES COVERED IN THIS CHAPTER

❑ *Federal Food, Drug, and Cosmetic Act* of 1938

❑ *Animal Medicinal Drug Use Clarification Act* of 1994

❑ *Animal Drug Availability Act* of 1996

❑ *Animal Drug User Fee Act* of 2003

❑ *Animal Drug User Fee Amendments* of 2008

❑ *Animal Generic Drug User Fee Act* of 2008

❑ *Minor Use and Minor Species Animal Health Act* of 2004

❑ *Generic Animal Drug and Patent Term Restoration Act* of 1988

❑ *Virus-Serum-Toxin Act* of 1913

❑ *Federal Insecticide, Fungicide, and Rodenticide Act* of 1972

❑ 9 CFR Subchapter E—Animals and animal products—viruses, serums, toxins, and analogous products; organisms and vectors

❑ 21 CFR 225–226 Current Good Manufacturing Practice for medicated feeds and Type A medicated articles

❑ 21 CFR 501 Animal food labeling

❑ 21 CFR 511 New animal drugs for investigational use

❑ 21 CFR 514 New animal drug applications

❑ 21 CFR 515 Medicated mill feed license

❑ 21 CFR 516 New animal drugs for minor use and minor species

❑ 21 CFR 530 Extralabel drug use in animals

❑ 21 CFR 558 New animal drugs for use in animal feeds

❑ *Guidance for Industry 61: FDA Approval of New Animal Drugs for Minor Uses and for Minor Species* (May 2008)

- *Guidance for Industry 82: Development of Supplemental Applications for Approved New Animal Drugs* (October 2002)

- *Draft Guidance for Industry 132: The Administrative New Animal Drug Application Process* (November 2002)

- *Guidance for Industry 170: Animal Drug User Fees and Fee Waivers and Reductions* (October 2008)

- *Guidance for Industry 173: Animal Drug Sponsor Fees under the Animal Drug User Fee Act (ADUFA)* (February 2005)

- *VS Memorandum No. 800.50: Basic License Requirements and Guidelines for Submission of Materials in Support of Licensure* (February 2011)

- *VS Memorandum No. 800.57: Market Suspensions* (September 1999)

- *VS Memorandum No. 800.78: Preparation and Submission of Facilities Documents* (November 2010)

- *VS Memorandum No. 800.91: Categories of Inspection for Licensed Veterinary Biologics Establishments* (May 1999)

- *VS Memorandum 800.101: US Veterinary Biological Product Permits for Distribution and Sale* (May 2002)

Introduction

Veterinary medical products are diverse, ranging from new animal drugs, vaccines, devices and diagnostic test kits to animal food additives, feed ingredients and animal grooming aids. Veterinary medical products may be used to prevent, treat or diagnose diseases in animals. They also include products that may be administered to or consumed by animals that produce food for humans, as well as those that may be consumed by pets or companion animals.

A veterinary medical product may be regulated by one of several US federal agencies, depending on the product type and its intended use. These regulatory bodies focus on ensuring that marketed products safely and effectively relieve animal pain and suffering, sustain animal health and improve farm animal productivity without compromising public health.

FDA

The US Food and Drug Administration's (FDA) Center for Veterinary Medicine (CVM) is responsible for ensuring that animal drugs and medicated feeds are safe and effective and that food from treated animals is safe to eat. CVM also is responsible for the regulatory oversight of medical devices used in veterinary medicine. CVM's authority is derived from the *Federal Food, Drug, and Cosmetic Act* of 1938 (*FD&C Act*) and amendments.

Animal Drugs

Since 1968, the *FD&C Act* has included provisions designed to ensure that animal drugs are safe and effective for their intended uses and do not result in unsafe residues in foods. Two main processes are involved in regulating the interstate shipment of animal drug products. The Investigational New Animal Drug exemption (INAD) allows the interstate shipment of experimental drugs for testing in animals. The New Animal Drug Application (NADA) process—and its variants, the Abbreviated New Animal Drug Application (ANADA) and Administrative NADA—allow the marketing of a new animal drug.

INAD

Typically, the new animal drug approval process begins when a drug sponsor submits a request for an INAD exemption to CVM. This exemption will allow the sponsor to use, ship and label a particular unapproved drug for experimental purposes without violating the *FD&C Act*.

Once CVM grants the INAD exemption, the sponsor must:
- ensure proper and safe investigational drug packaging and labeling
- report to CVM the names and locations of investigators to whom drugs are shipped
- maintain records of all drug shipments for at least two years after delivery
- maintain all reports received from investigators for at least two years after the termination of the investigation or approval of a new animal drug application
- ensure that the new animal drug or animal feed containing a new animal drug actually will be used for tests in animals and is not used in humans
- notify CVM immediately if a safety problem is observed (periodic safety reporting is not required, except as specified in 21 CFR 514.80(b)(4))
- notify FDA or the US Department of Agriculture (USDA) prior to slaughter of food animals treated with the investigational drug
- submit a request under the INAD for categorical exclusion under 21 CFR 25.30 or 25.33 (If such exclusion is not authorized, then an environmental

assessment (EA) must be submitted in accordance with 21 CFR 25.40.)

The sponsor may ask the Office of New Animal Drug Evaluation (ONADE) to review protocols for experimental work intended to support an NADA submission. Although such review is not required, it may help the sponsor obtain the necessary data.

NADA

The *FD&C Act* prohibits the introduction into interstate commerce of new animal drugs without an approved NADA. The NADA includes data demonstrating the drug's safety in the target animal and for humans who might consume products from the treated animal.

ONADE reviews the NADA to determine whether the animal drug should be approved for marketing and to evaluate the drug's effectiveness for the purposes claimed. If ONADE determines that the NADA information shows the product will be safe and effective for its intended use, it makes a recommendation to the CVM director. If the director agrees with the recommendation, the application is approved, and a notice of the approval is published in the *Federal Register*. CVM must take an appropriate action within 180 days after the filing of an NADA.

Section 512(b) of the *FD&C Act* and 21 CFR 514 describe information that must be submitted to FDA as part of an NADA. An NADA normally will be submitted to FDA in several sections or volumes:

- Identification (21 CFR 514.1(b)(1))
- Table of Contents and Summary (21 CFR 514.1(b)(2))
- Labeling (21 CFR 514.1(b)(3))—copies of each proposed label
- Components and Composition (21 CFR 514.1(b)(4))—a list of all drug product components, a statement of the drug product's composition and a complete description of antibiotic drug substances' fermentation
- Manufacturing Methods, Facilities and Controls (21 CFR 514.1(b)(5))—a detailed description of the manufacturer, personnel, facilities/equipment, new animal drug substance synthesis, raw material controls (specifications, tests and methods), manufacturing instructions, finished product analytical controls (specifications, tests and methods), stability program, container/packaging and lot-control number system
- Samples (21 CFR 514.1(b)(6))—only if requested by CVM
- Analytical Methods for Residues (21 CFR 514.1(b)(7))—method(s) and data for determining drug residues remaining in food-producing animals
- Evidence to Establish Safety and Effectiveness (21 CFR 514.1(b)(8))—data/information to permit evaluation of the drug product's safety and effectiveness for the claim(s) in the proposed species
- Applicant's Commitments (21 CFR 514.1(b)(11)) to label and market the new animal drug under the conditions stated in the NADA
- Good Manufacturing Practice Compliance (21 CFR 514.1(b)(12)(ii))—a statement that methods, facilities, and controls described in 21 CFR 514.1(b)(5) conform to current Good Manufacturing Practice (CGMP)
- Good Laboratory Practice Compliance (21 CFR 514.1(b)(12)(iii))—a statement of compliance or noncompliance with Good Laboratory Practices (21 CFR 58) for each nonclinical laboratory study
- Environmental Assessment (21 CFR 514.1(b)(14))—an EA (21 CFR 25.40) containing sufficient data/information to permit evaluation of the drug product's environmental safety, or a claim for a categorical exclusion from preparing an EA (21 CFR 25.33), as appropriate

  EAs focus on the use and disposal of veterinary drugs or feed additives. If CVM determines that the EA information indicates no significant environmental impact is expected, the center prepares a Finding of No Significant Impact (FONSI). In general, drugs for therapeutic use in companion animals receive a FONSI, whereas such drugs as broad-spectrum endoparasiticides in food-producing animals will require a full EA.
- Freedom of Information Summary (21 CFR 514.11)—a summary of the studies serving as the basis for drug approval; FDA will release these to the public, as requested, to comply with the *Freedom of Information Act* of 1966 (*FOIA*)

CVM must evaluate NADAs and ANADAs within 30 days of receipt to determine whether the submission meets the standards for filing, i.e., contains all required information. If CVM determines the application is not acceptable for filing, it must notify the applicant of the reason.

Like drugs intended for use in humans, new animal drugs must be produced under CGMP requirements. CVM's *Guidance for Industry: Drug Substance Chemistry, Manufacturing, and Controls Information*[1] describes the drug substance information sponsors must submit to ensure continued drug substance and drug product quality (identity, strength, quality, purity and potency) in support of NADAs and ANADAs. In an effort to support global harmonization, CVM's CGMP requirements are moving into alignment with the International Cooperation on Harmonisation of Technical Requirements for Registration of Veterinary Products (VICH).[2] The CVM guidance indicates that this chemistry, manufacturing and controls information can be presented in the format of the Common Technical Document—Quality (CTD-Q).[3]

The NADA also must be accompanied by a user fee.[4,5] The user fee system was initially put in place for animal drugs under the *Animal Drug User Fee Act* (*ADUFA*) of 2003, also known as *ADUFA I*, and is similar to those for human drugs and medical devices. Each fee category—sponsor, product, establishment and application—accounts for approximately 25% of the total fees collected. *ADUFA* was originally set to expire on 30 September 2008, but the *Animal Drug User Fee Amendments of 2008*, also known as *ADUFA II,* extended this user fee program until 30 September 2013, in addition to other enhancements. The law provides for fee waivers or reductions, upon request, when:

- the fee would present a significant barrier to innovation because of limited resources available to such person or other circumstance
- the fees to be paid under *ADUFA II* will exceed the anticipated present and future costs incurred by FDA in reviewing NADAs
- the NADA or supplement is intended solely to provide for the animal drug's use in a free-choice medicated feed
- the application is submitted under the provisions of the *Minor Use or Minor Species Act* (*MUMS*) (discussed below) and intended solely to provide for a minor use or minor species indication
- the applicant is a recognized small business submitting its first animal drug application to FDA for review

Provisions are provided within *ADUFA II* for the return of 75% of the user fee if the application is refused for filing.[6]

ADUFA, as written, does not apply to ANADAs submitted under Section 512(b)(2) of the *FD&C Act*. However, the *Animal Generic Drug User Fee Act* of 2008 (*AGDUFA*) amended the *FD&C Act* and authorized FDA to collect fees to support the review of generic new animal drugs. *AGDUFA* is set to expire 30 September 2013.

FDA completed negotiations with industry regarding reauthorization of *ADUFA* and the *AGDUFA* user fee programs and held a public meeting in December 2012 to hear the public's views on the proposed recommendations for reauthorization of *ADUFA II* and *AGDUFA*. Reauthorization of the two programs through Fiscal 2018, known as *ADUFA III* and *AGDUFA II*, respectively, is expected to be complete in 2013. FDA provides information about user fee programs, including *ADUFA* and *AGDUFA*, online at www.fda.gov/ForIndustry/UserFees/default.htm.

Each approved animal drug manufacturer must submit certain information to FDA regarding patents covering the animal drug or its method of use, and the agency is required to make this information public. In addition, FDA must publicize a list of all animal drug products approved for safety and effectiveness, and must update the list monthly. This list, entitled List of FDA-Approved Animal Drug Products and known as the *Green Book*,[7] is available online at www.fda.gov/AnimalVeterinary/Products/ApprovedAnimalDrugProducts/UCM042847.

The *Animal Drug Availability Act* of 1996 (*ADAA*) introduced several amendments to the *FD&C Act*, lending flexibility to the way CVM regulates animal drugs and medicated feeds. This law was designed to increase the number of animal drugs on the market through several means:

- amending the current definition of "substantial evidence of effectiveness," thereby permitting flexibility in the studies required to demonstrate a new animal drug's effectiveness and eliminating the requirement for field studies
- providing greater direct interaction between animal drug sponsors and FDA during the drug development process
- creating a new category of drugs—Veterinary Feed Directive Drugs—allowing new animal drug approval and use in animal feed, on a veterinarian's order, while incorporating safeguards to ensure the safe use of such drugs
- supporting "flexible labeling," permitting a range of acceptable or recommended doses to appear on animal drug product labeling rather than one optimum dose (This broadens the approval process to make available more drugs to treat minor species.)

Phased Review and Administrative NADAs

CVM does not require applicants to submit an NADA as one complete package. Instead, applicants may submit individual, completed technical sections or components to the INAD file for technical review. For instance, the applicant may submit data and information on the target animal safety, effectiveness, human food safety and labeling separately as they are each compiled. Overall NADA requirements remain the same as described above.

When each technical submission has been submitted for phased review and CVM has issued a "technical section complete" letter for each, the manufacturer submits an Administrative NADA.[8] CVM must review and respond to this submission within 180 days, but the review should be completed more quickly, as the scientific content already has been assessed.

Expedited Review

Under the CVM Expedited Review Status (ERS) program, certain products that offer important advances in animal health or in the reduction of human pathogens in food animals receive priority review.[9] Products approved for expedited review will receive higher priority and a faster review than routine applications. For instance, an expedited

NADA review generally should be completed within 90 days rather than 180. The standards for data quality and evaluation are unchanged.

A sponsor may apply for expedited review status at the INAD or NADA stage. ONADE will review and assess the request and should reach a decision on the status within 60 days of receiving the request.

MUMS

MUMS is similar in principle to the human *Orphan Drug Act* of 1983. It provides incentives to sponsors to address the shortage of FDA-approved drugs for treating relatively rare disorders of major veterinary species (minor use) and less-common animal species (minor species) under a veterinarian's care.[10]

MUMS defines minor species as all animals other than the major species (cattle, horses, swine, chickens, turkeys, dogs and cats). Minor species include zoo animals, ornamental fish, parrots, ferrets and guinea pigs. Some animals of agricultural importance also are considered minor species for the purposes of *MUMS*, e.g., sheep, goats, catfish and other food fish and honeybees.

MUMS creates three major incentives:

Conditional Approvals

A sponsor of a veterinary drug for a minor use or minor species can apply for "conditional approval," which allows the sponsor to market the drug before collecting all necessary effectiveness data, but only after proving the drug is safe in accordance with the full FDA approval standard and that there is a reasonable expectation of effectiveness. The drug sponsor can keep the product on the market for up to five years, through annual renewals, while collecting the remaining required effectiveness data. This provision is managed by ONADE, not by the Office of Minor Use and Minor Species Animal Drug Development (OMUMS).

Indexing

CVM can designate unapproved new drugs as legally marketed for a minor species. CVM may add the intended use to the Index of Legally Marketed Unapproved New Animal Drugs for Minor Species (the Index).[11,12] 21 CFR 516, Subpart C, provides standards and procedures to establish an index of legally marketed unapproved new animal drugs. Under the indexing rule, CVM:

- grants investigational exemptions for indexing purposes
- determines the eligibility of new animal drugs for indexing consideration
- approves the selection of qualified expert panels to review drug safety and effectiveness data
- reviews the findings of expert panels, issues final decisions and publishes the index

Designation

Similar to *Orphan Drug Act* provisions for human drugs with limited uses, CVM may designate a drug as eligible for monetary incentives and marketing exclusivity.[13,14] The manufacturer of the drug under development for a minor use or minor species is eligible for safety and effectiveness data development grants. The product is granted seven years of marketing exclusivity upon its approval or conditional approval for the minor use or minor species.

Abbreviated New Animal Drug Application (ANADA)

Products that are the same as an approved animal drug (the "pioneer" or reference product), have identical intended uses, and are demonstrated to be bioequivalent to the reference product may be approved through an ANADA. Broadly, the ANADA must contain information on the patent status of the reference product and the generic product's ingredients; labeling; bioequivalence; human food safety; chemistry, manufacturing and controls; and environmental impact.

CVM cannot approve generic versions of drugs that are still protected by patent or marketing exclusivity. Furthermore, the center will not approve ANADAs based on drugs that have been withdrawn from the market for safety or efficacy reasons.

The *Generic Animal Drug and Patent Term Restoration Act* of 1988 (*GADPTRA*) also provides for awarding of market exclusivity periods to products newly approved under NADAs, similar to the exclusivity awarded to certain newly approved drugs for human use. With *AGDUFA* of 2008, ANADAs submitted after 1 July 2008 are subject to a user fee program similar to that set forth by *ADUFA*. *AGDUFA* provides for fee waivers or reductions,[15] upon request, when the generic drug is intended solely to provide for a minor use or minor species indication.

Compendial Requirements

The *United States Pharmacopeia* (*USP*) and *National Formulary* (*NF*) are recognized as the official US compendia for human and animal drugs under the *FD&C Act*'s adulteration and misbranding provisions (Sections 501 and 502).[16] Since 1980, the two compendia have been published under the same cover (the *USP–NF*). Monographs for drug substances and preparations are featured in the *USP*; excipient monographs are in the *NF*.

Under *FD&C Act* requirements, ingredients, manufactured products and compounded preparations must have the strength, quality and purity specified in relevant *USP* and *NF* monographs. Monographs include the ingredient or preparation name; definition; packaging, storage and labeling requirements; and the specification. The specification is a series of analytical tests, test procedures and acceptance criteria. Certain tests and procedures require the use of official USP Reference Standards. *USP–NF* general chapters describe in detail analytical tests and procedures that are referenced in multiple monographs.

Animal Feeds, Medicated Feeds and Type A Medicated Articles

Feeds are either intended solely to meet an animal's nutritional requirements (non-medicated feeds) or as a means to orally administer drugs (medicated feeds). Animal feeds are defined under *FD&C Act* Section 201(w). CVM is responsible for both non-medicated animal feeds—including pet foods—and medicated feeds.

Animal feeds, like human foods, must be pure and wholesome, contain no harmful or deleterious substances and be truthfully labeled. Animal food labeling regulations are found in 21 CFR 501. Additionally, canned foods—including canned pet foods—must be processed in conformance with low-acid canned food regulations (21 CFR 113). Non-medicated animal feeds generally do not require FDA approval before they are marketed, provided they are made from ingredients that are either approved food additives or generally recognized as safe (GRAS) for their intended use. FDA is of the opinion that the *Dietary Supplement and Health Education Act* (*DSHEA*) does not apply to animal nutritional supplements and "nutraceuticals."[17] Substances marketed as human dietary supplements fall under the pre-*DSHEA* regulatory scheme when marketed for animals; they are considered food, food additives, GRAS items or new animal drugs, depending on the intended use. However, CVM often has exercised regulatory discretion and waived food additive petitions or NADAs for such articles when they are determined not to present animal or human safety concerns.

If a food substance is intended to treat or prevent disease or to affect the body's structure or function other than as a food, it falls within the *FD&C Act*'s definition of a drug. Thus, it must be the subject of an approved NADA, similar to that described above, before it can be marketed. Under 21 CFR 558, FDA recognizes Type A Medicated Articles, Type B Medicated Feeds and Type C Medicated Feeds.

Type A Medicated Articles are mixtures of one or more drug substance(s) with suitable vehicles. They are used to facilitate active drug component dilution and admixture with animal feed before administration. The manufacture of a Type A Medicated Article requires approval by CVM of either an NADA or ANADA for the medicated article. Type A Medicated Articles are divided into two categories. Category I includes those drugs that require no withdrawal period at the lowest use level in each species for which they are approved. Category II includes those drugs that require a withdrawal period at the lowest use level for at least one species for which they are approved, or are regulated on a "no-residue" basis or with a zero tolerance because of drug residue carcinogenic concerns. A Type A Medicated Article is intended solely for use in manufacturing another Type A Medicated Article (e.g., mixing two Type A Medicated Articles containing different active pharmaceutical ingredients to manufacture a third Type A Medicated Article) or a Type B or Type C Medicated Feed. Type A Article CGMPs are found in 21 CFR 226.

A Type B Medicated Feed contains either a Type A Medicated Article or another Type B Medicated Feed, plus a substantial quantity of nutrients (not less than 25% of the total weight), and is intended solely for use in manufacturing another Type B Medicated Feed or a Type C Medicated Feed. Before being fed to animals, a Type B Medicated Feed must be substantially diluted with one or more nutrients to produce a nutritionally appropriate and medically safe Type C Medicated Feed for administration to the patient.

A Type C Medicated Feed contains an active drug component(s) and is intended either to be offered as a complete animal feed or to be fed top-dressed or offered free-choice in conjunction with other animal feed to supplement the animal's total daily ration. A Type C Medicated Feed is produced by substantially diluting a Type A Medicated Article, a Type B Medicated Feed or another Type C Medicated Feed. Medicated feed CGMPs are found in 21 CFR 225.

A feed manufacturing facility must hold a medicated feed mill license to manufacture a Type B or Type C Medicated Feed from a Category II, Type A Medicated Article. No license is required if drug use is limited to Category I drugs (all types) and Type B sources of Category II drugs. FDA routinely inspects medicated feed mills and Type A Medicated Article manufacturers.

Postapproval Reporting

Under *FD&C Act* Section 506A and 21 CFR 514.8, the holder of an approved NDA or ANADA must notify FDA about each change in each condition established in an approved application beyond the variations already provided for in the application.[18] There are four reporting categories:

- Prior Approval Supplement—CVM must approve the supplement before the change can be implemented.
- Supplement—Changes Being Effected in 30 days (CBE-30)—The manufacturer may distribute the drug made using the change 30 days after CVM receives the supplement, unless CVM notifies the manufacturer that more information or prior approval is needed.
- Supplement—Changes Being Effected (CBE)—The manufacturer may begin distribution of the drug made using the change upon CVM's receipt of the supplement.

- Annual Report—The manufacturer may make minor changes during the year and document them in the Annual Report.

The change reporting category is based on the change's potential to adversely affect the drug product's identity, strength, quality, purity or potency, as these factors may relate to its safety or effectiveness. The sponsor also must submit a Manufacturing Changes and Stability Report (MCSR) annually.

Manufacturers must report serious, unexpected adverse drug events to CVM within 15 working days of becoming aware of the event. The manufacturer must investigate the event and submit a follow-up report. These events are reported on the Veterinary Adverse Drug Reaction, Lack of Effectiveness, Product Defect Report (Form FDA 1932).[19]

In addition, product and manufacturing defects that may result in serious adverse drug events are to be reported to CVM within three working days of the manufacturer's becoming aware that a defect may exist. The manufacturer should first inform CVM by telecommunication and then submit a Form FDA 1932.

Manufacturers also must submit a Transmittal of Periodic Reports and Promotional Material for New Animal Drugs (Form FDA 2301) periodically, reporting postmarketing surveillance experience and other information for new animal drugs.[20] As described in 21 CFR 14.80, this form must be submitted every six months for the first two years following NADA or ANADA approval and yearly thereafter. Form FDA 1932 also accompanies Form FDA 2301 as part of the periodic drug experience report and is used to report adverse drug events and product/manufacturing defects. Adverse drug reactions include lack of drug effectiveness and any adverse reaction occurring in humans from exposure during manufacture, testing, handling or use.

Extralabel Use

The *Animal Medicinal Drug Use Clarification Act* of 1994 (*AMDUCA*) allows veterinarians to prescribe certain approved animal drugs for extralabel uses and to prescribe approved human drugs for animals under certain conditions. Extralabel use refers to the use of an approved drug in a manner that is not in accordance with the approved label directions.

Under *AMDUCA*, any extralabel use must be by or on the order of a veterinarian in accordance with an appropriate medical rationale; must not result in violative residues in food-producing animals; and must be in conformance with additional restrictions in the implementing regulations in 21 CFR 530. Specific drugs identified in 21 CFR 530.41 are prohibited from extralabel use. To avoid volatile residues in food-producing animal products, veterinarians may obtain appropriate withdrawal times for drugs administered extralabel by consulting the Food Animal Residue Avoidance Databank (FARAD) at www.farad.org.[21]

Veterinary Devices

CVM has jurisdiction over medical devices for veterinary use; however, these devices are given regulatory discretion and are not subject to the same premarket approval requirements as medical devices intended for use in humans. Further, unlike medical devices for use in humans, veterinary devices are not subject to performance standards.

Veterinary medical devices that are not safe, effective or properly labeled are deemed to be adulterated and/or misbranded under *FD&C Act* Sections 501 and 502. Thus, it is the manufacturer's and/or distributor's responsibility to assure that these veterinary medical devices are safe, effective and properly labeled. Veterinary device labeling must not be false or misleading and must bear directions for use that are adequate for each target animal group for which the device is intended. Animal devices that do not comply with the *FD&C Act* may be subject to seizure, and firms and individuals responsible for marketing these illegal devices may be subject to other penalties under the act, including fines. While the *FD&C Act* authorizes imprisonment for certain violations, it is imposed only in extremely rare cases.

Although the Quality System Regulation in 21 CFR 820 applies to human devices only, CVM recommends that veterinary device manufacturers become familiar with these regulations and be guided by them in manufacturing and assembling their devices. CVM strongly recommends that labeling be sent in for Office of Surveillance and Compliance review to avoid misbranding.

Diagnostics used in safety testing of foods derived from animals may be regulated by the Center for Food Safety and Applied Nutrition (CFSAN) under product-specific regulations and guidelines. Additionally, veterinary electronic devices that emit radiation are subject to the *Radiation Control for Health and Safety Act* of 1968—which contains various performance and safety standards—and must be registered with the Center for Devices and Radiological Health (CDRH).

Animal Grooming Aids

Cosmetic articles intended to cleanse and beautify animals are referred to as "animal grooming aids." Grooming aids formulated only to cleanse or beautify animals are not subject to federal regulation, as the *FD&C Act* definition of "cosmetic" applies only to articles for use in humans. However, CVM still is concerned with the safety of such products, and tracks complaints and adverse reactions.

If animal grooming aids are labeled with direct or implied therapeutic claims, they may fall into the definition of drugs under *FD&C Act* Section 201(g) or the definition of new animal drugs under Section 201(v).

Chapter 32

USDA

Veterinary Biologics

Animal biologics are subject to both the *FD&C Act* and the *Virus-Serum-Toxin Act* (*VSTA*) of 1913, as amended. Veterinary biologics, including vaccines, bacterins, antisera, diagnostic kits and certain other products of biological origin, are regulated by the Center for Veterinary Biologics (CVB) in the Animal and Plant Health Inspection Service (APHIS) of USDA.

CVB implements *VSTA* provisions to ensure that pure, safe, potent and effective veterinary biologics are available for the diagnosis, prevention and treatment of animal diseases. CVB develops or approves appropriate product release standards and procedures; issues licenses and permits; monitors and inspects products and facilities; and controls veterinary biologic field tests and batch release.

To sell or manufacture a veterinary biologic product in the US, a manufacturer must hold both a Veterinary Biologics Product License for the product and a Veterinary Biologics Establishment License for the manufacturing facility. The Veterinary Biologics Product License application must include.[22]

- APHIS Form 2003, Application for United States Veterinary Biological Product License
- an outline of production (9 CFR 114.8–.9)
- master seed and cell reports for each microorganism and cell stock used in biological product manufacture, describing testing performed to demonstrate the purity, identity and safety of each (9 CFR 113)
- additional information regarding all master seeds used in the production of new live biological products and those created through recombinant technology (this must provide adequate data for the CVB laboratory to establish proper biocontainment requirements and conduct confirmatory testing)
- for vaccines, study protocols for host animal immunogenicity/efficacy, safety, back-passage, shed/spread, immunological interference and other relevant areas
- for diagnostic test kits, study protocols to assess diagnostic sensitivity and specificity, repeatability and reproducibility of results

Applicants also must submit such additional relevant product data and information as:
- in-process procedures and corresponding validation reports
- host animal immunogenicity/efficacy reports
- potency test development reports
- product safety reports
- stability reports
- Veterinary Biologics Production and Test Reports (APHIS Form 2008) for satisfactory pre-licensing serials (numbered lots) of product (three consecutive serials)
- labels and/or label sketches
- other data as necessary to support approval of label claims

Product samples must be selected and shipped to the CVB laboratory according to procedures described in 9 CFR 113.3.

The CVB Policy, Evaluation and Licensing unit (CVB-PEL) reviews production facility and biological product license applications and awards licenses. This unit also reviews product importation permit applications[23] and establishes licensing, testing and permit requirements and procedures.

Laboratories within CVB-PEL conduct pre-license testing and post-license quality-control monitoring. During pre-license testing, the laboratories assay parent materials (master seeds and cells) and final product. CVB-PEL tests master seed and master cell stock purity and identity (including identity of construct and expressed antigen for genetically engineered products) whether the intended final product is a live vaccine, inactivated vaccine or a diagnostic kit. Initial product serials (usually three) are tested for purity and potency to ensure quality product is reproducible and product tests are appropriate and transferrable.

The *VSTA* does not require that ingredients and manufactured products conform to standards for strength, quality and purity specified in relevant *USP* and *NF* monographs. Instead, the manufacturer must test all serials in accordance with the filed outline of production prior to sale and report results to CVB's Inspection and Compliance unit (CVB-IC). Results are compared with CVB-PEL check testing. Certain serials are selected for additional CVB-PEL testing. Each satisfactory batch is released by CVB-IC for marketing.

CVB-IC conducts random confirmatory potency and purity tests of serials as an additional manufacturing quality control program check. In addition, CVB-IC may test the marketed product's safety, purity, potency or efficacy in response to consumer or manufacturer concerns. CVB also monitors reports of suspected adverse events related to veterinary biologics.

Licensed veterinary biological manufacturing facilities must meet 9 CFR 108–116 requirements relating to sterilization/pasteurization processes, packaging and labeling, records and reports and other manufacturing practices. CVB-IC conducts periodic, unannounced, in-depth inspections of all licensed facilities.[24] Products imported from other countries must meet all US standards, and foreign facilities receive inspections similar to those of domestic firms.

If CVB has reason to believe a marketed product is unsatisfactory or presents a risk to the health of animals, to the public health or to the environment, it may notify the manufacturer to stop distribution and sale of the product.[25] If there are indications that raise questions regarding a product's purity, safety, potency or efficacy, or if there may be a problem regarding a product's preparation, testing or distribution, the manufacturer must inform CVB within three days of discovering the problem.

Similar to FDA's CVM guidance documents, CVB communicates guidance to industry through the use of Veterinary Services Memorandums and CVB Notices.

Phased Review of Product License Applications

CVB does not require applicants to submit a product license application as one complete package. Instead, applicants may submit individual, completed licensing deliverables for technical review. For instance, the applicant may submit the license application and outline of production, field safety and effectiveness reports and labeling separately when the necessary data and information have been compiled for each.

Tissue Residues

USDA's Food Safety and Inspection Service (FSIS) is responsible for inspecting meat and poultry products in slaughter and egg processing plants and establishments that further process meat and poultry products and has primary responsibility for the wholesomeness of these products. FSIS reports detection of violative drug residues in meat and poultry to FDA's CVM for regulatory follow-up.

Environmental Protection Agency— Animal Pesticides

Pesticides administered to animals—including topical flea products, fly sprays, ear tags and insecticide dips, and pesticidal feeds—are regulated by the Environmental Protection Agency (EPA) under the *Federal Insecticide, Fungicide, and Rodenticide Act* of 1947 *(FIFRA)*. According to *FIFRA*, pesticides include substances and mixtures of substances intended for preventing, destroying, repelling or mitigating any pest, if they are not considered to be new animal drugs under the *FD&C Act*. For example, articles having pesticidal qualities used to treat systemic macroinvertebrate parasite infestations are regulated as new animal drugs. Articles used to treat external macroinvertebrate parasites are regulated as pesticides.

Primary pesticide regulatory concerns are the safety of the worker who applies the product and the environmental effects caused by the product's manufacture, use and disposal. Actual product efficacy and safety are of lesser concern. Pesticide products are not required to be produced under CGMPs.

The *FD&C Act* authorizes EPA to set maximum pesticide residue levels for foods or animal feed. Pesticide residues in foods are monitored, and the tolerances enforced by FDA (fruits and vegetables, seafood) and USDA's Food Safety and Inspection Service (meat, milk, poultry, eggs and aquacultural foods).

Extralabel or unregistered pesticide use is prohibited unless EPA grants an emergency exemption.

Summary

- New animal drugs are reviewed and approved by the FDA's CVM through the submission of an NADA.
- *GADPTRA* requires that a generic animal drug product sponsor submit and receive approval of an ANADA prior to marketing.
- Animal drugs must be produced under CGMPs.
- The *VSTA* requires biological animal products and facilities to be licensed. Samples of all licensed biological products are submitted to USDA's CVB for testing and approval prior to sale.
- Veterinary medical devices are subject to regulatory discretion. While they are not subject to premarket approval requirements, it is the manufacturer's responsibility to ensure that these devices are safe, effective and properly labeled. Veterinary devices not meeting these requirements may be deemed adulterated and/or misbranded under the general provisions of *FD&C Act* Sections 501 and 502.
- Animal grooming aids with direct or implied therapeutic claims may be considered new animal drugs.
- Pesticides that are not new animal drugs are regulated by EPA.

References

1. *Guidance for Industry 169: Drug Substance Chemistry, Manufacturing, and Controls Information*. Rockville, MD: CVM;, 6 August 2010. FDA website. http://www.fda.gov/downloads/AnimalVeterinary/GuidanceComplianceEnforcement/GuidanceforIndustry/ucm052498.pdf. Accessed 20 May 2013.
2. International Cooperation on Harmonisation of Technical Requirements for Registration of Veterinary Products (VICH). VICH Guidelines. VICH website. www.vichsec.org/en/guidelines.htm. Accessed 3 March 2013.
3. The Common Technical Document for the Registration of Pharmaceuticals for Human Use: Quality—M4Q(R1) *(CTD-Q)*. ICH website. www.ich.org/products/ctd.html. Accessed 3 March 2013.
4. FDA User Fees. FDA website. www.fda.gov/ForIndustry/UserFees/default.htm. Accessed 3 March 2013.
5. *Guidance for Industry 173: Animal Drug Sponsor Fees under the Animal Drug User Fee Act (ADUFA)*. Rockville, MD: CVM; 7 February 2005. FDA website. http://www.fda.gov/downloads/AnimalVeterinary/GuidanceComplianceEnforcement/GuidanceforIndustry/ucm052490.pdf. Accessed 20 May 2013.
6. *Guidance for Industry 170: Animal Drug User Fees and Fee Waivers and Reductions*. Rockville, MD: CVM; 1 October 2008. FDA website. http://www.fda.gov/downloads/AnimalVeterinary/GuidanceComplianceEnforcement/GuidanceforIndustry/ucm052494.pdf. Accessed 20 May 2013.
7. The *Green Book*. FDA website. http://www.fda.gov/AnimalVeterinary/Products/ApprovedAnimalDrugProducts/default.htm. Accessed 3 March 2013.
8. *Draft Guidance for Industry 132: The Administrative New Animal Drug Application Process*. Rockville, MD: CVM; 6 November 2002.

FDA website. http://www.fda.gov/downloads/AnimalVeterinary/GuidanceComplianceEnforcement/GuidanceforIndustry/ucm052532.pdf. Accessed 20 May 2013.
9. *Guidance for Industry 28: Animal Drug Applications Expedited Review Guideline.* Rockville, MD: CVM; 19 January 2010. FDA website. http://www.fda.gov/AnimalVeterinary/GuidanceComplianceEnforcement/GuidanceforIndustry/ucm052902.htm. Accessed 20 May 2013.
10. *Guidance for Industry 61: FDA Approval of New Animal Drugs for Minor Uses and for Minor Species.* Rockville, MD: CVM; 29 May 2008. FDA website. http://www.fda.gov/downloads/AnimalVeterinary/GuidanceComplianceEnforcement/GuidanceforIndustry/ucm052375.pdf. Accessed 20 May 2013.
11. "Index of Legally Marketed Unapproved New Animal Drugs for Minor Species; Final Rule." *Federal Register,* 72:246, 69107–69131. 26 December 2007.
12. *Guidance for Industry 201: SECG for Index of Legally Marketed Unapproved New Animal Drugs for Minor Species* (1 September 2010). FDA website. http://www.fda.gov/downloads/AnimalVeterinary/GuidanceComplianceEnforcement/GuidanceforIndustry/UCM224589.pdf. Accessed 20 May 2013.
13. "Designation of New Animal Drugs for Minor Uses or Minor Species; Final Rule." *Federal Register,* 72:143, 41010–41022. 26 July 2007.
14. *Guidance for Industry 200: SECG for Designation of New Animal Drugs for Minor Uses or Minor Species* (1 September 2010). FDA website. http://www.fda.gov/downloads/AnimalVeterinary/GuidanceComplianceEnforcement/GuidanceforIndustry/UCM224588.pdf. Accessed 20 May 2013.
15. *Guidance for Industry 199: Animal Generic Drug User Fees and Fee Waivers and Reductions* (13 May 2009). FDA website. http://www.fda.gov/downloads/AnimalVeterinary/GuidanceComplianceEnforcement/GuidanceforIndustry/UCM150251.pdf. Accessed 20 May 2013.
16. United States Pharmacopeial Convention (USP). www.usp.org. Accessed 3 March 2013.
17. Docket number 95N–0308—Inapplicability of the Dietary Supplement Health and Education Act to Animal Products. *Federal Register* 61:78. 22 April 1996.
18. *Guidance for Industry 82: Development of Supplemental Applications for Approved New Animal Drugs* (28 October 2002). FDA website. http://www.fda.gov/downloads/AnimalVeterinary/GuidanceComplianceEnforcement/GuidanceforIndustry/ucm052411.pdf. Accessed 20 May 2013.
19. Form FDA 1932, "Veterinary Adverse Drug Reaction, Lack of Effectiveness, Product Defect Report" (January 2010). FDA website. http://www.fda.gov/downloads/AboutFDA/ReportsManualsForms/Forms/AnimalDrugForms/UCM048810.pdf. Accessed 20 May 2013.
20. Form FDA 2301, "Transmittal of Periodic Reports and Promotional Material for New Animal Drugs" (April 2012). FDA website. http://www.fda.gov/downloads/AboutFDA/ReportsManualsForms/Forms/AnimalDrugForms/UCM048810.pdf. Accessed 20 May 2013.
21. The Food Animal Residue Avoidance Databank (FARAD). www.farad.org. Accessed 3 March 2013.
22. Veterinary Services Memorandum No. 800.50: *Basic License Requirements and Guidelines for Submission of Materials in Support of Licensure* (9 February 2011). USDA website. http://www.aphis.usda.gov/animal_health/vet_biologics/publications/memo_800_50.pdf. Accessed 20 May 2013.
23. Veterinary Services Memorandum No. 800.101: *US Veterinary Biological Product Permits for Distribution and Sale* (28 May 2002). USDA website. http://www.aphis.usda.gov/animal_health/vet_biologics/publications/memo_800_101.pdf. Accessed 20 May 2013.
24. Veterinary Services Memorandum No. 800.91: *Categories of Inspection for Licensed Veterinary Biologics Establishments* (13 May 1999). USDA website. http://www.aphis.usda.gov/animal_health/vet_biologics/publications/memo_800_91.pdf. Accessed 20 May 2013.
25. Veterinary Services Memorandum No. 800.57: *Market Suspensions* (17 September 1999). USDA website. http://www.aphis.usda.gov/animal_health/vet_biologics/publications/memo_800_57.pdf. Accessed 20 May 2013.

Recommended Reading

- Center for Veterinary Medicine. US Food and Drug Administration guidance documents. www.fda.gov/AnimalVeterinary/GuidanceComplianceEnforcement/GuidanceforIndustry/default.htm. Accessed 3 March 2013.
- American Veterinary Medical Association. Available at: www.avma.org. Accessed 3 March 2013.
- Animal Health Institute. Available at: www.ahi.org. Accessed 3 March 2013
- Generic Animal Drug Alliance. www.gadaonline.org. Accessed 3 March 2013.
- Center for Veterinary Biologics Veterinary Services Memorandums. www.aphis.usda.gov/animal_health/vet_biologics/vb_regs_and_guidance.shtml. Accessed 3 March 2013.
- International Cooperation on Harmonisation of Technical Requirements for Registration of Veterinary Products. www.vichsec.org/en/guidelines.htm. Accessed 3 March 2013.
- American Feed Industry Association. www.afia.org/afia/home.aspx. Accessed 3 March 2013.
- "Guide for the Care and Use of Laboratory Animals." Washington, DC: National Research Council, National Academy Press; 1996. NIH website. http://grants.nih.gov/grants/olaw/Guide-for-the-care-and-use-of-Laboratory-animals.pdf. Accessed 20 May 2013.
- United States Pharmacopeial Convention (USP). www.usp.org. Accessed 3 March 2013.

Chapter 33

Food Products

Updated by Nigel Andre Sean Hernandez, PhD, MSc, MS, MBA, GCMD, GCIRA, RAC

OBJECTIVES

❏ Provide an overview of requirements for marketing an FDA-regulated food in the US

❏ Understand the basics of food labeling requirements and voluntary elements

❏ Develop a broad understanding of the mechanisms available for the use of new ingredients and color additives in compliance with regulatory requirements

❏ Explain food adulteration standards and major sanitation programs, including Good Manufacturing Practice and Hazard Analysis and Critical Control Point

❏ Describe administrative requirements for food facilities, such as facility registration, prior notice, recordkeeping and reporting of reportable foods

LAWS, REGULATIONS AND GUIDELINES COVERED IN THIS CHAPTER

❏ *Federal Food, Drug, and Cosmetic Act* of 1938, as amended (codified at 21 U.S.C. §301 et al)

❏ Section 321 Definitions

❏ Section 331 Prohibited Acts

❏ Sections 341–350f Food

❏ Section 374 Inspection

❏ Section 379e Color Additives

❏ *Food Allergen Labeling and Consumer Protection Act* of 2004 (P.L. 108-282)

❏ *Public Health Security and Bioterrorism Preparedness and Response Act* of 2002 (P.L. 107-188)

❏ *Food and Drug Administration Modernization Act* of 1997 (P.L. 105-115)

❏ *Food Safety Modernization Act* of 2011 (Public Law 111-353)

❏ *Dietary Supplement Health Education Act* of 1994 (P.L. 103-417)

❏ *Nutrition Labeling and Education Act* of 1990 (P.L. 101-535)

❏ *Orphan Drug Act* of 1983, §5 (P.L. 97-414)

❏ *Tariff Act* of 1930 (codified at 19 U.S.C. 1304)

❏ 9 CFR 317 Meat labeling, marking devices and containers

❏ 21 CFR 1 General enforcement regulations

❏ 21 CFR 7 Enforcement policy

- 21 CFR 70–82 Color additives
- 21 CFR 100–190 Food for human consumption
- FDA's Biotechnology Policy of 1992
- *Guidance for Industry: Regulation of Genetically Engineered Animals Containing Heritable Recombinant DNA Constructs* (January 2009)
- USDA's "A Guide to Federal Food Labeling Requirements for Meat and Poultry Products" (August 2007)
- *Food Action Defect Levels Handbook*
- *Guidance for Industry: A Food Labeling Guide* (Revised October 2009)
- *Guidance for Industry: Frequently Asked Questions About GRAS* (December 2004)
- *Foods Derived from Genetically Engineered Plants* (April 2013)
- *Summary of Qualified Health Claims Subject to Enforcement Discretion*
- *Guidance for Industry: Frequently Asked Questions About Medical Foods* (Revised May 2007)

Introduction

The US Food and Drug Administration (FDA) is the federal agency charged with regulation of most food and food-related products. FDA derives its authority to regulate foods primarily from the *Federal Food, Drug, and Cosmetic Act* of 1938 (*FD&C Act*), as amended.[1] The *FD&C Act* defines "food" broadly to mean

(1) articles used for food or drink for man or other animals, (2) chewing gum, and (3) articles used for components of any such article.[2]

As a result of this broad definition, FDA's regulation of food covers not just conventional human food, but also any individual component of food, ingredients, pet food and animal feed. Under the *Dietary Supplement Health Education Act* of 1994 (*DSHEA*),[3] dietary supplements also are regulated under the general umbrella of "foods," although they are subject to a number of labeling and ingredient requirements specific to dietary supplements. Regulation of dietary supplements is discussed in more detail in Chapter 30.

FDA implements the *FD&C Act* and establishes regulations to prevent food from adulteration, ensuring that foods are safe, wholesome and sanitary. FDA also regulates the misbranding of food labels and labeling, ensuring that products are honestly, accurately and informatively represented to the public. Within FDA, food regulation is managed by the Center for Food Safety and Applied Nutrition (CFSAN).

Although FDA regulates most foods, it does not regulate all foods. The US Department of Agriculture (USDA) has jurisdiction over meat, poultry and commercially processed egg products, as well as combination products (e.g., meat stew, pizza with meat toppings), depending on the meat or poultry content. Within USDA, the Food Safety and Inspection Service (FSIS) is responsible for the inspection, safety and labeling of these products. Further, although FDA regulates bottled water, the US Environmental Protection Agency (EPA) regulates tap water, and the US Alcohol and Tobacco Tax and Trade Bureau (TTB) regulates most alcohol products.

FDA also does not regulate all aspects of food products. For example, although FDA regulates food labeling, the agency works with the Federal Trade Commission (FTC) to regulate food advertising, with the FTC taking the lead on most enforcement actions.[4] Fruits, vegetables and other plants are regulated by USDA's Animal and Plant Health Inspection Service (APHIS) to prevent the introduction of plant diseases and pests into the US. The Agricultural Marketing Service (AMS) of USDA administers the National Organic Program, which develops, implements and administers national standards for organic agricultural products and accredits the certifying agents who inspect organic operations.

Moreover, FDA works jointly with numerous federal, state and local agencies to regulate various aspects of foods and specific food categories. For example, FDA works cooperatively with states and with other agencies, such as the Centers for Disease Control (CDC), to address outbreaks of foodborne illness. The following provides more detail on some of the agencies and other jurisdictions that are responsible for some aspect of food regulation or that work cooperatively with FDA on food matters:

- States are the primary regulators for restaurants, farms and retail establishments, including grocery stores. States work cooperatively with FDA to regulate milk and shellfish, and also are involved in the regulation of weights and measures.
- FTC works with FDA to regulate all advertising, ensuring that advertisements are truthful and not misleading for consumers. Within FTC, the Bureau of Consumer Protection has a mandate to protect consumers against unfair, deceptive or fraudulent practices.
- EPA establishes pesticide tolerances (acceptable residues) for food and animal feed, while FDA enforces compliance with pesticide tolerances. EPA also

establishes maximum contaminant levels in public drinking water.
- TTB, formerly the Bureau of Alcohol, Tobacco, and Firearms, enforces labeling and other regulatory requirements for beer, wine and distilled spirits.
- US Customs and Border Protection (CBP) works with FDA to regulate imported food (and other FDA-related imported products).

Food Ingredients and Packaging (Food Additives)

Unlike its regulation of drugs or medical devices, FDA has very limited authority to regulate food before it goes on the market. One significant exception is the regulation of food and color additives, which must be approved by FDA as safe for intended uses prior to marketing. The term "food additive" includes not just ingredients intentionally added to the food but also any substance used in the production process that could reasonably end up in the food, including packaging that could leach into food and even lubricants used on machinery that touches food during processing.

FDA approval of a new food additive must be by issuance of a regulation. For this reason, it can be important to determine whether a substance falls within any of the several exemptions from the definition of a food additive.

What is a Food Additive?

Stripping out the exclusions, the general definition of a food additive is broad:

> "Any substance the intended use of which results or may reasonably be expected to result, directly or indirectly, in its becoming a component or otherwise affecting the characteristics of any food...."[5]

The definition requires two key determinations. What is the intended use of the substance? When used as intended, can the substance be reasonably expected to end up in the food or affect the food in any way?

Substances such as cleaning solvents used on food processing machinery or packaging materials may be food additives if they could "reasonably be expected" to end up in the food in any amount or otherwise affect the food. The definition specifically states that "any substance intended for use in processing, manufacturing, packing, processing, preparing, treating, packaging, transporting or holding food" and "any source of radiation intended for any such use" can be a food additive.[6]

Regulations approving uses of direct food additives—that is, direct addition of a substance to food—can be found in 21 CFR 172 and 173. Regulations approving food additives that may indirectly become a component of food can be found at 21 CFR 175–178. Regulations approving the use of radiation on food can be found at 21 CFR 179.

What is Not a Food Additive?

The *FD&C Act* specifically excludes the following types of substances from the definition of food additive:
- any substance that is generally recognized as safe (GRAS) for its intended uses by scientific experts qualified to evaluate its safety
- pesticide chemical residues
- pesticides
- color additives
- new animal drugs
- new dietary ingredients (i.e., ingredients for use in dietary supplements)

Prior Sanction: any substance approved or sanctioned for use prior to 6 September 1958 under the *FD&C Act*, the *Federal Meat Inspection Act* of 1906 or the *Poultry Products Inspection Act* of 1957[7]

Any substance that falls within any of these seven exclusions need not be approved as a food additive prior to use, although it may be subject to other regulations, depending on the type of substance. For example, pesticides are approved for use by EPA,[8] and color additives must be approved by FDA under the color additive approval process in a different section of the *FD&C Act*.[9]

Most of the exclusions from the definition of food additive apply to defined categories of substances—a substance either is or is not an approved pesticide or color additive, and if not, it may be a food additive. The exclusion for GRAS substances, however, is more fluid; it depends on the available evidence supporting the safety of the intended use of the substance. Because a GRAS substance need not be approved by regulation prior to use in food, determining whether a substance is GRAS or is a food additive is important in developing new food products.

How is a Food Additive Approved?

A food additive is deemed unsafe, and cannot be used in food, unless FDA has issued a regulation setting out the conditions under which the food additive can be used safely.[10] For a food additive to be deemed "safe," FDA must determine that under the intended conditions of use, the additive presents a "reasonable certainty of no harm."

Once a substance is determined to be a food additive, it must be approved through the food additive process unless it falls in one of two limited categories: a food-contact substance (FCS) or a food additive intended solely for investigational use. The exception for investigational use is rarely used and requires FDA to issue a regulation allowing the exception.[11] The FCS substance notification process is discussed in more detail below.

Any person may petition FDA to issue a regulation approving a food additive for a particular use. A food additive petition must include:

Chapter 33

- the chemical identity and composition of the food additive
- the conditions of the additive's proposed uses
- data concerning the physical or technical effect the additive is intended to produce and the quantity of the additive required to produce such effect
- methods for determining the quantity of the additive in food
- full reports of investigations made with respect to the additive's safe use[12]

FDA also may request information on the production methods used for the additive and samples of the additive, its components or the food on which it will be used.

FDA must publish a notice in the *Federal Register* within 30 days of receiving a complete food additive petition. FDA then has 90 days (which may be extended to no more than 180 days) from the filing of the petition to publish a regulation approving the use of the food additive or to issue an order denying the petition.[13] Any person adversely affected by the approval or denial of a food additive petition may file objections within 30 days after publication of the order approving or denying the petition.[14] FDA must respond to the objections, including any request for a public meeting, "as soon as practicable."

FDA cannot approve a food additive petition if a fair evaluation of the data fails to establish that the proposed use of the additive will be safe, or if the data show that the proposed use of the food additive would promote consumer deception or otherwise result in adulteration or misbranding of food.[15] FDA has significant discretion to use its scientific judgment in evaluating the data to determine whether the use of a food additive is safe. For example, in determining safety, the agency may consider the probable level of consumption of the additive, the cumulative effect of the additive in the diet and other safety factors recognized by experts to be appropriate.

FDA has no discretion, however, if it determines that a food additive induces cancer. The so-called Delaney Clause in Section 409(c) of the *FD&C Act* states that FDA cannot approve the use of any food additive as safe if the food additive: (1) is found to induce cancer in man or animals when ingested; or (2) is found, by appropriate tests, to induce cancer in man or animals by methods other than ingestion.[16]

The Delaney Clause applies whenever FDA determines any risk exists that the additive may induce cancer, regardless of how small the risk.[17] Only two limited exceptions from the application of the Delaney Clause have been recognized. Courts have held that the Delaney Clause does not apply where a constituent of a food or color additive is deemed to be a carcinogen, unless the food or color additive itself is determined to induce cancer.[18] The Delaney Clause also does not apply to certain food additives intended for use as ingredients of feed for animals raised for food production.[19]

Food additive approvals apply to the additive generally and are not intended to be proprietary to a particular product. The food additive regulation will specify the conditions of use, which may include limits on the amounts of the additive, the types of foods in which the additive can be used or even labeling requirements for the use of the additive.

FCS Notifications

The *FD&C Act* was amended in 1997 to allow FCS products approved for use on food to go through a notification process rather than requiring FDA to issue a regulation.[20] An FCS is any substance used as a component of materials used in manufacturing, packing, packaging, transporting or holding food that is not intended to have a technical effect in the food. This definition includes such substances as paper, plastics, adhesives, lubricants and coatings used in food containers or packaging. It also includes food processing equipment, production aids, sanitizers, antimicrobials and colors used in packaging.

FDA requires that any FCS product be determined to be safe for its intended use before it is permitted for sale in the US. Safety is dictated by the regulatory status of each component that comprises the FCS. New components and uses of FCS products require premarket notification to FDA prior to marketing in the US.

The determination of how an FCS is regulated depends on its chemical composition. It is the responsibility of the FCS manufacturer to ensure that food contact materials comply with the specifications and limitations in all applicable authorizations. The identity, specifications and limitations of the individual FCS components are regulated by provisions in the Code of Federal Regulations, the *Federal Register*, Effective Food Contact Notifications, Prior Sanctioned Letters, GRAS Notices, Threshold of Regulations Exemptions, and FDA enforcement actions, such as import refusals, import alerts, Warning Letters, etc.

Anyone may submit a food contact notification to FDA. The agency has 120 days to review the notification. FDA may issue an objection or nonacceptance letter during the 120 days if it has safety concerns about the proposed use of the FCS. Before issuing an objection or nonacceptance letter, the agency typically contacts notifiers to request more information or to permit the notifier to withdraw the notification. If FDA does not issue an objection or nonacceptance letter within 120 days, the food-contact notification becomes effective on the 120-day date. At that point, FDA sends a letter to the notifier confirming the effective date. Approvals under the food-contact notification process are proprietary—that is, they extend only to the specific proprietary substance and use in the notification, not to other identical substances. During the 120-day review period, the information submitted in the notification cannot be publicly disclosed by FDA. Similarly, FDA cannot disclose information related to a notification that is withdrawn prior to the end of the 120-day review period.

FDA has a generous revision policy allowing submission of revisions for further reformulations of an FCS within 90 days at no extra cost.

GRAS Substances

As described above, any substance generally recognized as safe for its intended uses by scientific experts qualified to evaluate its safety is not a food additive and, therefore, does not have to be approved through the food additive process prior to use. Substances used in food prior to 1958 also can be deemed GRAS based on their common use in food, rather than requiring consensus on the scientific data,[21] but this basis for GRAS determination is rarely used anymore.

The *FD&C Act* does not set out how FDA is to determine whether a substance is GRAS. Moreover, the *FD&C Act* does not require that FDA approve a substance as GRAS prior to its use in food, so the agency only has authority to challenge whether a substance is, in fact, GRAS after it is used in food. As a result, a person may self-determine the GRAS status of a substance and use it in food. Many food manufacturers, however, will require suppliers to provide support for the assertion that a substance is GRAS to avoid the risk of FDA challenging the GRAS status of the substance after the product is on the market.

To help those seeking to determine whether a substance is GRAS, FDA issued *Guidance for Industry: Frequently Asked Questions About GRAS* in December 2004, discussing how the agency evaluates whether a substance is GRAS. The agency has also published regulations in 21 CFR Parts 182–186 affirming the GRAS status of certain substances. Due to limited resources, FDA rarely issues such regulations. Instead, FDA has implemented a voluntary GRAS notification process to provide manufacturers with some support for the assertion that a substance is GRAS.

FDA has taken the position that for a substance to be GRAS (other than substances used in food prior to 1958), the scientific data and information supporting its safe use must be of the same quantity and quality as needed for approval of a food additive petition, must be widely available, and there must be consensus among experts that the data establish the safe use of the substance. GRAS determinations cannot be based on private, proprietary data.

Under the GRAS notification program, FDA will review claims that a substance is GRAS. GRAS notifications should include a description of the substance (including chemical identity and properties), applicable conditions of use and the basis for the GRAS determination, including discussion of the scientific information supporting the safe use of the product and information supporting consensus of experts as to the safe use. FDA typically will consult with the notifier during its review of the notification. FDA does not approve GRAS notifications. However, at the conclusion of its review, FDA may issue a letter indicating the agency does not question the basis for the GRAS determination. Alternatively, the agency may issue a letter concluding that it does not believe the notification provides a sufficient basis for a GRAS determination. Because the GRAS notification process is voluntary, FDA is not bound by any timeline in completing its review but seeks to complete its review within 180 days.

Color Additives

A "color additive" is defined as any dye, pigment or other substance that can impart color to a food, drug or cosmetic, or to the human body, except that the term does not include any substance that FDA determines is intended solely for a use other than coloring.[22] All color additives (except cosmetic hair dyes[23]) are subject to premarket approval.[24] In addition, all color additives must be properly declared on food labels and beverage labels. Unlike food additives, there is no GRAS exemption from the definition of color additives.

FDA issues regulations listing color additives that have been approved as safe for their intended uses.[25] FDA's review of color additive petitions is similar to the review of food additive petitions. The petitioner must submit data demonstrating the safety and suitability of the new color additive for its intended uses. As is the case for food additives, there is a Delaney Clause for color additives that prohibits FDA from determining that a color additive is safe for any use that will result in ingestion of the additive if it is found by FDA to induce cancer when ingested by man or animals or if it is found by appropriate tests to induce cancer in man or animals through a method other than ingestion.

As a condition of use, some approved color additives are required to be certified by batch by FDA before they can be sold. Certification generally is required by FDA when the composition of the additive needs to be controlled to protect public health. Synthetic organic dyes, lakes[26] and pigments must be batch certified, whereas color additives derived from plant or mineral sources are generally exempt from batch certification.

As with food additives, the approved conditions of use for certain color additives may extend to labeling requirements. In addition, regulations governing labeling of color additives in foods can be found in 21 CFR 101.22.

Biotechnology and Genetically Modified Organisms

Biotechnology refers to the techniques used by scientists to modify the genetic material of microorganisms, plants or animals in order to achieve a desired trait. Common use of the terms "biotechnology" and "genetically engineered" in the US is limited to foods produced using recombinant DNA, or gene splicing.

FDA's Biotechnology Policy, published in 1992, is limited to foods derived from new plant varieties. FDA recommends that those developing a bioengineered food consult with the agency during development to discuss relevant safety, nutritional or other regulatory issues. FDA also recommends that developers submit a scientific and regulatory assessment of the food for review by the agency. FDA has proposed a rule that would require developers to submit such an assessment to FDA 120 days before a bioengineered food is marketed. The rule has not been finalized, so no requirement to this effect is currently in place. Bioengineered plants may also be subject to regulation by USDA's APHIS.

In January 2009, FDA issued *Guidance for Industry: Regulation of Genetically Engineered Animals Containing Heritable Recombinant DNA Constructs*. In the guidance, FDA takes the position that a recombinant DNA (rDNA) construct that is in a genetically engineered (GE) animal and is intended to affect the animal's structure or function meets the definition of an animal drug and is subject to premarket approval requirements. The guidance further states that developers of GE animals must demonstrate that the construct is safe for the health of the GE animals and, if they are food animals, that the construct and products of the construct are safe for human consumption.

In April 2013, FDA published *Foods Derived from Genetically Engineered Plants*; this covered Questions & Answers on Food from GE Plants, Background on GE Plants for Food and Feed, Draft Guidance on Voluntary Labeling, FDA Policy Statement on Foods Derived from New Plant Varieties and Consultation Procedures.

Misbranding: Food Labeling and Claims

Under Section 403(a) of the *FD&C Act*, a food is misbranded if its label or labeling is false or misleading in any particular, if it is offered for sale under the name of another food or if it is an imitation of another food without proper labeling.[27] A "label" is defined to include any "written, printed, or graphic matter upon the immediate container of any article."[28] "Labeling" is broader and includes "all labels and other written, printed, or graphic matter (1) upon any article or any of its containers or wrappers, or (2) accompanying such article."[29] Labeling has been interpreted by FDA and the courts to include flyers, brochures and displays that are proximate to the product in a store. FDA has further interpreted labeling to include information on a website from which a product can be purchased, and even information on websites reachable through links on a website where the product can be purchased.

In addition, FDA regulations include formal standards of identity for many kinds of food including: milk and cream; cheese and related cheese products; frozen desserts; bakery products; cereal flours and related products; macaroni and noodle products; canned fruits; canned fruit juices; fruit butters, jellies, preserves and related products; fruit pies; canned vegetables; vegetable juices; frozen vegetables; eggs and egg products; fish and shellfish; cacao products; tree nut and peanut products; beverages; margarine; sweeteners and table syrups; and food dressings; and flavorings. These regulations prevent the intentional substitution of ingredients without declaring those ingredients in labeling (e.g., using an unlisted, less-expensive ingredient to reduce the cost of manufacturing). The standards of identity require that products contain the ingredients mandated by the standard.

The *FD&C Act* prohibits misbranded foods from being introduced, delivered or received in interstate commerce.[30] FDA has authority to take action against a product if the label or labeling fails to identify "material facts."[31] Everything on a product's label or labeling must be truthful and cannot be misleading.

FDA regulates labeling for all foods, except those within USDA's jurisdiction (meat, poultry and cracked egg products). There is no label preapproval required by FDA; however, the agency has promulgated extensive regulations governing food labeling. The labeling rules governing foods regulated by USDA are similar to FDA's requirements; however, label preapproval is required for products within USDA's jurisdiction.

There are two primary areas of food labeling regulation: required elements and voluntary claims. All food labels must contain certain uniform elements to provide meaningful information to consumers in a manner that allows for easy comparison between products. Many products also bear voluntary claims promoting the benefits or usefulness of the products as they relate to either nutrition or health.

Mandatory Labeling Elements

The *FD&C Act* establishes requirements for numerous statements that must appear on a food product's label. Food labeling is required for most packaged foods, such as breads, cereals, canned and frozen foods, snacks, desserts and drinks. Labeling requirements are very specific, often requiring near-exact placement in a mandated size on a specific component of a certain label.

Food labels must contain five primary elements (unless subject to limited exemptions):
- statement of identity
- net quantity of contents
- nutrition facts
- ingredient statement
- manufacturer's statement

Additional labeling requirements are applicable to certain products; for instance, juice content, country of origin, use of irradiation, allergen declaration, mandated warnings and labeling of infant formulas. Certain label statements are prohibited, such as false or misleading statements or unapproved nutrient content or health claims.

The required information must appear on one of two label panels. The "principal display panel" (PDP), a product's primary label, is the "part of a label that is most likely to be displayed, presented, shown, or examined under customary conditions of display" for sale.[32] The PDP must contain the product's statement of identity and net weight. In addition, the PDP may include the ingredient statement, manufacturing statement and nutrition information. Many product labels also contain an "information panel," which is typically the "part of the label immediately contiguous and to the right of the principal display panel."[33] No intervening material is permitted between the PDP and the information panel unless the panel immediately to the right of the PDP is too small to accommodate the required information. The information panel generally includes the manufacturing statement, ingredient declaration and nutrition information.

Statement of Identity

All products must bear a product identity statement that is either a standard of identity, a common or usual name or an appropriately descriptive term or "fanciful" name.[34] Additionally, products that are deemed imitations of standardized foods must be labeled as such.

Standards of Identity

The *FD&C Act* authorizes FDA to establish standards of identity for certain foods.[35] Standards of identity define what a given food product is, its name and the ingredients that must be used, or may be used, in the manufacture of the food. Food standards ensure that consumers get what they expect when they purchase certain food products, providing predictability that a product labeled as "ice cream" is actually a frozen dairy product. Once a standard of identity is established, any food that purports to be the standardized food must comply with the standard of identity, and a food may not bear the standardized name if it does not comply with the standard. The standards of identity are codified in 21 CFR Parts 130–169.

Common or Usual Name

A standard of identity does not exist for all types of foods. To ensure consistency and predictability for consumers, the common or usual name of a product must "accurately identify or describe…the basic nature of the food or its characterizing properties or ingredients."[36] Regulations establish common or usual name requirements for particular foods, which are less rigid than standards of identity, but nonetheless must be followed when labeling these types of foods. These regulations are contained in 21 CFR 102.

Descriptive or Fanciful Name

When either a standard of identity or usual name is required for a food, and the nature of the food is obvious, the statement of identity is permitted to be a descriptive term or fanciful name.[37] For example, the brand name of many soft drinks serves as their statement of identity because such names are commonly used to refer to the products.

Imitation

If a food resembles a traditional food and is a substitute for the traditional food, but is nutritionally inferior to that food, it must be labeled as an imitation.[38] A food is considered nutritionally inferior if, for example, it contains less protein or a lesser amount of any essential vitamin or mineral. Products that are not nutritionally inferior and are a substitute for and resemble another food can use a fanciful name that is not false or misleading rather than using imitation labeling, such as using the phrase "Cool Whip" to identify a product that would otherwise be called "Imitation Whipped Cream."

Net Quantity of Contents

A net quantity of contents statement, expressed in terms of weight, measure, numerical count or a combination of numerical count and weight or measure, must appear in the lower 30% of the PDP.[39] The statement must declare the package's contents in both English and metric units, typically using pounds or grams for solids and ounces or milliliters for liquids. Detailed requirements mandate the type size and placement of the statement, which must appear as a "distinct item" separated from other printed label information. This statement must be accurate, although reasonable variations from stated weight are permitted for either statistical variations occurring during production under Good Manufacturing Practices or from loss or gain of moisture during distribution. As noted earlier, state and local authorities are also very active in regulating net quantity statements.

Nutrition Labeling

Regulations established to implement the *Nutrition Labeling and Education Act* of 1990 specify detailed substantive and technical requirements for the nutrition labeling of foods.[40] The embodiment of these detailed regulations is the Nutrition Facts panel. FDA places great importance upon maintaining uniformity in the presentation of information in the Nutrition Facts panel. Regulations dictate such details as font sizes, indentations, use of bolding and even the width of lines in the Nutrition Facts panel. Only those nutrients listed in FDA's nutrition regulations, as mandatory or voluntary components of the nutrition label, may be included in the Nutrition Facts label as directed in 21 CFR 101.9(c)). In addition to numerous other requirements, a food's nutrition label must:

- specify the serving size (based upon reference amounts customarily consumed)
- identify nutrients that must be declared
- follow specific formatting and type size requirements

Under the regulations, certain nutrients must be declared on the Nutrition Facts panel, while other nutrients may be declared voluntarily. FDA will evaluate products to confirm whether the product contains the level of nutrients that are declared on the nutrition panel, while recognizing that there will be some inherent variability in the nutritional composition of foods.

Ingredient Statement

The ingredients added to a product must be listed in the ingredient statement in descending order of predominance by weight.[41] Ingredients present at less than 2% of the total are exempt from the descending order of predominance requirement. Ingredients that are formulated from multiple components may either include the names of the components they combine to create followed by a parenthetical listing of each component or list each component in descending order in the ingredient statement without identifying the name of the multicomponent food itself. A small number of ingredients are eligible for "and/or" labeling when the ingredient may or may not be included in the product. There are also specific regulations governing the declaration of spices, flavors and colors.

Importantly, the *Food Allergen Labeling and Consumer Protection Act* of 2004 (*FALCPA*)[42] requires manufacturers to declare in English the presence of any major food allergen, specifically egg, wheat, milk, soy, fish, shellfish, peanuts and tree nuts.[43] The presence of the allergen may be declared in the ingredient statement or through the statement "Contains: (name of the allergen)" in bold immediately after the ingredient statement. The declaration for tree nuts, seafood and shellfish must indicate the particular species, while for other allergens, manufacturers are not required to specify the species (for example, Contains: Wheat, Milk, Cashews, Cod and Clams). FDA has not regulated the use of "May Contain" statements, such as "May contain milk" or implied "may contain" statements, such as "Processed in plant that also processes peanuts;" such statements are completely voluntary.

Manufacturer's Statement

The label must contain a manufacturing statement identifying the manufacturer, packer or distributor.[44] The company's actual corporate name must appear on the label, as well as its city, state and zip code. If the company is not listed in the city or telephone directory, its street address must also appear on the label. Unless it is misleading, it is acceptable to list the principal place of business instead of the actual place of manufacture. If the name on the label is not that of the manufacturer, it should be qualified with phrases such as "distributed by," "packed for" or "imported by."

Additional Requirements Imposed by USDA

Labeling for foods regulated by USDA must contain the above requirements, plus:
- an inspection legend and establishment number (in the form of a logo that looks like a USDA mark)[45]
- special handing instructions for products that require refrigeration or freezing[46]
- safe handling instructions for products that are not considered ready-to-eat[47]

Another distinction from FDA requirements is that labels for USDA-regulated products must be preapproved by FSIS prior to use.[48]

Country of Origin Labeling

USDA and CBP regulate separate country of origin labeling (COOL) requirements that affect many food products, including most imports. The *Farm Bills* of 2002 and 2008 mandated COOL for certain products. The final rule for all covered commodities (7 CFR Part 60 and Part 65) went into effect on 16 March 2009. The COOL program is administered by USDA's AMS. The rules require labeling at retail to indicate the country of origin for certain covered commodities (i.e., muscle cuts and ground beef, lamb, chicken, goat and pork; wild and farm-raised fish and shellfish; perishable agricultural commodities (specifically fresh and frozen fruits and vegetables); macadamia nuts; pecans; peanuts; and ginseng).[49] Excluded from USDA COOL requirements are "processed food items," defined as retail items derived from a covered commodity that has "undergone specific processing resulting in a change of character" or that has been "combined with at least one other covered commodity." For example, breaded fish sticks; fruit cups containing cantaloupe, watermelon and honeydew; and cured hams all are considered to be processed food items and are exempt from COOL requirements.

Almost all imported products, whether or not exempt from USDA COOL requirements, are still required to be marked with country of origin labeling under the *Tariff Act* of 1930,[50] enforced by CBP.[51] For example, although a bag of frozen peas and carrots is considered a processed food item and thus is exempt from USDA COOL requirements, if the peas and carrots are of foreign origin, CBP requires that the product's bag or its shipping container be marked with country of origin information. CBP's COOL requirements only apply until the product reaches its ultimate purchaser in the US, which may be a business that further manufactures the goods rather than a consumer. Thus, because CBP's restrictions allow labeling on shipping containers and do not transfer upon food processing, they do not have the same impact on consumers as USDA's requirements.

Voluntary Labeling Information

Manufacturers may choose to make claims on their food labels about the attributes or benefits of their products. FDA has comprehensive requirements regarding claims, requiring authorization prior to use of nutrient content claims, health claims and qualified health claims; and notification of health or nutrient content claims under the *Food and Drug Administration Modernization Act* of 1997 (*FDAMA*).[52] FDA also regulates structure/function claims, which do not require approval prior to use.

A product's intended use will determine whether it is subject to regulation as a food, dietary supplement or drug. Claims that are made for a product are key to determining its intended use. For example (and as explained in more detail below), a claim that a product treats or prevents a disease or abnormal health condition subjects it to regulation as a drug, while the claim that a product "maintains healthy cholesterol for people with normal cholesterol" is a permissible structure/function claim for a food. Because most drugs cannot be marketed until they have received premarket approval under the *FD&C Act*, food companies must avoid making claims that would subject their products to regulation as new drugs.

Nutrient Content Claims

A nutrient content claim describes the level of a nutrient using terms such as "free," "high" and "low," or compares the level of a nutrient in a food to that of another food, using terms such as "more," "reduced" and "lite."[53] For example, the statements "zero calorie" and "high in fiber" are nutrient content claims. Under the *FD&C Act*, a food is deemed misbranded if it bears a nutrient content claim, unless FDA has issued a regulation authorizing the claim and the claim is made in a manner consistent with the regulation.[54] Nutrient content claims can be express or implied and typically are based on the reference amount customarily consumed for the food at issue. There must be an established daily value for the nutrient that is the subject of the claim. Special labeling also is required for products that exceed designated "disclosure levels" for fat, saturated fat, cholesterol and sodium, using a statement such as "See nutrition information for fat content," for a food where the level of fat exceeds the disclosure level and a nutrient content claim is made.

Health Claims

A health claim describes the relationship between a substance (food or food component) and a disease or health-related condition.[55] For example, the statement, "While many factors affect heart disease, diets low in saturated fat and cholesterol may reduce the risk of this disease" is a model health claim. Health claims are limited to claims about reducing disease risk and cannot be claims about the cure, mitigation, treatment or prevention of disease. Since only drugs may bear claims that a product cures, mitigates, treats or prevents a disease (or unapproved health claims), such claims signal that the product is intended for use as a drug.[56] FDA will regard a food product bearing such claims as violative of the *FD&C Act* as both a misbranded food and as an unapproved new drug.

As noted, foods are deemed misbranded if they bear a health claim that is not authorized by FDA. Health claims must be supported by significant scientific agreement in order to be established. Foods are ineligible for health claims if they exceed disqualifying levels of certain nutrients (total fat, saturated fat, cholesterol and sodium), which are the same as the disclosure levels for nutrient content claims. Approved health claims are listed in the regulations at 21 CFR 101.72–101.83 and include claims relating such substances and diseases as calcium/osteoporosis and sodium/hypertension.

Qualified Health Claims

For claims for which there is not significant scientific agreement supporting the claim, manufacturers can petition to make "qualified health claims." The *FD&C Act* does not provide approval of health claims with less than significant scientific agreement. As a result of court decisions striking down FDA's denial of certain health claims on First Amendment grounds, the agency established a petition process for qualified health claims.

Though not requiring significant scientific agreement, such claims must be supported by scientific evidence. FDA has issued extensive guidance on how it evaluates scientific evidence for health claims and qualified health claims. If FDA agrees that the scientific evidence supports a qualified health claim, the agency will propose claim language for which it will exercise enforcement discretion. The claim language is tailored to accurately convey the level and quality of the science supporting the claim, e.g., "Supportive but not conclusive research shows that eating 1.5 ounces per day of walnuts, as part of a low saturated fat and low cholesterol diet and not resulting in increased caloric intake, may reduce the risk of coronary heart disease. See nutrition information for fat and calorie content." These statements often are so qualified as to not be useful. For example, in response to a petition for qualified health claims regarding a relationship between consumption of green tea and a reduced risk of certain cancers, FDA permitted the following claim:

> "Two studies do not show that drinking green tea reduces the risk of breast cancer in women, but one weaker, more limited study suggests that drinking green tea may reduce this risk. Based on these studies, FDA concludes that it is highly unlikely that green tea reduces the risk of breast cancer."

FDAMA Nutrient Content and Health Claims

FDAMA allows nutrient content and health claims to be made on the basis of statements issued by authoritative bodies such as the National Institutes of Health or the National Academy of Sciences.[57] FDA takes the position that these claims must meet the same standard of evidence (significant scientific agreement) as FDA-approved health claims. In order to make a *FDAMA*-based claim, a petition must be filed with FDA at least 120 days prior to introducing the food bearing the claim into interstate commerce. The petition must include the exact words of the claim, a copy of the authoritative government statement on which the claim is based and a balanced representation of the scientific literature supporting the nutrient/disease relationship. During the 120-day period, FDA may notify the person wishing to make the claim if any of the required information has not been submitted. After 120 days, the claim may be used until FDA either issues a regulation prohibiting or modifying the claim or takes enforcement action.[58]

Structure/Function Claims
Structure/function claims describe the role of substances intended to affect the normal structure or function of humans.[59] Such claims assume that a person is healthy and just wants to maintain that good health. For example, the statement "Calcium maintains strong bones" is a structure/function claim. FDA authorization is not required prior to use of structure/function claims; however, such claims cannot be false or misleading or fail to reveal any material facts. Additionally, the claims must derive from the nutritional value of the product bearing the claim. Structure/function claims may characterize the means by which substances act to maintain such structure or function (e.g., "Fiber maintains bowel regularity"), or they may describe general well-being from consumption of a nutrient or dietary ingredient.

Structure/function claims may not explicitly or implicitly link the relationship to a disease or health-related condition. For example, it is permissible to make the claim that a substance supports memory, but not to make the claim that the substance reduces memory loss. The one exception to this rule is that claims are permitted to describe a benefit related to a nutrient deficiency disease (e.g., Vitamin C and scurvy), as long as the statement also provides information about how widespread such a disease is in the US.

Dietary Guidance
Dietary guidance statements are made to assist and encourage individuals in making better food choices and establishing healthier eating patterns. For example, the statement, "Diets rich in fruits and vegetables reduce the risk of certain cancers" is an acceptable dietary guidance statement. Although a dietary guidance statement can mention a specific disease, the disease cannot be linked to a specific food or a specific substance in food. The recommendations of recognized government (e.g., US Surgeon General, National Cancer Institute) or private professional health organizations (e.g., American Heart Association) provide the basis for dietary guidance. FDA has never codified the requirements for these statements, but has addressed this issue in preambles to regulations and in guidance documents.

Medical Foods
A "medical food" is a food that is "formulated to be consumed or administered...under supervision of a physician and which is intended for the specific dietary management of a disease or condition for which distinctive nutritional requirements...are established by medical evaluation."[60] FDA has issued limited guidance on medical foods (see *Guidance for Industry: Frequently Asked Questions About Medical Foods* (Revised May 2007). In general, however, to be a medical food, the product must, at a minimum, be: a food for oral or tube feeding; labeled for the dietary management of a specific medical disorder, disease or condition with distinctive nutritional requirements; and must be intended for use under medical supervision.[61]

The main distinction between medical foods and other foods is in labeling. Medical foods are not subject to labeling requirements for nutrient content claims and health claims. In other words, medical foods may bear nutrient content claims and health claims without prior FDA approval, so long as the claims are truthful and not misleading. Medical food labels must bear a statement of identity, a statement of net quantity, a manufacturer statement, a list of ingredients and allergen labeling. Nutrition labeling requirements do not apply.

For more information on medical foods, see Chapter 35.

Foods for Special Dietary Uses
Foods for special dietary uses are foods "for supplying particular dietary needs which exist by reason of a physical, physiological, pathological or other condition, including but not limited to the conditions of diseases, convalescence, pregnancy, lactation, allergic hypersensitivity to food, underweight, and overweight."[62] Under 21 CFR 105.3, foods containing artificial sweeteners to reduce calories or available carbohydrate, or for use by diabetics are considered foods for special dietary use. These products must bear nutrition labeling as required for conventional foods.

Adulteration: Food Sanitation and Safety

The *FD&C Act* prohibits the adulteration of food. Conditions that can cause a food to be deemed adulterated are set out in Section 402 of the *FD&C Act*.[63] A food may be deemed adulterated if it bears or contains any:

- poisonous or deleterious added substance that may render it injurious to health
- poisonous or deleterious naturally occurring substance in a quantity that would ordinarily render it injurious to health

- unapproved pesticide chemical residue
- unapproved food additive
- unapproved new animal drug
- unapproved color additive

In addition, food may be deemed adulterated if it consists of any "filthy, putrid, or decomposed substance or if it is otherwise unfit for food," or if it has been "prepared, packed or held under insanitary conditions" whereby it may have been contaminated with filth or rendered injurious to health. The statute also lists a number of other conditions that may render a food adulterated that are less frequently raised.

A poisonous or deleterious substance is, basically, anything in food that could cause harm, whether the substance is physical (such as a shard of glass), chemical (lead) or biological (salmonella). Whether a substance in a food is an "added substance" or a naturally occurring substance will determine the standard FDA must meet to prove adulteration. Courts have essentially held that any act of man that causes the presence of the substance in the food renders the substance an "added substance." For example, the US Court of Appeals for the Fifth Circuit has affirmed that mercury in swordfish is an "added substance" where evidence established that any amount of the mercury resulted from industrial pollution.[64]

Unavoidable Poisonous or Deleterious Substances in Food

Some poisonous or deleterious substances in food are unavoidable, such as aflatoxins in peanuts. The *FD&C Act* recognizes that some such substances may be unavoidable, and the statute provides a mechanism for the agency to establish allowable tolerances for such substances.[65] However, because such tolerances must be established by resource-intensive formal rulemaking, the agency has not issued a new tolerance for decades. Instead, the agency has a procedure for establishing what it calls "regulatory limits," which set out levels at which an unavoidable added substance may render a food injurious to health.[66] Although regulatory limits can be established by notice and comment rulemaking, which is significantly easier than formal rulemaking, the agency has never set a regulatory limit. Instead, the agency has issued action levels for certain poisonous or deleterious substances. Action levels are unenforceable guidances that represent the agency's current thinking as to what level of the substance may render it injurious to health. An action level has no legal effect, so the agency must prove in any enforcement action that the level of the substance in the food may render it injurious to health—simply providing evidence that the action level was exceeded is not sufficient.

Current Good Manufacturing Practices (CGMPs)

FDA's CGMPs for the manufacturing, packing or holding of food are set out in 21 CFR 110. Failure to follow CGMPs is a determining factor in whether a food is adulterated in that it was manufactured under conditions that rendered it unfit for food[67] or whether it was prepared, packed or held under insanitary conditions whereby the food may have been contaminated with filth or rendered injurious to health.[68] The regulations set out CGMPs for personnel, buildings and facilities, equipment and production and process controls. 21 CFR 110 also provides for "defect action levels," which establish maximum allowable levels of certain types of contamination that may result despite compliance with CGMPs. For example, FDA's *Food Defect Action Level Handbook* sets out the maximum levels of insect fragments or rodent hair that may be present in wheat flour.[69] FDA also has separate CGMP regulations for bottled water in 21 CFR 129.

HACCP—Juice and Seafood Products

Whereas all USDA-regulated products (meat, poultry and processed eggs) are required to implement Hazard Analysis and Critical Control Point (HACCP) controls for the safety of their products, FDA currently requires HACCP only for producers of juice and seafood products. FDA's HACCP regulations require producers of juice and seafood products to conduct an analysis to identify food safety hazards that are reasonably likely to occur. If the analysis concludes such hazards exist, the producer is required to implement a HACCP plan that:
- identifies the possible hazards
- lists all critical control points (CCPs) for controlling each hazard while the product is in the producer's control
- lists critical limits that must be met at each CCP to control the hazard
- lists monitoring procedures and frequency for compliance with the critical limits
- includes any corrective actions to be taken in the event of a deviation from a critical limit
- lists verification procedures for the adequacy of the HACCP plan
- establishes a recordkeeping system that documents the monitoring of compliance with the critical limits

Under HACCP regulations, records must be maintained for a minimum of one year, and two years for some products with longer shelf lives. FDA has access to review and copy all records required to be maintained by HACCP regulations.

Acidified and Low-acid Canned Foods

Stringent processing controls are established for acidified and low-acid canned foods that present significant risks of contamination, such as from *Clostridium botulinum*. FDA requires manufacturers that produce certain shelf-stable, aseptically sealed, low-acid canned or acidified foods to obtain a Food Canning Establishment (FCE) registration. In addition, manufacturers must file documentation with FDA for each process used in the production of foods subject to these requirements. These submissions are known as "Process Filings" and each is assigned a unique "Submission Identifier" (SID).

The requirements for the manufacture of low-acid canned foods are set out in 21 CFR 113, and the requirements for acidified foods are in 21 CFR 114. In addition to the specific GMPs set out in 21 CFR 113 and 114, manufacturers of acidified and low-acid canned foods must register with FDA and file with the agency the scheduled processes they intend to use to ensure product safety.[70]

Food Safety Modernization Act of 2011

On 4 January 2011, President Obama signed the *Food Safety Modernization Act* (*FSMA*) into law.[71] This law was aimed at refocusing FDA's regulatory oversight of food production from a reactive stance to a preventive role, gave the agency recall authority and required that all food operations that were not already covered by HACCP or acidified and low-acid canned food regulations establish a program of hazard analysis and risk-based preventive controls. The law also required FDA to propose and enact regulations for ensuring the safe harvesting and handling of raw produce; increased FDA oversight of imported foods; required FDA to increase inspections; and allowed for a program of user fees for reinspections, recalls and import activities. The law assigned FDA the task of preparing various regulations, rulemakings and guidance documents to facilitate compliance with the act.

The act's provisions focus on three main areas of improvement:
- capacity to prevent food safety problems
- capacity to detect and respond to food safety problems
- safety of imported food

Perhaps the most significant change in the legislation is a requirement for food companies to take preventive steps to avoid food contamination. Manufacturers now are required to identify the critical points at which the food they are handling could become contaminated and implement procedures (documented in written food-safety plans) designed to prevent contamination.

Another significant change is that the law gave FDA the right to order companies to recall tainted food. Previously, the agency could only request that a company undertake a recall. Additionally, the bill contains provisions requiring:
- FDA to inspect food manufacturers more frequently
- FDA to create a pilot program to trace outbreaks quickly back to their source
- the federal government to oversee produce quality
- importers to verify that incoming foods meets US food-safety guidelines

Every food producer with more than $500,000 in sales is required to adopt a written food-safety plan that includes an internal inspection system with detailed recordkeeping. Facilities must spell out potential problems that could affect the safety of their products and outline steps the facility will take to lower the likelihood of those problems occurring.

This provision shifts the food safety onus to food producers and manufacturers and allows FDA's role to extend beyond simply responding to food safety problems when they arise.

First, the law calls for FDA to enforce science-based standards for the safe production and harvesting of fruits and vegetables. Those standards will consider both natural and man-made risks to the safety of fresh produce. Until the bill's passage, no agency had legal oversight of produce.

Next, the law calls for more frequent inspections and for the secretary of the Department of Health and Human Services to determine which food facilities are high risk. It also encourages the secretary to investigate compliance with the act through officials at the state and local level.

Foods and facilities that pose a greater risk to food safety will get the most attention—with inspections mandated at least once every three years. The secretary is charged with drafting new regulations for the sanitary transportation of food.

Finally, every two years, FDA is required to provide industry guidance on the most important food contaminants, based on evaluations (and re-evaluations) of data and other studies.

Inspections, Recalls, and Enforcement

FDA inspections, compliance, enforcement and recalls generally are covered in other chapters of this book. Addressed here are aspects of these FDA functions particular to foods.

FDA has the authority to inspect any factory, warehouse, establishment or vehicle in which food is manufactured, processed, packed or held for introduction into interstate commerce (excluding small farms and restaurants), as well as all pertinent equipment, finished and unfinished materials, containers and labeling therein.[72] FDA also may inspect and copy records relating to the manufacture, processing, packing, distribution, receipt, holding or importation of food if the agency has a reasonable belief that the food is adulterated and presents a threat of serious adverse health consequences or death (in other words, if the food meets the standard for a Class I recall).[73] FDA does not have the authority to inspect or copy financial data, sales data other than shipment data, pricing data, personnel data or research data.⁷⁴

FDA's recall authorities under 21 CFR 7 apply equally to food products as to other products. One aspect particular to foods is that failure to label the presence of a major food allergen in a food product is cause for a Class I recall. As noted above, *FSMA* gave FDA the authority to require food product recalls. This authority comes into effect if a food product is deemed to present "a reasonable probability that an article of food (other than infant formula) is adulterated under section 402 or misbranded under section 403(w) and the use of or exposure to such article will cause serious adverse health consequences or death to humans or animals" and if the manufacturer will not voluntarily recall the product.

FDA may take enforcement action to seize or enjoin the continued distribution of adulterated or misbranded food. In addition, the agency can charge each violation as a misdemeanor subject to imprisonment of not more than one year and a fine of up to $1,000. If the violation was committed with the intent to defraud or mislead, FDA can charge a criminal felony, with penalties of up to three years in prison and a fine of up to $10,000.

The Reportable Food Registry

In 2007, Congress amended the *FD&C Act* to provide for a Reportable Food Registry. Under the requirements, an owner, operator or agent in charge of a registered food facility who determines that an article of food (other than infant formula or pet food or feed) that has been in the facility meets the standard for a Class I recall (reasonable probability of serious adverse health consequences or death) is required to file a report with the registry with 24 hours of the determination. The only exception to the reporting requirement is if the adulteration originated in the facility, was detected prior to transfer of the food to any other person and was corrected or the food destroyed. The report must be filed electronically through FDA's MedWatchPlus portal and must provide certain information regarding the food and the adulteration, including contact information for the immediate previous source of the food and the immediate subsequent recipient in the supply chain. FDA then may require notification of the identified persons in the supply chain. The Reportable Food Registry requirements were effective as of 8 September 2009.

Food Defense

The *Public Health Security and Bioterrorism Preparedness and Response Act* of 2002 (*Bioterrorism Act*)⁷⁵ amended the *FD&C Act* to provide several new authorities for FDA to protect against the possibility of an attack on the food system or other food safety emergency. Provisions of the *Bioterrorism Act* include facility registration, prior notice of imports and administrative detention authority.

Facility Registration

All food facilities must be registered with FDA. A "food facility" subject to the registration requirement is any facility engaged in manufacturing, processing, packing or holding food for consumption in the US.⁷⁶ The requirement extends to foreign facilities that are the last foreign facilities to engage in manufacturing or packaging of food to be imported to the US, provided such processing is more than *de minimis*.⁷⁷ The requirement does not apply to farms, retail food establishments (such as supermarkets), restaurants, fishing vessels or facilities regulated exclusively by USDA.⁷⁸

The registration must provide, among other information, the types of food manufactured, packed or held at the facility and a 24-hour emergency contact for the facility. FDA issues each facility a unique registration number.⁷⁹ Failure to register is a prohibited act under the *FD&C Act*. The information provided with each registration is exempt from public disclosure under the *Freedom of Information Act*.

FSMA requires food facilities to renew their FDA Food Facility Registrations between 1 October 2012 and 31 December 2012, and biennially thereafter.

Prior Notice of Imported Food

Notice must be given to FDA prior to the import of any food into the US, except meat, poultry and egg products regulated by USDA; food imported for export; and foods imported for personal use only.⁸⁰ The amount of prior notice required depends on how the food is being imported: two hours if by road, four hours if by rail, four hours if by air and eight hours if by water.⁸¹ Prior notice must be submitted electronically through links on FDA's website www.fda.gov/. Food submitted without prior notice may be refused for import.⁸²

Administrative Detention

FDA has the authority, upon issuance of a detention order, to detain any article of food found to present a threat of serious adverse health consequences or death during an inspection, examination or investigation.⁸³ The detention may not exceed 20 calendar days, but up to 10 more days may be authorized if necessary to institute a seizure or injunction action.⁸⁴ Any person who can claim the detained food can appeal a detention order challenging the determination that the food presents a threat.⁸⁵

Summary

- FDA regulates most foods. Exceptions include meat, poultry and processed egg products, which are regulated by USDA, and tap water and alcohol, which are regulated by EPA and TTB, respectively. FDA also does not regulate all aspects of food; for example, it regulates food labeling, and FTC regulates food advertising. EPA sets pesticide tolerances, and FDA enforces them. FDA primarily regulates food processing and manufacturing, whereas states are the primary regulators of restaurants, farms and retail establishments.

- Under the *FD&C Act*, FDA's regulatory authority over foods can be divided into two major categories: adulteration of food and misbranding of food labels and labeling.
- Food may be deemed adulterated for a variety of reasons set out in the *FD&C Act*, including poisonous or deleterious substances in the food, filthy or insanitary conditions under which the food was produced, or use of unapproved food additives in the food. FDA has set out CGMPS for sanitation in the production of food. The production of seafood and juice product is regulated through HACCP principles set out by regulation.
- In general, food labeling is misbranded if it is false or misleading in any particular. FDA's food labeling regulations set out detailed requirements governing mandatory labeling, such as ingredient, nutrition and allergen labeling. FDA's regulations also govern how certain types of voluntary labeling—primarily claims such as structure/function claims and nutrient content claims—may be made. Nutrient content and health claims cannot be made on foods unless FDA has approved the claims.
- Food additives must be approved by regulation for specific uses prior to use. GRAS substances are exempted from the definition of food additives and, therefore, do not require premarket approval for use. FDA provides a voluntary GRAS notification program for persons seeking some assurance that the agency agrees a substance is GRAS.
- Color additives must also be premarket approved by FDA for specific uses prior to use in any FDA-regulated product. FDA requires batch approval of certain types of color additives.
- Recent food defense amendments require all food facilities to be registered with FDA. In addition, FDA must be provided with prior notice of any food imports being shipped to the US for distribution. Since September 2009, food facilities also are required to report to FDA whenever the facility determines that food manufactured, processed, packed or held there presents a reasonable probability of a serious adverse health consequence or death.

References
1. The *FD&C Act* is codified at 21 U.S.C. § 301 *et al.*
2. 21 U.S.C. §321(f).
3. P.L. 103-417 (Oct. 25, 1994).
4. The distinction between "labeling" and "advertising" is discussed in more detail under Misbranding: Food Labeling and Claims. Generally, "labeling" includes the food label and all materials "accompanying" the food where sold (such as brochures, displays, or information on websites where the product can be purchased). "Advertising" is, broadly, any marketing of the product that is not labeling.
5. 21 U.S.C. §321(s).
6. Ibid.
7. Ibid.
8. See 21 U.S.C. §346a.
9. See 21 U.S.C. §379e.
10. 21 U.S.C. §348(a).
11. See 21 U.S.C. §348(j).
12. 21 U.S.C. §348(b).
13. 21 U.S.C. §348(c)(1)-(2).
14. 21 U.S.C. §348(f).
15. 21 U.S.C. §348(c)(3).
16. 21 U.S.C. §348(c)(3)(A).
17. *Les v. Reilly*, 968 F.2d 985 (9th Cir. 1992) (food additives); *Public Citizen v. Young*, 831 F.2d 1108 (D.C. Cir. 1987) (color additives).
18. See *Scott v. Food and Drug Administration*, 728 F.2d 322 (6th Cir. 1984); *Public Citizen v. Young*, 831 F.2d 1108, 1118-19 (D.C.Cir. 1987).
19. See 21 U.S.C. §348(c)(3)(A).
20. Codified at 21 U.S.C. §348(a)(3).
21. See 21 U.S.C. §321(s).
22. 21 U.S.C. §321(t).
23. See 21 U.S.C. §361(e). Cosmetics are discussed in detail in Chapter 28.
24. 21 U.S.C. §379e(a).
25. See generally 21 CFR 70–82.
26. In the context of color additives, a "lake" is a form of color additive that is extended on a substratum to make it water insoluble.
27. 21 U.S.C. §343.
28. 21 U.S.C. §321(k).
29. 21 U.S.C. §321(m).
30. *FD&C Act*, Section 331(a), (b), (c).
31. *FD&C Act*, Section 321(n).
32. 21 CFR 101.1.
33. 21 CFR 101.2(a).
34. 21 CFR 101.3.
35. *FD&C Act*, Section 401.
36. 21 CFR 102.5(a).
37. 21 CFR 101.3(b)(3).
38. 21 CFR 101.3(e).
39. 21 CFR 101.105.
40. 21 CFR 101.9.
41. 21 CFR 101.4.
42. Pub. L. No. 108-282.
43. *FALCPA* §203.
44. 21 CFR 101.5.
45. 9 CFR 317.2(c)(5).
46. 9 CFR 317.2(k).
47. 9 CFR 317.2(l).
48. 9 CFR 317.4; see also "A Guide to Federal Food Labeling Requirements for Meat and Poultry Products," FSIS, August 2007.
49. The final rule became effective on 16 March 2009 and is codified in 7 CFR 60 and 65. 74 *Fed Reg.* 2658 (15 January 2009).
50. 19 U.S.C. 1304.
51. 19 CFR 134.11
52. *FDAMA* refers to the *Food and Drug Administration Modernization Act* of 1997, which, among other amendments, provided for health and nutrient content claims based on statements issued by authoritative government bodies, like the National Academies of Science or the National Institutes of Health.
53. 21 CFR 101.13.
54. *FD&C Act*, Sections 403(r)(1)(A) and 403(r)(2).
55. 21 CFR 101.14.
56. 21 U.S.C. §321(g).

57. 21 U.S.C. §343(r)(3)(C).
58. 21 U.S.C. §343(r)(3)(D).
59. 21 CFR 101.93.
60. *Orphan Drug Act* §5, codified at 21 U.S.C. 360ee(b)(3).
61. Food Labeling; Reference Daily Intakes and Daily Reference Values; Mandatory Status of Nutrition Labeling and Nutrition Content Revision proposed rule (56 *Fed. Reg.* 60366 at 60377, November 27, 1991.
62. Op cit 60.
63. 21 U.S.C. §342.
64. *United States v. Anderson Seafoods, Inc.*, 622 F.2d 157, 159-60 (5th Cir. 1980)
65. 21 U.S.C. §346.
66. 21 CFR 109.
67. 21 U.S.C. §342(a)(3).
68. 21 U.S.C. §342(a)(4).
69. FDA. Defect Levels Handbook. FDA website. http://www.fda.gov/Food/GuidanceRegulation/GuidanceDocumentsRegulatoryInformation/SanitationTransportation/ucm056174.htm. Accessed 8 May 2013.
70. 21 CFR 108.25 (acidified foods) and 108.35 (low acid canned foods).
71. Public Law 111-353 (4 January 2011).
72. 21 U.S.C. §374.
73. 21 U.S.C. §350c.
74. 21 U.S.C. §374.
75. P.L. 107-188.
76. 21 U.S.C. §415.
77. 21 CFR 1.226(a).
78. 21 CFR 1.226.
79. 21 CFR 1.232.
80. 21 CFR 1.277.
81. 21 CFR 1.279.
82. 21 CFR 1.283.
83. 21 CFR 1.378.
84. 21 CFR 1.379.
85. 21 CFR 1.401.

Appendix A. Major Federal Food Safety Agencies and Selected Laws

Agency	Major Responsibilities and Activities	Primary Authorities
Department of Health and Human Services		
Food and Drug Administration (FDA)[a]	Ensures that all domestic and imported foods, except processed egg products and major types of meat and poultry, are safe, wholesome and properly labeled by setting safety and sanitation standards, periodically inspecting manufacturing facilities, reviewing records of and spot-checking imports. Also oversees the safety of animal drugs and feeds, including those used in food-producing animals.	*Federal Food, Drug, and Cosmetic Act* (*FD&C Act*; 21 U.S.C. §§301–399a) as amended; *Public Health Service Act* (42 U.S.C. §201), *Egg Products Inspection Act* (21 U.S.C. §1031); *Federal Import Milk Act* (21 U.S.C. §§141–149); *Fair Packaging and Labeling Act* (15 U.S.C. §§1451–1461); *Federal Anti-Tampering Act* (18 U.S.C. §1365); *Pesticide Monitoring Improvements Act* of 1988 (21 U.S.C. §1401)	
Centers for Disease Control and Prevention (CDC)	Monitors, identifies and investigates foodborne diseases; develops and evaluates improved epidemiological and laboratory methods.	*Public Health Service Act* (42 U.S.C. §201)	
Department of Agriculture		
Food Safety Inspection Service (FSIS)a	Regulates the safety, wholesomeness and proper labeling of most commercial types of both domestic and imported meat and poultry, catfish products and processed egg products by approving establishment designs, safety plans; inspecting every animal and carcass in slaughtering plants and daily inspecting all meat and poultry processing plants; determining the equivalency of importing countries' meat and poultry safety systems.	*Federal Meat Inspection Act* (21 U.S.C. §§601–695); *Poultry Products Inspection Act* (21 USC §§451–472); *Egg Products Inspection Act* (21 U.S.C. §§1031–1056); *Humane Methods of Slaughter Act* of 1978 (7 U.S.C. §§1902, 1904, 21 U.S.C. §§603, 610, 620); *Federal Anti-Tampering Act* (18 U.S.C. §1365); *Agricultural Marketing Act* of 1946 (7 U.S.C. §1622); *Richard B. Russell National School Lunch Act* (42 U.S.C. §§1751–1770), as amended by *Child Nutrition and WIC Reauthorization Acts* (42 U.S.C. §1762a(h))	
Animal and Plant Health Inspection Service (APHIS)	Oversees animal and plant health, including the prevention of foreign diseases and pests, and eradication and containment of such problems domestically (including those that threaten public health).	*Animal Health Protection Act* (7 U.S.C. §§8301–8322); *Plant Health Protection Act* (7 U.S.C. §§7701–7721); *Agricultural Bioterrorism Act* of 2002 (7 U.S.C. §8401)	
Agricultural Marketing Service (AMS)	Establishes quality and marketing grades and standards for dairy products, fruits and vegetables, livestock, meat, poultry, seafoods and shell eggs; certifies quality programs; conducts quality grading services, generally user fee-funded.	*Agricultural Marketing Act* of 1946 (7 U.S.C. §§1621–1638d), *Perishable Agricultural Commodities Act*, 1930 (7 U.S.C. §§499a–499s); *Federal Seed Act* (7 U.S.C. §§1551–1611)	
Food and Nutrition Service (FNS)	Encourages and coordinates efforts to ensure the safety of foods in school lunch and other domestic programs	Program subsidies authorized by *Richard B. Russell National School Lunch Act* (42 U.S.C. §§1751–1770), as amended by *Child Nutrition and WIC Reauthorization Acts* (42 U.S.C. § 1762a(h))	
Grain Inspection, Packers and Stockyards Administration (GIPSA)	Sets quality standards for and tests grains and related commodities, primarily for marketing purposes.	*US Grain Standards Act* (7 USC §§71–87k), *Agricultural Marketing Act* of 1946 (7 U.S.C. §§1622, 1624)	
Agricultural Research Service (ARS)	Conducts in-house USDA research on agricultural and food topics, of which food safety is one of many.	Numerous laws dating to the *Department of Agriculture Organic Act* of 1862 (7 U.S.C. §2201 note), up through and including recent omnibus farm laws	
National Institute of Food and Agriculture (NIFA) (formerly Cooperative State Research, Education, and Extension Service)	Coordinates and administers federal funding of land grant and other institutions to conduct agricultural and food research, education and extension activities; food safety is one of many subject areas.	Numerous laws dating to the *Department of Agriculture Organic Act* of 1862, up through and including recent omnibus farm laws	

Food Products

Department of Commerce			
National Oceanic and Atmospheric Administration (NOAA)	Offers a variety of voluntary seafood safety and quality inspection services on a fee-for-service basis.	*Agricultural Marketing Act* of 1946 (7 U.S.C. §§1622, 1624); *Lacey Act* (16 U.S.C. §3371); *Fish and Wildlife Act* of 1956 (16 U.S.C. §742)	
US Environmental Protection Agency (EPA)	Regulates the use of certain chemicals and substances that present an unreasonable risk of injury to health or the environment. Regulates pesticide products; sets maximum allowable tolerances for residue levels on food commodities and animal feeds. Sets national drinking water standards and consults with FDA. Sets scientific water quality criteria for rivers, lakes and streams that are protective of human health and wildlife.	*FD&C Act* (21 U.S.C. §§301–399a), as amended; *Federal Insecticide, Fungicide, and Rodenticide Act* (7 U.S.C. §§136-136y), as amended by the *Food Quality Protection Act* of 1996 (21 U.S.C. §346a); *Clean Water Act* (33 U.S.C. 1251-1387); *Safe Drinking Water Act* of 1974 (21 U.S.C. §349 and 42 U.S.C. §§300f–300j-26); Toxic Substance Control Act (15 U.S.C. §§2601-2697)	
Federal Trade Commission (FTC)	Enforces federal prohibitions against unfair or deceptive acts or practices in trade, including consumer deception regarding foods.	*Federal Trade Commission Act* (15 U.S.C. §§41–58)	
Department of the Treasury			
Alcohol and Tobacco Tax and Trade Bureau (TTB)	Administers and enforces laws on the production, safety, distribution and use of alcoholic beverages.	*Federal Alcohol Administration Act* (27 U.S.C. §§201–219a); Internal Revenue Code (26 U.S.C. Ch. 51)	
Department of Homeland Security			
U.S. Customs and Border Protection (CBP)	Coordinates many food security activities, including inspecting imports of food, plants, and animals at the border. Conducts agricultural border inspection activities formerly done by APHIS.	*Homeland Security Act* of 2002 (6 U.S.C. §101); *Tariff Act* of 1930 (19 U.S.C. §§1202–1654)	

Source: Prepared by CRS based in part on various reports by the Government Accountability Office, including GAO, *Federal Food Safety Oversight*, GAO-11-289, March 2011. Does not include two USDA agencies included by GAO (Research, Education, and Economics (REE) agencies: National Economic Research Service (ERS) and National Agricultural Statistics Service (NASS).

a. These agencies have the leading food safety regulatory authorities.

Chapter 33

Appendix B. Selected Comparison of FSIS and FDA Responsibilities

Activity	Food Safety and Inspection Service	Food and Drug Administration (Foods Program only)
Primary Authorizations	*Federal Meat Inspection Act* (21 U.S.C. 601), *Poultry Products Inspection Act* (21 U.S.C. 451), *Egg Products Inspection Act* (21 U.S.C. 1031)	As may be amended by the *FDA Food Safety Modernization Act* (*FSMA*): *Federal Food, Drug, and Cosmetic Act* (*FD&C Act*); 21 U.S.C. 301; *Public Health Service Act* (42 U.S.C. 201); *Egg Products Inspection Act* (21 U.S.C. 1031); *Public Health Security and Bioterrorism Preparedness and Response Act* (21 U.S.C. 341)
Foods Regulated	Major types of domestic and imported meat and poultry and their products; catfish products; processed (dried, frozen, liquid) egg products (20% of at-home US food spending)	All other domestic and imported foods, also animal drugs and feeds including those used in food-producing animals (80% of at-home US food spending)
Funding (enacted Fiscal 2012)	Appropriated: $1.004 billion for Fiscal 2012. Expected user fees are estimated to include another $150 million. Including authorized fees, total available funding is estimated at about $1.154 billion.	Appropriated: $866.1 million for FDA's Foods Program, not including funding from expected user fees. Expected user fees are estimated to include another $79 million. Including authorized fees, total available funding is estimated at about $945 million.
Staff (2011)	9,600 FTEs	3,400 FTEs
Domestic facilities	6,300 slaughter and/or processing establishments	68,000 subject to inspection
Inspection Approach	Ante- and post-mortem inspection of every animal, carcass and part; traditionally organoleptic (but see "Food safety plans" below); only USDA inspected and passed products may enter commerce	Prohibits adulteration or misbranding; relies on facilities that manufacture, process, pack or hold food for humans or animals to meet prescribed standards (e.g., regarding additives, contaminants, etc.); all facilities must register, report changes in timely manner.
Required inspection frequency	Slaughter plants: all times of operation; processing plants: at least once daily	*FSMA* requires increased inspection rates for any registered facility, particularly those identified as "high-risk." Domestic high-risk facilities are to be inspected not less than once in the five-year period after enactment, and not less than once every three years thereafter. Domestic non-high-risk facilities are to be inspected not less than once in the seven-year period after enactment, and not less than once every five years thereafter.
Food safety plans	Requires all establishments to prepare and have preapproved "HACCP" (hazard analysis and critical control point) plans determining risks, controlling them (with documentation)	Prior to *FSMA*, facilities followed general regulations on Good Manufacturing Practices (GMPs) to address safe handling and plant sanitation—except a form of HACCP required for seafood, low-acid canned foods, juices. *FSMA* §103 created new requirements for facilities to evaluate hazards, implement preventive controls, monitor controls and maintain records. FDA rulemaking is clarifying requirements under new written HACCP-type and/or broader written food safety plans as part of its so-called Hazard Analysis and Risk-Based Preventive Controls.
Imports	Specified products only from countries where FSIS has determined "equivalence" of foreign safety system, with annual verification; imports exempt from prior notice but subject to reinspection at 150 import establishments (est. 10% reinspected)	Prior to *FSMA*, food safety system equivalence was not determined beforehand; reliance on inspections was at 300 ports (est. 1% of notified entries inspected). *FSMA* provides for tighter controls and use certification or verification systems for imported foods (to be determined by FDA rulemaking). At least 600 foreign facilities must be inspected the year following enactment, and in each of the subsequent five years the number of foreign facilities inspected is to double.
Third-party certification	Private labs accredited for chemical testing of meat and poultry (for imports, see above)	Prior to *FSMA*, there was no accreditation for food testing labs or use of third parties for import oversight. *FSMA* §202 requires FDA to establish a program for testing of food by accredited laboratories and to recognize accreditation bodies to accredit labs. *FSMA* §303 creates a system of accreditation of third-party auditors and audit agents to certify importing entities. FDA's rulemaking is ongoing.

		Food Products
On-farm oversight	FSIS inspection authority begins at slaughter plant	Prior to *FSMA*, those engaged solely in harvesting, storing or distributing raw agricultural commodities generally were exempt from registration, GMP regulations, and recordkeeping. *FSMA* §105 created new farm-level requirements, particularly for fresh produce determined to be higher-risk (FDA rulemaking is ongoing). Some small farm businesses are exempt from regulation.
Labeling	Review and preapproval required for all labels	All foods must adhere to food labeling requirements such as statement of identity, declaration of net contents, nutrition labeling; labels cannot be false or misleading.
Notification Requirements	P.L. 110-246 §11017 amended meat and poultry laws to require an establishment to notify USDA if it has reason to believe that an adulterated or misbranded product has entered commerce	P.L. 110-85 (amended by *FSMA*) requires FDA to maintain a reportable food registry for industry to report food safety cases in order to help FDA better track patterns and target inspections. *FSMA* §204 provided for an enhanced tracing system for foods that FDA determines to pose a higher food safety risk. As part of the ongoing rulemaking process, FDA has launched product tracing pilots.
Recall Authority	No authority to mandate recalls; relies on voluntary efforts	Prior to *FSMA*, FDA had no authority to mandate recalls (except infant formula). *FSMA* §206 provides for mandatory recall authority where there is a reasonable probability that a food is adulterated or misbranded, and its use or exposure to it will cause serious adverse health consequences or death. Civil/criminal penalties apply for failure to comply with a recall order.

Source: Congressional Research Service

Chapter 34

Companion Diagnostics

By Mya Thomae, RAC

OBJECTIVES

❑ Understand what companion diagnostics are

❑ Understand the responsibilities of both diagnostic (Dx) and drug (Rx) companies in the development and FDA approval of companion diagnostics

❑ Understand the requirements for companion diagnostics during the investigational phase

❑ Understand how companion diagnostics obtain regulatory approval in relation to drug approval

❑ Understand the postapproval responsibilities of both Dx and Rx companies in relation to the companion diagnostic

LAWS, REGULATIONS AND GUIDANCE DOCUMENTS COVERED IN THIS CHAPTER

❑ *Draft Guidance for Industry and Food and Drug Administration Staff: In Vitro Companion Diagnostic Devices Draft Guidance (July 2011)*

Note: This chapter assumes the reader has read Chapter 21 In Vitro Diagnostics Submissions and Compliance.

Introduction

As defined by the President's Council on Advisors on Science and Technology, "Personalized Medicine" refers to the tailoring of medical treatment to the individual characteristics of each patient. It does not mean the literal creation of drugs or medical devices that are unique to a patient, but rather the ability to classify individuals into subpopulations that differ in their susceptibility to a particular disease or their response to a specific treatment.[1]

The products created to "classify individuals into subpopulations" are often in vitro diagnostics (IVDs). When IVDs are used to inform doctors about whether a drug or other intervention can be used in a safe and effective manner, they are specifically classified by the US Food and Drug Administration (FDA) as in vitro companion diagnostic devices.[2]

This chapter summarizes the current FDA approach to regulation of IVD companion diagnostic devices. In addition, information is presented regarding the roles and responsibilities of both the diagnostic (Dx) and therapeutic (Rx) partner when a companion diagnostic project is undertaken.

What is a Companion Diagnostic?

FDA's definition of an IVD companion diagnostic (CoDx) device is: "an in vitro diagnostic device that provides information that is essential for the safe and effective use of a corresponding therapeutic product."[3] FDA specifically does not include other tests in the definition, including Laboratory Developed Tests (LDTs) that provide information to a physician on therapeutic choices. Rather, CoDx products are very specifically products on which safe and effective use of a specific therapeutic depends on the information from the IVD companion diagnostic device.

Early Days

The early stages of FDA's policies around companion diagnostics can be traced to the 1998 approval of Dako's Herceptest (an assay for detection of HER2, a genetic marker linked to Genetech's Herceptin). The Herceptest approval was the first instance where FDA linked the intended use of a specific assay to a specific drug and required contemporaneous approval of both products. Over the next several years, other diagnostic companies followed Dako in obtaining approval on HER2 assays including Ventana, Life Technologies and Leica Biosystems. FDA also approved kits to measure EGFR (linked to the drugs Erbitux and Vectibix) as well C-Kit (linked to the drug Gleevec).

After the early HER2 approvals but before the release of a formal CoDx guidance, FDA made a few decisions that no longer are considered to represent FDA policy. Although it is important to be aware of these interim decisions, it is just as important to understand that FDA policy has changed and it may not consider these decisions as a binding precedent for future decisions.

The most significant example of an interim decision by FDA involves use of the Monogram HIV Tropism test with Pfizer's Selzentry (maraviroc). The labeling on Selzentry states that "Tropism testing must be conducted with a highly sensitive tropism assay that has demonstrated the ability to identify patients appropriate for use of Selzentry." Despite this requirement on the drug label, no HIV Tropism assay is currently cleared or approved by FDA. This is due, in part, to the fact that FDA did not require such an approval or clearance to be obtained in concert with the drug approval. Monogram's labeling states that the Monogram test was used in Selzentry's Phase 3 trials, noting "… the assay has been used to screen over 5100 patients to characterize baseline tropism, and at subsequent time points to provide an understanding of why patients may experience treatment failure on the drug." The HIV Tropism assay situation is widely discussed, but it reflects a specific moment in the evolution of FDA's policy. FDA representatives have stated publicly that the agency does not intend to repeat this decision.[4]

Policy Established

In 2011, FDA policy around CoDx took shape more clearly and consistently. In addition to releasing the first CoDx draft guidance document, FDA approved several companion diagnostics that conform to the key thinking contained in the guidance, including Roche Molecular Systems' COBAS 4800 BRAF V600 Mutation Test (P110020), Abbott Molecular's VYSIS ALK Break Apart FISH Probe Kit (P110012) and Qiagen's Therascreen KRAS RGQ PCR Kit (P110030). These approvals represent FDA's latest thinking on companion diagnostic requirements and policy and are appropriate to reference when considering a companion diagnostic project.

Exceptions to Policy

There are also recent cases where FDA decided that existing cleared or approved IVDs are sufficient for the purpose of ensuring safe and effective use of a drug. One example of such a finding is the approval of Vertex's Kayldeco. Kayldeco is approved for the treatment of cystic fibrosis (CF) for patients that have a mutation in their CF gene called the G551D mutation. Kayldeco is not effective in patients with CF with two copies of the F508del mutation (F508del/F508del) in the CF gene. If the patient's genotype is unknown, the labeling of the drug states that an FDA-cleared CF mutation test should be used to detect the presence of the G551D mutation.

In this case, several FDA-cleared CF tests included detection of these mutations in their indications. As a result, FDA decided it was not necessary to submit a separate application for a diagnostic with a specific companion diagnostic intended use. Although FDA determined it was in the interest of public health to not require a separate device approval in the case of Kayldeco, the agency has determined in other cases that an existing 510(k) clearance is not sufficient to ensure safe and effective use of the device as a companion diagnostic. If a 510(k)-cleared product will be used to select patients during a pivotal trial, it is important for the study sponsor to have a discussion with both CDER and CDRH to ensure any requirements for a companion diagnostic device are known early in the development process.

Policy on LDTs

FDA's approach to LDTs as companion diagnostics is consistent with its approach to IVDs used for CoDx and not modeled on its approach to LDTs more generally (see Chapter 21 on In Vitro Diagnostics for more information on LDTs). Although FDA currently is exercising "enforcement discretion" regarding most LDTs (i.e., not requiring clearance or approval prior to marketing), that policy does not extend to the use of LDTs as companion diagnostics. FDA has stated publically that if an LDT meets the definition of a companion diagnostic, the enforcement discretion approach will not be taken. An example of a CoDx LDT clearance is the Focus Diagnostics test for Anti-JCV antibody detection (k112394) that should be performed for patients being considered for treatment with natalizumab (Biogen Idec's therapy for multiple sclerosis).

FDA has been clear in public statements that it believes it is important for safe and effective use of drugs for companion diagnostics to be cleared or approved contemporaneously with drugs. Even so, FDA has given itself room for negotiation in the CoDx co-development guidance document: "FDA may decide that it is appropriate to approve a therapeutic product even though the IVD companion diagnostic device for which it is labeled for use is not being approved or cleared contemporaneously." It is unclear from current approvals what case or condition might form the basis of such a finding.

For reference and convenience, FDA has included a page on the website of approved IVD Companion Diagnostics Devices:

www.fda.gov/MedicalDevices/ProductsandMedicalProcedures/InVitroDiagnostics/ucm301431.htm.

Regulatory Roles of Dx and Rx Companies in CoDx Projects

A few companies produce both drugs and diagnostic products (e.g., Roche and Abbott). Generally, however, diagnostic products and therapeutic products come from separate companies (the Dx partner and Rx partner, respectively). Since the establishment of FDA policy on CoDx, it has become very important for Rx and Dx partners to work closely together so both products are cleared or approved for the US market at the same time.

Selecting Partners

Most CoDx projects begin with an Rx company identifying a need for a diagnostic and deciding to seek out the assistance of a Dx partner. Typically, the Rx company provides substantial funds for the project and controls project scheduling. Business and economic factors make this the most likely case, but regulatory factors also are involved. For example, there is an imbalance under current FDA policy between the labeling requirements of a CoDx drug and diagnostic. A CoDx drug generally requires an "FDA-approved diagnostic" in its labeling, but a CoDx diagnostic's labeling refers to a specific drug. As a consequence, Rx companies have some latitude to work with multiple partners or no partner at all; it is difficult for Dx companies to proceed beyond early development with a CoDx project without identifying an Rx partner (the exception is for follow-on assays after the first Premarket Approval Application (PMA) is approved as noted with HER2 example earlier).

Much of the early work on a CoDx project consists of the Rx company finding the right partners to work with and establishing the right agreements. Many criteria may shape the Rx company's final decision; at minimum, the right Dx partner will have both the technical ability and the appropriate rights to test for a particular analyte or gene. For example, an Rx company may discover that it needs to test for a particular gene, but the rights to test for this gene (or the bulk of the information pertaining to the gene) are owned exclusively by one Dx company or by a small number of companies. If this is the case, the Rx partner is unlikely to have broad latitude in who its Dx partner will be; essentially, it will be impossible to submit a regulatory application without securing the rights-holder's permission. For most analytes and genes, however, there are no such ownership claims. When this is the case, the Rx company will need to choose a Dx partner that has the technical ability to detect the marker that is linked to use of the drug and the right infrastructure and business relationships to support the drug postapproval.

Role of Rx Partner

The Rx company must provide as much information as possible on both the disease biology and the action of the drug to allow the Dx company to understand precisely what the test needs to measure and what performance characteristics (such as cut-offs) the test needs to demonstrate. It will be very important for the biomarker scientists at the Rx company to work closely with the Dx development scientists to ensure the proper requirements are captured prior to use in a pivotal clinical trial. If additional development activities are performed after the diagnostic is used in a pivotal trial, the results from that trial could be compromised and additional studies might be required. It is not always practical to complete diagnostic development prior to the pivotal trial, but it is highly advisable to know what impact development may have on project schedule and budget.

Role of Dx Partner

The role of the diagnostic partner is to develop a test that will measure an analyte or analytes at a level of precision appropriate for informing treatment decisions for the drug. This work will need to be performed in a manner and to standards that will facilitate approval by FDA. Specifically, the diagnostic company must develop the product under design control and comply with the other portions of the Quality System Regulation (QSR, 21 CFR Part 820), including software validation. QSR compliance will be required for all types of CoDx assays, including those developed as single laboratory assays.

Presubmission Activities

Meetings With Drug Review Branch (CDER or CBER)

Early meetings about the companion diagnostic typically happen in the context of the review of the drug. It is the responsibility of the drug review branch (Center for Drug Evaluation and Research (CDER) or Center for Biologics Evaluation and Review (CBER)) to determine whether the investigational study design is appropriate for eventual approval of the therapy. One key discussion point will be whether the drug should be studied in a "selected" group of patients (either marker-negative *or* marker-positive) or an "unselected" group (both marker-negative and marker-positive patients). Selected designs are becoming more common, as this type of design often allows for a more efficient selection process. FDA tends to prefer unselected designs, however, making it possible to meaningfully determine whether marker status usefully predicts the drug's efficacy. Generally, FDA is inclined to resist a selected design unless selection addresses a specific safety issue.

Meetings with the drug review branch typically include personnel from the device review branch (usually the Center for Devices and Radiological Health (CDRH), but in certain cases, CBER). Device review personnel are invited to early stage drug review meetings so there is broad understanding across the relevant groups at FDA regarding issues with both the drug and the diagnostic test.

Meetings With Device Review Branch (CDRH or CBER)

Once a drug moves past Phase 2 and it appears the marker may be important to safe and effective use of the drug, the drug review branch typically will recommend to the Rx company that a meeting should be set up with the device review branch (CDRH or CBER). The device review branch will be responsible for ensuring the diagnostic product performs appropriately and all studies demonstrating both nonclinical and clinical performance have been completed to the appropriate standard. Early discussions will include the required analytical studies (i.e., Limit of Detection (LoD), precision, linearity, interfering substances, cross-contamination). The LoD study is nearly always a key issue of discussion. The detection limit of the assay needs to be determined by the biology of the disease and the drug. The final determination of the LoD will require coordination and agreement between both FDA review branches.

It is now the norm to have the drug review branch attend early meetings with the device review branch. Depending on the situation, an Rx company may choose to have a meeting with the device review group prior to selecting a diagnostic partner. These meetings may help the Rx company understand regulatory requirements and thus make a more informed partner choice. In other situations, it may be more efficient to engage device review personnel after a Dx partner is selected.

Investigational Device Exemptions vs. Investigational New Drugs

An Investigational Device Exemption (IDE) is not required for many diagnostic studies, but is often required in a companion diagnostic study. In the early days of companion diagnostics, the drug company incorporated the relevant device information into its Investigational New Drug (IND) application in lieu of submitting a parallel IDE. More recently, device review branches have been requesting that device companies prepare a separate IDE that is approved in parallel with the IND. Submitting a parallel IDE appears to address challenges with information-sharing across the centers and provide some efficiency for each center in tracking reviews and approvals separately.

The key information to include in a CoDx are the data that support use of the investigational product to select patients for the trial. This is typically a subset of the analytical testing that will ultimately be required for PMA approval. The IDE also must contain the drug study protocol and key study documentation such as the informed consent form. Although the protocol will be for the drug study (not a separate device study), the IDE must provide information on the site(s) that will perform the assay (rather than the investigators who will administer the drug). By restricting the scope of the IDE to the assay-running sites, it will be easier to know whether the IDE or IND needs to be updated as the trial proceeds.

The ultimate responsibility for adhering to Good Clinical Practices (GCPs) falls to the study sponsor, typically the Rx partner. Even so, the Dx partner may take on some responsibility to ensure the test is being run appropriately and that the test does not change during the trial.

PMA and NDA

The diagnostic information from the trial will need to be incorporated into the NDA or Biologics License Application (BLA) for the therapy. Since the study sponsor handles the clinical database, the Rx partner typically has the diagnostic information needed for an NDA or BLA once the trial is completed. However, the Dx partner should be prepared to respond to requests if any issues are noted with diagnostic testing during or after the trial. Apart from providing incidental support, it is not typical for the Dx partner to be involved with the Rx submission.

Although the Dx partner does not have much involvement with the Rx partner's submission, typically, the reverse is not true. The Dx partner will need several key pieces of information from the Rx partner before filing the PMA or 510(k). Because the diagnostic's clinical utility involves the safe and effective use of the drug, the Rx partner's safety analysis is germane to documenting that use. In some cases, the diagnostic may have undergone additional development or revision subsequent to the pivotal trial. If this is the case, it will be necessary to conduct a bridging study to show concordance between the clinical trial assay and the assay being submitted for approval. Meeting this requirement will involve the Rx partner, because the safety analysis must be performed again with the assay to be commercialized to ensure that the change in versions has not affected the basis for clinical utility.

Normally, companion diagnostics are Class III (high risk) devices requiring a PMA and new therapies typically require an NDA or BLA. To ensure FDA has adequate time to review both submissions, diagnostics companies typically submit a modular PMA. The modular PMA approach allows the diagnostic company to submit the PMA in pieces (modules) while the clinical trial is ongoing. For example, the diagnostic information on quality systems and manufacturing, software and analytical studies could be submitted and reviewed during the study. Then, when the clinical data are ready, the final clinical PMA module is submitted at the same time as the NDA. This approach allows FDA to keep the reviews in sync and, hopefully, be ready to approve both the drug and device at the same time.

Currently, if either the drug or device falls behind in the review process, there is a high risk that the paired products will be held up for review until both can be approved contemporaneously. However, the risks are not the same for both parties and delays can realign incentives dramatically. A CoDx device cannot be approved without the drug, but the reverse is not always true.

There is no formal process yet for resolving CoDx submission sync issues. The "correct" policy answer is that both approvals must wait, as each product is only safe and effective in the context of the other. Practically speaking, FDA faces political and public health pressures to approve certain therapies that can lead to "creative" thinking on such policies.

Postapproval

At the time of publication, companion diagnostics are still new enough that there is not enough definitive information to determine how postapproval responsibilities and issues will be handled. The labeling of both the Rx and Dx components of a CoDx assume that both products will be available commercially at the same time. It is not clear yet what would happen if FDA were to pull one of these paired products off the market. It is even more challenging to contemplate what should happen if one product were voluntarily removed from the market or was not meaningfully offered for sale in the first place.

The Rx and Dx partners may wish to co-promote the drug, diagnostic or their pairing. In this case, the normal issues of promoting within the labeling of both of the Rx and Dx product will apply. The usual rules surrounding changes to either product also apply. Because the diagnostic likely will be a Class III device, most changes will require a PMA amendment.

As previously mentioned, CoDx drug labels do not generally reference a specific diagnostic product, but rather require an FDA-approved diagnostic. This labeling policy explicitly leaves open the possibility that additional diagnostic products may be approved for the same marker after the drug is approved. In cases such as HER2, multiple companies have successfully gained approval to market diagnostics that are intended for use with a drug, but have done so well after the initial drug approval.

References

1. Priorities for Personalized Medicine; President's Council of Advisors on Science and Technology (September 2008). The White House website. www.whitehouse.gov/files/documents/ostp/PCAST/pcast_report_v2.pdf. Accessed 22 April 2013.
2. *Draft Guidance for Industry and Food and Drug Administration Staff: In Vitro Companion Diagnostic Devices* (July 2011). FDA website. www.fda.gov/downloads/MedicalDevices/DeviceRegulationandGuidance/GuidanceDocuments/UCM262327.pdf. Accessed 22 April 2013.
3. Ibid.
4. Thomae M. Companion Diagnostics: LDTs Need Approval Too (June 2012). Myraqa Inc. website. www.myraqa.com/blog/companion_diagnostics_ldts_app. Accessed 22 April 2013.

Chapter 35

Medical Foods

By Maruthi Prasad Palthur

OBJECTIVES

❑ Develop a broad understanding of the medical foods regulation

❑ Understand the basics of medical food labeling requirements

❑ Understand the basic regulatory requirements for medical food manufacturing and adverse event reporting

LAWS, REGULATIONS AND GUIDELINES COVERED IN THIS CHAPTER

❑ *Food Allergen Labeling and Consumer Protection Act* of 2004 (Public Law 108-282)

❑ *Fair Packaging and Labeling Act* of 1966 (Public Law 89-755)

❑ *Federal Food, Drug, and Cosmetic Act* of 1938 (codified as amended at 21 U.S.C. § 301 et al)

❑ *Health Research and Health Services Amendments* of 1976 (Public Law 94-278)

❑ *Orphan Drug Amendments* of 1988 (Public Law 100-290)

❑ *Nutrition Labeling and Education Act* of 1990 (Public Law 101-53)

❑ *Food Allergen Labeling and Consumer Protection Act* of 2004 (Public Law 108-282)

❑ *Food Safety Modernization Act* of 2011 (Public Law 111-353)

❑ *Food and Drug Administration Amendments Act* of 2007 (Public Law 110-085)

❑ 21 CFR 350 Vitamins and minerals

❑ 21 CFR 101 Food Labeling

❑ 21 CFR 343 Misbranded food

❑ 21 CFR 101.9 Nutrition labeling of food

❑ 21 CFR 110 Current Good Manufacturing Practice in manufacturing, packing, or holding human food

❑ 21 CFR 113 Thermally processed low-acid foods packaged in hermetically sealed containers

❑ 21 CFR 108 Emergency permit control

❑ 21 CFR 1, Subpart H Registration of food facilities

❑ 21 CFR Part 106 Infant formula quality control procedures

❑ 21 CFR Part 107 Infant formula

Chapter 35

- 21 CFR 350f Reportable food registry

- 21 CFR 107.240 Notification requirements

- *Compliance program 7321.002. Medical Foods Program – Import and Domestic* (24 August 2006)

- *Compliance Program 7321.006: Infant Formula Program – Import and Domestic* (31 July 2006)

- *Guidance for Industry: Frequently Asked Questions about Medical Foods* (May 1997; Revised May 2007)

- *Guidance for Industry: Questions and Answers Regarding Food Allergens, including the Food Allergen Labeling and Consumer Protection Act of 2004 (Edition 4); Final Guidance* (October 2006)

- *Guidance for Industry: Acidified Foods* (September 2010)

- *Guidance for Industry: Submitting Form FDA 2541 (Food Canning Establishment Registration) and Forms FDA 2541a and FDA 2541c (Food Process Filing Forms) to FDA in Electronic or Paper Format* (July 2012)

- *Guidance for Industry: Questions and Answers Regarding Food Facility Registration (Fifth Edition)* (December 2012)

- *Guidance for Industry: Frequently Asked Questions about FDA's Regulation of Infant Formula* (1 March 2006)

- *Draft Guidance for Industry: Questions and Answers Regarding the Reportable Food Registry as Established by the Food and Drug Administration Amendments Act of 2007 (Edition 2)* (May 2010)

- *Guidance for Industry: Questions and Answers Regarding the Reportable Food Registry as Established by the Food and Drug Administration Amendments Act of 2007* (September 2009)

Introduction

Traditionally, food has been viewed as a means of providing basic calories and nutrients to maintain homeostasis. As a response to advances in food sciences and health-related research, some foods have adopted a different connotation of promoting health and reducing the risk of disease, beyond meeting basic nutritional needs. In the course of this evolution, a special category of foods with an emphasis on nutritional intervention to meet the distinctive nutritional requirements or metabolic deficiencies of a particular disease state have emerged. These foods are distinguished from the broader category of foods and are specially formulated for the specific dietary management of a disease or condition. These foods are unique in that they cannot be classified as either conventional foods or prescription drugs, thereby requiring the creation of a distinct class of foods. At the global level, the approach to defining and regulating this unique category of foods is heterogeneous. In the US, these products are regulated as "medical foods."

Historical Regulation of Medical Foods

In the *Federal Register* of 22 November 1941 (6 FR 5921), the US Food and Drug Administration (FDA) for the first time promulgated a regulation stating the term "special dietary uses." "Special dietary uses," as applied to food for man, means particular (as distinguished from general) uses of food, and means, among other things, "uses for supplying particular dietary needs which exist by reason of a physical, physiological, pathological or other condition, including but not limited to the conditions of disease, convalescence, pregnancy, lactation, allergic hypersensitivity to food, underweight, and overweight."

Before 1972, FDA regulated the products for dietary management in disease condition as drugs under Section 201(g)(1)(B) of the *Federal Food, Drug, and Cosmetic Act* (*FD&C Act*) because of their role in mitigating serious adverse effects of the underlying diseases.[1] An infant formula, Lofenalac, was one of the first products to be developed for use in the dietary management of a rare genetic condition known as phenylketonuria and was regulated as a drug. FDA reassessed its position to foster innovation in the development of products for the dietary management of diseases and conditions. In 1972, FDA stated that Lofenalac would no longer be regulated as a drug but rather as a "food for special dietary use."[2] In addition, the agency began to follow a policy of regulating similar types of products as "foods for special dietary use." When FDA made nutrition labeling mandatory for certain foods in 1973, it exempted certain types of foods for special dietary use from this requirement.

The vitamin-mineral amendments of the *Health Research and Health Services Amendments* of 1976 (Pub. Law No. 94-278) prohibited FDA from classifying vitamin and mineral supplements as drugs based solely on their combinations or potency, unless drug claims were made.[3] This legislation also incorporated the statutory definition of "special dietary use."[4] Congress amended the *Orphan Drug Act* (Pub. Law. 97-114 of 1983) to formally define medical foods in 1988. The *Orphan Drug Amendments* of 1988 (Pub. Law. 100-290) enacted for the first time a statutory definition of "medical food." Although Congress provided a statutory definition for medical foods, the legislative history of the *Orphan Drug Amendments* does not discuss the definition and, therefore, does not provide any further information regarding the types of products the definition was intended to cover.

The *Nutrition Labeling and Education Act* (*NLEA*) of 1990 (Pub. Law 101-53) incorporated the definition of medical foods contained in the *Orphan Drug Amendments* of 1988 into *FD&C Act* Section 403(q)(5)(A)(iv) (21 U.S.C. 343(q)(5)(A)(iv)), and exempted medical foods from the nutrition labeling, health claim and nutrient content claim requirements applicable to most other foods. The final rule on mandatory nutrition labeling (58 FR 2079 at 2151, 6 January 1993) exempted medical foods from the nutrition labeling requirements and incorporated the statutory definition of a medical food into the regulations at 21 CFR 101.9(j)(8). In this regulation, FDA enumerated criteria that were intended to clarify the characteristics of medical foods.[5] In 1996, FDA proposed an advance notice of proposed rulemaking on regulation of medical foods, which was subsequently withdrawn due to lack of activity, lack of resources and change in priorities.[6] FDA provided a guidance on medical foods in May 1997 and revised the same in May 2007.[7] Effective 24 August 2006 FDA issued a *Compliance Program* specific to medical foods.[8]

Since 1972, the legislative and regulatory history of medical foods has reflected FDA's efforts to develop a regulatory framework to ensure the safety and nutritional adequacy of medical foods to manage the distinctive nutritional requirements resulting from diseases or health conditions.

Definition

"Medical food," as defined in Section 5(b) of the *Orphan Drug Act* (21 U.S.C. 360ee(b)(3)), is "a food which is formulated to be consumed or administered enterally under the supervision of a physician and which is intended for the specific dietary management of a disease or condition for which distinctive nutritional requirements, based on recognized scientific principles, are established by medical evaluation."[9] The agency advises that it considers the statutory definition of medical foods to narrowly constrain the types of products that fit within this category of food.

The criteria that clarify the statutory definition of a medical food can be found at 21 CFR 101.9(j)(8).[10] A food is a medical food and exempt from nutrition labeling only if:
  i. It is a specially formulated and processed product (as opposed to a naturally occurring foodstuff used in its natural state) for the partial or exclusive feeding of a patient by means of oral intake or enteral feeding by tube.
  ii. It is intended for the dietary management of a patient who, because of therapeutic or chronic medical needs, has limited or impaired capacity to ingest, digest, absorb, or metabolize ordinary foodstuffs or certain nutrients, or who has other special medically determined nutrient requirements, the dietary management of which cannot be achieved by the modification of the normal diet alone.
  iii. It provides nutritional support specifically modified for the management of the unique nutrient needs that result from the specific disease or condition, as determined by medical evaluation.
  iv. It is intended to be used under medical supervision.
  v. It is intended only for a patient receiving active and ongoing medical supervision wherein the patient requires medical care on a recurring basis for, among other things, instructions on the use of the medical food.

Medical foods are distinguished from the broader category of foods for special dietary use and foods that make health claims by the requirement that medical foods are intended to meet distinctive nutritional requirements of a disease or condition, be used under medical supervision and are intended for the specific dietary management of a disease or condition. The term "medical foods" does not pertain to all foods fed to sick patients. Medical foods are foods that are specially formulated and processed for the patient who is seriously ill or who requires the product as a major treatment modality.[11]

Labeling

Medical foods are regulated, as are other foods, under the provisions of the *FD&C Act* and the *Fair Packaging and Labeling Act* (*FPLA*) of 1966 (Pub. Law 89-755).[12] As a part of the broader category of foods, medical foods must comply with the general food labeling requirements of 21 CFR 101.[13] Medical foods must contain the following mandatory label information and conformation requirements:
- label must contain a statement of identity (21 CFR 101.3)
- an accurate statement of the net quantity of contents (21 CFR 101.105)
- name and place of business of the manufacturer, packer or distributor (21 CFR 101.5)
- complete list of ingredients, listed by their common or usual name and in descending order of predominance (21 CFR 101.4)
- all words, statements and other information required by or under authority of the act to appear on the label or labeling shall appear thereon in the English language (21 CFR 101.15(c)(1))
- any representation in a foreign language requires all mandatory label information be repeated in each foreign language used on the label (21 CFR 101.15(c)(2))

- conformance with the principal display panel requirements (21 CFR 101.1), the information panel requirements (21 CFR.101.2) and the misbranding of food requirements (21 CFR 101.18)

In addition, to be considered a medical food, the product must be labeled for the dietary management of a specific medical disorder, disease or condition for which there are distinctive nutritional requirements. Furthermore, medical foods must be labeled for use under medical supervision.[14]

As part of the broader category of packaged foods regulated under the *FD&C Act*, the *Food Allergen Labeling and Consumer Protection Act* (*FALCPA*) of 2004 (Pub. Law 108-282) requires that medical foods labeled after 1 January 2006 must comply with *FALCPA*'s food allergen labeling requirements.[15] However, medical foods are exempted from the labeling requirements for health claims and nutrient content claims under the *NLEA*.[16]

Under the *FD&C Act*, the manufacturer or distributor is responsible for ensuring that the medical food is not adulterated or misbranded. Medical foods are misbranded within the meaning of *FD&C Act* Section 403(a)(1) if their labeling is false and misleading.[17] Claims may be misleading not only because of affirmative representations made in the labeling, but also because the labeling fails to reveal material facts in the light of such representations with respect to consequences that may result from the use under the conditions of use prescribed in the labeling. FDA also regards medical foods to be misbranded if they are labeled and marketed as medical foods but do not meet the statutory definition of a medical food in Section 5(b) of the *Orphan Drug Act* (21 U.S.C. 360ee(b)(3)) or the criteria set forth in 21 CFR 101.9(j)(8).[18,19] Due to their intended use in supplying the distinctive nutritional needs of patients who are ill or otherwise medically vulnerable, it is essential that medical foods be appropriately formulated for the particular disease or condition for which they are labeled. If the product, as formulated and consumed, does not actually meet those distinctive requirements, it would violate the act. Medical foods claims should be specific for the dietary management of a disease or condition for which distinctive nutritional requirements are based on recognized scientific principles and are established by medical evaluation.

Manufacturing and Facilities Registration

Medical foods must be comprised of components designated as Generally Recognized as Safe (GRAS). Ingredients used in medical foods must be approved as food additives or as food additives that are the subject of exemptions for investigational use (21 U.S.C. 321 and 348) if the ingredient is not GRAS. FDA has several lists of GRAS substances codified in 21 CFR 182, 21 CFR 184 and 21 CFR 186.[20-22] Importantly, these lists are not all-inclusive. Because the use of a GRAS substance is not subject to premarket review and approval by FDA, it is impracticable to list all substances that are used in food on the basis of the GRAS provision. Other ingredients may achieve GRAS through GRAS affirmation or the GRAS notification program.[23]

Medical foods must comply with the requirements for food manufacturing, including the current Good Manufacturing Practice (CGMP) regulations in manufacturing, packing or holding human food (21 CFR 110).[24] If applicable, medical foods must comply with the low acid canned food regulations (21 CFR 113),[25] and *Emergency Permit Control* regulations (21 CFR 108).[26] The commercial processor, when first engaging in the manufacture, processing or packing of acidified foods or low-acid canned foods shall register and file information with FDA, including the name of the establishment, principal place of business, the location of each establishment in which processing is conducted, the processing method and a list of foods so processed in each establishment (21 CFR 108.25(c)(1) and 21 CFR 108.35(c)(1)).[27] A commercial processor engaged in processing acidified foods shall provide FDA with information, using Form FDA 2541a, on the scheduled processes for each acidified food in each container size (21 CFR 108.25(c)(2)). In addition, commercial processors engaged in the processing of low-acid canned foods shall provide FDA the process filing information using either Form FDA 2541a or Form FDA 2541c (21 CFR 108.35(c)(2)).[28]

Medical foods do not have to undergo premarket review or approval by FDA. Individual medical food products do not have to be registered with FDA; however, food facilities must be registered (21 CFR Part 1 Subpart H).[29] *FD&C Act* Section 415 (21 U.S.C. 350d) requires domestic and foreign facilities that manufacture, process, pack or hold food for human or animal consumption in the US to register with FDA.[30] Medical foods are "food" and, accordingly, a facility that manufactures/processes, packs or holds a medical food or a component of medical food (i.e., a raw material) is required to be registered as a food facility.[31] Only facilities that manufacture/process, pack or hold food for consumption in the US are required to be registered. Thus, facilities that manufacture/process, pack or hold food that will be consumed outside the US do not need to be registered.

Registrants must register using Form FDA 3537.[32] Registrations can be submitted in paper format by mail, electronically via the Internet, on CD-ROM or by fax. Instructions for completing Form FDA 3537 and additional information on registration of food facilities can be found at the FDA registration of food facilities webpage[33] and the FDA online registration of food facilities portal.[34] In the future, FDA may require registration, including the initial registration, renewals, updates and cancellations, to be submitted in an electronic format. The requirement for the electronic format cannot take effect before 4 January 2016.

The *Food Safety Modernization Act* (*FSMA*) (Pub. Law 111-353), enacted on 4 January 2011, amended the food facility registration requirements in *FD&C Act* Section 415.[35] Following is the general outline of *FSMA* food facility registration requirements. The outline is not intended to be complete or all-inclusive, but does provide some key points:

- provides authority for FDA to require registration to be submitted in an electronic format (This authority does not take effect until 5 years from the date of enactment of *FSMA* (i.e., 4 January 2016)
- requires biennial renewal of food facility registrations
- provides for an abbreviated biennial renewal process for facilities without information changes
- provides authority for FDA to suspend a food facility's registration
- requires registrant to include in registration the e-mail address for the facility's contact person (For a foreign facility, the registration must include the e-mail address of the facility's US agent.)
- provides authority for FDA to determine and identify appropriate additional food categories to be included in the registration
- requires the registration to include an assurance that FDA will be permitted to inspect the facility
- provides that food offered for import from a foreign facility with a suspended registration can be held at the port of arrival
- requires FDA to promulgate regulations to implement changes to Section 415 regarding suspension of food facility registrations

The adulteration provisions of *FD&C Act* Section 342 are applicable to medical foods.[36] If the medical food product also is intended for use as an infant formula, additional statutory and regulatory requirements apply. These additional requirements are found in *FD&C Act* Section 412 and FDA's implementing regulations in 21 CFR 106 and 21 CFR 107.[37,38] *FD&C Act* Section 412(c)(1) requires a person who plans to introduce or deliver any new infant formula into interstate commerce to register with FDA the name of the person (manufacturer) and their place of business and all establishments at which the person intends to manufacture the new infant formula.[39] *FD&C Act* Section 412(d)(1) requires persons responsible for the manufacture of infant formula to submit information relative to the manufacture of the new infant formula at least 90 days before marketing their product.[40]

Provisions of the Reportable Foods

Medical foods are subject to the provisions of reportable foods. A "reportable food" is an article of food (other than dietary supplements or infant formula) for which there is a reasonable probability that the use of, or exposure to, such article of food will cause serious adverse health consequences or death to humans or animals.[41] The populations that consume medical foods, often as the sole or a major source of nutrition, are extremely vulnerable, e.g., pediatric patients in periods of growth and development, the elderly, patients who have serious illnesses and patients in intensive care units. FDA interprets the definition of reportable food to include those foods that would meet the definition of a Class I recall situation. A Class I recall situation is one in which there is a reasonable probability that the use of, or exposure to, a violative product will cause serious adverse health consequences or death (21 CFR 7.3(m)(1)).[42]

Registered food facilities that manufacture, process, pack or hold food for human or animal consumption in the US under Section 415(a) of the *FD&C Act* (21 U.S.C. 350d) are required to report when there is a reasonable probability that the use of, or exposure to, an article of food will cause serious adverse health consequences or death to humans or animals.[43] A responsible party is required to submit a report to FDA through the reportable food electronic portal as soon as practicable, but in no case later than 24 hours after determining that an article of food is a reportable food (*FD&C Act* Section 417(d) (1)). The responsible party is the person who submits the registration under *FD&C Act* Section 415(a) (21 U.S.C. 350d) for a food facility that is required to register under Section 415(a), at which such article of food is manufactured, processed, packed or held. The Reportable Food Registry (RFR) was established by Section 1005 of the *Food and Drug Administration Amendments Act* of 2007 (Pub. Law 110-085).[44] The RFR is an electronic portal for industry to report when there is reasonable probability that an article of food will cause serious adverse health consequences. As of 24 May 2010, the reportable food electronic portal is a part of the FDA-National Institutes of Health (NIH) safety reporting portal.[45] The RFR helps FDA to better protect public health by tracking patterns and targeting inspections. The RFR applies to all FDA-regulated categories of food and feed, except dietary supplements and infant formula. If the adulteration of the food article has originated with the responsible party, the responsible party is required to investigate the cause of the adulteration and report their findings when known. The responsible party shall maintain records related to each report received, notification made and reports submitted to the FDA for two years.[46] If the medical food product also is intended for use as an infant formula, manufacturers must comply with notification requirements for violative infant formula as established in 21 CFR 107.240.[47]

Compliance Program

FDA has a specific Compliance Program for medical foods.[48] The Compliance Program enables FDA inspectors to: obtain information regarding the manufacturing/control processes and quality assurance programs employed by domestic manufacturers of medical foods through establishment inspections; collect domestic and import surveillance samples of medical foods for nutrient and microbiological analyses; and take action when significant violations of the *FD&C Act* (or related regulations) are found.

Due to the susceptible population for which medical foods are intended, FDA is committed to assuring their continued safety and integrity through annual inspections of all medical foods manufacturers in the US and other countries. If the medical food product also is intended for use as an infant formula, the domestic and foreign establishments are inspected annually for compliance with the requirements of *FD&C Act* Section 412 as well.[49]

Adverse Event Reporting

Reporting of serious adverse events, product quality problems, product use errors, or therapeutic nonequivalence/failure suspected to be associated with the use of medical food in the course of clinical care is voluntary. Form FDA 3500 should be used by healthcare professionals and consumers for voluntary reporting of adverse events, product use errors and product quality problems with medical foods. The three routes available to submit voluntary adverse event reports to FDA include MedWatch online reporting, reporting by telephone and submitting Form FDA 3500A in hard copy by either mail or fax. Instructions for Completing Form FDA 3500 can be found at www.fda.gov/Safety/MedWatch/HowToReport/DownloadForms/ucm149236.htm. MedWatch Online Voluntary Reporting 3500 Form can be found at https://www.accessdata.fda.gov/scripts/medwatch/medwatch-online.htm.

Summary

- Medical foods are distinguished from the broader category of foods by the requirement that medical foods are intended to meet distinctive nutritional requirements of a disease or condition, be used under medical supervision and are intended for the specific dietary management of a disease or condition.
- Medical foods should meet the statutory definition of a medical food in the *Orphan Drug Act* (21 U.S.C. 360ee(b)(3)) and the criteria set forth in 21 CFR 101.9(j)(8).
- Medical foods are regulated, as are other foods, under the provisions of the *FD&C Act* and the *Fair Packaging and Labeling Act*.
- Medical foods do not have to undergo premarket review or approval by FDA.
- As part of the broader category of foods, medical foods must comply with the mandatory food labeling requirements of 21 CFR 101. In addition, the product must be labeled for the dietary management of a specific medical disorder and for use under medical supervision.
- Under the *FD&C Act*, the manufacturer or distributor is responsible for ensuring that the medical food is not adulterated or misbranded.
- Medical foods must be comprised of components designated as Generally Recognized as Safe (GRAS).
- Medical foods must comply with the requirements for the manufacture of foods, including the current Good Manufacturing Practices regulations in manufacturing, packing or holding human food (21 CFR 110).
- Individual medical food products do not have to be registered with FDA; however, food facilities must be registered.
- Medical foods are subject to the provisions of reportable foods.
- FDA has a compliance program specific to medical foods.
- Reporting of serious adverse events, product quality problems, product use errors or therapeutic nonequivalence/failure suspected associated with the use of medical food in the course of clinical care is voluntary.
- If the medical food product also is intended for use as an infant formula, additional infant formula statutory and regulatory requirements apply.

References
1. 21 U.S.C. 321(g)(1)(B). Cornell University Law School website. www.law.cornell.edu/uscode/text/21/321. Accessed 8 April 2013.
2. 37 FR 18229 at 18230, 8 September 1972.
3. 21 U.S.C. 350. Cornell University Law School website. www.law.cornell.edu/uscode/text/21/350. Accessed 9 April 2013.
4. 21 U.S.C. 350(c)(3). GPO website. www.gpo.gov/fdsys/pkg/USCODE-2010-title21/pdf/USCODE-2010-title21-chap9-subchapIV-sec350c.pdf. Accessed 9 April 2013.
5. 21 CFR 101.9(j)(8). GPO website. www.gpo.gov/fdsys/pkg/CFR-2012-title21-vol2/pdf/CFR-2012-title21-vol2-sec101-9.pdf. Accessed 8 April 2013.
6. Regulation of Medical Foods, Advance notice of proposed rulemaking. *Federal Register* Vol. 61, No. 231, 60661–60671. Available at www.gpo.gov/fdsys/pkg/FR-1996-11-29/pdf/96-30441.pdf. Accessed 8 April 2013.
7. *Guidance for Industry: Frequently Asked Questions About Medical Foods* (May 1997; Revised May 2007). FDA website. www.fda.gov/Food/GuidanceRegulation/GuidanceDocumentsRegulatoryInformation/MedicalFoods/ucm054048.htm. Accessed 8 April 2013.
8. Compliance program 7321.002. Medical Foods Program (August 24, 2006) – Import and Domestic. Available at www.fda.gov/downloads/Food/GuidanceComplianceRegulatoryInformation/ComplianceEnforcement/ucm073339.pdf. Accessed 9 April 2013.
9. 21 U.S.C. 360ee(b)(3). GPO website. www.gpo.gov/fdsys/pkg/USCODE-2011-title21/pdf/USCODE-2011-title21-chap9-subchapV-partB-sec360ee.pdf. Accessed 9 April 2013.
10. Op cit 5.
11. Op cit 7.
12. Fair Packaging and Labeling Act (Pub. Law 89-755). FTC website. www.ftc.gov/os/statutes/fpla/fplact.shtm. Accessed 9 April 2013.
13. 21 CFR 101. FDA website. www.accessdata.fda.gov/scripts/cdrh/cfdocs/cfcfr/CFRSearch.cfm?cfrpart=101. Accessed 9 April 2013.
14. Op cit 7.

15. *Guidance for Industry: Questions and Answers Regarding Food Allergens, including the Food Allergen Labeling and Consumer Protection Act of 2004 (Edition 4); Final Guidance* (October 2006). Available at www.fda.gov/downloads/Food/GuidanceComplianceRegulatoryInformation/GuidanceDocuments/FoodLabelingNutrition/UCM301394.pdf. Accessed 9 April 2013.
16. 21 U.S.C. 343(q)(5)(A)(iv). Cornell University Law School website. www.law.cornell.edu/uscode/text/21/343. Accessed 9 April 2013.
17. 21 CFR 343. FDA website. www.accessdata.fda.gov/scripts/cdrh/cfdocs/cfcfr/CFRSearch.cfm?CFRPart=343&showFR=1&subpartNode=21:5.0.1.1.18.2. Accessed 9 April 2013.
18. NeuroScience Inc. Warning Letter. FDA website. www.fda.gov/ICECI/EnforcementActions/WarningLetters/2011/ucm284391.htm. Accessed 9 April 2013.
19. Bioenergy Inc. Warning Letter. FDA website. www.fda.gov/ICECI/EnforcementActions/WarningLetters/2010/ucm232086.htm. FDA website Accessed 9 April 2013.
20. 21 CFR 182. FDA website. www.accessdata.fda.gov/scripts/cdrh/cfdocs/cfcfr/cfrsearch.cfm?cfrpart=182. Accessed 9 April 2013.
21. 21 CFR 184. FDA website. www.accessdata.fda.gov/scripts/cdrh/cfdocs/cfcfr/cfrsearch.cfm?cfrpart=184. Accessed 9 April 2013.
22. 21 CFR 186. FDA website. www.gpo.gov/fdsys/pkg/CFR-2000-title21-vol3/pdf/CFR-2000-title21-vol3-part186.pdf. Accessed 9 April 2013.
23. *Guidance for Industry: Frequently Asked Questions About GRAS* (December 2004). FDA website. www.fda.gov/Food/GuidanceRegulation/GuidanceDocumentsRegulatoryInformation/IngredientsAdditivesGRASPackaging/ucm061846.htm. Accessed 9 April 2013.
24. 21 CFR 110. FDA website. www.accessdata.fda.gov/scripts/cdrh/cfdocs/cfcfr/cfrsearch.cfm?cfrpart=110. Accessed 9 April 2013.
25. 21 CFR 113. FDA website. www.accessdata.fda.gov/scripts/cdrh/cfdocs/cfcfr/CFRSearch.cfm?CFRPart=113. Accessed 9 April 2013.
26. 21 CFR 108. FDA website. www.accessdata.fda.gov/scripts/cdrh/cfdocs/cfCFR/CFRSearch.cfm?CFRPart=108&showFR=1. Accessed 9 April 2013.
27. *Guidance for Industry Acidified Foods* (September 2010). FDA website. www.fda.gov/downloads/Food/GuidanceComplianceRegulatoryInformation/GuidanceDocuments/AcidifiedandLow-AcidCannedFoods/UCM227099.pdf. Accessed 9 April 2013.
28. *Guidance for Industry: Submitting Form FDA 2541 (Food Canning Establishment Registration) and Forms FDA 2541a and FDA 2541c (Food Process Filing Forms) to FDA in Electronic or Paper Format* (July 2012). FDA website. www.fda.gov/downloads/Food/GuidanceComplianceRegulatoryInformation/GuidanceDocuments/AcidifiedandLow-AcidCannedFoods/UCM309379.pdf. Accessed 9 April 2013.
29. 21 CFR 1, Subpart H. FDA website. www.accessdata.fda.gov/scripts/cdrh/cfdocs/cfCFR/CFRSearch.cfm?CFRPart=1&showFR=1&subpartNode=21:1.0.1.1.1.6. Accessed 9 April 2013.
30. 21 U.S.C. §350d. GPO website. www.gpo.gov/fdsys/pkg/USCODE-2011-title21/pdf/USCODE-2011-title21-chap9-subchapIV-sec350d.pdf. Accessed 9 April 2013.
31. *Guidance for Industry: Questions and Answers Regarding Food Facility Registration (Fifth Edition)* (December 2012). FDA website. www.fda.gov/downloads/Food/GuidanceComplianceRegulatoryInformation/GuidanceDocuments/FoodDefenseandEmergencyResponse/UCM332460.pdf. Accessed 9 April 2013.
32. Form FDA 3537. FDA website. www.fda.gov/downloads/AboutFDA/ReportsManualsForms/Forms/UCM071977.pdf. Accessed 9 April 2013.
33. Registration of Food Facilities. FDA website. www.fda.gov/Food/GuidanceRegulation/FoodFacilityRegistration/default.htm.. Accessed 9 April 2013.
34. FDA registration of food facilities. FDA website. http://www.fda.gov/Food/GuidanceRegulation/FoodFacilityRegistration/ucm2006831.htm. Accessed 7 May 2013.
35. *Food Safety Modernization Act* (Public Law 111–353). GPO website. www.gpo.gov/fdsys/pkg/PLAW-111publ353/pdf/PLAW-111publ353.pdf. Accessed 9 April 2013.
36. 21 U.S.C. 342. GPO website. www.gpo.gov/fdsys/pkg/USCODE-2011-title21/pdf/USCODE-2011-title21-chap9-subchapIV-sec342.pdf. Accessed 9 April 2013.
37. 21 CFR Part 106. FDA website. www.accessdata.fda.gov/scripts/cdrh/cfdocs/cfcfr/CFRSearch.cfm?CFRPart=106. Accessed 9 April 2013.
38. 21 CFR Part 107. FDA website. www.accessdata.fda.gov/scripts/cdrh/cfdocs/cfCFR/CFRSearch.cfm?CFRPart=107. Accessed 9 April 2013.
39. *Guidance for Industry: Frequently Asked Questions about FDA's Regulation of Infant Formula* (March 1, 2006). FDA website. www.fda.gov/Food/GuidanceRegulation/GuidanceDocumentsRegulatoryInformation/InfantFormula/ucm056524.htm. Accessed 9 April 2013.
40. *Guidelines Concerning Notification and Testing of Infant Formulas*. Available at www.fda.gov/Food/GuidanceRegulation/GuidanceDocumentsRegulatoryInformation/InfantFormula/ucm169730.htm. Accessed 9 April 2013.
41. 21 U.S.C. 350f. Cornell University Law School website. www.law.cornell.edu/uscode/text/21/350f. Accessed 9 April 2013.
42. 21 CFR 7.3(m). FDA website. www.accessdata.fda.gov/scripts/cdrh/cfdocs/cfcfr/CFRSearch.cfm?fr=7.3. Accessed 9 April 2013.
43. *Draft Guidance for Industry Questions and Answers Regarding the Reportable Food Registry as Established by the Food and Drug Administration Amendments Act of 2007* (Edition 2) (May 2010). FDA website. www.fda.gov/downloads/Food/GuidanceComplianceRegulatoryInformation/GuidanceDocuments/FoodSafety/UCM213214.pdf. Accessed 9 April 2013.
44. *Guidance for Industry: Questions and Answers Regarding the Reportable Food Registry as Established by the Food and Drug Administration Amendments Act of 2007* (September 2009). FDA website. www.fda.gov/Food/GuidanceRegulation/GuidanceDocumentsRegulatoryInformation/RFR/ucm212793.htm. Accessed 9 April 2013.
45. Reportable Food Registry for Industry, FDA-NIH Safety Reporting Portal. FDA website. www.fda.gov/Food/ComplianceEnforcement/RFR/default.htm. Accessed 9 April 2013.
46. Op cit 43.
47. 21 CFR 107.240. GPO website. www.gpo.gov/fdsys/pkg/CFR-2011-title21-vol2/pdf/CFR-2011-title21-vol2-sec107-240.pdf. Accessed 9 April 2013.
48. Op cit 8.
49. Food and Drug Administration, Compliance Program 7321.006: Infant Formula Program – Import and Domestic (July 31, 2006). FDA website. www.fda.gov/downloads/Food/GuidanceComplianceRegulatoryInformation/ComplianceEnforcement/ucm073349.pdf. Accessed 9 April 2013.

Recommended Reading

- *Guidance for Industry: Frequently Asked Questions about Medical Foods* (May 1997; Revised May 2007). FDA website. www.fda.gov/Food/GuidanceRegulation/GuidanceDocumentsRegulatoryInformation/MedicalFoods/ucm054048.htm Accessed 9 April 2013
- *Compliance program 7321.002. Medical Foods Program – Import and Domestic* (July 31, 2006). FDA website. www.fda.gov/downloads/Food/GuidanceComplianceRegulatoryInformation/ComplianceEnforcement/ucm073339.pdf. Accessed 9 April 2013
- 21 CFR 101 Food Labeling. FDA website. www.accessdata.fda.gov/scripts/cdrh/cfdocs/cfcfr/CFRSearch.cfm?cfrpart=101. Accessed 9 April 2013.

- 21 CFR 101.9 Nutrition labeling of food. FDA website. www.accessdata.fda.gov/scripts/cdrh/cfdocs/cfcfr/cfrsearch.cfm?fr=101.9. Accessed 9 April 2013.
- *Guidance for Industry: Questions and Answers Regarding Food Allergens, including the Food Allergen Labeling and Consumer Protection Act of 2004 (Edition 4); Final Guidance* (October 2006). FDA website. www.fda.gov/downloads/Food/GuidanceComplianceRegulatoryInformation/GuidanceDocuments/FoodLabelingNutrition/UCM301394.pdf. Accessed 9 April 2013.
- *Guidance for Industry: Frequently Asked Questions about GRAS* (December 2004). FDA website. www.fda.gov/Food/GuidanceRegulation/GuidanceDocumentsRegulatoryInformation/IngredientsAdditivesGRASPackaging/ucm061846.htm. Accessed 9 April 2013.
- 21 CFR 110 Current Good Manufacturing Practice in Manufacturing, packing, or holding human food. FDA website. www.accessdata.fda.gov/scripts/cdrh/cfdocs/cfcfr/cfrsearch.cfm?cfrpart=110. Accessed 9 April 2013.
- *Guidance for Industry: Questions and Answers Regarding Food Facility Registration (Fifth Edition)* (December 2012). FDA website. www.fda.gov/downloads/Food/GuidanceComplianceRegulatoryInformation/GuidanceDocuments/FoodDefenseandEmergencyResponse/UCM332460.pdf. Accessed 9 April 2013.
- *Guidance for Industry: Frequently Asked Questions about FDA's Regulation of Infant Formula* (March 1, 2006). FDA website. www.fda.gov/Food/GuidanceRegulation/GuidanceDocumentsRegulatoryInformation/InfantFormula/ucm056524.htm. Accessed 9 April 2013.
- *Draft Guidance for Industry Questions and Answers Regarding the Reportable Food Registry as Established by the Food and Drug Administration Amendments Act of 2007 (Edition 2)* (May 2010). FDA website. www.fda.gov/downloads/Food/GuidanceComplianceRegulatoryInformation/GuidanceDocuments/FoodSafety/UCM213214.pdf. Accessed 9 April 2013.
- *Guidance for Industry: Questions and Answers Regarding the Reportable Food Registry as Established by the Food and Drug Administration Amendments Act of 2007* (September 2009). FDA website. www.fda.gov/Food/GuidanceRegulation/GuidanceDocumentsRegulatoryInformation/RFR/ucm212793.htm. Accessed 9 April 2013.
- *Food and Drug Administration, Compliance Program 7321.006: Infant Formula Program – Import and Domestic* (July 31, 2006). FDA website. www.fda.gov/downloads/Food/GuidanceComplianceRegulatoryInformation/ComplianceEnforcement/ucm073349.pdf. Accessed 9 April 2013.
- Alpers DH, Stenson WF, Taylor B and Bier DM. *Manual of nutritional therapeutics.* Lippincott Williams & Wilkins, 2008.
- Schmidl MK, Labuza TP, Schmidt RH and Rodrick GE. "Medical foods." *Food Safety Handbook*, 571–606, 2005.
- Thomas B. *Manual of dietetic practice.* No. Ed. 3. Blackwell Science, 2001
- *Medical Foods Equity Act* of 2011. GovTrack.us website. www.govtrack.us/congress/bills/112/hr1311. Accessed 9 April 2013.

Chapter 36

FDA Inspection and Enforcement

By William Kitchens, JD and Alan Minsk, JD

OBJECTIVES

❑ Understand FDA inspectional authority

❑ Understand prohibited acts under the *Federal Food, Drug, and Cosmetic Act* and FDA's implementing regulations

❑ Understand FDA enforcement options and objectives

LAWS, REGULATIONS AND GUIDELINES COVERED IN THIS CHAPTER

❑ *Federal Food, Drug, and Cosmetic Act* of 1938 (FD&C Act)

❑ Applicable Parts of 21 CFR

Introduction

The US Food and Drug Administration (FDA) is, first and foremost, a public health organization. Whether evaluating a product for potential marketing authorization, inspecting a manufacturing site or deciding whether to take enforcement action against a noncompliant company, FDA's primary mission is to protect the consumer. This chapter reviews FDA's inspectional authority, prohibited acts and the agency's enforcement options in response to unlawful activity.

FDA Inspections

Overview of FDA's Inspectional Authority

FDA conducts inspections for many reasons, such as a directed inspection for a specific reason (e.g., notice of a complaint about a product); a routine audit to ensure company compliance with current Good Laboratory Practices (CGLPs), Good Clinical Practices (GCPs), current Good Manufacturing Practices (CGMPs) or Quality System Regulation (QSR) requirements; a reinspection after a Warning Letter or other enforcement action; a recall effectiveness check; a preapproval inspection (PAI); or to evaluate prospective suppliers of products to US government agencies. The parameters of FDA's inspectional authority are set forth in Section 704 of the *Federal Food, Drug, and Cosmetic Act* of 1938 (*FD&C Act*), as amended.[1] FDA may enter a factory, warehouse, establishment or vehicle in which regulated products are manufactured, processed, packed or stored. The inspection is to occur at a reasonable time and in a reasonable manner, and "shall extend to all things therein (including records, files, papers, processes, controls, and facilities)" bearing on whether the products comply with the *FD&C Act* and FDA's implementing regulations. FDA is required to inspect at least once every two years but, due to limited financial and personnel resources, the agency focuses its efforts primarily on high-risk products, new facilities not yet inspected and sites with poor compliance histories.

Before the domestic inspection may begin, FDA investigators must present their credentials and issue a properly signed and completed Form FDA 482, Notice of Inspection. Credentials consist of two identification cards held in a carrying case: one describes the authorities of the credential bearer, while the other contains the investigator's photograph and personal description. The identification card also contains a badge number and bears an expiration date. A person from the facility being inspected should carefully examine an inspector's credentials to ensure the individual is, indeed, a government official and to verify which agency is represented (e.g., federal or state, FDA, Environmental Protection Agency (EPA), Drug Enforcement Administration (DEA)).

FDA may conduct routine inspections without a search warrant. However, the agency may seek to utilize a search warrant, for example, to carry out an inspection in a timely and effective manner, if a firm refuses to be inspected or if FDA anticipates that the firm will refuse inspection. A search warrant from a federal court may be sought by any federal enforcement officer pursuant to statutory and constitutional requirements. FDA may obtain a search warrant if it demonstrates to a federal magistrate that there is probable cause to believe that a crime is being committed by a person who is being served the search warrant, or that there are records or other evidence at the facility that relate to the commission of a crime.

A routine inspection may cover the premises and all pertinent equipment, finished and unfinished materials, containers and labeling within an establishment or vehicle in which products are manufactured, processed, packed, held or transported.[2] The *FD&C Act* provides broader inspector powers in the case of plants that manufacture prescription drugs, nonprescription drugs for human use, restricted devices and infant formulas.[3] FDA also is given authority under the *FDA Food Safety Modernization Act* of 2010 (*FSMA*), which amends the *FD&C Act*, to inspect all records relating to an article of food and any other food that FDA "reasonably believes" is adulterated and prevents a threat of serious adverse health consequences or death to humans or animals.[4]

The overall scope of an inspection by FDA generally will be determined, in part, by the reason for the inspection and any deficiencies encountered during the current or prior investigation. FDA's Investigations Operations Manual (IOM) describes an inspection as a careful, critical, official examination of a facility to determine compliance with FDA rules and regulations. Evidence of violations gathered during inspections may be used to support an enforcement action in federal court.

Limitations on Inspections

While FDA may gather evidence during an inspection, there are limits as to what inspectors are entitled to review or gather. As a routine matter, FDA may not gather the following during an investigation:
- financial data
- pricing data
- personnel data (other than information regarding qualifications of technical and professional personnel performing FDA-related functions)
- sales data (other than shipment information)
- research data (other than information relating to new drugs and antibiotic drugs and subject to reporting to and inspection by FDA)

Further, FDA has no authority to require individuals to sign affidavits or attest to the accuracy of any observations or statements, although it may attempt to secure such evidence. FDA's legal authority to take photographs is not expressly cited in the law. There are two court cases FDA frequently cites to assert its authority to take photographs. One case involved EPA's aerial photography of open fields.[5] Another case involved a company that did not stop FDA from taking photographs, but later challenged the admissibility of the photographs as evidence in an enforcement action. In this case, the court held that, because no objection was made when the photographs were taken during the inspection, there had been full consent by the company.[6] FDA believes it has the authority to take photographs, but it will typically respect a corporate policy against it. However, if the company will not allow the taking of photographs and FDA insists on them, the agency might seek court intervention. If the company decides to permit the taking of photographs after consulting with counsel, it should document that it protested and make its objection clear to FDA.

Pharmacies licensed by state law that do not manufacture, prepare, propagate, compound or process drugs and/or medical devices are exempt from FDA inspections, although that may change if proposed federal legislation, currently under consideration, is enacted to provide increased FDA regulation and oversight over pharmacy compounding.[7]

Extraterritorial Jurisdiction Over Products Intended for Import and Authority to Detain Imported Products

FDA's authority to inspect is limited generally to sites within the US, but the *Food and Drug Administration Safety and Innovation Act* (*FDASIA*), which was enacted on 9 July 2012 and amends the *FD&C Act*, provides extraterritorial jurisdiction over any violation of the *FD&C Act* relating to any drug, device, food or other article regulated under the *FD&C Act* if such product is intended for import into the US or if any act in furtherance of the violation was committed in the US.[8] Moreover, *FDASIA* authorizes FDA to enter into agreements with foreign governments to recognize inspections of FDA-registered foreign establishments to facilitate risk-based inspections.[9]

It is also important to recognize that FDA, with US Customs and Border Protection, can detain imported products that appear to be noncompliant, and the agency may delay product approval if data are generated or products are manufactured at a foreign site it has not inspected. Therefore, foreign companies or sites typically do not object to FDA inspections even if the agency lacks express authority to proactively inspect. Moreover, FDA has opened posts in certain countries to expedite foreign inspections.

Types of Inspections

Inspections may be comprehensive, abbreviated, directed or conducted for the purpose of preapproval. A comprehensive inspection covers all aspects of a facility's FDA-regulated products and processes. This may include coverage of all major areas of a company's quality system in accordance with the QSR for medical devices or CGMPs for pharmaceuticals. An abbreviated inspection is performed on a specific area or at a depth described in the inspection assignment or compliance program. It may include coverage of one product or a specific aspect of the company's operations, such as complaints received by FDA or a limited number of subsystems/systems for QSR and GMP inspections. A directed inspection is usually in response to a product failure or contamination and is focused on the conditions that led to the violation.

Preapproval inspections (PAIs) cover the product preapproval process for three FDA centers: the Center for Devices and Radiological Health (CDRH), the Center for Drug Evaluation and Research (CDER) and the Center for Biologics Evaluation and Research (CBER). There are two primary components of a PAI:

- a rigorous, scientific review of required data by the applicable center's review division to ensure the product's safety and effectiveness; the application content and process vary by center
- comprehensive compliance evaluation of production facilities to ensure the company is capable of manufacturing the product in accordance with information submitted in the application and quality-related standards

New Inspection Authority Under FDASIA

FDASIA maintains the biennial inspection schedule for Class II and Class III medical devices and replaces the biennial inspection schedule for drugs with a "risk-based" inspection schedule.[10] In establishing this new requirement, Congress determined that a risk-based inspection schedule would focus resources on high-risk drug manufacturing facilities, both domestic and foreign, that present the greatest risk and help ensure inspection parity of domestic and foreign drug establishments.[11] *FDASIA* sets out certain risk factors that FDA must consider in determining whether to inspect a drug establishment, including:

- the compliance history of the establishment
- the record, history and nature of recalls linked to the establishment
- the inherent risk of the drug manufactured, prepared, propagated, compounded or processed at the establishment
- the inspection frequency and history of the establishment, including whether the facility has been inspected within the past four years;
- whether the establishment has been inspected by a foreign government or an agency of a foreign government
- any other criteria deemed necessary and appropriate for purposes of allocating inspection resources[12]

In applying this criteria, FDA will not consider whether the drugs manufactured, prepared, propagated, compounded or processed by the establishment are prescription drugs.

With regard to device inspections, *FDASIA* reauthorizes until 1 October 2017 a voluntary third-party inspection program for eligible manufacturers of Class II and Class III medical devices. Under this program, device manufacturers may elect to have an accredited person perform the equivalent of an FDA Quality System inspection. The Accredited Person must meet prescribed requirements[13] and will prepare and forward the inspection report to FDA, which makes the final classification determination (see the Possible Outcomes section later in this chapter).[14]

FDASIA also provides a new inspection authority for FDA regarding records of facilities that manufacture, prepare, propagate, compound or process drugs. Upon request, such establishments must provide to FDA, in advance of or instead of an inspection, sufficiently described records either electronically or in physical form.[15] FDA must provide a "sufficient description of the records requested," and establishments must provide the records "within a reasonable time frame, within reasonable limits, and in a reasonable manner."[16] Establishments are responsible for the costs of producing such records but may challenge record requests they consider to be overly broad or vague that would not meet the "sufficient description" requirement in the new law.[17]

Finally, *FDASIA* amends the *FD&C Act* by authorizing FDA to detain a drug found in a facility being inspected if, during the inspection, FDA has reason to believe that the drug is adulterated or misbranded.[18] FDA already had this authority with respect to devices found during the inspection of a device manufacturing facility that it believes are adulterated or misbranded.[19]

FDA Procedures to Inspection

Investigators use the IOM as a guide when conducting investigations. It describes what evidence an investigator may obtain during an investigation and what issues should be investigated. There are many other guidance documents and materials available on FDA's website (www.fda.gov/) to assist investigators in conducting inspections. These include but are not limited to:

- Compliance Policy Guides (CPG)
- Compliance Program Guidance Manuals (CPGM)
- FDA/Office of Regulatory Affairs (ORA) Guide to International Inspections and Travel

- Inspector's Technical Guide
- Regulatory Procedures Manual (RPM)

Systems Approach to Investigations

The systems approach was developed by FDA to effectively ensure products are manufactured in compliance with CGMP and QSR requirements while saving agency resources during inspections by streamlining the inspection process. The systems approach is based on the idea that a system is out of control if the product's quality, identity, strength and purity resulting from that system cannot be assured adequately. Documented CGMP deficiencies demonstrate that a system is not in a state of control. Thus, under the systems approach, FDA focuses on seven quality subsystems:
- management responsibility
- design control
- corrective and preventive action, frequently referred to as CAPA
- production and process controls
- records/document change controls
- material controls
- facilities and equipment controls

A deficiency in any one of these areas acts as a red flag to FDA that a company is not operating under a state of control. If a company cannot handle big issues, it is unlikely that it has addressed more specific, implementing measures.

Discussions With Management

When an inspection has concluded, the investigator will discuss, both verbally and in writing, the observations believed to be deficiencies, citing the appropriate regulation for each deficiency. Written observations are documented on a Form FDA 483 (FDA 483), Inspectional Observations. In some cases, an FDA 483 will not be issued.

Form FDA 483

At the conclusion of an FDA inspection, an FDA 483 may be issued to company management. It contains observations made by the investigator during the inspection that represent potential violations of the law or regulations. FDA 483s are not mentioned in the law and are not considered a final agency action. FDA 483s are available for review under the *Freedom of Information Act* (*FOIA*), although they may be redacted to protect confidential information.

At the conclusion of an inspection, if an FDA 483 is presented, the FDA investigator will explain the observations and solicit responses from the company. This is an important time for the company to identify any perceived errors that may appear on the form, to seek clarification and to indicate any corrective actions it plans to take. If the investigator has made an error, a correction will be made. Once the FDA 483 is issued and the investigator has left the facility, no changes may be made to the form.

A company generally responds to the agency regarding corrective action it plans to take and FDA has recently increased pressure on manufacturers to respond within 15 working days of a facility inspection. The agency will accept responses after the 15-day mark, but has noted it may not take those late responses into consideration before issuing a Warning Letter. The FDA 483 response should show that the company is working in good faith to address FDA's observations, explain what has been implemented and provide a reasonable timeframe for other corrections. If the observations are serious and if the corrective action plan is going to take months to complete, a company should consider committing to submit periodic status updates to FDA until the company has met the action plan outlined in the response.

An effective response to an FDA 483 typically will minimize the risk that the agency will pursue other enforcement actions, such as issuing a Warning Letter. FDA is not required to issue an FDA 483 before proceeding to a Warning Letter; the particular facts of a case will dictate the agency's course of action. If FDA issues a Warning Letter, it is typically because the agency has expressed its concerns previously, does not consider the company's response to the 483 sufficient or does not believe the company intends to resolve the issues. FDA also might consider the deficiencies so important and basic to quality control that it wants to signal to senior management that it expects these fundamental observations to be addressed expeditiously and such lack of quality oversight was sufficiently serious to warrant the Warning Letter. Unlike the procedure used for issuing an FDA 483, before a Warning Letter is issued, several groups within FDA review the issues and company responses, so the decision to send a Warning Letter is not taken lightly and is a collective one. FDA publicizes and posts Warning Letters on its website (with some exceptions, the agency does not typically post FDA 483s online). While most companies consider a Warning Letter to be a wake-up call and take appropriate action at this point, FDA will consider court action, such as product seizure or injunctive relief (discussed later), if the violations persist. FDA is not required to issue a Warning Letter before proceeding to court.

Voluntary Corrections

FDA is more likely to consider a company's voluntary plan of compliance when the violations are not sufficiently serious or significant to warrant other enforcement action. Voluntary plans can take several forms. They may include the company's commitment to make corrections according to a defined timeframe. FDA frequently will offer suggestions or comments, particularly when discussing proposed timeframes. FDA rarely provides any commitments other than those implied by the recognition of the plan as an alternative to enforcement action. FDA also makes clear that its comments or suggestions are not binding and do not reflect endorsement or assurance that the company's efforts will be successful. FDA normally will not engage in any discussions of this type if it has already decided to pursue other enforcement action.

Establishment Inspection Report (EIR)

An EIR is a narrative report, prepared by the investigator after the inspection is completed, that describes the investigator's inspectional findings. The EIR will include the reason for the inspection; the dates, classification and findings of the previous inspection; the scope of the inspection; the type of inspection (e.g., comprehensive or directed); and a brief description of products, processes or systems covered during the inspection.

Inspection reports describe and discuss each objectionable condition or practice cited on the FDA 483. The reports also include samples, photographs and documents collected during the inspection that support the deficiencies observed. These documents are attached as exhibits to the EIR. The EIR and all supporting documents serve as evidence for any regulatory/compliance action FDA may consider against a company. EIRs, after redaction of sensitive information, can be disclosed under *FOIA*, although there are notable exceptions. For example, if FDA is considering taking enforcement action, it may delay disclosure of the EIR.

Possible Outcomes

At the end of all inspections and following completion of the EIR, FDA will classify the inspection using one of three primary classifications:
1. NAI—No Action Indicated
2. VAI—Voluntary Action Indicated
3. OAI—Official Action Indicated

These classifications are assigned in accordance with inspectional findings and agency policy. FDA will not take further action on investigations classified as VAI unless the company cannot achieve compliance. Appropriate enforcement actions and dates for the next inspection will be recommended for the OAI designation.

Enforcement

Section 301 Prohibited Acts

The commission of a prohibited act, as defined by the *FD&C Act*, gives FDA the authority to exercise its enforcement remedies of seizure, injunction, civil penalties, criminal prosecution or import or export restrictions, to name a few.[20] For purposes of this chapter, the enforcement provisions apply to pharmaceuticals and medical devices, but FDA's enforcement authority reaches other product categories, such as food, color additives, cosmetics and biologics. Prohibited acts under Section 301 of the *FD&C Act* include, but are not limited to:
- introducing or delivering an adulterated or misbranded product into interstate commerce
- adulterating or misbranding a product while it is in interstate commerce
- receiving an adulterated or misbranded product in interstate commerce or delivering it for pay or otherwise
- refusing to permit FDA entry or inspection
- manufacturing a product that is adulterated or misbranded
- failing to register the facility establishment
- failing to register or list drugs or devices with FDA
- altering, mutilating, destroying, obliterating or removing the labeling of, or doing of any act with respect to, a product held for sale after shipment in interstate commerce that results in such product being adulterated or misbranded

The most common violations cited by FDA in the inspectional context are adulteration and misbranding. Adulteration typically focuses on quality-related deficiencies, and misbranding includes, but is not limited to, false or misleading labeling or other information (e.g., advertising and promotion). The sale or promotion of an unapproved new drug is a separate violation.[21] While other chapters in this publication define "adulteration" and "misbranding" in more detail, a drug, device or biologic is considered adulterated if, among other things:
- It consists of a filthy, putrid or decomposed substance or has been produced under unsanitary conditions whereby it may have been so contaminated.
- It has not been manufactured in compliance with GMPs.
- Its container is composed of any poisonous or deleterious substance that may render the contents injurious to health.
- Its strength, quality or purity differs from an official compendium or that which it purports or is represented to possess.
- It is a Class III medical device and does not have an approved Premarket Approval Application and is not otherwise exempt.
- It is a banned device.

A product is misbranded if, among other things:
- Its labeling is false or misleading.

- Its label fails to include the manufacturer, packer or distributor's name and place of business, and an accurate statement of the quantity of contents.
- It is a drug and its label does not contain the established name of the drug and the established name and quantity or the proportion of each active ingredient.
- Its label fails to bear adequate directions for use and such warnings as are necessary for the protection of users.
- It is dangerous to health when used in the dosage or manner recommended by the labeling.
- It is not listed with FDA or is manufactured in a facility not registered with FDA.
- It is a device for which premarket notification was not provided as required by Section 510(k) of the *FD&C Act*.

Separately, for those products defined as biologics (e.g., serums, toxins, blood products), FDA has enforcement authority under the *Public Health Service Act*. For example, FDA may suspend or revoke product licensure for unlawful activities.[22]

US Code Title 18

The intentional submission of certain false declarations or statements to a federal government agency such as FDA is a prohibited act under Sections 301 (w) and (x) of the *FD&C Act* and is a violation of Section 1001 of Title 18 of the US Code and may subject a person to possible criminal sanctions. Under 18 USC §1001, anyone who makes a materially false, fictitious or fraudulent statement to the US government is subject to criminal penalties. Specifically, a false statement is made when a person knowingly and willfully: falsifies, conceals or covers up by any trick, scheme or device a material fact; makes any materially false, fictitious or fraudulent statement or representation; or makes or uses any false writing or document, knowing the same to contain any materially false, fictitious or fraudulent statement or entry. A person who makes any such statement, "shall be fined, imprisoned not more than five years."[23]

Enforcement Discretion

FDA has broad enforcement discretion in deciding whether to use its power and resources to pursue, investigate or penalize specific activities. The US Supreme Court has held that FDA has wide prosecutorial discretion to decide whether to exercise its discretionary powers in individual cases and that this discretion is unreviewable.[24] However, apart from the language in Section 309 of the *FD&C Act*, which states that FDA is not required to pursue minor violations when it believes "that public interest will be adequately served by a suitable written notice or warning," there is no statutory provision dictating how FDA is to use its resources to remedy all the violations that are reported to or discovered by the agency. FDA has the authority to publicize the actions it takes and, in certain circumstances, to seek civil monetary penalties and other administrative sanctions. For example, civil penalties may be sought for violations relating to the sale or trade of drug samples, for violations of postmarketing drug safety provisions and for offenses relating to clinical trials.

Debarment

"Debarment" is the legal exclusion of an individual or company from certain rights, privileges or practices. Under the *Generic Drug Enforcement Act* of 1992, FDA may debar an individual or company convicted of certain types of felonies. The statute also imposes sanctions of debarment of individuals from the pharmaceutical industry, debarment of corporations from the drug approval process and withdrawal and suspension of product approvals for certain prohibited conduct. The practical effect is that the individual or firm can no longer provide services in any capacity to a company that has approved drug product applications, unless FDA decides otherwise (21 U.S.C. § 355a–335c). The act also authorizes FDA to impose civil penalties for fraud relating to generic drug approval applications.

Enforcement Jurisdiction

FDA's authority to apply its resources to enforce compliance with the *FD&C Act* is directly related to movement or possible movement of an article in interstate commerce. Section 201(b) of the *FD&C Act* defines interstate commerce as: commerce between any state or territory and any place outside thereof, and commerce within the District of Columbia or within any other territory not organized with a legislative body. Thus, any product that is not manufactured in any "state" or "territory" as defined in the *FD&C Act* and not distributed to the US is not subject to FDA's jurisdiction. "Territory" is defined as any territory or possession of the US, including the District of Columbia, and excluding the Commonwealth of Puerto Rico and the Panama Canal Zone. A product that is manufactured in another country and distributed in interstate commerce also is subject to FDA's jurisdiction, but if the product is not distributed in the US, it cannot be seized or subjected to a request for injunctive relief. No provision of the *FD&C Act* or any regulation promulgated under the authority of the act is applicable to regulated products that do not enter into US interstate commerce. Finished products that have been shipped in interstate commerce or have been manufactured using components that have been shipped in interstate commerce are subject to FDA jurisdiction.

FDA may initiate enforcement action if it establishes certain elements of proof. It must establish jurisdiction, interstate commerce, violation and responsibility. To satisfy the jurisdictional element, the product must be subject to the provisions of the *FD&C Act* (e.g., it meets the law's definition of a drug or medical device). The interstate commerce element is satisfied if the product or any of its components is shipped across state lines, within the limitations described above. In 1997, Congress amended the *FD&C Act* so that FDA no longer has the initial burden to demonstrate a connection to interstate commerce (21 U.S.C. 379a). The violation element is satisfied if the product is adulterated, misbranded or otherwise in violation of the act (e.g., unapproved new drug). Finally, enforcement actions directed at individuals or companies also must establish responsibility for the violation.

Penalties

FDA's Administrative Sanctions (separate from judicial actions)

When a problem arises with a product regulated by FDA, the agency can take a number of actions to protect public health. It is important to note that a risk to public health is not the only requirement for FDA to act; a violative act is punishable. Normally, the agency works with the manufacturer to correct the problem voluntarily. If that fails, FDA may utilize administrative or judicial enforcement tools. FDA may initiate administrative enforcement outside the court system and without the involvement of the Department of Justice (DOJ). This enforcement may be specifically authorized by a statute or developed by the agency under broad statutory authority. FDA uses the following administrative sanctions:

- recalls
    - voluntary
    - mandatory (only applicable to medical devices, infant formulas and food when there is a reasonable probability that the food is adulterated or misbranded and the use of or exposure to the food will cause serious adverse health consequences or death)
- administrative detentions
- Application Integrity Policy
- device ban or repair, replacement or notification requirements
- import detention
- debarment
- clinical investigator disqualification
- license suspension or revocation
- product approval suspension, withdrawal or delay
- restitution and disgorgement
- civil money penalties
- Notice(s) of Violations
    - inspectional findings (Form FDA 483)
- compliance correspondence
    - Warning Letters
    - Untitled Letters (frequently used for advertising or promotional violations)
- publicity

When the agency uses administrative means to achieve enforcement, the process generally starts from an FDA field office or a center at FDA headquarters. Most administrative actions identified above require center concurrence and approval and, in some cases, consultation with FDA's Office of Chief Counsel.

Judicial Actions

The agency generally will attempt to achieve compliance through administrative means. However, in certain instances, FDA will pursue judicial actions. In pursuing judicial action, FDA may use the judicial tools of seizure, injunction or criminal prosecution. It is noteworthy that FDA, with the assistance of the Department of Justice, may bring an enforcement action; the law does not allow an individual to bring a private cause of action to enforce the *FD&C Act*.

Seizures

Seizure actions are authorized by Section 304 of the *FD&C Act*.[25] A product in violation of the *FD&C Act* is subject to seizure, a civil action providing for government "arrest" of the goods. A seizure action is against the products that are alleged to be in violation of the *FD&C Act* rather than against a company or individual. Thus, a seizure is a civil action that is intended to remove adulterated or misbranded goods from interstate commerce and accessibility by consumers. Seizure actions can occur at a company's own facilities or wherever the product is located. Seizure actions are published in FDA's Enforcement Report on its website.

FDA can initiate, through DOJ, three types of seizure actions against an industry participant: lot, multiple and mass.[26] Lot seizures generally involve one (or more) lot of product in one location that is or has become adulterated or misbranded during interstate commerce. Multiple seizures involve more than one action to arrest goods located in different jurisdictions where the goods are adulterated or lack required approval. Multiple seizures may be filed against allegedly misbranded product when it has been the subject of a prior court judgment, presents a danger to health or contains a fraudulent or materially misleading label that may injure a purchaser. Mass seizures involve a warehouse full of products usually manufactured at one location and deemed adulterated or misbranded. FDA can accomplish injunctive-type relief through a mass seizure on the basis that the scope of the violations render every article in the facility adulterated.

The seizure process normally is triggered by the collection of a sample found to be in violation of the law. FDA requests the appropriate US Attorney's office to file a Complaint for Forfeiture in the jurisdiction where the goods to be seized are located. If the US Attorney files the complaint, a judge or magistrate signs an order for arrest for the goods and the US Marshals Service executes the warrant. Once the warrant is served by a US marshal, the goods fall under the custody of the federal government. A return is usually made to the court by the US marshal indicating the success of the seizure, including the quantity seized and its location. Anyone having an interest in the goods must file a claim within specified timeframes.

A claimant may appear and propose that the goods be reconditioned to bring them into compliance. If FDA agrees to the method of reconditioning, the court issues a Decree of Condemnation permitting reconditioning under the supervision of FDA after a bond is posted. Alternatively, the claimant can file an answer denying the allegations and seek a court trial to contest the government's assertion that the goods are in violation of the law. To argue against the seizure, the claimant must prove the product is not adulterated or misbranded. To support its case, FDA normally produces evidence gathered through facility inspections. If no claim is filed, however, the US Attorney will file a motion for a Default Decree of Condemnation and Forfeiture, ultimately resulting in the destruction of the goods by the US Marshals Service.

No prior judicial finding that a violation of the *FD&C Act* has occurred is necessary prior to the institution of a seizure action. Once a seizure action is instituted by the government, it is well established that the affected company's remedy is to contest the seizure action by filing a claim and answer; no separate suit seeking to enjoin the seizure action can be brought.

Injunctions

Injunctions are authorized by Section 302 of the *FD&C Act* and are utilized to enjoin conduct (i.e., proactively do something or refrain from doing something) where there is a likelihood that violations will continue or recur. FDA initiates three types of injunctions:

1. temporary restraining order
2. preliminary
3. permanent[27]

FDA seeks an injunction in two circumstances: when there have been chronic violations and efforts by the agency to obtain voluntary compliance have been unsuccessful; or when immediate court intervention is needed to address an imminent public health hazard. In the latter situation, FDA will seek a temporary restraining order. Unlike injunction proceedings brought by private litigants, FDA does not have to prove in an injunction action that there will be "irreparable injury," but merely that the violative conduct is likely to continue.[28]

When the agency's efforts to obtain correction of violative conduct over a period of time have failed, DOJ will file a Complaint for Injunction asking the court to restrain further violations and allow FDA oversight and control of the company's conduct. A Complaint for Preliminary Injunction may be sought to enjoin the company until a hearing and/or trial can be held on a Complaint for Permanent Injunction. Because most injunctions require the company to suspend all or most of its operations, judges have tended to encourage FDA and the company to agree on a plan to correct the problems. Companies also generally prefer a negotiated settlement rather than a protracted and public legal battle. Thus, FDA's inclination has been to negotiate a Consent Decree of Permanent Injunction with the company and then file it simultaneously with an abbreviated Complaint for Permanent Injunction.

Consent decrees of permanent injunctions, once granted, continue in perpetuity unless one party or the other petitions the court to vacate the injunction. Commonly, a company negotiates a sunset provision for dissolution of the injunction conditioned upon the company meeting all of the consent's provisions.

Criminal Prosecution
The Decision to Prosecute
FDA does not prosecute its own criminal cases. Rather, DOJ must bring the criminal case to court. FDA, however, does recommend cases to DOJ for criminal prosecution. Generally, FDA decides to recommend criminal prosecution in cases where there are: gross violations that evidence management's disregard for compliance with the *FD&C Act*; obvious and continuing violations where management has not exercised appropriate care; life-threatening violations or those where injuries already have occurred; and deliberate attempts to circumvent the law, such as the submission of false information to the agency.[29] Once FDA has decided to seek criminal prosecution against a corporation or an individual, it proceeds through DOJ to obtain a criminal information or an indictment, depending on whether a misdemeanor or felony charge is involved. Recently, FDA has stated its intent to target more executives with misdemeanor prosecutions when their companies have violated the *FD&C Act*. FDA has legal authority to bring these criminal cases under a 36-year-old Supreme Court precedent.[30]

FDA has established the Office of Criminal Investigations (OCI), which conducts the majority of criminal investigations related to the *FD&C Act*. OCI, working with DOJ, obtains and executes search warrants and arrest warrants, conducts physical surveillance, obtains and serves grand jury subpoenas, obtains and reviews telephone toll records, bank records and other materials to support a case against an individual, company or conspiracy.

Standard of Liability Under the FD&C Act
The *FD&C Act* is a "strict liability" criminal misdemeanor statute. People who commit prohibited acts can be criminally convicted notwithstanding their intent (or lack thereof) to commit a crime. Thus, the fact that a corporate officer has no direct involvement in the conditions that give rise to a criminal violation does not excuse that officer from liability. Case law makes it clear that an individual in a position of responsibility may face personal criminal accountability if he or she fails to seek out and remedy violations when they occur or implement measures that ensure violations will not occur.[31] Evidence that the individual played a role in or had knowledge of the violation is not necessary. Before pursuing criminal actions against individuals, FDA normally considers many factors, including the individual's position and authority within the company; whether a violation is likely to have harmed the public; the obviousness of the violation; whether a violation reflects a pattern of illegal behavior; and whether the proposed prosecution is a prudent use of agency resources.

Guaranty Clause
Sections 303(c)(2) and (3) of the *FD&C Act* provide a safe harbor from criminal prosecution under the general criminal penalty provisions of Section 303(a)(1). A guaranty received by a corporation, individual or employee of a corporation that states the articles delivered by the guarantor are not adulterated or misbranded within the meaning of the *FD&C Act*, and (as applicable) that they are not unapproved food additives, color additives, drugs or Class III devices subject to an approval requirement, protects the recipient of the guaranty from criminal liability. Guaranties may be limited to a specific shipment or may be general and continuing.[32]

In its enforcement regulations covering guaranties, FDA provides that a "guaranty…will expire when, after the covered products are shipped or delivered by the guarantor, the products become adulterated or misbranded, or become unapproved products" under the *FD&C Act*.[33] Thus, the original guarantor's guaranty will not serve as a "safe harbor" if the products covered by the guaranty are subsequently adulterated, misbranded or become a violative, unapproved product.

Furnishing a false guaranty is a separate prohibited act under the *FD&C Act* and can result in criminal liability. Under the *FD&C Act*, however, a company that receives a guaranty and then, in good faith, provides a subsequent guaranty premised on the original guarantor's representations, is not guilty of a prohibited act.

Section 305 Hearings
In most cases, the person against whom criminal proceedings are being contemplated will be given an opportunity to present his or her views with regard to such criminal proceedings. This usually is done in the form of a Section 305 hearing.[34] FDA is instructed by Section 305 of the *FD&C Act* to hold a hearing to give the target company or individual(s) opportunities to present views orally or in writing before any violation is reported by the secretary to any US Attorney for institution of a criminal proceeding. A 305 hearing will not be provided, however, if the agency has reason to believe that the opportunity for a hearing may result:
- in the alteration or destruction of evidence; or
- in the prospective defendant's fleeing to avoid prosecution; or
- if a grand jury investigation of a possible felony prosecution is planned[35]

The Section 305 hearing is held pursuant to a formal notice. The hearing is usually an informal meeting, often held in an FDA district office, and its purpose is to provide a party an opportunity to furnish information that will dissuade FDA from making a criminal referral to DOJ.

Other Federal and State Regulatory Agencies
FDA primarily takes the initiative for enforcing unlawful activities relating to product manufacture, safety and quality-related issues or labeling and promotion.[36] However, there are other regulatory agencies that have the authority to take action. For example, the Consumer Product Safety Commission regulates child-resistant packaging for certain types of FDA-regulated products. The Securities and Exchange Commission can take action for misleading investor-related materials (e.g., press releases or financial statements) involving products sold by publicly traded companies. Customs and Border Protection can sample, detain or refuse imports and exports. The Federal Trade Commission regulates over-the-counter drug, food, cosmetic and most medical device advertising to ensure promotional claims are truthful, substantiated and fair.

In addition to enforcement by federal agencies, state regulatory agencies may choose to take enforcement action, typically to ensure compliance with state consumer protection laws.

Summary
FDA has broad authority to inspect establishments and facilities under its jurisdiction to protect the public health. However, the reach and scope of the inspection power is not unlimited, and firms should make their employees aware of these limitations through training and internal standard

operating procedures. FDA's primary purpose in conducting inspections is to determine whether regulated products have been manufactured, packed and held under conditions that may result in such products being adulterated or misbranded, or whether products lacking required FDA approval are being distributed and sold. There are various types of FDA inspections, ranging from a comprehensive review of manufacturing controls and practices to a targeted review of a specific practice in the facility. The agency's approaches during an inspection will depend on the scope of the inspection and the circumstances presented. Likewise, whether the agency will take administrative action or institute legal proceedings following an inspection will depend on what FDA discovers during the inspection.

The agency has broad discretion to decide what enforcement action it will take against companies, individuals and products that violate the law, and, as a general rule, FDA attempts to choose the enforcement tool that is commensurate with the unlawful conduct. These options range from administrative sanctions, such as a Warning Letter, to a seizure, injunction or criminal prosecution in federal court with the approval and assistance of DOJ. Nevertheless, FDA prefers companies to comply voluntarily and take proactive steps to ensure regulatory compliance.

References
1. 21 U.S.C. §374.
2. 21 U.S.C. §374(a)(1).
3. Ibid.
4. 21 U.S.C. §§350c(a), 374(a)(1).
5. Dow Chemical v. U.S., 476 U.S. 227 (1986).
6. *U.S. v. Acri Wholesale Grocery Co.*, 409 F. Supp. 529 (S.D. Iowa 1976).
7. Statement of Margaret A. Hamburg, MD, Commissioner of Food and Drugs, Food and Drug Administration, 15 November 2012. FDA website. www.fda.gov/NewsEvents/Testimony/ucm327667.htm. Accessed 17 May 2013.
8. 21 U.S.C. §338.
9. 21 U.S.C. §384e.
10. 21 U.S.C. §360(h)(2),(3).
11. See H.R.Rep. No. 112-495, at 31.
12. 21 U.S.C. §360(h)(4)
13. 21 U.S.C. § 374(g)(3)
14. 21 U.S.C. §374(g)(11)
15. 21 U.S.C. §374(a)(4)
16. Ibid.
17. Ibid.
18. 21 U.S.C. §334(g). FDA is required to promulgate regulations to implement administrative detention authority with respect to drugs within two years of enactment of *FDASIA* and must consult with stakeholders in developing these regulations.
19. 21 U.S.C. §334(g)(1)
20. 21 U.S.C. §331 et seq.
21. 21 U.S.C. §355(a).
22. 42 U.S.C. §262.
23. 18 U.S.C. §1001.
24. *Heckler v. Chaney*, 470 U.S. 821 (*1985*).
25. 21 U.S.C. §334.
26. Parker FR. *FDA Administrative Enforcement Manual* (2005).
27. 21 U.S.C. §332.
28. Parker FR. *FDA Administrative Enforcement Manual* (2005).
29. Fine SD. "The Philosophy of Enforcement." 31 *FOOD DRUG COSM. L.J.* 324 (1976).
30. *United States v. Park*, 421 U.S. 658 (1975).
31. Ibid.
32. 21 U.S.C. §333(c)(2)–(3); 21 CFR 7.13(a)(2).
33. 21 CFR 7.13.
34. 21 U.S.C. §335. FDA, *Regulatory Procedures Manual*, Part 6: Judicial Action, Chapter 6-5 (March 2008). FDA website. www.fda.gov/ICECI/ComplianceManuals/RegulatoryProceduresManual/default.htm. Accessed 17 May 2013.
35. 21 CFR 7.84(a)(2)–(3).
36. FDA initiated a "Bad Ad Program" that encourages healthcare providers to report potential false and misleading prescription drug advertising and promotion.

Chapter 37

Healthcare Fraud and Abuse Compliance

Updated by Ojas Chandorkar

OBJECTIVES

❑ Introduce and explain state and federal laws directed at preventing waste, fraud and various other abuses by life sciences firms

❑ Explain types of fraud

❑ Provide overview of amendments to the existing laws

❑ Provide examples of circumstances that might trigger concerns under these laws

❑ Identify consequences of a violation of these laws

❑ Identify compliance methods and tools to combat healthcare fraud and abuse

---

LAWS, REGULATIONS AND GUIDELINES COVERED IN THIS CHAPTER

❑ *Federal Food, Drug, and Cosmetic Act* of 1938

❑ *Guidance for Industry: Good Reprint Practices for the Distribution of Medical Journal Articles and Medical or Scientific Reference Publications on Unapproved New Uses of Approved Drugs and Approved or Cleared Medical Devices* (January 2009)

❑ *False Claims Act* of 1863 (Lincoln Law)

❑ Federal and state Anti-Kickback Laws

❑ Federal and state Physician Self-Referral Laws (*Stark Law*)

❑ Pharmaceutical Research and Manufacturers of America Code on Interactions with Healthcare Professionals

❑ Price Reporting Laws

❑ Medicaid Drug Program

  o Federal Upper Limit

  o Public Health Service Program

  o Federal Government Ceiling Price

  o Medicare Part B

  o Medicare Part D

❑ State sales and marketing compliance laws

❑ *Physician Payment Sunshine Act* of 2009

❑ *Patient Protection and Affordable Care Act* of 2010

Introduction

Healthcare fraud and abuse have become a primary focus of regulators in recent years, and they have led to the loss of billions of dollars annually. Since Medicare and

Medicaid programs make up approximately 20% of the federal budget, it is obvious these systems are susceptible to fraudulent activities.

Life sciences firms selling items that are ultimately utilized in the healthcare industry are subject to laws directed at preventing waste, fraud and various other abuses. Any company that provides goods or services reimbursed under Medicare, Medicaid or any other federal healthcare program may be subject to civil or criminal penalties under federal laws including the *Medicare and Medicaid Patient Protection Act* of 1987 (*Federal Anti-Kickback Statute*), the *Stark Law*, the *False Claims Act* (*FCA*) and various US Food and Drug Administration (FDA) regulations. Companies that provide goods or services reimbursed by state healthcare programs, or even by individuals or private payors, may find themselves subject to similar, but usually not identical, state statutes. This chapter introduces several key risk areas for pharmaceutical and medical device manufacturers, with the aim of identifying illustrative, but not exhaustive, patterns that may, if not properly managed, lead to allegations of fraud, waste or abuse. It also discusses the various types of frauds that are being reported every year and talks about the proactive measures the federal government is taking to curb these activities.

Off-label Promotion

FDA seeks to ensure the safety and efficacy of drugs and devices. This means that most drugs and devices must be approved or cleared by FDA prior to promotion or marketing. As part of this process, FDA approves or clears drugs and devices for certain uses or indications. The agency generally prohibits manufacturers of new drugs or medical devices from promoting or marketing products for any use that FDA has not approved or cleared. According to FDA, an approved new drug marketed for an unapproved use is an unapproved new drug with respect to that use. Specifically, an approved drug or device or an uncleared device that is marketed for an unapproved use is considered to be misbranded. If the manufacturer promotes a drug or device for any unapproved or uncleared indication, it is commonly called "off-label promotion" and may violate both FDA laws and the *FCA*.

FDA recognizes that off-label use can be appropriate and valuable to patient care, and thus the statutes allow for off-label use by physicians as part of the professional practice of medicine. In fact, drugs and devices are commonly used for off-label indications with good results. Also, FDA understands that there must be some room for free exchange of educational and scientific information in order to advance the cause of science and healthcare. For example, in FDA's *Guidance for Industry: Good Reprint Practices for the Distribution of Medical Journal Articles and Medical or Scientific Reference Publications on Unapproved New Uses of Approved Drugs and Approved or Cleared Medical Devices* (January 2009), the agency allows dissemination of certain scientific information by manufacturers, with constraints designed to ensure that these exchanges are not used as subterfuges for off-label promotion. Most companies have special processes and procedures that must be followed when disseminating off-label information to ensure adherence to FDA guidance on this point.

The *False Claims Act* may be invoked by off-label promotion. This law prohibits the filing of a false or fraudulent claim to be reimbursed by the government. It imposes civil liability on persons who knowingly submit a false or a fraudulent claim or engage in various activities or wrong practices that involve federal government money or property. Penalties under this act include treble damages, plus an additional penalty of $5,000 to $11,000 for each false claim filed. This law also allows any person or party who has knowledge of the wrongdoing and brings it to court to receive between 15% and 30% of the monetary proceeds of the action or settlement recovered by the government. In addition, the law encompasses companies that "cause" the filing of such a claim." Because the general rule is that Medicare and Medicaid will provide reimbursement for a drug or device only when it is prescribed for an approved use, when a company markets a drug or device for an unapproved use, the government may argue that such marketing "caused" a healthcare professional to file a claim with Medicare or Medicaid for an off-label use. The *FCA* has steep per-claim civil monetary penalties and treble damages, meaning that a low-valued claim can quickly result in significant fines.

The federal government takes an aggressive stance regarding the enforcement of off-label promotion and has obtained some significant judgments against manufacturers for the practice. These cases tend to emanate from sales and marketing practices designed to persuade healthcare providers to prescribe products for off-label uses. For example, in January 2009, the Department of Justice (DOJ) accepted a guilty plea from Eli Lilly and Co. and fined the company $515 million. This fine was in addition to a civil settlement of approximately $800 million. These billion dollar-plus in criminal and civil settlements resulted from a claim that Eli Lilly was promoting its drug Zyprexa for the treatment of dementia, Alzheimer's, depression, anxiety, sleep problems and behavioral symptoms such as agitation, aggression and hostility, despite the fact that the drug was approved only for the treatment of psychotic disorders and bipolar disorder. Similarly, in April 2009, Nichols Institute Diagnostics, a subsidiary of Quest Diagnostics Inc., pled guilty to a felony misbranding charge in violation of the *Food, Drug, and Cosmetic Act* of 1938 (*FD&C Act*) and agreed to pay a criminal fine of $40 million as part of a $302 million global settlement with the federal government. In its guilty plea, Nichols Institute Diagnostics admitted that, over approximately a six-year period beginning in May 2000, it marketed a misbranded test. The misbranding claim was premised on the allegation that Nichols Institute Diagnostics distributed marketing materials describing the Advantage Intact PTH Assay as having "excellent correlation" to another assay—despite the fact that Nichols Institute Diagnostics was aware that the Advantage Intact PTH Assay was not consistently providing equivalent results.

In addition to monetary relief, FDA may seek an injunction to prohibit a company from manufacturing and distributing an unapproved drug. For example, in April 2009, FDA announced that it was barring Neilgen Pharmaceuticals Inc., its parent company Advent Pharmaceuticals Inc. and two of its officers from manufacturing and distributing any unapproved, adulterated or misbranded drugs. According to FDA, the unapproved drugs (primarily prescription cough and cold products) manufactured by Neilgen and Advent had not undergone the agency's drug approval process. Accordingly, the companies failed to establish the drugs' safety and effectiveness, and FDA had not reviewed the adequacy and accuracy of the directions for use and related label warnings. As part of the consent decree with FDA, Neilgen and Advent were ordered to destroy their existing drug supply and were expressly prohibited from commercially manufacturing and distributing any new drugs without the agency's approval. The companies also were required to consult with outside experts who could provide guidance regarding appropriate compliance standards and to obtain written authorization from FDA before resuming operations. They face the prospect of steep financial penalties for any future violations. While the failure to obtain FDA approval makes this an extreme case, the enforcement action demonstrates the significant business disruption that can result from violations of FDA regulatory requirements.

It is also important to note that claims of off-label promotion are not levied exclusively against manufacturers. For example, in 2006, DOJ charged a psychiatrist with conspiring with the manufacturer of a drug called Xyrem to promote the drug for off-label uses. According to the indictment, the manufacturer of Xyrem, Orphan Medical Inc., paid the psychiatrist thousands of dollars for promoting Xyrem for off-label uses at various speaking engagements. As a result, both the company and the physician were charged. Orphan Medical paid $20 million to settle civil and criminal charges, and in 2008, the physician pled guilty to misbranding.

Kickbacks

Patients rely on their physicians to recommend the best treatments, drugs and devices. Indeed, patients cannot obtain prescription medical products and services without a referral or order from a medical professional. Thus, the physician-patient relationship is regarded as a special, fiduciary relationship in which the physician is obliged to act with the best interest of the patient as the motivating concern. Remunerative relationships (such as consulting arrangements) between manufacturers and physicians who make referrals for or order the manufacturers' products can create an apparent or real conflict of interest, thereby potentially tainting referral decisions.

This is the underlying concern of the federal *Anti-Kickback Statute*. Generally, the statute prohibits intentionally soliciting, offering or receiving any remuneration (including any kickback, bribe, discount or rebate) in return for referring an individual to a person for the furnishing of any item or service for which payment may be made under a federal or a federally-funded state healthcare program such as Medicare or Medicaid. For example, the *Anti-Kickback Statute* would prohibit the provision of remuneration to a physician to induce or reward the physician for writing prescriptions for a particular product. The mandatory penalties for violations of this statute are severe, and a party guilty of violating the *Anti-Kickback Statute* is guilty of a felony and may be subject to a prison term of up to five years. In addition, a party that has violated the statute is excluded from participation in Medicare, Medicaid and other federal healthcare programs. For life sciences companies, this means that Medicare and Medicaid will no longer provide reimbursement for the company's products.

The application of the *Anti-Kickback Statute* is complex. Many common situations involving remuneration between manufacturers and referral sources can be structured to comply with the statute. For example, there is a "safe harbor" to the *Anti-Kickback Statute* that can protect arrangements with consultants, speakers and advisory board members providing services to companies. It is important that all remunerative relationships (i.e., transfers of value through compensation or otherwise) between manufacturers and their customers and others in a position to generate business for the manufacturer be properly vetted for compliance with the *Anti-Kickback Statute*.

There are many examples of investigations and prosecutions under the *Anti-Kickback Statute*. These actions typically arise from cases where a device or pharmaceutical manufacturer gives something, such as excessive compensation, to a physician or another person in a position to recommend its product, and it appears that the reason behind the transfer was to induce the recipient to recommend or order the manufacturer's product. Notably, it is not unusual to see a prosecution involving allegations that a company made improper payments to a physician to induce the physician to prescribe products for off-label uses, thereby violating both the prohibition against off-label promotion and the *Anti-Kickback Statute*.

These cases often involve payments to physicians, but can also involve payments to other parties in a position to promote the manufacturer's product. For example, one fairly recent prosecution involved a large pharmacy benefit manager, Medco. The government alleged that Medco violated the *Anti-Kickback Statute* by soliciting and accepting payments from pharmaceutical companies for favorable formulary placement, and by paying kickbacks to induce health plans to award Medco contracts to provide mail order pharmacy benefits for the plans' beneficiaries.

Many states have adopted their own versions of the *Anti-Kickback Statute*. These statutes also may affect arrangements involving items or services that are not covered under a governmental program. Also, these state laws may implicate slightly different behavior than is implicated by the federal statute. The existence of these state anti-kickback statutes means that remunerative relationships with referral sources must be scrutinized for compliance with both state and federal law.

Physician Self-referrals

Historically, physicians have branched out from the practice of medicine to provide ancillary services to their patients, such as laboratory tests, pharmaceuticals, durable medical equipment, imaging and lithotripsy. Some physicians may own interests in hospitals or other facilities to which they refer patients, or in device companies producing products used by their patients. While this practice seems like a natural evolution—and is beneficial to the extent that it increases accessibility or quality or spurs innovation—it also has the potential for creating a conflict of interest. The financial interest provides the physician with an incentive to direct patients to purchase services or products from an entity in which he or she has an interest, despite the fact that these products or devices may not be the best or cheapest available to the patient. The conflict of interest may also provide an incentive toward over-utilization.

The *Stark Law* (named for its primary sponsor, US Representative Pete Stark of California) and its associated regulations address this concern by prohibiting physician self-referrals for certain "designated health services" reimbursed by Medicare or Medicaid, except in certain specified circumstances. As with the *Anti-Kickback Statute*, many states have adopted their own variant of the *Stark Law* and prohibit self-referrals in the same or similar circumstances as prohibited by the federal law. Of course, not all of these arrangements will be problematic; rather they may fall under one of numerous statutory or regulatory exceptions. However, all of these arrangements require careful attention.

Of particular interest to device manufacturers is the question of whether the *Stark Law* should apply to prohibit physician-owned companies (POCs) that produce medical devices from selling those devices to hospitals and other facilities for ultimate use by the physician-owner's patients. The Centers for Medicare & Medicaid Services (CMS) currently is considering how to properly regulate POCs, and recently has solicited comments from the public on this issue. The ultimate decision could impact manufacturers that enter into arrangements with POCs.

PhRMA Code and AdvaMed Code

In addition to laws that govern manufacturers' conduct, trade organizations have also adopted voluntary codes of ethics. The Pharmaceutical Research and Manufacturers of America (PhRMA) adopted a voluntary marketing code to govern the pharmaceutical industry's relationships with physicians and other healthcare professionals. The PhRMA Code on Interactions with Healthcare Professionals (the PhRMA Code) originally took effect in 2002 and was revised and made more stringent in 2009. Similarly, the Advanced Medical Technology Association (AdvaMed) issued its Code of Ethics on Interactions with Health Care Professionals (the AdvaMed Code) in 2005 and revised it in 2009 to coincide with the PhRMA Code revisions.

Both the PhRMA Code and the AdvaMed Code have established standards for manufacturers' interactions with healthcare professionals. For example, the codes discuss gifts, entertainment, the use of consultants, support of third-party conferences and grants. As discussed at the end of this chapter, a number of states have enacted laws that require or recommend compliance with the codes.

Bad Reimbursement Advice

Manufacturers of complex or innovative products often provide reimbursement advice to their customers. Liability can arise from advice that is faulty or perceived as promoting over-utilization. For example, in *United States v. Augustine Medical Inc.*, the government alleged that a manufacturer directed its customers to bill Medicare in a manner that obscured the true nature of its product, because it believed that if Medicare knew exactly what product was being billed, it would reimburse for the product at a less-favorable rate. Augustine Medical and various individuals associated with the company faced criminal and civil enforcement actions. The company eventually settled all claims against it. However, certain Augustine Medical executives pled guilty to criminal charges related to withholding facts used to determine rights to Medicare payments, and each received probation and incurred a significant fine. Companies should take care to provide only objective and accurate reimbursement information and remind customers about their own duty to confirm reimbursement policies before submitting claims so as to avoid a similar investigation.

Price Reporting Fraud

Pharmaceutical manufacturers report drug prices under a number of different programs using several different methodologies (e.g., Average Manufacturer Price, Best Price, Average Sales Price, Average Wholesale Price and Wholesale Acquisition Cost). Additionally, sponsors of programs operating under Medicare Part D are required to report all price concessions obtained from manufacturers to CMS (e.g., rebates or discounts). Allegations that a pharmaceutical manufacturer defrauded Medicare or Medicaid (or another government program) are often premised on the alleged inaccuracy of the various pricing reports. Charges of misconduct can arise in connection with, for example, inaccurate reporting or characterization of discounts or rebates. Allegations of "marketing the spread"—where manufacturers report their Average Wholesale Price to Medicare as "x" but sell to physicians at "x-y," thereby yielding a windfall gain to physicians—have been prosecuted aggressively. Similarly, causes of action based on concealment of Best Price (where manufacturers do not report certain discounts to the states in connection with their Best Price reporting obligations under Medicaid) also have been popular theories for prosecution.

Beyond ensuring the integrity of data generated and submitted for government reimbursement purposes, accurate compliance with the various price reporting programs requires attention to periodic filing and reporting requirements. The key federal programs to which pharmaceutical manufacturers may need to submit price reporting data include the Medicaid Drug Program, Federal Upper Limit (applicable to multiple source drugs under Medicaid), Public Health Service Program, Federal Government Ceiling Price (applicable only to single source and innovator multiple source drugs), Medicare Part B and Medicare Part D (outpatient drug program).

Patient Protection and Affordable Care Act

The *Patient Protection and Affordable Care Act* (*PPACA*) commonly known as the Affordable Care Act, Health Insurance Reform, Healthcare Reform or the Obamacare Act is a US federal statute that was signed by President Obama on 23 March 2010. The main goal of this act is to reduce the number of uninsured people in the US and help reduce healthcare costs. It also aims to combat healthcare fraud, waste and abuse.

New rules have been implemented to help reduce fraud and waste and also to increase federal sentencing guidelines for people involved in fraud. The law has strengthened screenings and checks on providers and suppliers who pose high risks. CMS has started using enhanced tools and technologies to understand and analyze trends and predict fraudulent areas in a more precise manner. There is also major funding provided (approximately $350 million over a period of 10 years) to boost anti-fraud efforts.

Other Types of Frauds

Phantom Billing

This type of fraud includes the billing for tests that were never performed on the patient. It also may include inappropriate or unnecessary billing of procedures that were never conducted. There may be cases where the patient is billed for equipment that was not ordered during the course of treatment. Charging Medicare or Medicaid higher prices while providing the patient with cheaper and lower quality products is also an aspect of phantom billing. Additionally, there may be instances where a Certificate of Medical Necessity (CMN) may be completed by the drug or equipment supplier instead of the physician.

Code Jamming

This involves a laboratory inserting a fake diagnosis code to make a patient eligible for Medicare or Medicaid coverage (http://medicarefraudcenter.org).

Upcoding

This fraud involves inflating bills by using diagnosis billing codes that show the patient suffers from medical complications and/or needs more expensive treatment. In this instance, the provider intentionally uses a higher paying code on the claim form for a patient that also asserts that the patient was treated with a more expensive procedure or required the use of more costly devices during the treatment than were actually used.

A $31 million settlement was reached in 2000 with Community Health Systems, arising from allegations of upcoding by a hospital in Brentwood, TN stemmed from misuse of eight different codes, including those for pneumonia, septicemia, certain cardiac conditions, and respiratory failure and ventilators between 1 January 1994 and 31 December 1997 (Source: http://medicarefalseclaims.com/?page_id=358).

Unbundling

This type of fraud is usually found in laboratory billing, where the bills are submitted in parts thus making the overall amount billed higher than the original required total. Certain types of tests are priced less because they are used frequently by physicians and are supposed to be billed together for reduced cost. Under unbundling, the healthcare provider artificially increases the total bill amount by billing each test separately. This type of fraud is also known as "fragmentation."

Reflex Testing

In this type of fraud, the laboratory runs certain tests automatically and bills the amount to Medicare. These tests are run even though the physician never prescribed or requested them. These cases are discovered when proper documentation from the physician is not sent to the laboratories.

Defective Testing

This type of fraud results when the physician has prescribed certain tests to be carried out but the laboratory or clinic is unable to conduct them due to a lack of the appropriate technology or the absence of necessary equipment. The laboratory or clinic still bills these tests to Medicare.

Use of Medicare or Medicaid Numbers

In some instances, agencies are providing free services and products in exchange for the recipients' Medicare or Medicaid numbers. The numbers are used to conduct fraudulent activities.

Overbilling

Hospices and rehabilitation centers are sometimes found to be overbilling Medicare and Medicaid authorities for the patients staying in these centers and the caretakers. In some cases, medical bills are inflated and submitted to the authorities to get higher reimbursements than the actual amount spent. Nursing homes have been discovered to be overbilling their staff hours to obtain higher reimbursements.

State Laws Relating to Sales and Marketing

A number of state legislatures have sought new approaches to contain healthcare costs, track interactions between manufacturers and healthcare practitioners and generally reduce healthcare fraud. These approaches include laws requiring the reporting of marketing activities and expenditures and regulating interactions between manufacturers and healthcare professionals. As of April 2011, eight states—California, Connecticut, Maine, Massachusetts, Minnesota, Nevada, West Virginia and Vermont—and the District of Columbia had such laws:. For the most part, these laws are triggered when a manufacturer interacts with a healthcare professional that is licensed in that state, meaning these laws must be considered if a manufacturer interacts with a healthcare professional licensed by one of those states at a national conference (e.g., may wish to invite a physician licensed in Maine to attend a dinner after a conference in another state) or may engage a healthcare professional licensed in one of the states to serve on an advisory board or speaker's bureau.

Following is a summary of the laws of the nine jurisdictions mentioned above. Companies are cautioned to monitor these laws for revisions and to watch for the promulgation of new laws by other states.

California

Pharmaceutical and device manufacturers are required to adopt a Comprehensive Compliance Program (CCP). The CCP must include a specific dollar limit on "gifts, promotional materials, or items or activities" the manufacturer gives or provides to "medical or healthcare professionals." The manufacturer must declare annually in writing that it is in compliance with the provisions of the law and its CCP. The CCP and annual written declaration must be available on the company's website and through a toll-free number. Although the California law does not provide for specific penalties, violators of the law may face civil enforcement actions under other state laws.

Connecticut

Pharmaceutical and device manufacturers were required to implement, at a minimum, the PhRMA Code on or before 1 January 2011. Manufacturers are also required to adopt a comprehensive compliance program that contains all of the requirements prescribed in the PhRMA or AdvaMed Codes as such codes were in effect on 1 January 2010. The Commissioner of Consumer Protection may impose a civil penalty of not more than $5,000 for any violation of the compliance law.

District of Columbia

Any person engaged in the practice of pharmaceutical detailing in DC must obtain and maintain a license with the District's Board of Pharmacy and must agree to adhere to a code of ethics promulgated by the DC city council, which includes compliance with the PhRMA Code.

Maine

Drug manufacturers must report the value, nature, purpose and recipient (persons/entities licensed to provide healthcare in the state) of expenses associated with educational or information programs. Specifically, manufacturers must report: support for continuing medical education and charitable grants; printing design and product costs for patient education materials; consulting fees, speakers' bureaus and market research; and expenses for food, entertainment and gifts, that are greater than $25. A civil penalty of $1,000 may be imposed for failure to report and for each false report or omission of required information.

Massachusetts

Drug and device manufacturers must adopt a code of conduct that complies with the requirements of the Massachusetts regulations. The code of conduct must address a number of areas, including Massachusetts' strict rules on the provision of meals to customers. Under the law, manufacturers may provide modest meals as an occasional business courtesy in connection with informational presentations of scientific, educational or business information, but only if those meals are provided in the customer's office or a hospital setting. A manufacturer must establish a program that provides for regular training of appropriate employees, including sales and marketing staff, on the marketing code of conduct. A manufacturer must adopt policies and procedures for investigating noncompliance with the regulations, taking corrective action, and reporting instances of noncompliance to appropriate state authorities. Upon request, a manufacturer must provide a copy of the marketing code of conduct, training program and policies, as well as a certification that the company is in compliance with the law to the Department of Public Health. Further, a manufacturer must disclose annually the value, nature, purpose and recipient of any fee, payment, subsidy or other economic benefit with a value of $50 or more provided directly or through its agents to a covered recipient in connection with its sales and marketing activities. A fine of not more than $5,000 per transaction, occurrence or event may be imposed for failure to comply with the law.

Minnesota

Minnesota has a gift-ban law applicable to drug manufacturers. Under the law, a drug manufacturer is prohibited from giving "any gift of value" to a healthcare professional. The following are not gifts under Minnesota law: (1) free samples, publications and educational materials; (2) items with a total combined retail value of not more than $50 per year; (3) salaries or benefits to employees; (4) payments to conference sponsor or for other educational programs; (5) reasonable honoraria/expenses for faculty; and (6) compensation for substantial professional or consulting services. Notably, only items 4–6 are required to be disclosed annually (i.e., payments to conference sponsor, reasonable honoraria/expenses and compensation for substantial professional or consulting services). Minnesota's gift-ban law does not address penalties for failure to comply with the law.

Nevada

Under Nevada's law, drug and device manufacturers are required to adopt a written marketing code of conduct and develop a program to provide regular training to appropriate employees. A copy of the code of conduct must be provided to the Nevada Board of Pharmacy. Note that if a company uses, without modification, the PhRMA Code as its marketing code of conduct, it is permitted to so indicate on its submission to the Board of Pharmacy in lieu of submitting its marketing code of conduct. In addition, a manufacturer must adopt policies for investigating instances of noncompliance with the marketing code of conduct and must conduct an annual audit to monitor compliance with the code of conduct and certify annually to the Board of Pharmacy that an audit has been completed. Notably, Nevada's compliance law does not address penalties for failure to comply with the law.

West Virginia

Drug manufacturers must report the total number of prescribers by dollar amount categories to whom the company provides gifts, grants or payments of any kind in excess of $100 for the purpose of advertising prescription drugs. West Virginia's disclosure law does not address penalties for failure to comply with the law.

Vermont

Vermont prohibits drug and device manufacturers from offering or giving any gift to persons authorized to prescribe or recommend drugs or devices, their employees, agents or contractors and certain healthcare entities (e.g., hospitals, nursing homes). A gift is defined as anything of value provided to a healthcare provider for free or any payment, food, entertainment, travel, subscription, advance, service or anything else of value provided to a healthcare provider unless: (1) it is an allowable expenditure as defined by the law; or (2) the healthcare provider reimburses the cost at fair market value. A manufacturer must annually disclose to the Vermont Office of the Attorney General the value, nature, purpose and recipient of any allowable expenditure made to Vermont healthcare providers as well as any academic institution and any professional or patient organization representing or serving healthcare professionals or patients. Anything of value provided by a manufacturer to a healthcare professional that is not an "allowable expenditure" or otherwise exempt from the gift ban may subject the manufacturer to a civil penalty of up to $10,000 per violation. In addition, Vermont's Attorney General may seek injunctive relief, costs and attorney's fees. Violators of the disclosure rules are also subject to civil penalties of up to $10,000 per violation.

The Physician Payment Sunshine Act

On 23 March 2010, President Obama signed into law H.R. 3590, the *PPACA*. A section of that law, known as the *Physician Payment Sunshine Act*, requires drug and device manufacturers to make an annual public disclosure of certain payments or other transfers of value to a physician or a teaching hospital.

By 1 October 2011, the entity charged with collecting such reports, the Department of Health and Human Services (DHHS), was required to establish procedures for submitting information and making public disclosure. The first annual reports, covering the 2012 calendar year, were due 31 March 2013. The information will be made available on an Internet website, in a searchable format, no later than 30 September 2013.

Under the law, the transfer of anything with a value greater than $10 must be reported (or if the aggregate amount for the calendar year exceeds $100). However, there are a number of exemptions to this reporting obligation.

Figure 37-1. Fraud Detection Technology

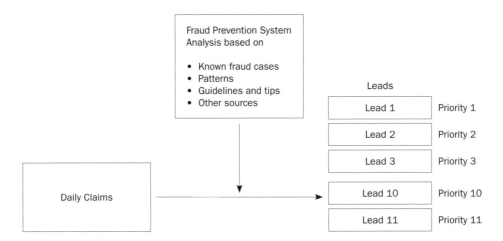

For example, gifts of educational materials that directly benefit patients or are intended for patient use need not be reported. Failure to report is subject to significant civil monetary penalties ranging from $1,000 to $100,000 per transfer that is not disclosed.

Notably, the *Sunshine Law* preempts state reporting requirements that are duplicative in their requirements to make reports. However, any additional and more stringent reporting requirements that states may choose to impose are not preempted.

The details of the federal *Sunshine Law* are not yet known, as (at the time of publication) the implementing regulations have not yet been published. Companies are cautioned to follow developments in this area.

Compliance Methods Enacted to Prevent Fraudulent Activities

Office of Inspector General (OIG)
The OIG was organized to combat waste, abuse and fraud taking place in the Medicare and Medicaid programs. Following are some of the duties carried out by the OIG, which investigates instances of fraud, waste and mismanagement that may constitute either criminal wrongdoing or violation of DHHS and Broadcasting Board of Governors regulations.

Health Care Fraud Prevention and Enforcement Action Team (HEAT)
The Health Care Fraud Prevention and Enforcement Action Team (HEAT) has played a vital role in preventing fraudulent activities. One vital component of HEAT, the Medical Strike Force, includes a team of analysts, investigators and prosecutors who are constantly on the lookout for and target emerging or migrating fraud schemes. The Medical Strike Force filed charges against 107 individuals in May 2012 who were allegedly involved in fraud schemes amounting to $452 million, and 91 individuals in October 2012 involved in $432 million in false billing http://www.healthcare.gov/news/factsheets/2011/03/fraud03152011a.html.

HEAT's mission activities include, but are not restricted to mustering resources across the government to help prevent fraud and waste, to crack down on people and organizations who abuse the system, reduce overall healthcare costs and improve quality of care by preventing fraud.

Tough Rules and Sentences for Criminals
Operation HEAT has led to a significant increase in the number of individuals charged with healthcare fraud. Criminals convicted of fraudulent activities are facing tougher and longer sentences. It also has established penalties for obstructing fraud investigations and audits.

Fraud Detection Technology
Fraud Detection Technology—Fraud Prevention Systems (FPS) employ predictive analytic technology to identify and track suspicious or fraudulent billing patterns. They use sophisticated mathematical and statistical algorithms and models to identify suspicious behavior. The systems analyze information from multiple data sources such as Medicare. FPS systems run predictive models against all Medicare claims nationwide before the final payment is made to detect any deviation in billing patterns and other suspicious activities. When an FPS system detects irregularities or any suspicious activities it generates reports that provide leads and further data to investigate. The system automatically prioritizes the leads that help in conducting the investigation of high risk zones or entities (See **Figure 37-1**).

Senior Medicare Patrols

Since 1997, the Administration on Aging (AoA) has funded Senior Medical Patrols (SMP) projects that recruit and train senior citizens and retired personnel to help the government recognize and report fraudulent activities to authorities. The Obama administration has expanded the Senior Medicare Patrol taskforce by providing more funding for these groups. These patrols educate and authorize their colleagues to identify, prevent and report healthcare fraud.

Summary

Life sciences firms selling items that ultimately are utilized in the healthcare industry are subject to laws directed at preventing waste, fraud and various other abuses. While a multitude of scenarios exist under which a life sciences company can find itself in trouble, attention should be focused on avoiding activities that are common enforcement targets, including: engaging in off-label promotion; giving illegal kickbacks; involvement in prohibited physician self-referrals; distributing misleading reimbursement advice; failing to comply with price reporting obligations; and failing to adhere to state sales and marketing laws. This chapter is designed to increase awareness of these risk areas, so the regulatory professional can help his or her company avoid them. It also aims to depict the latest countermeasures the federal government is taking to combat fraud, abuse and waste.

Recommended Reading
- DHHS Administration on Aging website. http://www.aoa.gov/. Accessed 5 May 2013.
- Medicare & Medicaid Fraud Reporting Center website, http://medicarefraudcenter.org/. Accessed 5 May 2013.
- STOP Medicare Fraud website, http://www.stopmedicarefraud.gov/. Accessed 5 May 2013.
- HealthCare.gov website, http://www.healthcare.gov/. Accessed 5 May 2013.

Chapter 38

Regulatory Information Resources in Review

By Diane R. Whitworth, MLS

OBJECTIVES

❑ Become familiar with print and electronic information resources relevant to the regulatory healthcare industry

❑ Understand how to access and retrieve publicly available, Internet-based government agency and association resources to support the regulatory intelligence process

❑ Recognize the value of industry associations to expand professional knowledge and develop regulatory core competencies

❑ Learn how to access selected Web 2.0 tools (blogs and social networks) to increase professional effectiveness

LAWS, REGULATIONS AND GUIDELINES COVERED IN THIS CHAPTER

❑ *Federal Register (FR)* and Code of Federal Regulations (CFR)

Introduction

Regulatory professionals have significantly improved their productivity, effectiveness and expertise in the workplace through access to the ever-increasing array of Internet-based regulatory information resources. The ease with which regulatory information may now be obtained is profound compared to the days when the only way to acquire this documentation was via telephone, fax or mail. This chapter provides a detailed review of a broad range of electronic industry, government and association resources available to regulatory professionals. The value of each of these tools in supporting product substantiation, regulatory review analysis, strategic planning and increasing professional knowledge are assessed.

Print and Electronic Publications

Print and electronic information resources play an essential role in a regulatory professional's ability to gain, maintain and advance knowledge and understanding of various healthcare industry product sectors. The regulatory profession is characterized by repeated job changes among professionals as well as by frequent mergers among the pharmaceutical, medical device and biologics companies themselves. For example, it is not uncommon for a regulatory professional's career to begin in the pharmaceutical industry and transition into the device area due to a job change, lateral move into another division within a company or perhaps to a work assignment in an area that requires an understanding of combination products. There are many and varied reasons why a professional may require additional regulatory information. Fortunately, print and electronic tools to fulfill this requirement are increasingly abundant.

Book Publishers

A number of publishers specialize in print and electronic publications focused on healthcare regulatory topics. This section reviews industry, government, association and standards publishers that target the regulatory healthcare profession and explains how regulatory professionals can retrieve the most relevant resources using the publishers' online catalogs. Because regulatory affairs is an interdisciplinary profession, publishers that primarily concentrate on

Chapter 38

scientific research and development (R&D), law, medicine, business or government, or possibly all of the above, may also feature publications focused specifically on the regulatory aspects of these subjects.

CRC Online Press, John Wiley & Sons, Lippincott Williams & Wilkins/Wolters Kluwer Health, Majors.com and Springer are major publishing firms that provide broad subject coverage and also feature a significant number of publications directed at the regulatory profession.

The CRC Online Press website contains numerous regulatory books within the general category of pharmaceutical science. Users can locate these publications within the following subcategories: biotechnology/biopharmaceutical; cleaning and sterilization; clinical trials; computer software; drug delivery and development; drug discovery; laboratory; manufacturing and engineering; medical devices; quality assurance; regulations and standards; and training and validation. Similarly, John Wiley & Sons produces regulatory publications on drug submissions, clinical trials, drug safety evaluation, pharmaceutical manufacturing regulations, quality and preclinical development.

Lippincott Williams & Wilkins, a division of Wolters Kluwer Health, also produces several publications on drug development, clinical trials and pharmaceuticals. Majors.com's publications focus on regulatory compliance; quality assurance; risk management; the *Health Insurance Portability and Accountability Act* (*HIPAA*); coding and reimbursement; administrative law and regulatory practice; pharmaceutical research; medical devices; biotechnology; chemistry, manufacturing and controls compliance; laboratory auditing; validation; and clinical research. Springer, by comparison, covers regulatory and toxicology issues such as pharmaceutical safety evaluation in its pharmaceutical science area.

The following keywords are effective for searching these online catalogs:
- regulatory
- regulatory affairs
- regulatory healthcare
- pharmaceutical
- biotechnology
- medical device
- pharmacology

Other industry publishers concentrate on specific regulatory areas such as quality assurance and standards. For example, the American Society for Quality's (ASQ) Quality Press publishes books, standards and training materials relating to quality issues, and the Bureau of National Affairs (BNA) concentrates on the legal aspects of regulatory affairs. Selected topics covered by BNA publications include pharmaceutical, biotechnology and health law, intellectual property and patent law.

In the same manner, the United States Pharmacopeia (USP), an official public standards-setting authority for prescription, over-the-counter (OTC) medicines and US-manufactured healthcare products, develops documentary and quality reference standards. Its key publications include the *US Pharmacopeia–National Formulary* (*USP–NF*) and the *Food Chemical Codex*. *USP–NF* monographs contain standards and procedures that are enforceable by the US Food and Drug Administration (FDA). The *USP–NF* contains public pharmacopeial standards for medicines, dosage forms, drug substances, excipients, medical devices and dietary supplements.[1]

Another valuable standards resource for regulatory professionals is IEEE, formerly the Institute of Electrical and Electronics Engineers, which develops and publishes conference proceedings, training materials, standards and publications central to regulatory research. It is the leading global professional association for the advancement of technology and the authority on biomedical engineering and medical devices.

The International Organization for Standardization (ISO), similarly, is a key nongovernmental standards-producing organization, consisting of a network of national standards institutes representing 159 countries and a coordinating Central Secretariat in Geneva, Switzerland. ISO's catalog comprises more than 175,000 published international standards.

The American Society of Testing and Materials (ASTM) is an additional example of a standards organization that produces Special Technical Publications, compilations, manuals, monographs, journals and handbooks on regulatory topics.

Standards publications focused on healthcare regulatory issues may be found through a search of the following terms:
- biological
- biotechnology
- clinical
- pharmaceutical
- medical device
- medical instrumentation
- quality management
- regulatory

Several industry publishers specialize in publications that focus entirely or largely on regulatory and compliance issues. Barnett International is one such company; it publishes regularly updated reference manuals, industry compendiums and job aids to assist regulatory professionals in complying with federal regulations. It also prepares regulatory industry executive analyses, question and answer guides on regulatory topics and a study site training series for regulatory professionals. FDAnews is another publisher that prepares reference tools specifically aimed at the pharmaceutical, biologics and medical device regulatory industry. Its products include the Code of Federal Regulations (CFR) compilations, an adverse event compliance series and publications on biologics, biosimilars and combination drug products. Similarly, GMP Publications targets the regulatory industry through its CFR pocket guides and good clinical practice and good manufacturing practice handbooks.

The Government Printing Office (GPO) serves as the country's official online bookstore for US government publications. GPO is the primary resource for gathering, cataloging, producing, providing, authenticating and preserving published information in all its forms for the executive, legislative and judicial branches of the federal government.[2] Publications pertaining to regulatory healthcare topics may be accessed by searching with the keywords "FDA" or "Food and Drug Administration" and "DHHS" or "Department of Health & Human Services" combined with more specific terms such as "pharmaceutical," "clinical" or "drug industry." GPO Access operates within the GPO to provide free electronic access to legislative resources, including Congressional bills, the *Congressional Record*, public and private law, the US Code; executive sources, such as the CFR, the *FR* and presidential materials; and judicial sources, including the Supreme Court, trial and appellate court cases, opinions, oral arguments and decisions.

Another type of publication of particular value to regulatory professionals is the market research report. Piribo, which brands itself as "online business intelligence for the BioPharma Industry,"[3] specializes in this type of resource. The UK-based publisher prepares detailed and costly global market research reports, handbooks, strategic analysis profiles and regulatory overviews. Report subject categories range from biotechnology, drug delivery and medical devices to prescription drugs, regulatory policy and pricing and reimbursement. Urch Publishing, like Piribo, is a UK-based publisher of market intelligence reports covering the global pharmaceutical and healthcare industry. Urch covers topics including chemicals, drug discovery/R&D, generics, pharmaceutical industry trends, pricing and reimbursement, regulatory, sales and marketing and therapeutics.

Thompson Publishing, by comparison, dedicates an entire product line to food and drug regulatory materials. Thompson's products are primarily subscription-based and are available in print or electronically. These products generally consist of two-volume manuals containing regularly updated newsletters, an archive and special reports, in conjunction with access to additional online resources. Topics covered include Good Clinical Practice, FDA advertising and promotion, FDA enforcement and medical device regulation. Aspen Publishers, another division of the aforementioned Wolters/Kluwer, also publishes a complete line of food, drug and medical device publications. It provides detailed coverage of the FDA approval process and expert guidance on generic drugs. The majority of Aspen's manuals are loose-leaf formatted, and subscribers automatically receive documentation updates, supplements and/or new editions.

Many associations, such as the Regulatory Affairs Professionals Society (RAPS) and the Food and Drug Law Institute (FDLI), publish materials intended for regulatory professionals that are available in their online bookstores. This book is a key example of one such product produced by RAPS. In addition, RAPS publishes regulatory affairs certification (RAC) preparatory materials for the US, Canadian, EU and Global exams; self-assessment exams for each certification; and books on topics key to the development of regulatory professionals. Also included in RAPS' bookstore are some third-party publications of interest to regulatory professionals. FDLI, similarly, markets its own publications as well as third-party products addressing regulatory and legal topics.

Free Industry Resources (Electronic Newsletters (e-Newsletters)

In addition to books, reports and standards, a number of industry resources are available to regulatory professionals to monitor current events and advance their knowledge of healthcare product regulation. This section reviews both free and fee-based sources. However, the free publications will be discussed in greater detail, as there are several valuable free sources of which regulatory professionals may be not be aware. The fee-based resources, by comparison, tend to encompass the more widely recognized monthly journals and association publications made available as a membership benefit. The sources reviewed in this section cover a range of drug, device and biologics regulatory publications. Although not comprehensive, they may give regulatory professionals a solid basis for further independent research.

Many publishers produce multiple newsletters aimed at different healthcare product sectors. For example, FDAnews publishes the following free e-newsletters: *FDAnews Device Daily Bulletin*, *FDAnews Drug Daily Bulletin* and *The QMN Weekly Bulletin*. *FDAnews Device Daily Bulletin* monitors FDA regulatory, legislative and business news developments as well as selected international news affecting the medical device industry. *FDAnews Drug Daily Bulletin* provides parallel coverage for the pharmaceutical industry. *The QMN Weekly Bulletin* covers current quality management news, regulatory developments and inspection trends. The summaries provided by these publications offer brief but valuable perspectives on current regulatory management issues for drugs, devices and quality. A link to the full-text article is listed below each summary; some of the cited sources require subscriptions to fee-based publications. These links afford regulatory professionals an opportunity to obtain further information on a particular subject as well as learn about new resources.

SmartBrief, an independent e-newsletter publisher, produces 25 industry-specific daily newsletters that are available free of charge by subscription. This company

Chapter 38

partners with trade associations and professional societies to publish its newsletters. *AdvaMed SmartBrief* is issued in conjunction with the Advanced Medical Technology Association (AdvaMed) and targets medical device, diagnostic product and health information system professionals. *BIO SmartBrief*, produced in cooperation with the Biotechnology Industry Organization (BIO), focuses on biotechnology industry professionals, and *FDLI SmartBrief* works with FDLI to reach food and drug industry professionals. The summaries in all three publications are based on original information from news organizations and are repackaged by SmartBrief's editorial staff. Each newsletter typically covers top stories: healthcare in transition; hot topics; business and market trends; science and health or science and health policy; emerging technologies; and product-specific and association-specific news. Regulatory professionals can use these publications to track current regulatory developments in time-saving compilations and obtain valuable competitive intelligence.

In a similar manner, VertMarkets has established 68 online community marketplaces for eight industry groups to connect buyers and suppliers. For each of its online industry communities, VertMarkets produces free bi-weekly email bulletins that provide not only product offerings, but also industry updates and the latest news to its members. The newsletters directed to regulatory professionals fall into the life sciences category and include the *Bioresearch Online Newsletter*, *Drug Discovery Online Newsletter*, *Laboratory Network Community Newsletter*, *Medical Device Online Community Newsletter* and *Pharmaceutical Online Newsletter*. Typical content includes top news stories, featured articles, featured downloads and a product showcase.

FierceMarkets is a digital media company that also specializes in supporting business-to-business marketing in the life sciences, healthcare, IT, telecom and finance industries through its e-newsletters, websites, webinars and live events. *FiercePharma is a daily e-newsletter focused on* pharmaceutical company news and market development of FDA-approved products. Regulatory professionals can stay informed and save time by reviewing these types of industry-specific publications. Categories included in *FiercePharma* are: pharmaceutical company news and reports; FDA rulings; regulations; recalls and warnings; drug launches and safety; pharmaceutical sales; and marketing news and activities of key industry professionals. *FierceBiotech* is another daily e-newsletter in the FierceMarkets' digital product family. It concentrates on drug discovery and clinical trials news as well as the latest biotechnology trends, breakthroughs and FDA approval updates. *FierceBioResearcher* reports on biotechnology research news, information and tools, with a special focus on the science of drug discovery. *FierceVaccines*, *FierceHealthcare* and *FierceSarbox* are the company's other three e-newsletters within the healthcare division.

F-D-C Reports, an Elsevier subsidiary, is a newsletter publisher that has been serving the healthcare product industry since 1939. Although the majority of its publications are fee-based, it does offer a complimentary subscription to a few of its weekly e-newsletters. One of these publications, *Medical Devices Today*, provides strategy, regulation, innovation and investment coverage from *The Gray Sheet*, *Medtech Insight*, *IN VIVO*, *Start-Up*, *The Silver Sheet* and *Strategic Transactions*. The articles cover drug and business development, finance, strategy, regulation and reimbursement. Summaries and reprints are excerpted from recognized publications including F-D-C Reports' *The Pink Sheet*, *The Gold Sheet*, *Pharmaceuticals Approval Monthly* and *PharmAsia News* and Elsevier Business Intelligence's *Start-Up* and *The RPM Report*.

A few other free electronic resources worth briefly mentioning are *Pharma Marketing News*, the *Pharmaceutical Technology Weekly Update*, *Pharmaceutical Technology Weekly Round-up*, *Pharmaceutical Technology Magazine*, and *PharmaFocus*. VirSci Corporation's *Pharma Marketing News* is a monthly newsletter for pharmaceutical and marketing professionals designed to keep subscribers informed about industry trends and innovations. It also offers a professional network for career advancement. Frequently covered topics include: physician marketing; sales and education; regulatory compliance; patient education; and direct-to-consumer advertising and marketing.

Pharma Technology Daily Update, *Pharmaceutical Technology Weekly Round-up* and *Pharmaceutical Technology Magazine* are produced by a UK-based company, SPG Media. These publications are dedicated to pharmaceutical professionals working with technology. Subscribers have access to the latest developments in global industry projects, company profiles, industry events and recruitment information that provides career assistance and the latest job vacancies. *PharmaFocus* is also published in the UK, but unlike *Pharma Technology Newsletter*, its primary focus is on news affecting the pharmaceutical industry and the UK's National Health Service. This publication is a bit more exclusive in that it is only sent free of charge to selected permanent employees of companies that manufacture ethical and OTC pharmaceuticals and biotechnology companies. The complete version of the latest issue, however, is accessible on the website.

Canon Communications Pharmaceutical Media Group also publishes a free e-newsletter, *PharmaLive Daily Advantage*. This publication is another great source of industry intelligence, providing summaries of industry events and trends affecting pharmaceutical and clinical professionals, accompanied by a link to the full text and related articles. Information is categorized by business and therapeutic area, and the news and information focus on clinical research, product marketing and pharmaceutical business.

In addition to their fee-based resources, a few associations, including RAPS and the Drug Information Association (DIA), have recently launched free daily electronic publications available by subscribing on the association websites. RAPS' *RF Today*, launched in January 2012, features summaries of the top regulatory news stories from around the world relating to pharmaceuticals, medical devices, biotechnology and the agencies that regulate them. DIA's daily e-newsletter highlights breaking news and information about the pharmaceutical, biotechnology and medical device fields from thousands of global news sources.

Clinical monitoring news is another area covered in a free weekly e-newsletter entitled *BioPharm Insight Clinical Newsletter*. Infinata, the publisher, is also the developer of BioPharm Insight, a commercial, fee-based database discussed later in this chapter. The newsletter covers the latest information on clinical enrollments, clinical results, drug approvals, drug licensing and medical devices. An additional free electronic resource providing current news for the clinical research community is the Association of Clinical Research Professionals' (ACRP) biweekly e-newsletter, *ACRP Wire*.

The medical device industry also receives excellent web coverage through a number of free publications. *Medical Device & Diagnostic Industry (MD&DI)* is one of 13 magazines published by Canon Communications that focuses on the medical technology industry. *MD&DI* is a monthly magazine written exclusively for original equipment manufacturers of medical devices and in vitro diagnostic products. For more than 25 years, it has supported the industry's efforts to comply with regulations, keep up-to-date on current events, improve manufacturing and design processes and understand market demand. *QMed Daily* is a Canon publication available free of charge with membership to QMed, formerly Medical Device Link. Members can sign up for all of Canon Communications' publications. *QMed Daily* is a daily e-newsletter that reports on top industry headlines and important FDA announcements and features articles on technology breakthroughs in the medical device industry worldwide.

TradePub.com is another excellent source for free healthcare and medical magazines, publications and newsletters covering the pharmaceutical and medical device industries, and more. Some of TradePub.com's more widely known publications include *Pharmalot Daily Newsletter* and *medtechinsider newsletter – Global Edition*. It is also possible to subscribe to some of the FierceMarkets publications through this website.

Fee-Based Industry Resources

The list of fee-based regulatory publications is long and varied, ranging from industry newsletters and peer-reviewed journals to association magazines. Key publishers in the regulatory sphere include Canon Communications, Dickinson, F-D-C Reports, PJB Publishers and Thompson Publishing.

The previously mentioned Canon Communications Pharmaceutical Media Group also publishes two fee-based magazines: *Med Ad News* and *R&D Directions*. *Med Ad News* is an established resource for competitive business intelligence and marketing strategy information. *R&D Directions* provides extensive coverage of pharmaceutical product development and insight into successful R&D strategies. Canon also publishes special reports on biotechnology; company analysis; drug delivery and development; healthcare sales and marketing; pipeline data; strategic issues and therapeutic areas.

Dickinson's FDAReview is a monthly newsletter published by Ferdic Inc. that provides in-depth analyses of the medical device and drug industries as well as FDA inspection and enforcement activities, including *Freedom of Information Act* (*FOIA*) daily logs and Warning Letter summaries. *FDAUpdate* is a weekly fax document containing *FR* updates pertaining to FDA rules and regulations; newly released Warning Letters; weekly filed citizen petitions; Advisory Committee proceedings and calendar; and late-breaking FDA and pharmaceutical product news. Free items also available on Dickinson's interactive website, *FDAWebview*, include FDA Warning Letters, *FR* notices and an FDA calendar.

In addition to the free e-newsletters published by FDAnews, this company distributes 10 fee-based subscription newsletters. The publications are: *Clinical Trials Advisor, Devices & Diagnostics Letter, Drug GMP Report, Drug Industry Daily, Generic Line, International Medical Device Regulatory Monitor, International Pharmaceutical Regulatory Monitor, The Food & Drug Letter, The GMP Letter* and *Washington Drug Letter*. As mentioned above, F-D-C Reports publishes newsletters designed to clarify developments affecting US healthcare product and services marketing and regulation for industry executives, policymakers and analysts. Newsletters published by F-D-C Reports include: *The Pink Sheet/The Pink Sheet DAILY, Pharmaceutical Approvals Monthly, The Gold Sheet* and *PharmAsia News* in the pharmaceuticals and biotechnology category; *The Silver Sheet* and *The Gray Sheet* in the medical devices and diagnostics category; *The Tan Sheet* and *The Rose Sheet* in the consumer products category; and *Health News Daily* in the health policy and biomedical research category.

Another well-recognized, fee-based publisher is Informa Healthcare, which is one of the largest publishers of business information for the pharmaceutical, biotechnology, medical devices and diagnostics industries. Its two key regulatory publications are *Regulatory Affairs Journal (RAJ) Pharma* and *Regulatory Affairs Journal (RAJ) Devices*. *RAJ Pharma* has served as a key source of global news, commentaries and analyses of regulation in the pharmaceutical

Chapter 38

Table 38-1. Publisher Resources

Publisher	Website	Resources
AdvaMed	http://advamed.org/	News Alerts (Fee-based)
American Society for Quality (ASQ Quality Press)	http://asq.org/quality-press/	Books, Standards, Training Materials & Journals (Fee-based)
American Society of Testing and Materials (ASTM)	www.astm.org/Standard/books_journals.shtml	Books, Standards, Technical Publications, Manuals, Handbooks, Journals (Fee-based)
Aspen Publishers	www.aspenpublishers.com	Books, Journals & Newsletters (Fee-based)
Association of Clinical Research Professionals (ACRP)	www.acrpnet.org/	Newsletters and Bimonthly Journal (Free & Fee-based)
Barnett International	www.barnettinternational.com/EducationalServices/Publications.aspx	Books, Reference Manuals & Compendiums (Fee-based)
Bureau of National Affairs (BNA)	www.bna.com/products/books.htm	Books, Directories & Handbooks (Fee-based)
Canon Communications	http://globalriskcommunity.tradepub.com/free/pdan/	Newsletters (Free)
Canon Communications Pharmaceutical Media Group	https://eforms.kmpsgroup.com/paidpub/pharmalive_signup.aspx	Newsletters (Free & Fee-based)
CRC Online Press	www.crcpress.com	Books & Journals (Fee-based)
Drug Information Association (DIA)	www.diahome.org/en/Resources/Publications/AboutPublications	Directories, Compilations, Journals & Newsletters (Free & Fee-based)
Elsevier Business Intelligence	http://www.elsevierbi.com/eletters-and-blogs	Newsletters (Free & Fee-based)
FDAnews	www.fdanews.com/	Books, White Papers & Newsletters (Free & Fee-based)
Ferdic Inc.	www.fdareview.com/	Newsletters (Fee-based)
FierceMarkets	www.fiercemarkets.com/advertise/publications	Newsletters (Free)
Food and Drug Law Institute (FDLI)	www.fdli.org/	Books, Directories, White Papers, CDs, Journals & Newsletters (Free & Fee-based)
Global Regulatory Press	www.globalregulatorypress.com/	Quarterly Journal (Fee-based)
GMP Publications	www.gmppublications.com/	Books, Handbooks & Manuals (Fee-based)
Government Printing Office (GPO)	http://bookstore.gpo.gov/	Books, Handbooks, Manuals, Guides, Journals & Newsletters (Fee-based)
Infinata	http://www.biopharminsight.com/company/press.html	Newsletters (Free)
Informa Healthcare	http://informahealthcare.com/action/showPublications?display=bySubject&category=area-regulatory	Journals (Fee-based)
Institute for Electrical and Electronics Engineers (IEEE)	www.ieee.org/index.html	Books, Standards, Conference Proceedings & Journals (Fee-based)
International Organization for Standardization (ISO)	www.iso.org/iso/home.htm	Standards, Handbooks, CDs & Journals (Fee-based)
John Wiley & Sons	www.wiley.com/WileyCDA/	Books & Journals (Fee-based)
Lippincott Williams & Wilkins	www.lww.com/	Books, Journals & Newsletters (Fee-based)
Majors.com	www.majors.com/wws/home.htm	Books (Fee-based)
Medical Device Manufacturers Association (MDMA)	www.medicaldevices.org/	Newsletters, White Papers & Special Reports (Fee-based)
Medtech Insight	www.medtechinsight.com	Newsletters (Fee-based)
Parenteral Drug Association (PDA)	www.pda.org	Books, Handbooks, Technical Bulletins, CDs & Journals (Fee-based)
Pharmaceutical-technology.com (Net Resources International)	www.pharmaceutical-technology.com/register/	Newsletters (Free)
Piribo	www.urchpublishing.com/publications/regulatory/index.html	Market Reports (Fee-based)
Regulatory Affairs Professionals Society (RAPS)	www.raps.org	Books, Journals, CDs & Newsletters (Fee-based)
SmartBrief	www.smartbrief.com/index.jsp	Newsletters (Free)

Publisher	Website	Resources
Society of Clinical Research Associates (SoCRA)	www.socra.org/	Journals (Fee-based)
Springer	www.springer.com	Books, Handbooks & Journals (Fee-based)
Thompson Publishers	www.thompson.com/public/library.jsp?cat=FOODDRUG	Books, Reports, CDs & Newsletters (Fee-based)
The Organisation for Professionals in Regulatory Affairs (TOPRA)	www.topra.org/TOPRA-Publishing	Newsletters (Fee-based)
Tradepub.com	http://thefreesite.tradepub.com/category/healthcare-and-medical/1205/	Newsletters (Free)
United States Pharmacopeia (USP)	www.usp.org	Books, Compendiums, & Standards (Fee-based)
VirSci Corporation	www.virsci.com/pharmamarketing.html	Newsletters (Free)

Note: Website urls are current at time of publication.

and biotechnology industries since 1990. Pharmaceutical regulatory intelligence on worldwide rules governing the development, launch and postmarket surveillance of medicines and combination products is provided. Areas of coverage include: regulatory agencies and legislation; application requirements and guidelines; R&D; patents and intellectual property; international harmonization; pediatric legislation; pharmacovigilance; pharmacoeconomics; and drug safety. Since 1995, *RAJ Devices* has also reported on current worldwide news and provided analyses of worldwide medical device regulatory affairs. Some unique areas of focus include: trade and environmental issues; healthcare systems and their impact on regulation and marketing; vigilance; and approval requirements and guidelines. Informa Healthcare also produces a broad range of fee-based industry news sources (e.g., *Scrip World Pharmaceutical News*); business and market research reports; R&D analytical tools and databases (e.g., Pharmaprojects and TrialTrove); contact directories (e.g., Scrip Directory); and research journals (e.g., *Clinical Research & Regulatory Affairs, Drug Development and Industrial Pharmacy*).

Elsevier Business Intelligence distributes several e-newsletters that monitor business information and intelligence trends, technologies and companies in the medical device, diagnostics and biotech industry. The company's fee-based newsletters include *Medtech Insight, IN VIVO: The Business and Medicine Report, START-UP: Emerging Medical Ventures* and *The RPM Report*. *Medtech Insight* is particularly useful to regulatory professionals for its clinical and industry perspectives on products, procedures and technologies shaping the global medical technology market. *IN VIVO* provides in-depth analyses of marketing, R&D and regulatory and finance strategies in the biopharmaceutical, medical technology and diagnostics industries. *START-UP* examines new product and leading-edge company and investment trends in the pharmaceutical, biotechnology, medical device and in vitro diagnostics industries. *The RPM Report* is a useful business resource for the biopharmaceutical regulatory professional. Its primary focus is on FDA, the Centers for Medicare and Medicaid Services (CMS) and public sector issues. Global Regulatory Press' *Journal of Medical Device Regulation* is yet another important resource for medical device regulatory professionals. This is a quarterly publication currently only available in electronic format. Regulatory professionals can monitor global regulatory developments through legislative changes summarized in each issue and obtain guidance from review articles analyzing current medical device regulatory and compliance issues.

Fee-Based Association Resources

The majority of association publications are free with membership but require nonmembers to pay an annual subscription fee. RAPS is one example of an association that publishes a monthly electronic magazine, *Regulatory Focus*, that is available to its members, with limited online guest access to selected articles. This magazine focuses on current regulatory issues affecting the drug, medical device and biological healthcare product sectors. Another member-based resource that RAPS offers is a weekly e-newsletter, *RAPS Weekly Update*. Similarly, The Organisation for Professionals in Regulatory Affairs (TOPRA) publishes a members-only international journal, *Regulatory Rapporteur*, which provides current news and analyses on regulatory and legislative topics. In addition, TOPRA issues a quarterly member newsletter, *In Touch*, which serves as an association news digest covering member and organizational activities. FDLI publishes a quarterly magazine, the *Food and Drug Law Journal*, which is also available free to members and by subscription to the public. The journal features articles on food, drug, cosmetic, medical device and healthcare technology industry regulation and legislation, implications of proposed regulations, policy trends and analyses of judicial decisions in food and drug law. Its members-only resource,

Update, is issued bimonthly and contains the latest association and industry news, viewpoints on industry-specific trends, FDA agency developments and articles on various regulatory topics.

Similarly, DIA publishes its official monthly journal, *Therapeutic Innovation & Regulatory Science*, formerly the *Drug Information Journal*. This newly launched journal encompasses drug, device and diagnostic innovations, global regulatory topics as well as pharmaceutical research and development issues. In addition to publishing a monthly journal, DIA also produces *Global Forum*, a bimonthly, four-color print and digital magazine dedicated to global coverage of pharmaceutical and medical products from discovery and development to regulation, marketing and surveillance. *Global Forum* also delivers up-to-date association and member news. Finally, DIA offers professionals a quarterly newsletter, the *Global Pharmaceutical Forum*, developed in collaboration with the Chinese Pharmaceutical Association, focusing on China's current regulatory news.

The Parenteral Drug Association (PDA) has a membership publication entitled *PDA Letter* that reports on science, technology, quality, regulatory affairs, association news and updates relevant to the PDA community. The *PDA Journal of Pharmaceutical Science and Technology* is a bimonthly publication that contains peer-reviewed scientific and technical papers covering the pharmaceutical and biotech industries. The journal is distributed as a member benefit and is also available by subscription. *PDA Technical Reports* are global consensus documents addressing a range of topics relating to pharmaceutical production, validation and quality assurance. Expert task forces prepare the reports, which are then reviewed by technical forums and ultimately evaluated and approved by an advisory board and the PDA board of directors. *PDA Technical Bulletins* are short, scientific position papers responding to issues raised during worldwide regulatory inspections. These board-reviewed and approved papers address a single issue in one or two pages and can be used to support an industry response to a regulatory concern.

Within the biologics/biotechnology sphere, BIO supports professionals engaged in R&D of new healthcare technology, biotechnology and related fields through its advocacy, business development and communications services. Its members-only publication, *BIO News*, is published six times a year and reports on organizational activities, professional perspectives on industry issues and member activities. The Society for Biomaterials is another biologics-focused organization that promotes progress in biomedical materials R&D. The society also publishes members-only resources to foster an understanding of current industry and regulatory developments among regulatory professionals. Members are afforded free access to its official news magazine, *Biomaterials Forum*, which is available by subscription to nonmembers as well. The forum reports on current biomaterials community activities and includes book reviews, technical briefs and professional services information. The *Journal for Biomedical Materials Research* is the official journal of the society and is a peer-reviewed publication provided free to members. It features clinical studies and research reports on a range of topics including the preparation, performance and development of new biomaterials. *Applied Materials* is published as Part B of the journal. It contains peer-reviewed articles on device development; implant retrieval and analysis; manufacturing; regulation of devices; liability and legal issues; standards; reviews of devices; and clinical applications. Nonmembers may subscribe directly by contacting John Wiley & Sons.

In the medical device and technology field, AdvaMed is a lobbying/advocacy organization that supports the industry's goals of advancing global healthcare and increasing patient access to medical technology. AdvaMed also promotes policies that encourage high ethical standards, rapid product approvals, appropriate reimbursement and international market access. Its members-only publications include three alerts: the *Member Advisory Program (MAP) Alerts* to follow the latest payment policy changes; the *Technology and Regulatory News Alert* to stay informed about key FDA regulatory developments; and the *International News Alert* to monitor global medical technology sales and operations developments. By comparison, the Medical Device Manufacturers Association (MDMA) represents the interests of smaller, innovative medical technology companies through its advocacy and educational services. Its members-only publications include the *Weekly MDMA Update* and the *Monthly Member Services Newsletter*.

Two key associations in the clinical research area are the aforementioned ACRP and the Society of Clinical Research Associates (SoCRA). In addition to its free biweekly e-newsletter, ACRP publishes a bimonthly journal, *The Monitor*, featuring peer-reviewed articles, association news and a guide to certification preparation courses and exams available only to members. SoCRA, like ACRP, is dedicated to the continuing education and development of its members and publishes the *SoCRA Research Journal*, a members-only quarterly publication that contains scientific and professional articles; society news and events; and professional opportunities and services. Selected articles from past issues of the journal are available to the public on SoCRA's website. A comprehensive list of all the fee-based and free publisher resources reviewed and their corresponding website addresses is provided in **Table 38-1.**

Online Commercial and Government Databases

Commercial Databases—Regulatory Intelligence

A number of commercial, fee-based databases are available to support the regulatory professional's legislative tracking and regulatory analysis responsibilities. These tools are extremely valuable when used in conjunction with other sources of regulatory expertise, from networking with colleagues to contacting consultants and/or directly communicating with government agency authorities.

Tarius Regulatory Database, an independent fee-based subscription database service, is included among these database providers. The Tarius database enables regulatory and quality professionals to stay informed about the latest legislative developments worldwide and to interpret regulations and guidelines applicable to global healthcare products. Tarius offers two types of products: customized regulatory and quality databases and predefined base modules on drugs and devices. The customized database solution prescreens data from multiple global government and legislative websites according to searches defined by a particular company or individual. The predefined drug and device modules, by comparison, contain continuously updated reference documents compiled from US and EU regulatory authorities and key international regulatory bodies. As part of its database subscription service, Tarius also offers users a complimentary daily electronic summary of published *FR* proposed rules, notices and regulations pertaining to CFR Titles 9, 21 and 40 relevant to drugs, biologics and devices. Other users may pay a nominal fee to subscribe.

Thomson-Reuters' IDRAC is another fee-based global regulatory intelligence database of regulatory, legal and scientific information accessed by professionals who develop and register human drug and biologics products. As is true of Tarius, IDRAC frequently updates its documents and provides expert analyses on key regulatory topics for more than 60 countries. The database also provides excellent coverage of FDA Advisory Committee activities through its AdComm Bulletins, summaries of new pharmaceutical legislation and summary bases of approvals (SBAs). In addition, subscribers can choose to receive the *IDRAC Weekly Alert*, covering current global regulatory developments, or customize an email alert with saved queries structured to meet their own information preferences.

Wolters Kluwer's MediRegs is also a provider of healthcare research products and software solutions for regulatory professionals. Its healthcare compliance software and risk management solutions product, ComplyTrack Suite, enables risk and compliance professionals to restructure their compliance programs and risk management initiatives to achieve greater efficiency. Revenue Cycle Solutions software targets coding and reimbursement healthcare professionals while the Life Science Regulatory Solutions online portal supports regulatory compliance professionals in the pharmaceutical, device and food industries. US and European database resources include regulatory publications, policy manuals, guidance documents, commission reports and automatic updates from domestic and international regulatory bodies.

MediRegs' US-focused regulatory resources include the Pharmaceutical Regulation Suite and the Device Regulation Library. The Pharmaceutical Regulation Suite provides access to enforcement materials; Establishment Inspection Reports (EIRs), 483s and Warning Letters dating back to the 1970s; SBAs dating back to 1964; US Code and public law legislation; the CFR; the *FR* back to 1991; FDA and NIH manuals and guidelines; and *FOIA* logs. The Device Regulation Library also affords regulatory professionals access to enforcement materials and EIRs, 483s and Warning Letters, as well as establishment registration and product listings, premarket approval (PMA) summaries back to 1945 and FDA product safety information.

Founded in 1975, FOI Services Inc., is an additional source for *FOIA* documents. The FOI online library contains more than 150,000 FDA-related documents, including: New Drug Application and Abbreviated New Drug Application approval letters; drug reviews; drug and biologics SBAs; dissolution reviews; device and biologics premarket notifications; 510(k)s; PMAs; device Summaries of Safety and Effectiveness; EIRs; 483s; company/FDA inspection correspondence; Warning Letters; Advisory Committee minutes; guidance manuals; internal FDA meetings; color and food additive petitions; and veterinary FOI summaries. *FOIA* documents may also be identified using the online commercial database, DIOGENES FDA Regulatory Updates. Available through the database vendor, the Dialog Corporation, this resource provides data from FDA's Enforcement Reports, 510(k)s, PMAs, medical device reports (MDRs) and the new drug list. Clients can request documents not already available in FOI's library. This fee-based FDA document service offers an excellent path for professionals seeking essential competitive regulatory intelligence while wishing to be discreet about their research.

Commercial Databases—Business Intelligence

In addition to the regulatory intelligence tools available to support regulatory professionals' surveillance, analysis and strategic planning responsibilities, numerous commercial business intelligence databases now may be obtained to increase their understanding of industry competition. Originally, these resources were only accessible to professional information searchers, but now the databases are specifically designed for users without prior search experience. It is currently possible to independently access these invaluable resources through company database subscriptions.

Infinata's BioPharm Insight, briefly mentioned earlier in the chapter, is a fee-based online database that provides global biotechnology and pharmaceutical industry competitive intelligence. This resource covers the entire drug product lifecycle from discovery and development through the drug approval stages, as well as licensing deals, pharmaceutical sales/projections, management contacts and medical devices. BioPharm Insight partners with Pharmawire journalists, a part of the Financial Times Group, to report on key items including drug pipelines; patent expirations and litigation issues; licensing pipelines; and merger and acquisition pipelines. The BioPharm Insight database consists of Pharmawire Intelligence, the Clinical Trials Network, Drug Profiles, Drug Forecasts and Drug Licensing Deals. The BioPharm Devices database, in turn, affords users detailed coverage of the medical device pipeline. Each company profile contains a review of the organization and its markets; product forecasts and launches; manufacturing facilities; and key management contacts. Profiles of devices currently in distribution also are included in the database, as well as clinical trial and Investigational Device Exemption daily updates. And lastly, BioPharm Outsource is a database containing detailed profiles of contract service providers for the pharmaceutical and biotechnology industry.

Another pharmaceutical industry competitive intelligence resource is eKnowledgebase, an interactive online pharmaceutical database. eKnowledgebase is produced by Canon Communications Pharmaceutical Media Group, the publisher of *MedAdNews*, *R&D Directions* and *Trend Reports*. This fee-based database provides extensive company coverage as well as pipeline information for each stage of a drug's development. eKnowledgebase is updated daily and contains more than 26,000 compounds in development and drugs currently on the market. A user can choose to subscribe to the entire eKnowledgebase database or purchase either the Pipeline portion to search drugs in development or the Brands portion to search drugs on the market.

Informa Healthcare's Pharmaprojects database also serves as a valuable source of pharmaceutical intelligence. This tool tracks more than 36,500 drugs in active development with a drug, company and therapy profile for each. The drug profile contains product data, including therapies and indications by phase; originator and licensees; chemical data and structure; clinical trials; pharmacologies; country information; licensing opportunities and more. The company profile consists of addresses; subsidiaries; overview of operations; financial results; joint ventures and agreements; a licensing contact; and a direct link to the corporate website. The therapy profile is comprised of incidence, prevalence and market data; trends and forthcoming events; pharmacological strategies in progress; and links to related websites. Pharmaprojects enables drug regulatory professionals to analyze competitor performance, review R&D pipeline data to assess trends and evaluate potential business partnerships. Data sources include the companies themselves, Pharmaprojects' sister publication, *Scrip World Pharmaceutical News* and interviews with company personnel who attend global conferences.

Another Informa Healthcare product that contributes to the wealth of available pharmaceutical intelligence database resources is Pipeline. This database consists of all the novel drugs and formulations developed since 1980. These drugs are tracked throughout their product lifecycle and are kept in the database even if they fail at any stage. What makes Pipeline unique is that it not only affords web-based access to an unlimited number of employees under one site license, but also includes free, unlimited research support from expert analysts and offers free training. Regulatory professionals can use this global drug resource to monitor competitors' R&D programs, discover new competitors, evaluate the competitive landscape for a specific drug, benchmark product performance and identify potential collaborators.

Elsevier's PharmaPendium database, by comparison, provides drug safety data on FDA-approved drugs. This online resource affords researchers searchable access using the *Medical Dictionary for Regulatory Activities* search terminology. It also incorporates animal and human study data from the FDA Adverse Events Reporting System (FAERS); drug monographs from *Mosby's Drug Consult*; *Meyler's Side Effect of Drugs*; preclinical, clinical and postmarket data from FDA approval packages/SBAs; Registry for Toxic Effects of Chemical Substances toxicity data; and metabolite data for approved drugs. Regulatory professionals can use this database to obtain pharmacovigilance data to evaluate the full scope of projected risks early in the drug development process.

While the pharmaceutical intelligence databases discussed earlier focus on drug pipelines and R&D data, Life Science Analytics' MedTRACK concentrates on worldwide private and public biomedical company intelligence data. MedTRACK's key areas of focus are company profiles and financials, product data, R&D spending, patents, corporate deals, venture financing, industry statistics and epidemiology.

Clinical trial surveillance information is also accessible through Citeline's TrialTrove. This database contains a comprehensive repository of global ongoing clinical trials information. Clinical and regulatory professionals have access to competitive trial information organized by 90 disease groups through analyst monitoring of more than 12,000 data sources. As is true of the Pipeline database product, TrialTrove offers users a research support service with direct access to Citeline analysts for no extra charge. A comprehensive list of all the commercial databases reviewed and their corresponding website addresses is provided in **Table 38-2**.

Government Databases—Legislative and Regulatory Tracking

An integral component of a regulatory professional's work is to stay informed about the latest regulatory and legislative developments. The resources reviewed in this section highlight noteworthy governmental and nongovernmental database tools to support these monitoring and surveillance responsibilities. GPO Access, discussed at the beginning of this chapter, operates within the GPO to provide electronic access to legislative reference tools. The *FR*, published by the Office of the Federal Register, National Archives and Records Administration, serves as the official daily publication for rules, proposed rules, executive orders, presidential documents, and federal agency and organization notices. The *FR* volume for 2013 is Volume 78, and it may be searched separately or in conjunction with prior years dating back to 1994, Volume 59. Users may also sign up for a free daily email containing the *FR* table of contents. The CFR codifies the general and permanent rules published in the *FR*. The CFR is divided into 50 titles representing broad areas subject to federal regulation. Each CFR volume is updated once a year and issued quarterly. Titles are divided into chapters, usually bearing the issuing agency's name. Chapters, in turn, are subdivided into parts covering specific regulatory areas (e.g., 21 CFR 316.24 = Title 21 - Food and Drugs, Chapter I-Food and Drug Administration, Department of Health and Human Services, Subchapter D-Drugs for Human Use, Part 316-Orphan Drugs, Subpart C-Designation of an Orphan Drug, Section 316.24 - Granting orphan-drug designation.). Some CFR records on GPO Access date back to 1996; all titles are available from 1997 to the current year. Documents are available as ASCII text and PDF files.[4] In addition to the *FR* and CFR, GPO Access contains links to numerous databases to search Congressional bills, the *Congressional Record*, the US Code, statutes at large and public and private laws.

Unveiled in 1995, the Library of Congress' THOMAS database was created at the direction of the 104th Congress to make federal legislation publicly available. THOMAS offers a vast range of government resources, including databases to search bill resolutions; bill and amendment summaries; bills across multiple Congresses; public laws searchable by number; House and Senate roll call votes; legislation by sponsor; Congressional activity databases; the *Congressional Record*; days-in-session calendars; committee reports; and treaties. GovTrack.us, an independent, nonpartisan, non-commercial and open-source website launched in September 2004, provides access to some of the same tools available on THOMAS and GPO Access. This website is an extremely useful tool for regulatory professionals who need to monitor the status of federal legislation or Congressional events. Users can subscribe to RSS feeds (commonly referred to as really simple syndication) throughout the site or use trackers to create customized feeds and receive email updates. RSS feeds are a family of Internet feed formats used to publish frequently updated works—such as blog entries, news headlines, audio and video—in a standardized format.[5]

Government Databases—Federal Agency Resources

In addition to the legislative and regulatory tracking databases discussed previously, many federal agencies have built their own specialized databases to monitor specific regulatory issues and provide public access to biomedical, clinical and other useful government resources. This section focuses primarily on the databases created within FDA's centers. The Center for Drug Evaluation and Research (CDER) and the Center for Devices and Radiological Health (CDRH) have developed the largest number of database systems, with some overlap between CDER and the Center for Biologics Evaluation and Research (CBER). The Center for Veterinary Medicine (CVM) and the Center for Food Safety and Applied Nutrition (CFSAN) have also developed some unique databases. Due to chapter length constraints, however, this summary will review only selected center databases. A comprehensive list of all the agency's databases and corresponding website addresses is provided in **Table 38-2**.

CDER and CBER share the responsibility for reviewing postmarket safety reports submitted to FAERS, a database containing voluntarily submitted reports on approved drugs or therapeutic biologics products. CBER's other database systems include one for storing incoming Biological Product Deviation Reports and a Vaccine Adverse Event Reporting System (VAERS). Like the FAERS database, VAERS is based on a cooperative agency program between CBER and the Centers for Disease Control (CDC) to address vaccine safety.

Two of CDER's most heavily searched databases focus on drug product approvals: the Approved Drug Products with Therapeutic Equivalence Evaluations (*Orange Book*) database, which lists drugs approved on the basis of safety and effectiveness; and the Drugs@FDA database, a searchable catalog of brand-name and generic prescription and OTC human drugs and biological therapeutic products approved since 1939. Drug manufacturing firms are required to register their sites with Drugs@FDA within five days of commercial distribution and re-register annually at the Drug Establishments Current Registration Site database. The National Drug Code Directory is a database of marketed prescription drugs listed by universal product identifiers. CDER's two clinically oriented databases are the Bioresearch Monitoring Information System, which identifies personnel engaged in Investigational New Drug (IND) studies; and the Clinical Investigator Inspection List Database, which contains data relevant to IND studies gathered by clinical investigator inspections.

CDRH has built and maintains more than 18 databases to monitor medical device and radiological products. Its 510(k) Premarket Notification (PMN) database, which contains releasable 510(k)s, and its Premarket Approval (PMA) database, which provides manufacturer premarket approval status, are critical tools for device regulatory professionals. CDRH has also developed two adverse event reporting systems similar to CDER's FAERS database: the MAUDE (Manufacturer and User Facility Device Experience) database and the Medical Device Reporting (MDR) (formerly CDRH's Device Experience Network)

Chapter 38

Table 38-2. Commercial & Government Databases

Databases	Website	Subject Coverage
Commercial		
BioPharm Insight	www.infinata.com/biopharma-solution/by-product/biopharm-insight.html	Drug/Biotech & Device Business & Regulatory Intelligence
e-Knowledgebase	www.pharmalive.com/content/neweKB/	Drug/Biotech Business & Regulatory Intelligence
FOI Services	http://www.foiservices.com/	Regulatory Intelligence
IDRAC	www.idrac.com/FrontPage.aspx	Drug/Biotech Regulatory Intelligence
MediRegs	www.mediregs.com/	Regulatory Intelligence
MedTRACK	www.citeline.com/products/medtrack/overview/	Drug/Biotech Business Intelligence
Pharmaprojects	www.pharmaprojects.com	Business & Regulatory Intelligence
Pipeline	http://sites.informahealthcare.com/	Drug/Biotech Business Intelligence
Tarius	www.tarius.com	Drug/Biotech & Device Regulatory Intelligence
TrialTrove	http://www.citeline.com/products/trialtrove/	Drug/Biotech Clinical Trial Intelligence
Government		
Business.gov	www.sba.gov/	Federal Agency Information Portal for Small Businesses
Code of Federal Regulations (CFR)	www.gpo.gov/fdsys/browse/collectionCfr.action?collectionCode=CFR	Drug/Biotech & Device Regulatory & Legislative Intelligence
Forms Catalog	www.usa.gov/Topics/Reference-Shelf/forms.shtml?locale=en&m=false	Federal Agency Form Resource
Federal Register (FR)	www.gpo.gov/fdsys/browse/collection.action?collectionCode=FR	Drug/Biotech & Device Regulatory & Legislative Intelligence
FDA Warning Letter Database	www.fda.gov/ICECI/EnforcementActions/WarningLetters/default.htm	Drug/Biologics & Device Regulatory Intelligence
FDA/CBER On-Line: Establishment Registration & Biological Product Deviation Reporting	www.accessdata.fda.gov/scripts/cber/CFApps/Login/Index.cfm?CFID=19739204&CFTOKEN=4b5801a44b35d755-36EF1D27-1372-5AE1-6AA44EA2CBE290EA	Biologics/Biotech Regulatory Intelligence
FDA/CBER Vaccine Adverse Event Reporting System (VAERS)	http://vaers.hhs.gov/index	Biologics/Biotech Regulatory Intelligence
FDA/CDER FDA Adverse Event Reporting System (FAERS)	www.fda.gov/Drugs/GuidanceComplianceRegulatoryInformation/Surveillance/AdverseDrugEffects/default.htm	Drug/Biologics Regulatory Intelligence
FDA/CDER Approved Drug Products with Therapeutic Equivalence Evaluations (Orange Book) Database	www.accessdata.fda.gov/scripts/cder/ob/default.cfm	Drug/Biologics Regulatory Intelligence
FDA/CDER Bioresearch Monitoring Information System (BMIS)	www.accessdata.fda.gov/scripts/cder/bmis/	Drug/Biologics Regulatory Intelligence
FDA/CDER Clinical Investigator Inspection List Database	www.accessdata.fda.gov/scripts/cder/cliil/	Drug Regulatory Intelligence
FDA/CDER Drug Establishments Current Registration Site Database	www.accessdata.fda.gov/scripts/cder/drls/default.cfm	Drug/Biologics Regulatory Intelligence
FDA/CDER Drugs@FDA Database	http://www.fda.gov/Drugs/InformationOnDrugs/ucm135821.htm	Drug/Biologics Regulatory Intelligence
FDA/CDER National Drug Code Directory	www.accessdata.fda.gov/scripts/cder/ndc/default.cfm	Drugs Regulatory Intelligence
FDA/CDRH Advisory Meeting Materials Archive	www.accessdata.fda.gov/scripts/cdrh/cfdocs/cfAdvisory/search.cfm	Device Regulatory Intelligence
FDA/CDRH Clinical Laboratory Improvement Amendments (CLIA) Database	www.accessdata.fda.gov/scripts/cdrh/cfdocs/cfCLIA/clia.cfm	Device Regulatory Intelligence
FDA/CDRH MAUDE (Manufacturer and User Facility Device Experience) Database	www.accessdata.fda.gov/scripts/cdrh/cfdocs/cfMAUDE/search.CFM	Device Regulatory Intelligence

Databases	Website	Subject Coverage
FDA/CDRH Medical Device Reporting (MDR) Database	www.accessdata.fda.gov/scripts/cdrh/cfdocs/cfmdr/search.CFM	Device Regulatory Intelligence
FDA/CDRH Premarket Approval (PMA) Database	www.accessdata.fda.gov/scripts/cdrh/cfdocs/cfPMA/pma.cfm	Device Regulatory Intelligence
FDA/CVM Animal Drugs@FDA Database	www.accessdata.fda.gov/scripts/animaldrugsatfda/	Drug Regulatory Intelligence
GovTrack.us	www.govtrack.us/	Drug/Biotech & Device Regulatory & Legislative Intelligence
GPO Access	http://www.gpo.gov/fdsys/	Drug/Biotech & Device Regulatory & Legislative Intelligence
NIH ClinicalTrials.gov	http://clinicaltrials.gov/	Clinical Research
NLM—PubMed	www.ncbi.nlm.nih.gov/pubmed	Biomedical research
NLM—TOXNET	http://toxnet.nlm.nih.gov/	Biomedical/Toxicological Research
OMB/GSA RegInfo.gov	www.reginfo.gov/public/	OMB Regulatory Reviews/GSA Regulatory & Deregulatory Actions
Regulations.gov	www.regulations.gov/#!home;tab=search	Federal Agency Published Regulations & Public Comments
Thomas	http://thomas.loc.gov/home/thomas.php	Drug/Biotech & Device Regulatory & Legislative Intelligence
USA.gov	www.usa.gov	Federal Agency Information Portal

Note: Website urls are current at time of publication.

database. MAUDE presents voluntarily submitted user facility medical device adverse event reports since 1991, distributor reports since 1993 and manufacturer reports since 1996. The MDR database consists of reports on devices that may have malfunctioned or caused a death or serious injury from 1984–96, when it was replaced by MAUDE. Other noteworthy CDRH databases include the Advisory Committee/Panel Meetings database containing both information about upcoming meetings and historical information with links to summaries and/or transcripts of recent past meetings; the *Clinical Laboratory Improvement Amendments* (*CLIA*) database, which represents commercially marketed FDA- and CDC-categorized in vitro diagnostic test systems; and the Establishment Registration database, which comprises domestic establishments engaged in the manufacture, preparation, propagation, compounding, assembly or processing of medical devices intended for human use and commercial distribution.

CVM's Animal Drugs@FDA is comparable to CDER's Drugs@FDA and CDRH's 510(k) and PMA databases. This database allows users to search for approved animal drug products, suitability petitions, sponsors, the *Green Book*, CFR, *FR*, patents and exclusivity. In addition, FDA maintains its own Warning Letter database through its FOI office. The Warning Letter collection covers documents issued from November 1996 to the present. The database can be searched by company, subject, issuing office or date.

In addition to the regulatory information available through FDA's databases, regulatory professionals requiring biomedical research can access PubMed, the National Library of Medicine's (NLM) biomedical database, which includes more than 18 million citations from MEDLINE and other life science journals dating back to 1948.[6] NLM also produces TOXNET, the toxicology data network, which consists of databases on toxicology, hazardous chemicals, environmental health and toxic releases. For molecular biology information, NLM's National Center for Biotechnology Information (NCBI) offers a comprehensive resource. Established in 1988, NCBI has created numerous public databases covering genetic sequencing and molecular processes affecting human health and disease and has developed software tools for analyzing genome data. Lastly, the National Institutes of Health's (NIH) ClinicalTrials.gov site contains current information to identify federally and privately supported clinical trials for a range of diseases and conditions. The database includes 104,582 trials sponsored by NIH, other federal agencies and private industry conducted in all 50 states and 165 countries.[7]

A few additional recommended federal databases are the Forms Catalog and RegInfo.gov. Branded as "the US government's official hub for federal forms," the Forms Catalog contains many, though not all, of the citizen and business forms issued by federal agencies. Forms may be searched by agency, agency list or form number and are alphabetically listed by form name or keyword. A direct link to forms published on specific agency websites is also available if the form being searched is not available through the Forms Catalog. The Office of Management and Budget (OMB) and the General Services Administration (GSA), in turn, jointly produce RegInfo.gov. This website contains a catalog

Table 38-3. Agencies Associated with Healthcare Product Regulation

Agency	Website	Subject Coverage
Consumer Product Safety Commission (CPSC)	www.cpsc.gov/	Poisoning, Packaging, Labeling, Prescription/OTC Drug Products
Environmental Protection Agency (EPA)	www.epa.gov/	Environment & Public Health, Chemicals, Air Pollutants, Medical Waste
Federal Trade Commission (FTC)	www.ftc.gov/	Business Competition & Consumer Protection
Food & Drug Administration (FDA)	www.fda.gov	Food, Drugs, Medical Devices, Biologics/Blood & Vaccines, Animal & Veterinary, Cosmetics, Radiation-Emitting Products, Combination Products
Center for Biologics Evaluation and Research (CBER)	www.fda.gov/BiologicsBloodVaccines/default.htm	
Center for Drug Evaluation and Research (CDER)	www.fda.gov/Drugs/default.htm	
Center for Devices and Radiological Health (CDRH)	www.fda.gov/MedicalDevices/default.htm	
Center for Food Safety and Applied Nutrition (CFSAN)	www.fda.gov/Food/default.htm	
Center for Veterinary Medicine (CVM)	http://www.fda.gov/AnimalVeterinary/default.htm	
Office of Combination Products (OCP)	www.fda.gov/CombinationProducts/default.htm	
Freedom of Information Act (FOIA) Reading Room	www.fda.gov/RegulatoryInformation/foi/default.htm	
Information for the FDA-Regulated Industry	www.fda.gov/ForIndustry/default.htm	
Department of Health & Human Services (DHHS)	www.hhs.gov	Public Health, Food & Drug Safety, Grants & Funding, Research, Health Insurance
Administration for Children & Families (ACF)	www.acf.hhs.gov/	
Administration on Aging (AOA)	www.aoa.gov/	
Agency for Healthcare Research & Quality (AHRQ)	www.ahrq.gov/	
Agency for Toxic Substances & Disease Registry (ATSDR)	www.atsdr.cdc.gov/	
Centers for Disease Control & Prevention (CDC)	www.cdc.gov/	
Centers for Medicare & Medicaid Services (CMS)	www.cms.gov/	
Health Resources & Services Administration (HRSA)	www.hrsa.gov/	
Indian Health Service (IHS)	www.ihs.gov/	
National Institutes of Health (NIH)	www.nih.gov/	
Substance Abuse & Mental Health Services Administration (SAMHSA)	www.samhsa.gov/	
International Medical Device Regulators Forum (IMDRF), formerly Global Harmonization Task Force (GHTF)	http://www.imdrf.org/	Medical Devices
International Conference on Harmonisation of Technical Requirements for Registration of Pharmaceuticals for Human Use (ICH)	www.ich.org/	Drugs & Biologics
World Health Organization (WHO)	http://www.who.int/en/	Public Health, Drugs & Biologics
WHO Biologicals Program	www.who.int/biologicals/en	
WHO Essential Medicines & Pharmaceutical Policies	www.who.int/medicines/about/en/index.html	

Note: Website urls are current at time of publication.

searchable by government agency to locate all the regulatory reviews conducted by OMB's Office of Information and Regulatory Affairs (OIRA). It also has a catalog of the GSA's Regulatory Information Service Center's (RISC) semiannually published *Unified Agenda of Federal Regulatory and Deregulatory Actions* dating back to late 1995. The *Regulatory Plan* is part of the fall edition of the *Unified Agenda*. The *Regulatory Plan* serves as a defining statement of the administration's regulatory and deregulatory policies and priorities, while the *Unified Agenda* provides information about regulations that the government is considering or reviewing. RISC is responsible for gathering and publishing information on federal regulations through the semiannual *Unified Agenda of Federal Regulatory and Deregulatory Actions* and the annual *Regulatory Plan*, both required by Executive Order 12866, "Regulatory Planning and Review." The same executive order mandates that OIRA review federal regulations and information collections. OIRA also develops and oversees the implementation of government-wide policies on information technology, information quality, privacy and statistics.[8]

Reginfo.gov also provides links to several other government resources that will be briefly mentioned in this section. The first is USA.gov, the government's official portal to federal agency websites and information. This website is the product of an interagency initiative administered by the GAO's Office of Citizen Services and Communications. It provides a centralized database to locate information on US local, state and federal government agency websites. Regulations.gov is another resource that can be accessed from Reginfo.gov's website. It is an extremely valuable tool for locating government agency regulations, rulemakings or notices, and is also useful for finding, submitting and obtaining public comments on proposed *FR* regulations. In addition, a comment can be submitted directly via the website by accessing documents that are still open for public comment. Business.gov, the US government's official website for small businesses, provides information on regulatory compliance and other information for small business owners. Managed as a partnership by 22 government agencies, Business.gov offers a wealth of information on regulatory compliance, legal issues surrounding running a business and registration, license and permit requirements. For example, a pharmaceutical or biotech small business can click on the industry link and find a page dedicated to providing information on complying with laws and regulations applicable to producers, distributors and marketers of human and veterinary drugs, medicines, biologics, medical devices and equipment and controlled substances.

Government Resources Related to Healthcare Product Regulation

The previous section reviewed federal agency databases useful for legislative tracking and healthcare product approval review and reporting. This section features government agency websites that offer additional healthcare product regulatory information.

US Government Agencies

In addition to FDA's wealth of databases, the agency, to its credit, provides users with many handy navigational tools to obtain information from its website. Upon launching the agency's homepage, users are introduced to numerous ways to access information including the search box and A–Z index browsing feature. Moreover, users can select one of the broad subject categories (food, drugs, medical devices, vaccines/blood/biologics, animal/veterinary, cosmetics, radiation-emitting products and tobacco products) to be directed to an agency center or office. Within each of these links, additional navigational tools are provided to locate information. The CDER, CBER, CDRH, CFSAN and CVM homepages all offer drug, device, biologic, food and animal/veterinary-specific topical coverage, spotlighted center links, recalls/alerts, approvals/clearances, news/announcements, resources targeting industry, consumers and healthcare professionals, links to program area coverage, a search box and contact information. The radiation-emitting products, tobacco products and cosmetics categories listed on FDA's homepage follows a format comparable to the previously described centers.

A few other particularly helpful resources within the FDA website are the Office of Regulatory Affairs (ORA) and the Office of Combination Products (OCP) pages. The ORA page features a spotlight section, ORA news, links to resources and requested documents, recalls/alerts and a link to the ORA Freedom of Information Act (FOIA) electronic reading room. The Freedom of Information (FOI) page contains links to frequently asked questions; how to make a *Freedom of Information Act (FOIA)* request; *FOIA* fees; online payments; an electronic reading room; annual reports; the *Privacy Act;* reference materials; and contacts and links to other *FOIA* requester centers within the US Department of Health and Human Services (DHHS). The OCP website plays a role in all of the centers in which combination products are reviewed. Its links are designed to assist users in defining their own products. Consequently, this page provides an overview of OCP, a section providing links to further information, including the combination products page, guidance documents, information pertaining to the request for designation process, performance reports and contact information.

DHHS is the US federal agency whose mission is to protect the health of all US citizens and provide essential human services. The office of the secretary and its subdivisions carry out DHHS' initiatives while 11 operating agencies perform a broad range of tasks and services, from conducting research and ensuring food and drug safety to funding grants and programs and managing health insurance. The specific operating agencies are: the Administration for Children and Families, the Administration on Aging, the Agency for Healthcare Research and Quality (AHRQ), the Agency for Toxic Substances and Disease Registry, the Center for Medicare & Medicaid Services, CDC, FDA, the Health Resources and Services Administration, the Indian Health Service, NIH and the Substance Abuse and Mental Health Services Administration. Due to chapter length limits, DHHS operating agencies other than FDA are not discussed in detail. However, they are listed with their corresponding website addresses in **Table 38-3**.

An especially valuable feature of the DHHS website is the ability to subscribe to multiple DHHS and partnering agency publications with a single email address. Once a user selects the Official HHS Email Updates envelope icon at the top of the page and enters the appropriate email address, he or she can check the boxes next to all preferred publications. These preferences will then be forwarded to the appropriate agencies within DHHS. The partnering agencies that list publications are the National Institute of Allergy and Infectious Diseases, AHRQ, CDC, FDA, Disabilityinfo.gov, the Department of Defense Military Health System, the President's Malaria Initiative and USAID Health.

It is also worth mentioning a few other government agency websites that are helpful to professionals conducting healthcare product regulatory reviews and designing strategic product development plans. The first is the US Environmental Protection Agency, which examines the potential environmental, chemical and medical waste regulatory concerns related to developing various healthcare products. The second is the US Federal Trade Commission (FTC), which addresses issues related to enforcing appropriate business competition and monitoring anticompetitive practices. The FTC's Bureau of Consumer Protection is specifically responsible for handling fraudulent and dishonest consumer protection activities, which encompass advertising and e-commerce oversight. Advertising and consumer safety are also key priorities for healthcare product regulatory professionals. The US Consumer Product Safety Commission (CPSC) is another agency that deeply impacts a regulatory professional's product development decisions. CPSC's primary mission is to protect the public from unreasonable risks of injury or death from a broad range of consumer products. For example, its poison prevention packaging standards and testing procedures, as well as its child-resistant and senior-friendly packaging guidelines, determine how OTC and prescription drugs and physician samples must be packaged. Although a regulatory professional's decision making process is shaped by several other federal agency regulations and guidelines, this chapter will not go into detail about these governmental bodies. However, an in-depth and instructive discussion on this subject appears in a 2007 *Regulatory Focus* article by Novales-Li and Temple.[9]

Global Organizations

Although this chapter centers on US regulatory information resources, a few global organizations are too important to overlook given the critical role the US plays within each of these groups. The International Conference on Harmonisation (ICH) is one of these global bodies. ICH brings together the regulatory bodies of the EU, US and Japan and experts from the pharmaceutical industry in the three regions to discuss scientific and technical aspects of product registration.[10] The organization's safety, efficacy, quality and multidisciplinary guidelines are indispensable to pharmaceutical regulatory professionals as they evaluate proposed products to ensure regulatory compliance.

The International Medical Device Regulators Forum (IMDRF), formerly the Global Harmonization Task Force on Medical Devices (GHTF), is another international organization in which US regulatory representatives actively participate. IMDRF was conceived in 2011 as a voluntary group of medical device regulators from around the world who have joined forces to build on the foundation laid by the GHTF and to accelerate international medical device regulatory harmonization and convergence. Its representatives include medical device regulatory authorities from Australia, Brazil, Canada, the EU and the US, as well as the World Health Organization (WHO) which serves as an official observer.[11] The membership of China and the Russian Federation currently is being confirmed. The documents originally created by the GHTF study groups are finalized and current and embody harmonized regulatory practices for safety, effectiveness, performance and quality in medical device development. Medical device regulatory professionals review these documents as they evaluate device conformity assessment, quality management systems and postmarket surveillance issues surrounding their device products.

WHO is the final intergovernmental body to be considered in this section. WHO provides leadership on health matters, shapes the health research agenda and sets norms and standards within the United Nations. The US actively participates in WHO activities, particularly within its Essential Medicines and Pharmaceutical Policies Department, which is involved in developing, implementing and monitoring national medicines policies and guidelines. Another WHO program in which the US participates is the Biologicals Program. The goal of this program is to ensure that national regulatory authorities implement effective systems to ensure the quality and safety of blood products and in vitro diagnostic devices. **Table 38-3** lists websites for these global organizations.

Industry Associations

Print and electronic publications, online commercial and government databases and other Internet-based government agency resources unquestionably have an integral place in a regulatory professional's work. These resources enable him or her to monitor the latest news; track the status and development of laws, regulations and guidelines; and engage in effective strategic product development. It is, however, industry associations that function as indispensable educational resources for regulatory professionals themselves. The organizations mentioned earlier in the chapter, including RAPS, DIA, TOPRA, BIO, AdvaMed, FDLI and ACRP, offer a broad variety of learning opportunities to their members. Regulatory professionals can begin their education or update their knowledge of the regulatory healthcare industry and fulfill core competency requirements by participating in classroom and online courses, self-paced home study, audio and web-based training and certificate programs and attending workshops and conferences. In addition to offering formal learning options, associations enable professionals to engage in networking and to exchange information with their colleagues through forums and online communities.

Web 2.0 Tools

The second generation of Internet-based services, commonly referred to as Web 2.0, has enabled Internet users to participate in more dynamic and interactive information sharing. To complement the networking benefits of industry association memberships, regulatory professionals now can connect with colleagues through blogs and social networking websites. The rapidly growing number of blogs, or weblogs, which are regularly updated journal entries designed to be read by a professional audience and represent the unique personality of the author or website,[12] is remarkable. Some of the more popular blogs worth reviewing within the regulatory healthcare sector are: FDA Law Blog (Hyman, Phelps & McNamara PC); Biotech Blog; Eye on FDA (RX for Pharma Industry Communications and Planning); Medical Device and Diagnostic Industry (MDDI) blogs, including Device Talk and Transforming FDA; HTAi Blog (Health Technology Assessment International); and Pharmalive Blogs, including PharmaBlogReview, MedAdNewsInsider and R&D Directions Insider. This list does not begin to scratch the surface of the widely available information for this profession; however, it is a good starting point.

Social networking sites are another widely used Web 2.0 Internet service. Regulatory professionals can participate in sites such as LinkedIn, the Quality and Safety Regulatory Network and reg-info.com to establish a public professional profile, search for jobs, interact with colleagues, search for other regulatory professionals, review uploaded presentations and read member interviews. LinkedIn operates the world's largest professional network on the Internet with more than 200 million members in over 200 countries and territories.[13] Joining the network is free and simply requires the user to create a profile summarizing his or her professional experience and accomplishments. The information a user chooses to make publicly available can then be searched by other professionals within the LinkedIn network and used for the purpose of meeting and collaborating with other members. Similarly, the Quality and Safety Regulatory Network supports professionals working in quality assurance, regulatory affairs and compliance in highly regulated industries. This group was established to allow professionals to share experiences and expand their network of people and ideas in quality, regulatory, safety, health, sustainability, risk and compliance for continuous improvement across multiple industries.[14] Lastly, reg-info.com is another professional group created to allow pharmaceutical professionals to share ideas and initiate a forum for issues related to regulatory intelligence and information gathering. This community also assists pharmaceutical professionals in finding regulatory intelligence information through links to key regulatory and related information sources.[15]

Summary

This chapter has reviewed a wide range of print and electronic information resources and selected social networking tools available to regulatory professionals. From this review, it is clear that the wealth of publications, databases and government, association and industry web-based tools, as well as social networking opportunities that have sprouted up in just the past few decades is truly staggering. The new challenge for regulatory professionals is to distill the essential knowledge they require from the vast storehouse of information available to perform their jobs as effectively as possible. This will call for carefully managing electronic and print subscriptions, becoming skilled in using relevant government and industry databases, making use of associations' educational resources to advance professional knowledge and, finally, using social networking tools with discipline and discrimination. In this way, regulatory professionals will be certain to reap the greatest benefit from the abundant resources available, thereby increasing their productivity, effectiveness and overall expertise.

References
1. About USP – An Overview. US Pharmacopeia website. www.usp.org/about-usp. Accessed 19 March 2013.
2. About GPO. GPO website. www.gpo.gov/about/. Accessed 19 March 2013.
3. About Us. Piribo. Pharmaceutical Market research website. www.pharmaceutical-market-research.com/about_us/index.html. Accessed 19 March 2013.
4. Code of Federal Regulations (CFR) main page. GPO Access website. www.gpo.gov/fdsys/browse/collectionCfr.action?collectionCode=CFR. Accessed 19 March 2013.
5. "RSS." Wikipedia. http://en.wikipedia.org/wiki/RSS. Accessed 19 March 2013.
6. PubMed home page. NCBI website.: www.ncbi.nlm.nih.gov/pubmed/. Accessed 19 March 2013.
7. ClinicalTrials.gov Background. ClinicalTrials.gov website. http://clinicaltrials.gov/ct2/info/about. Accessed 19 March 2013.
8. Reginfo.gov homepage. www.reginfo.gov/public/jsp/Utilities/index.jsp. Accessed 20 March 2013.
9. Novales-Li P, Temple L. "Non-FDA Agencies Involved in US Healthcare Regulation." *Regulatory Affairs Focus*. Vol 12. No 8, pp 8-15 (August 2007).
10. ICH homepage. www.ich.org/. Accessed 20 March 2013.
11. About IMDRF. IMDRF website. www.imdrf.org/about/about.asp. Accessed 20 March 2013.
12. "Glossary." bytown Internet. Available at: www.bytowninternet.com/glossary. Accessed 20 March 2013.
13. About LinkedIn. LinkedIn.com website. http://press.linkedin.com/about/. Accessed 20 March 2013.
14. Quality and Regulatory Network. Linkedin.com website. www.linkedin.com/groups/Quality-Regulatory-Network-80327/about. Accessed 20 March 2013.
15. reg-info.com–Regulatory intelligence for pharma. Linkedin.com website. www.linkedin.com/groups/reginfocom-Regulatory-intelligence-pharma-833547?home=&gid=833547&trk=anet_ug_hm&goback=%2Econ. Accessed 20 March 2013.

Chapter 38

Regulatory Affairs Comparative Matrix of the Regulations Across Product Lines

FDA Centers		
	Source	**Centers**
Biologics	www.fda.gov/BiologicsBloodVaccines/default.htm	• Center for Biologics Evaluation and Research (CBER) • Center for Drug Evaluation and Research (CDER) for therapeutic protein and monoclonal antibody products
Cosmetics	www.fda.gov/Cosmetics/default.htm	• Center for Food Safety and Applied Nutrition (CFSAN)
Devices	www.fda.gov/MedicalDevices/default.htm	• Center for Devices and Radiological Health (CDRH) • Center for Biologics Evaluation and Research (CBER) for 510(k)s that involve blood and other biologics
Drugs	www.fda.gov/Drugs/default.htm	• Center for Drug Evaluation and Research (CDER)
Foods	www.fda.gov/Food/default.htm	• Center for Food Safety and Applied Nutrition (CFSAN)
Tobacco	www.fda.gov/TobaccoProducts/default.htm	• Center for Tobacco Products (CTP)
Veterinary	www.fda.gov/AnimalVeterinary/default.htm	• Center for Veterinary Medicine (CVM)

Regulatory Affairs Comparative Matrix of the Regulations Across Product Lines

FDA Requirements—Authority	
Acts	
Devices	• Pure Food and Drugs Act of 1906 • Federal Food, Drug, and Cosmetic Act of 1938 *(FD&C)* • Fair Packaging and Labeling Act of 1966 • Medical Device Amendments of 1976 • Safe Medical Devices Act 1990 *(SMDA)* • Medical Device Amendments of 1992 • FDA Export Reform and Enhancement Act of 1996 *(FDERA)* • FDA Modernization Act of 1997 *(FDAMA)* • Medical Device User Fee and Modernization Act of 2002 *(MDUFMA)* • Food and Drug Administration Amendments Act of 2007 *(FDAAA)* • Food and Drug Administration Safety and Innovation Act *(FDASIA)* of 2012
Drugs	• Pure Food and Drugs Act of 1906 • Federal Food, Drug, and Cosmetic Act of 1938 *(FD&C)* • Fair Packaging and Labeling Act • Durham-Humphrey Amendment of 1951 • Kefauver-Harris Drug Amendments of 1962 • Orphan Drug Act of 1983 • Drug Price Competition and Patent Term Restoration Act of 1984 • Prescription Drug User Fee Act of 1992 *(PDUFA)* • FDA Modernization Act of 1997 *(FDAMA)* • The Pediatric Research Equity Act (PREA) of 2003 • Food and Drug Administration Amendments Act of 2007 *(FDAAA)* • Food and Drug Administration Safety and Innovation Act *(FDASIA)* of 2012
Biologics	• Biologics Control Act (also known as the *Virus-Toxin Act*) of 1902 • Federal Food, Drug, and Cosmetic Act of 1938 *(FD&C Act)* • Public Health Service Act of 1944 • FDA Modernization Act of 1997 *(FDAMA)* • The Pediatric Research Equity Act (PREA) of 2003 • Food and Drug Administration Amendments Act of 2007 *(FDAAA)* • Biologics Price Competition and Innovation Act of 2009 • Food and Drug Administration Safety and Innovation Act *(FDASIA)* of 2012

Major Guidelines

	Source	Major Guidelines
Devices	www.fda.gov/MedicalDevices/DeviceRegulationandGuidance/GuidanceDocuments/default.htm	• Blue Book Memoranda • Write It Right • Premarket Approval Application (PMA), 510(k) and Investigational Device Exemption (IDE) preparation manuals • Medical Device Quality Systems Manual
	www.fda.gov/MedicalDevices/DeviceRegulationandGuidance/default.htm	• CDRH Device Advice website
Drugs	www.fda.gov/Drugs/GuidanceComplianceRegulatoryInformation/default.htm www.fda.gov/AboutFDA/CentersOffices/OfficeofMedicalProductsandTobacco/CDER/ManualofPoliciesProcedures/default.htm	• Guidance documents • Guidelines • Manual of Policies & Procedures (MaPPs) (CDER) • Current Good Manufacturing Practices (CGMP) for Drugs: Reports, Guidances and Additional Information
	www.ich.org/products/guidelines.html	International Conference on Harmonisation (ICH) Guidelines
Biologics	www.fda.gov/BiologicsBloodVaccines/GuidanceComplianceRegulatoryInformation/default.htm www.fda.gov/BiologicsBloodVaccines/GuidanceComplianceRegulatoryInformation/ProceduresSOPPs/default.htm	• Guidance documents • Guidelines • ICH Guidelines • Standard Operating Procedures and Policies (SOPPs)—CBER • Other Recommendations - Points to Consider (PTC)

Regulatory Affairs Comparative Matrix of the Regulations Across Product Lines

Meetings with FDA		
	Source	**Content**
Devices	*Guidance for Industry and CDRH Staff: Early Collaboration Meetings Under the FDA Modernization Act*	Types of Meetings: • Agreement Meetings—purpose is to reach concurrence on the key parameters of the investigational plan • Determination—limited to PMAs/PDPs, purpose is to determine the type of valid scientific evidence required to demonstrate that a device is safe and effective for its intended use • Pre-IDE—established, formal collaboration meetings, whose purpose is to expedite the regulatory review process and minimize product development delays • Pre-PMA—intended to help guide the development of PMA submissions, they include the result of preclinical testing not included in the IDE submission, reliability testing, CMC issues and clinical results. • PMA day 100—scheduled to occur 100 days after a PMA is accepted for filing, they provide an opportunity to discuss the application's review status and obtain additional information to complete the PMA review
Drugs	*Guidance for Industry: Formal Meetings Between the FDA and Sponsors or Applicants*	Type A meetings are those that are immediately necessary to address and resolve issues with a product submission—one that is delaying FDA's review. Type A meetings generally are reserved for dispute resolution, discussion of clinical holds or Special Protocol Assessments. A Type A meeting should be held within 30 days of FDA's receipt of a written request. A meeting package should be submitted to FDA at least two weeks before the meeting. Type B meetings are pivotal development meetings that occur prior to progression to the next development stage. FDA will schedule Type B meetings within 60 days of receipt of a written request. FDA expects the sponsor to submit a meeting package at least four weeks before the formal meeting. Type B meetings include: Pre-IND meetings, certain End-of-Phase 1 meetings; End of Phase 2 meetings/Pre-Phase 3 meetings and Pre-NDA/BLA meetings. Type C meetings are any other product development meeting not included in Type A or B. According to FDA guidance, the agency will schedule Type C meetings within 75 days of receipt of a written request. Type C meeting packages should be submitted to FDA at least four weeks before the formal meeting
Biologics	*Guidance for Industry: Formal Meetings Between the FDA and Sponsors or Applicants*	Same as Drugs

Product License, Listing Requirements and Establishment Registration

	Source	Forms	Product Classification
Devices	21 CFR 807	FURLS website	• Initial establishment registration • Annual registration of device establishment • Product listing • Device Classification: Class I, Class II or Class III • Combination Products (Device/Biologic or Device/Drug) Who must register: All owners/operators of any establishment, foreign or domestically-owned, engaged in the manufacture, preparation, compounding or processing of a medical device; those who initiate and develop specifications, manufacture, repackage, relabel, restore and commercially distribute a device; and initial distributors (US agents of foreign manufacturers), but not domestic distributors. All registration and listing information (Annual, Initial or Updates) must be submitted electronically unless FDA grants a waiver. There is a device facility user fee requirement associated with registration.
	21 CFR 807		
	21 CFR 860		
Drugs	21 CFR 207	Electronic Submission Gateway (ESG)	• Drug establishment registration • Annual update of drug/biologic establishment • Drug product listing • Registered establishments' Reports of Private Label Distributors • Groups within FDA: topical, oncology, etc. • Prescription Drugs • Generic Drugs • Over-the-Counter Drugs • Orphan Drugs • Combination Products (Drug/Device or Drug/Biologic) Who must register: Unless specifically exempted by law or regulation, all establishments, foreign or domestic, that manufacture or process drugs in the US are required to be registered with FDA and all drugs marketed within the US, including imported drugs, are required to be listed with the agency. All registration must be submitted electronically using the SPL format, unless FDA grants a waiver. There are user fees associated with registration and/or listing for prescription and generic drugs
	21 CFR 300 21 CFR 320 21 CFR 328-369 21 CFR 316		

Biologics	21 CFR 207
	21 CFR 207
	21 CFR 207
	21 CFR 601
	21 CFR 607
	
	21 CFR 1271
		Electronic Submission Gateway (ESG)
		2830—Blood
		3356—HCT/Ps
			• Establishment registration
			• Annual update of drug/biologic establishment
			• Drug product listing
			• Product licensing Biologics License Application (BLA) • Blood and blood product establishment registration and product listings
			• Combination products (biologic/device or biologic/drug)
			Who must register:
			  – All manufacturers of biological drug products
			  – All owners and operators of human blood and blood product establishments must register their establishment annually
			  – Human cells, tissue, and cellular and tissue-based product establishments
			Registration for some products must be submitted electronically using the SPL format, unless FDA grants a waiver.
			
			There are user fees associated with registration and/or listing for some products.

Regulatory Affairs Comparative Matrix of the Regulations Across Product Lines

Premarket Approval Submissions			
	Source	**Forms**	**Premarket Approval (PMA) Submissions**
Devices	21 CFR 814	3514 Premarket Submission Cover Sheet	**PMA Required for:** • Any Class III device that was not on the market prior to 28 May 1976 • Pre-1976 devices after FDA "calls" for PMA
			PMA Sections: • CDRH Submission Cover Sheet/table of contents (optional) • Summary of submission • Indications for use • Device description • Description of intended existing alternative practices and procedures for device • Description of marketing history (foreign) • Summary of nonclinical and clinical data • Discussion of safety and efficacy • Device Master Record • Performance standards • Technical section • Published and unpublished reports on device • Sample of device(s) • Proposed labeling • Environmental assessment • Financial Certification of Disclosure
			PMA Approval Criteria: Substantial evidence of safety and efficacy, which includes adequate and well-controlled investigations User fees apply to original PMAs and certain types of PMA supplements. Small businesses are eligible for reduced or waived fees
			Approval Time Frames: • 45-day administrative review preliminary to "filing" of PMA • Must be reviewed (initially) within 180 days after filing PMA
			Possible Outcomes: • Approval order, approvable letter, not approvable letter, order denying approval • Summary of safety and effectiveness (S&E) written with FDA approval for public dissemination

Drugs	21 CFR 314	356h	**NDA or Abbreviated New Drug Application (ANDA) Required for:**
			• Any new drug:
			  - A new drug is any drug that was not generally recognized as safe and effective before 1938
			• An approved drug may be considered a new drug if
			  - Contains a new substance (active ingredient, excipient, carrier, coating or other component)
			  - New combination of already approved drugs
			  - Proportion of ingredients has been changed
			  - New intended use of drug
			  - Dosage, method or duration of administration or application is changed

			ANDA versus NDA: The ANDA is an abbreviated new drug submission. The ANDA submission does not include preclinical (animal) and clinical (human) data to establish safety and effectiveness.
			NDA or ANDA Sections: • Summary volume • Chemistry, manufacturing and controls • Samples, methods validation and labeling • Nonclinical pharmacology and toxicology • Human pharmacokinetics and bioavailability • Microbiology • Clinical data • Statistical section

Premarket Approval Submissions

	Source	Forms	Premarket Approval (PMA) Submissions
			• Case reports and tabulations • Patent information • Patent certification • Debarment certification • Field copy certification • User fee cover sheet
			Common Technical Document Sections: • Module 1: Regional information (forms, waivers, patent information, etc.) • Module 2: Table of Contents, Introduction, Quality Overall Summary, Nonclinical Overview and Summaries, Clinical Overview and Summary • Module 3: Quality • Module 4: Nonclinical Study Reports • Module 5: Clinical Study Reports (and ISS/ISE for US submissions) User fees are applicable for both NDAs and ANDAs A fee waiver or reduction for: • The first NDA of a small business • Applications for orphan products • Applications for drugs providing a benefit to public health, or applications where the fees constitute a barrier to innovation NDA may be submitted as paper or electronically—electronic preferred Content of label must be submitted electronically in Structured Product Label (SPL) format
			NDA Approval Criteria: Substantial evidence of safety and efficacy, based on adequate and well-controlled investigations

			Approval Time Frames:
			• Within 60 days of receipt, FDA must determine whether an NDA can be filed
			• PDUFA V review goals:
			  - Priority NDA: six months from FDA's filing date (rather than six months from receipt date, as in previous PDUFAs)
			  - Standard NDA: 10 months from FDA's filing date

			Possible Outcomes: • Approval Letter • "Complete Response" letter that states the product is: approvable or not approved • Refusal to file letter • Notification that the application is withdrawn • Summary Basis of Approval (SBA) is available to public
Biologics	21 CFR 601	356h	**BLA:** Similar to NDA, filed for all biologics
	21 CFR 601.2		The following specified categories have modified requirements: • Therapeutic DNA plasmid products • Therapeutic synthetic peptides of 40 or fewer amino acids • Monoclonal antibodies for in vivo use • Therapeutic recombinant DNA-derived products
	21 CFR 601.25		User fees are applicable
			Approval Time Frames: Same as Drugs
			Possible Outcomes: same as Drugs

Regulatory Affairs Comparative Matrix of the Regulations Across Product Lines

Premarket Notification Submission		
	Source	**Premarket Notification Submission**

Devices	21 CFR 807, Subpart (e)	**510(k) Premarket Notification:**
		• Pertaining to Section 510(k) of *Medical Device Amendments* (1976) to *FD&C Act*
		• Preamendment devices on the market prior to 28 May 1976 are grandfathered
		• Required for devices introduced into commercial distribution after 28 May 1976 that have been classified as Class I or Class II devices when the device is:
		  - First introduced into market (not substantially equivalent to predecessor)
		  - Already marketed but introduced for the first time by manufacturer
		  - Already marketed but has a change or modification to the device that could significantly affect safety or effectiveness of the device such as changes in design, material, chemical composition, energy source, manufacturing process
		  - Has new intended use

	21 CFR Parts 862-892	**Exemptions From Premarket Notification:** • Almost all Class I devices, except Restricted Devices • Many Class II devices • Custom devices (devices not commercially available and created for a specific patient, physician or dentist) • Distributors of 510(k)-cleared devices with written permission of the manufacturer or 510(k) holder • Initial postamendment distribution of a pre-1976 Class III device requires a 510(k)—until FDA calls for a PMA; the 510(k) must include Class III certification and summary of safety and effectiveness
		Substantial Equivalence (SE) compares a new device to a legally marketed "predicate" device. **Requirements:** • Same technological characteristics as predicate device or • Different technological characteristics but raises no new or different questions of safety or effectiveness and • Same intended use as predicate device
		510(k) Content/Format CDRH Submission Cover Sheet (Optional): • Trade, common or classification name • Establishment registration number of submitter • Device classification
	www.fda.gov/MedicalDevices/DeviceRegulationandGuidance/GuidanceDocuments/default.htm	**Application Contents:** • Device User Fee Cover Sheet (Form 3601), Certification of Compliance with ClinicalTrials.gov (Form 3674) • Proposed labeling (device description, specifications, intended use, directions for use) • Substantial equivalence information (comparison to predicate device) • Data demonstrating what effect modification or new intended use has on safety and effectiveness • 510(k) summary or statement
		Data Requirements: • The need for performance data depends on complexity of device and ability to demonstrate equivalence to predicate based on use and technological • FDA may require human clinical data in a 510(k) to demonstrate SE for certain higher-risk devices
		***SMDA* Provisions:** • Manufacturer must receive written SE order before commercial distribution • 510(k) must include 510(k) summary or statement • Summaries and statements are made public 30 days after SE notice
		510(k) Review: • Review begins when CDRH logs in the submission • 90-day statutory requirement for FDA review (often exceeded) • Request for additional information puts submission on hold—30 days to respond. If no response, the 510(k) is withdrawn unless an extension is requested. The 90-day clock restarts when FDA receives additional data

Regulatory Affairs Comparative Matrix of the Regulations Across Product Lines

Premarket Notification Submission		
	Source	**Premarket Notification Submission**
		510(k) Paradigm: • Traditional 510(k): standard filing • Special 510(k): option where device modification does not affect its intended use • Abbreviated 510(k): alternative to traditional 510(k) where a guidance document exists that provides reasonable assurance that the device's safety and effectiveness have been established
		Possible Outcomes: • SE, NSE, request additional information, withhold decision until financial disclosure statement is submitted, advise the 510(k) is not required • SE determination implies "clearance" to market device, not "approval" to market device
Drugs		No comparable mechanism
Biologics		**510(k):** some products regulated by CBER are by definition "medical devices."
		Appropriate biologic "devices" are submitted as 510(k)s to CBER.
		See Devices for procedure

Regulatory Affairs Professionals Society

Regulatory Affairs Comparative Matrix of the Regulations Across Product Lines

Reporting/Recordkeeping Requirements for PMA, NDA or BLA Submissions and Application Maintenance and Changes

	Source	Forms	Reporting/Recordkeeping Requirements

Devices	21 CFR 814		• *PMA Amendment* adds information or modifies a pending application:
			  - Resets 180-day "clock" for a major addition or change; and
			  - Includes additional voluntary information or additional information requested by FDA
			• *PMA Supplement* is used for changes or modifications to a PMA approved device:
			  - Normal 180-day review cycle
			• *Special PMA Supplement—Changes Being Effected*
			Limited supplement changes can be made once FDA has acknowledged the submission is being processed
			• *Alternate PMA Supplement (30-day):*
			FDA will have indicated that the alternate submission would be permitted (if information is insufficient, FDA will instruct the applicant what is needed and the supplement will become a 135-day supplement)
			• *Periodic Reports* are updates or changes post-approval, which do not affect S&E; submitted after approval letter, in annual report or as by FDA

Drugs	21 CFR 314.60
	
	21 CFR 314.70
		356h	• *NDA Amendment* adds information or modifies a pending application
			  - Extension of up to 180-day review clock for a major amendment
			  - Minor amendments do not extend the review time
			• NDA Supplements submit changes to an approved NDA
			• Manufacturing supplements/changes are submitted as:
			  - Changes requiring prior approval
			  - Changes Being Effected (CBE)
			  - Supplements (may be made before FDA approval) or
			  - Changes via Annual Report (minor changes)

	21 CFR 314.50 (d)(5)(vi)(b)
	
	21 CFR 314.80
	
	21 CFR 314.81
	
	21 CFR 314.80 (c)(2)
		3500A
		
		2252
			Reporting:
			• 120-day Safety Report Amendment: Due 120 days after NDA filing
			• Postmarketing 15-day Alert Report: (15 calendar days) for serious and unexpected adverse event
			• NDA Annual Report:
			  - Due within 60 days of anniversary of date of approval;
			  - Includes distribution data, labeling, CMC changes, nonclinical data and clinical data
			• NDA Field Alert: Three working days for failed batches, mistaken identification, contamination, etc.
			• Periodic Adverse Drug Experience Reports: Quarterly for three years after approval and then annually

Biologics			Same as Drugs • Amendment: Submission of additional information to an unapproved license application • Supplement: Submission of changes to an approved license application • Manufacturing Supplement: Same as drugs • Biologics Deviation Report
	21 CFR 600.80	3500A VAERS-1 – for vaccines	**Reporting:** • 15-day Alert Report (15 calendar days) for serious and unexpected adverse events • BLA/NDA Annual Reports
			• Periodic Adverse Experience/Event Reports: Quarterly for three years after approval and then annually
			• Distribution Reports: Quantity of product distributed in US; due every six months

Requirements and Submissions for Clinical Investigations

	Source	Forms	Requirements and Submissions for Clinical Investigations
Devices	21 CFR 812 21 CFR 50 21 CFR 56	3674—ClinicalTrials.gov Data Bank 3514—CDRH Premarket Review Submission Cover Sheet	• Investigational Device Exemption (IDE) • Informed Consent • Institutional Review Board (IRB) Review and Approval of Protocol and Informed Consent • Good Clinical Practice (GCP) • An IDE permits a device to be shipped in Interstate commerce for clinical investigations to determine its safety and effectiveness. The IDE regulation exempts the device from: - Misbranding and adulteration - Establishment registration and device listing - 510(k)/PMA - Performance standards - Banned devices - Restricted devices - QSRs/GMPs (except for 820.30 requirements) - Records and reports All clinical investigations of devices to determine safety and effectiveness require an approved IDE (from IRB, or IRB and FDA, depending upon risk).
	21 CFR 812.2(b)		**IDE Time Frame:** FDA will review and approve, approve with modification, or disapprove an IDE application within 30 days of receipt. Requirements vary based on risk level. The determination of significant risk versus nonsignificant risk is made by the sponsor and approved by the IRB, but may be decided by FDA.
			Nonsignificant Risk Device Studies Require: • An abbreviated IDE • IRB approval (IDE submission to FDA is not required) • Labeling: "CAUTION-Investigational Device. Limited by Federal (or US) Law to Investigational Use" • For IVDs: "For Investigational Use Only. The performance characteristics of this product have not been established."
	21 CFR 812.2(a)		**Significant Risk Device Studies Require:** • All of the requirements above for nonsignificant risk devices • IDE application and approval from FDA • Final report to FDA and IRB
	21 CFR 812.2(c)		**Exempted Investigations:** • IVDs if for laboratory research or if for human patients, provided a legally marketed IVD is used for confirmation • Custom devices • Devices shipped for animal research • Consumer preference testing if not for determining safety or efficacy • Devices intended for veterinary use only
	21 CFR 812.40-46 21 CFR 54.4		**Sponsor Responsibilities:** • Select qualified investigators • Control distribution of devices • Monitor studies • Ensure that investigator receives IRB approval • Submit IDE to FDA (if required) • Ensure that any IRB and FDA are promptly informed of significant new investigation information
	21 CFR 812.60-66 and 21 CFR 56 21 CFR 812.100		**IRB Responsibilities:** • Review and approve studies • Review and approval of informed consent • Protect the safety and welfare of subjects • Determine if the device is either significant or nonsignificant risk
	21 CFR 812.110 21 CFR 54.4		**Investigator Responsibilities:** • Get IRB approval before study • Conduct study per agreement • Follow protocol and FDA regulations • Control and supervise device use • Obtain informed consent

Regulatory Affairs Comparative Matrix of the Regulations Across Product Lines

Requirements and Submissions for Clinical Investigations			
	Source	**Forms**	**Requirements and Submissions for Clinical Investigations**
Drugs	21 CFR 312 21 CFR 50 21 CFR 56	1571 3674	• Investigational New Drug Application (IND) • Informed Consent • IRB Review and Approval of Protocol and Informed Consent • Good Clinical Practice (GCP) An IND is submitted to FDA for notification of the intention to conduct clinical studies with a new drug or biologic and to request an exemption for shipping unapproved drug or biologic. Required for new dosage form, new route of administration, new concentrations, new sponsor or manufacturer, or new indication.
	21 CFR 310 21 CFR 320		**IND Types:** • Commercial (routine) • Physician (Sponsor-Investigator) • Treatment • Emergency
			Important IND Sections: • Introductory statement • General investigational plan • Investigator's brochure • Protocol • CMC information • Pharmacology and toxicology • Previous human experience
			IND Time Frame: Effective in 30 days from FDA receipt unless clinical hold is placed on the study.
	21 CFR 312.50–53 and 21 CFR 54.4	1572	**Sponsor Responsibilities:** • Select qualified investigators • Obtain investigator records (including Statement of Investigator Protocol Signature Page, CVs, Financial Disclosure) • Control distribution of drugs • Monitor studies • Ensure that investigator receives IRB approval • Submit IND/Protocol to FDA (if required)
	21 CFR 56.108–110		**IRB Responsibilities:** • Review and approve studies • Review and approval of informed consent • Protect the safety and welfare of subjects • Ensure risk to subjects is minimized
	21 CFR 312.60		**Investigator Responsibilities:** Same as Devices
Biologics	21 CFR 312 21 CFR 50 21 CFR 56	1571 3674	• Investigational New Drug Application (IND) • Informed Consent • IRB Review and Approval of Protocol and Informed Consent • Good Clinical Practice (GCP)
			IND Time Frame: Same as Drugs
			Sponsor Responsibilities: Same as Drugs
			IRB Responsibilities: Same as Drugs
			Investigator Responsibilities: Same as Devices

Reporting/Recordkeeping Requirements for Clinical Investigations

	Source	Forms	Requirements and Submissions for Clinical Investigations

Devices	21 CFR 812.140		**Investigator Records:**
			• Correspondence
			• Device receipt, use, disposition
			• Subject records including
			  - Informed consent
			  - Adverse device effects
			  - Device exposure date and times
			  - Protocol and other records

	21 CFR 812.140		**Sponsor Records:** • NSR/SR decision • Correspondence • Device shipment and disposition • Investigator agreements and financial disclosure • Adverse device effects • Investigator list • IRB list and other records
	21 CFR 812.150		**Investigator Reports:** • Unanticipated Adverse Device Effects (10 working days) • Withdrawal of IRB approval • Progress reports • Deviations from investigational plan • Informed consent • Final report (due to sponsor and IRB within three months of study termination or completion)
	21 CFR 812.150		**Sponsor Reports:** • Unanticipated ADE (10 working days) • Withdrawal of IRB approval • Withdrawal of FDA approval • Current Investigator list • Progress reports • Recall and device disposition • Final report (for SR, notify FDA within 30 working days of the completion or termination and submit final report to FDA and all reviewing IRBs and investigators within 6 months. For NSR final report to all reviewing IRBs within 6 months.) • Significant risk determination
	21 CFR 812.140		**Record Retention:** For two years after the latter of • Date of study completion or termination or • Date that records are no longer needed to support a 510(k), PMA or notice of completion of a PDP

Drugs	21 CFR 312.62		**Investigator Records:**
			• Correspondence
			• Investigational drug receipt, use, disposition
			• Case histories
			  - Informed consent
			  - Source documentation (case report forms and medical records)
			  - Safety reports
			  - Protocol and other records
			  - Laboratory information

	21 CFR 312.57		**Sponsor Records:** • Correspondence • Investigational drug shipment and disposition • Investigator agreements and financial disclosure • Protocol and amendments • Clinical study report and publications • Monitoring and safety reports (serious adverse events) • Investigator list • IRB list and other records • Decoding and randomization records (if applicable)

Regulatory Affairs Comparative Matrix of the Regulations Across Product Lines

Reporting/Recordkeeping Requirements for Clinical Investigations			
	Source	Forms	Requirements and Submissions for Clinical Investigations
	21 CFR 312.64		**Investigator Reports:** • Progress reports (to sponsor and IRB; at least annually) • Safety reports • Final (study closure) report • Financial disclosure reports

	21 CFR 312.31
	
	21 CFR 312.32
	
	21 CFR 312.33
		1571
		3674
		
		1571
		3500A
		
		1571
			Sponsor Reports:
			• IND Amendments
			  - Amendments to an IND, such as new investigator or new information, must be submitted not more than every 30 days.
			• IND Safety Reports
			  - Telephone report—7 calendar days (either by phone or fax)
			    » Unexpected fatal or life-threatening adverse experience (AE) associated with the use of the drug
			  - Written reports—15 calendar days
			    » Serious and unexpected AE associated with the use of the drug
			• IND Annual Reports
			  - Must be submitted within 60 days of the anniversary date of when the IND became effective

	21 CFR 312.57 21 CFR 312.62		**Record Retention:** • Sponsor: two years after NDA approval or, if no application is to be filed or if the application is not approved for such indication, two years after the investigation is discontinued and FDA is notified. • Investigator: same as sponsor
Biologics			**Sponsor and Investigator Records:** Same as Drugs
			Reporting: Same as Drugs
			Record Retention: Same as Drugs

Regulatory Affairs Comparative Matrix of the Regulations Across Product Lines

Labeling Requirements

	Source	Labeling Requirements
Devices	21 CFR 801	**General Requirements:** • Name and place of business • Intended use • Adequate directions (in layman terms) • Prominence of statements • English language (exceptions: product solely distributed in Puerto Rico or territories in which English is not the predominant language)
	21 CFR 809 16 CFR 1500	**IVD Labeling:** • Proprietary and established names • Intended use • Statement of warnings or precautions • Name and place of business of manufacturer, packer or distributor. • Lot or control number • For reagents, storage instructions, ingredients, and quantity of contents • For laboratory phase IVD, not represented as effective, label must include "For Research Use Only" • For products undergoing testing prior to full commercial release, label must include "For Investigational Use Only. The performance characteristics of this product have not been established." • Directions for Use Exemption for general use laboratory reagents where the product is labeled "For Laboratory Use"
	21 CFR 801	**Exemptions from Directions for Use:** • Prescription devices require this statement on the label: "Caution: Federal Law restricts this device to the sale by or on the order of a physician" • Retail exemption (devices delivered to end user by or on order of a physician) • Devices having commonly known directions to the ordinary individual • Devices for processing, repacking, or manufacturing if the label bears the statement: "Caution: For manufacturing, processing or repacking" • In vitro diagnostic products • Devices used in teaching, research, law enforcement (nonclinical use)
	21 CFR 812.5	**IDE Labeling:** • Label must bear prominently name and place of manufacturer • Contents of package • Statement: "Caution: Investigational Device. Limited by Federal (or US) Law to Investigational Use" • No representation that device is safe and effective for its investigational use
	21 CFR 820, Subpart K	**QSR/GMP Labeling Requirements:** • Label integrity (maintain legibility) • Separation of operations • Label inspections (for accuracy) and release • Storage (prevent mix-ups)
Drugs	21 CFR 201–202 21 CFR 208	**General Requirements:** • Label must bear prominently name and place of manufacturer, packer or distributor • Identify the quantity and dosage • National Drug Code requested to appear on all drug labels and labeling • Adequate directions for lay persons to use • No misleading statements misrepresenting drug • Statement of all ingredients with accurate names and proportions • Claims must be supported with clinical data • Label must state "Rx Only" for approved prescription drugs • Drugs scheduled by DEA must bear classification on label • English language (exceptions: product solely distributed in Puerto Rico or territories in which English is not the predominant language)

Regulatory Affairs Comparative Matrix of the Regulations Across Product Lines

Labeling Requirements

	Source	Labeling Requirements
	21 CFR 201.100	**Exemptions From Directions for Use:** • In the possession of a person regularly and lawfully engaged in the manufacture, transportation, storage or wholesale distribution of prescription drugs • In the possession of a retail, hospital or clinic pharmacy, or public health agency, that is regularly and lawfully engaged in dispensing prescription drugs • In the possession of a practitioner licensed by law to administer or prescribe such drugs • New drugs under IND exemption • Drugs having commonly known directions • Inactive ingredients • Prescription chemicals and other prescription components (label must include "For prescription compounding") • Drugs for processing, repacking or manufacturing if the label bears the statement: "Caution: For manufacturing, processing or repacking" • Drugs used in teaching, research, law enforcement (nonclinical use)
	21 CFR 312.26	**IND Labeling:** Immediate package of Investigational Drug must have label "Caution—New drug limited by Federal (or US) law to Investigational Use"
	21 CFR 211, Subpart G	**GMP Label Requirements:** • Label integrity (meets specifications) • Storage (prevent label mix-ups; limited access to labels) • Separation of operations (between drug products or dosage forms) • Labeling materials (inspection) • Gang printing of labels for different drug products is prohibited • Area Inspections (prior to labeling operation) • Reconciliation of labels issued and labels used • Destruction of Labels (after batch and lot are complete or obsolete/outdated)
Biologics	21 CFR 600, 606, 610 21 CFR 208	**General Requirements:** • Proper name of the product • Name, address and license of manufacturer or distributor • Lot number and other lot identification (including expiration date and recommended individual dose) • Adequate directions for lay persons to use (Medication Guide) • Statement of all ingredients with accurate names and proportions • Label must state "Rx only" for approved prescription biologics Additional information and precautionary measures are required of labels for biologics, depending on the product.
	21 CFR 211, Subpart G	**GMP Label Requirements:** Same as Drugs

Regulatory Affairs Comparative Matrix of the Regulations Across Product Lines

Promotion and Advertising			
	Source	**Form**	**Promotion and Advertising**
Devices	*FTC Act* Section 5, 15 US Code 45		**Advertising Regulated by Federal Trade Commission (FTC):** FTC covers nonrestricted device advertising and requires • Claim substantiation and • Ads that are fair and not misleading FDA covers restricted medical devices FDA can deem the device misbranded if advertising promotes an intended use that is inconsistent with or not included in the device labeling.
	21 CFR 820.120		**PMA:** • Labeling approved in PMA • Restricted medical devices must bear the statement "Caution: Federal law restricts this device to sale, distribution, and use by or on the order of a (indicate type of practitioner and, if applicable, required training/experience, and facilities to which the use is restricted)." • "Full disclosure" in ads (warnings, cautions, adverse effects, etc.)
Drugs	21 CFR 202		**Advertising Regulated by:** • Rx Drugs: CDER's Office of Prescription Drug Promotion (OPDP) • OTC Drugs: FTC Noncompliance with the advertising regulations causes the drug to be "misbranded"
	21 CFR 314.81 21 CFR 314.550	2253	**NDA:** • All advertising and promotional labeling must be filed to the NDA at the time of initial dissemination/publication. • For drugs approved for serious and life-threatening diseases under accelerated approval launch materials are reviewed by FDA prior to dissemination; after 120 days following market approval, promotional material must be submitted at least 30 days prior to dissemination. • Changes in labeling are reported in the Annual Report to an approved NDA or a supplemental NDA.
			Rx Drug Advertising: • Cannot make safety or efficacy claims before product approval • Can promote that a new product is coming unless product carries a boxed warning • Cannot promote use of a product for an indication not in the labeling • Promotional items cannot suggest off-label uses • Cannot be false, misleading or lacking in fair balance • Product comparisons must be supported by substantial clinical experience • Advertising must include a brief summary of side effects, contraindications and effectiveness • Promotional labeling must include a copy of the instructions for use. • Reminder advertisements are exempt from the brief summary requirement.
Biologics	21 CFR 601.45	2253 2567	Advertising Regulated by CBER's Advertising and Promotional Labeling Branch (APLB)
	21 CFR 601.12		**BLA:** Same as Drugs
			Biologics Advertising: • Concurrent notification rather than preapproval required. Exception: products under Accelerated Approval.

Regulatory Affairs Comparative Matrix of the Regulations Across Product Lines

Postmarketing Adverse Experience/Event and Medical Device Reporting

	Source	Form	Postmarketing Adverse Experience/Event and Medical Device Reporting
Devices	21 CFR 803	3500A	**MDR Reportable Event:** • Information that reasonably suggests that a device may have caused or contributed to a death or serious injury, or • A malfunction has occurred that would be likely to cause or contribute to a death or serious injury if the malfunction recurred
	21 CFR 803.50-803.56	3500A	**Manufacturers and Initial Distributors Must Report Within:** • Five work days of an event that requires remedial action to prevent unreasonable risk of substantial harm to public health or after becoming aware of a reportable event for which FDA has made a written request, or • 30 calendar days after the manufacturer becomes aware of a reportable event
	21 CFR 803.30-803.33	3500A 3419	**User Facility Reporting:** • Report death to FDA and manufacturer within 10 work days • Report serious injury to manufacturer only or to FDA if manufacturer is unknown within 10 work days, and • Report annually to FDA the total number of deaths and serious injuries
			Domestic Distributor Requirements: Recordkeeping only
Drugs	21 CFR 314.80		**Serious Adverse Drug Experience (SADE):** Any adverse drug experience occurring at any dose that results any of the following outcomes: • Causes death • Threatens life • Requires or prolongs existing hospitalization • Causes persistent or significant disability or incapacity • Induces congenital anomaly/birth defect • Important medical event
			Adverse Drug Experience (ADE): Any adverse event associated with the use of a drug, whether or not drug-related including: • Use of drug in professional practice • Drug overdose • Drug abuse or withdrawal • Failure of expected pharmacological action

		3500A
		
		356h
		356h
			Postmarketing 15-day Alert Reports
			• Needs to be filed for ADE that is:
			  - Both serious and unexpected (not in labeling)
			  - Foreign or domestic
			  - No later than 15 calendar days after initial notification
			• Sources of ADE/SADE
			  - Manufacturer
			  - Healthcare professional
			  - Consumer
			  - Distributor
			  - Foreign use
			  - Literature
			  - User facility
			• Periodic Reports: quarterly for the first three years after approval. Reports to be submitted within 30 days of the close of the reporting period.
			• Annual Reports thereafter, with the reports to be submitted within 60 days of the anniversary of the issuance of the product approval.

Biologics	21 CFR 314.80, 600.80		**Adverse Experience (AE):** AE reporting is any event associated with the use of a biological product in humans, whether or not it is considered product-related including: • Use of the biological product in professional practice • Biological product overdose • Biological product abuse or withdrawal • Failure of expected pharmacological action
			Serious Adverse Drug Experience: Same as Drugs
		3500A VAERS-1	**Postmarketing 15-day Alert Reports:** Same as Drugs • Reporting requirements are the same as for drugs except that vaccine AEs are reported on Vaccine Adverse Event Reporting System (VAERS) form.

Regulatory Affairs Comparative Matrix of the Regulations Across Product Lines

Good Manufacturing Practice (GMP)/ Quality System Regulation (QSR)		
	Source	**GMP**

Devices	21 CFR 820	**Quality System Regulation (QSR):**
		QSR aligns US requirements with international quality standards (ISO 13485), including management responsibility and review, design controls, purchasing controls, process validation, service record keeping and review, corrective and preventative action, and statistical techniques. Eliminates the distinction for critical devices.
		Subparts:
		  A. General Provisions (scope, definitions, quality system)
		  B. Quality System Requirements (management responsibility, quality audit, personnel including consultants)
		  C. Design Controls
		  D. Document Controls
		  E. Purchasing Controls
		  F. Identification and Traceability
		  G. Production and Process Controls (production and process controls; inspection, measuring and test equipment; process validation)
		  H. Acceptance Activities (receiving, in-process and finished device acceptance, acceptance status)
		  I. Nonconforming Product
		  J. Corrective and Preventive Action
		  K. Labeling and Packaging Control (device labeling, device packaging)
		  L. Handling, Storage, Distribution and Installation
		  M. Records (general requirements, Device Master Record, Device History Record, Quality System Record, complaint files)
		  N. Servicing
		  O. Statistical Techniques
		Failure to comply renders the device adulterated

Drugs	21 CFR 210–211	**Current GMP for Finished Pharmaceuticals:**
		  A. General Provisions (scope, definitions)
		  B. Organization and Personnel (responsibilities of quality control unit, personnel qualifications, personnel responsibilities, consultants)
		  C. Buildings and Facilities (design, construction, lighting, air filtration, HVAC, plumbing, sewage and refuse, washing and toilet facilities, sanitation, maintenance)
		  D. Equipment (design, size, location, construction, cleaning and maintenance, automatic, mechanical, and electronic equipment, filters)
		  E. Control of Components and Drug Product Containers and Closures (receipt and storage; testing and approval/rejection; use of approved components, containers, and closures; retesting rejected components, containers, and closures)
		  F. Production and Process Controls (written procedures, deviations, charge-in of components, yield calculation, equipment identification, sampling and testing of in-process materials and products, time limitations on production, control of microbiological contamination, reprocessing)
		  G. Packaging and Labeling Control (materials examination and usage criteria, labeling issuance, packaging and labeling operations, tamper-resistant packaging, drug product inspection, expiration dating)
		  H. Holding and Distribution (warehousing procedures, distribution procedures)
		  I. Laboratory Controls (general requirements, testing and release for distribution, stability testing, special testing requirements, reserve samples, laboratory animals, penicillin contamination)
		  J. Records and Reports (general requirements, equipment cleaning and use log, component and drug product container, closure and labeling records, master production and control records, batch production and control records, production record review, laboratory records, distribution records, complaint files)
		  K. Returned and Salvaged Drug Products

Biologics	21 CFR 210–211	**Same as Drugs Plus Additional Requirements:**

	21 CFR 600, 606, and 610	**Biological Products—Subparts:**
		  A. General Provisions (definitions)
		  B. Establishment Standards (personnel, physical establishment, equipment, animals and care, records, retention samples, reporting of product deviations, temperatures during shipment)
		  C. Establishment Inspections (inspectors, time of inspection, duties of inspector)
		  D. Reporting of Adverse Experiences (postmarket reporting of adverse experiences, distribution reports, waivers)

Regulatory Affairs Comparative Matrix of the Regulations Across Product Lines

Good Manufacturing Practice (GMP)/ Quality System Regulation (QSR)

Source	GMP
21 CFR 610	**General Biological Products Standards—Subparts:** A. Release Requirements (Tests prior to release required for each lot. Requests for samples and protocol, official release.) B. General Provisions (equivalent methods and processes, potency, general safety, sterility, purity, identity, constituent materials, total solids in serums, permissible combinations, cultures) C. Standard Preparations and Limits of Potency D. Mycoplasma (test for mycoplasma) E. Testing Requirements for Communicable Disease Agents (test requirements, donor deferral, restrictions on use for further manufacture of medical devices, use of reference standards by makers of test kits, HIV and HCV "lookback" requirements) F. Dating Period Limitations (date of manufacture, dating periods for licensed biologics) G. Labeling Standards (container label, package label, proper name, legible type, divided manufacturing responsibility to be shown, name of selling agent or distributor, products for export, bar code label requirements)
21 CFR 606	**Current GMP for Blood and Blood Components—Subparts:** A. General Provisions (definitions) B. Organization and Personnel C. Plant and Facilities D. Equipment (equipment, supplies and reagents) E. Reserved F. Production and Process Controls (standard operating procedures, plateletpheresis, leukapheresis, plasmapheresis) G. Additional Labeling Standards for Blood and Blood Components (labeling, general requirements, container label, instruction circular) H. Laboratory Controls (laboratory controls and compatibility testing) I. Records and Reports (records, distribution and receipt, procedures and records, adverse reaction file, reporting of product deviations)

Complaint Files

	Source	Complaint Files
Devices	21 CFR 820.198	**Written Procedures Required for:** • Receiving, reviewing and evaluating complaints by a formally designated unit • Processing all complaints uniformly in a timely manner • Documenting oral complaints upon receipt • Evaluating complaints to determine whether an MDR reportable event has occurred • Reviewing and investigating device service reports that identify a reportable MDR event immediately

		Requirements:
		• The written record shall include the following information, if known
		  - Name of the device
		  - Date complaint was received
		  - Any device identification and control numbers
		  - Name, address and phone number of complainant
		  - Nature and details of complaint
		  - Date and results of investigation
		  - Any corrective action taken
		  - Reply to complainant
		  - Complaints that are MDRs must be clearly identified

	21 CFR 820.180	**Complaint Retention:** All records shall be retained for a period of time equivalent to the design and expected life of the device, but in no case less than two years from the date of release for commercial distribution by the manufacturer. Complaint file must be available during GMP inspection
Drugs	21 CFR 211.198	**Written Procedures Required for:** • Handling both written and oral complaints • Review to determine whether the complaint represents a serious and unexpected adverse drug experience.

		Requirements:
		• The written record shall include the following information, if known
		  - Name and strength of the drug product
		  - Lot number
		  - Name of complainant
		  - Nature of complaint
		  - Reply to complainant
		  - Finding of an investigation or reason an investigation was not necessary

		Complaint Retention: • Written records involving a drug product shall be maintained until at least one year after the expiration date of the drug product, or one year after the date that the complaint was received, whichever is longer. Complaint file must be available during an FDA GMP inspection
Biologics		Same as Drugs

Regulatory Affairs Comparative Matrix of the Regulations Across Product Lines

FDA Inspections

	Source	Form	FDA Inspections
Devices	*FD&C Act* Section 704 21 CFR 814.44–45		**FDA May Inspect All Companies That Manufacture, Process, Pack or Hold FDA-Regulated Products Including:** • Domestic manufacturing companies Contract testing laboratories • Clinical study sponsors, monitors and investigator sites • IRBs • Contract Research Organizations (CROs) • Foreign companies
			Types of Inspections (routine or for cause): • GMP/QSR Compliance (routine surveillance, establishment license, or pre-approval) • GLP Compliance • GCP Compliance (Sponsor or investigational site)
			FDA May Not Inspect: • Sales or pricing data • Retail or hospital pharmacies regulated by state law • Financial data • Personnel files (other than qualifications) • Internal audit files
		482	**Present Credentials** **Notice of Inspection**
		483	**Inspectional Observations**
		484	**Receipt for Samples**
			Establishment Inspection Report
Drugs	*FD&C Act* Section 704		**Same as Devices**
Biologics	*PHS Act* Section 262 21 CFR 600.20		**Same as Devices**

Lot and Batch Release Requirements		
	Source	**Lot and Batch Release Requirements**
Devices	21 CFR 820.80	Review and sign-off, with date, of finished device acceptance by a designated individual. Sterile devices require review of sterility test results before release
Drugs	21 CFR 211.165	Lot must comply with release specifications in compendia or as negotiated and approved by FDA during the application review and approval process.
Biologics	21 CFR 610.1	Same as Drugs. If product is subject to lot release (e.g., vaccines), lots cannot be distributed until they are released by CBER, which reviews samples and protocols.

Regulatory Affairs Comparative Matrix of the Regulations Across Product Lines

Traceability Requirements		
	Source	**Traceability Requirements**
Devices	21 CFR 820.65 21 CFR 821	Traceability required for devices intended for surgical implant or a device to support or sustain life whose failure to perform when properly used in accordance with the instructions for use provided in the labeling can be reasonably expected to result in a significant injury. Procedures, documented in the Device History Record, established to identify unit, lot or batch of finished devices and, where appropriate, key components with a control number that facilitates corrective action. In addition to traceability requirement, FDA has identified specific devices that require tracking, as specified in 21 CFR 821.1(a): the failure of the device would be reasonably likely to have serious adverse health consequences; or the device is intended to be implanted in the human body for more than 1 year; or the device is a life-sustaining or life-supporting device used outside a device user facility.
Drugs	21 CFR 211, Subpart J	All manufacturing records and QC test results, forward and backward traceability from raw materials to finished product
Biologics	21 CFR 211, Subpart J 21 CFR 600.12 21 CFR 606.160 21 CFR 1271.290	Same as Drugs Tracking of blood-derived products from collection through processing, storage and distribution Tracking of human cells, tissues, and cellular and tissue-based products requires establishing and maintaining a system to track all HCT/Ps from: (i) The donor to the consignee or final disposition; and (ii) The consignee or final disposition to the donor.

Regulatory Affairs Comparative Matrix of the Regulations Across Product Lines

Retention of Product Samples		
	Source	**Retention of Product Samples**
Devices	21 CFR 58	No requirement for devices except where required by specific company procedures or GLP
Drugs	21 CFR 211.170	**Active Ingredient:** • Reserve sample consists of at least twice the quantity necessary for all tests required (except sterility and pyrogen testing) • Retention time depends upon the active ingredient; in general, one reserve sample from each lot shall be retained for one year after expiration date of the last lot of the drug product containing it
		Radioactive Active Ingredient: • Three months after the last lot if expiration is less than 30 days or • Six months after the last lot if expiration if more than 30 days • OTC drugs that are exempt from bearing an expiration date should be retained three years after distribution of the last lot
		The reserve sample of each lot of drug product must be stored under the same conditions as the label indicates and must be visually examined once per year
Biologics	21 CFR 600.13	• At least six months after the expiration date unless a different time period is specified in additional standards • Stored at temperatures and conditions to maintain identity and integrity • The quantity must be sufficient for examination and testing of potency • At least one final container as a final package

Regulatory Affairs Comparative Matrix of the Regulations Across Product Lines

Import and Export Requirements			
	Source	**Form**	**Import and Export Requirements**
Devices	FDERA		**Import for Domestic Distribution:** Foreign establishments must meet applicable US medical device regulations, including establishment registration, device listing, QSR manufacturing, MDs and 510(k) or PMA, if applicable. Foreign manufacturers also must designate a US Agent who: assists FDA communicating with the foreign establishment, responds to questions about the foreign establishment's devices imported to the US assists FDA in scheduling inspections of the foreign establishment if FDA unable to contact the foreign establishment directly or expeditiously, FDA may provide documents to the US agent An initial importer must register its establishment with FDA, follow MDRs, corrections and removals and tracking, if applicable.
	FD&C Act Sections 801–802		**Export:** Devices that are legally marketed in the US may be exported to anywhere in the world without prior FDA notification or approval. All devices not cleared for marketing in US must: • Meet the specifications of the purchaser • Not conflict with laws of the importing country • Be labeled for export only • Not be sold in domestic commerce • May require Certificate of Exportability (COE) or Certificate of Foreign Government (CFG) Class III devices with no PMA require FDA approval to export Alternative (Section 802) for Class III devices with no PMA does not require FDA approval to export; only require "simple notification"—with restrictions
Drugs	21 CFR 312.110 21 CFR 314.410		**Import for Domestic Distribution:** • Imports comply with requirements if subject to IND • In US, the sponsor, a qualified investigator or a domestic agent of foreign sponsor, can be consignee • New drug may be imported if it is the subject of an approved application • Foreign manufacturers of drug substances and drug products that wish to import products must have a US agent and are required to register with FDA.
	FDERA		**Export of Investigational Drug:** • Exports can be done under IND but not required • Each person who received drug should be an investigator named in application
			Export of Approved Drug: • New drug may be exported if it is the subject of an approved application • Exporter must be listed as supplier in approved application, and the drug substance intended for export meets the specifications of—and is shipped with—a copy of the labeling required for the approved drug product
Biologics	FDERA		Same as Drugs

FDA Enforcement Options

	Source	Form	FDA Enforcement Options
Devices	*FD&C Act* Sections 301–304 21 CFR 812.119 *Safe Medical Devices Act* of 1990	483	• Withdrawal of product approval • Criminal actions against investigator • Disqualified investigator • Inspections • Warning Letters • Adverse publicity • Recalls (mandatory and voluntary) • Alert List • Import alert • Civil penalties • Application Integrity Policy (AIP) investigation and enforcement (third-party review of data) • Injunctions, seizures, criminal actions • Request to state agencies to take action
Drugs	*FD&C Act* Sections 301–304 *Generic Drug Enforcement Act*	483	Same as Devices, also: • Debarment of individuals or corporations • Dear Doctor letter
Biologics	*FD&C Act* Sections 301–304	483	Same as Devices and Drugs

Regulatory Affairs Comparative Matrix of the Regulations Across Product Lines

Field Corrections and Recalls

	Source	Field Corrections and Recalls
Devices	21 CFR 7 21 CFR 806 21 CFR 810	Enforcement/Recall Policy Medical Device Corrections and Removals Medical Device Recall Authority
	21 CFR 806	**Recall:** Recall Classification: Class I, II or III (assigned by FDA) Device recalls may be either voluntary (firm initiated or at FDA request) or mandatory by FDA order Mandatory reports of corrections/removals required for any firm-initiated removal/correction conducted to: • Reduce risk to health posed by a device or • Remedy a violation of the *FD&C Act* caused by a device, which may present risk to health Written report required within 10 working days of removal/correction
	21 CFR 810	**Mandatory Medical Device Recall:** Cease Distribution and Notification order is issued by FDA if the agency finds a reasonable probability that a distributed device would cause serious adverse health consequences or death. The order requires a manufacturer to • Cease distribution • Notify healthcare professionals and user facilities • Instruct professionals and user facilities to cease use of the device If after a chance for hearing and further review, FDA determines that devices in distribution pose a risk, the agency may amend the order and require a recall.
		Recall Strategy Elements Must Include: • Depth of recall • Public warning • Effectiveness checks
Drugs	21 CFR 7 21 CFR 314.81	**Same as Devices Except:** NDA Field Alert: Within three working days, a field alert must be sent to FDA district office for distributed product that has contamination, change, deterioration or labeling causing mistaken identity. Recalls are voluntary and may be firm-initiated or requested by FDA. "FDA-requested" recall must begin immediately. For firm-initiated recall, notify district office, and it will assign the recall to a class.
Biologics	21 CFR 7 21 CFR 600.14	**Same as Drugs Except:** Biologic Product Deviation Report: Filed within 45 calendar days concerning any event, and information relevant to the event, associated with the manufacturing, to include testing, processing, packing, labeling or storage, or with the holding or distribution, of a licensed biological product, if that event meets all the following criteria: (1) Either: (i) Represents a deviation from current good manufacturing practice, applicable regulations, applicable standards, or established specifications that may affect the safety, purity, or potency of that product; or (ii) Represents an unexpected or unforeseeable event that may affect the safety, purity, or potency of that product; and (2) Occurs in your facility or another facility under contract with you; and (3) Involves a distributed biological product.

Regulatory Affairs Comparative Matrix of the Regulations Across Product Lines

Corrective and Preventive Action Requirements

	Source	Corrective and Preventive Action Requirements
Devices	21 CFR 820.100	Requires manufacturers to establish procedures for: • Analyzing processes, operations, audit reports, quality and service records, complaints, returned devices and other information to identify existing potential causes of nonconforming product • Investigating the cause of nonconformities • Identifying the corrective and preventive action needed to prevent recurrence of nonconforming product • Verifying and validating that the corrective and preventive action is effective • Implementing changes in methods and procedures needed to effect the corrective and preventive action • Ensuring that information related to nonconforming product and corrective and preventive action is disseminated to persons responsible for ensuring quality and preventing such problems • Submitting relevant information for management review
Drugs	21 CFR 211.22 *Guidance for Industry: Quality Systems Approach to Pharmaceutical CGMP Regulations*	Same as Devices Quality control unit approves or rejects all components and drug products and investigates errors or out-of-specification lots.
Biologics		Same as Drugs

Regulatory Affairs Professionals Society

Regulatory Affairs Comparative Matrix of the Regulations Across Product Lines

Misbranding		
	Source	**Misbranding**
Devices	*FD&C Act 501-502*	**Failure to:** • File a 510(k) • Provide information as required • Have advertisements approved by FDA if required • List device • Register establishment • Comply with notification or recall order or • Comply with postmarket surveillance order
	FD&C Act Section 518	**Misbranding:** • False or misleading labeling including advertising and promotional materials • Label does not contain manufacturer's name and address in required prominence • Label does not contain quantity of contents • Required wording is not prominently displayed • Label does not contain adequate directions for use • Device is dangerous to health when used as prescribed • Product does not comply with color additive provision of Act • Device does not adhere to performance standard if applicable • Failure to comply (notification, reporting, record keeping) • Impression of official approval, based on registration and clearance of 510(k)
Drugs	*FD&C Act 501-502* 21 CFR 201	**Misbranding** • Labeling is false or misleading • Packaged form does not bear name of manufacturer, packer or distributor • Required information does not appear or is not prominently placed • Habit-forming substance does not bear habit-forming warning • Generic established name is less than one half the size of the trade/brand name • Not listed in official compendium • Packaging is misleading • Subject to deterioration without precautions • Labeling does not bear adequate directions for use • Drug is dangerous to health when used as suggested in the accompanying labeling • Antibiotic certificate of release, if required, was not issued • False or misleading advertisements or descriptive printed materials • Manufacturer not registered or drug not listed • Packaging or labeling does not comply with the *Poison Prevention Packaging Act* • Container is misleading
Biologics		Same as Drugs

Adulteration

	Source	Adulteration

Devices	*FD&C Act* Section 501(a)–(d)	• Not manufactured under GMPs
		• Contaminated and defective product
		• Class III device for which PMA:
		  - is not filed
		  - is not approved or
		  - has been suspended or withdrawn
		• Marketed Class III device without a PMA before FDA down-classified the device as Class I or II
		• Banned device
		• Strength, purity or quality fall below what they are represented to be
		• Not in conformance with a performance standard.
		• Contains unsafe color additives
		• Failure to comply with approved IDE requirements

Drugs	*FD&C Act* Section 501(a)–(d)	**If the Drug:** • Consists of filthy, putrid or decomposed substance • Has been prepared, packed or held under unsanitary conditions • Methods used in, or facilities or controls used for its manufacture do not conform to GMPs or • Strength differs from or purity is less than stated in the labeling • Mixture with or substitution of another substance
Biologics		Same as Drugs

Regulatory Affairs Comparative Matrix of the Regulations Across Product Lines

Glossary

30-day hold
Time period between filing a protocol under an IND and FDA approval to proceed with enrollment. Also, the time period between when a company submits an IND and when it can initiate a protocol. This timeline may be extended if FDA does not agree with the proposed protocol. (See "Clinical Hold.")

120-day Safety Report
Amendment to an NDA containing a safety update due 120 days after the NDA is filed.

180-day Exclusivity
Protects an ANDA applicant from competition from subsequent generic versions of the same drug product for 180 days.

505(b)(2) Application
An application submitted under section 505(b)(2) of the *FD&C Act* for a drug for which one or more of the investigations relied on by the applicant for approval of the "application were not conducted by or for the applicant and for which the applicant has not obtained a right of reference or use from the person by or for whom the investigations were conducted" (21 U.S.C. 355(b)(2)).

510(k)
- Traditional 510(k): A premarket notification submitted to FDA to demonstrate that the medical device to be marketed is as safe and effective or "substantially equivalent" to a legally marketed device. 510(k) refers to the section of the *FD&C Act* authorizing the submission of the premarket notification.
- Special 510(k): For use where device modifications neither affect the intended use nor alter its fundamental scientific technology. FDA processing time is 30 days.
- Abbreviated 510(k): A type of 510(k) submission that is supported by conformance with guidance document(s), special controls or standards.

515 Program Initiative
Created to facilitate reclassification action on the remaining pre-amendments Class III 510(k)s.

A

AABB
American Association of Blood Banks

Accelerated Approval
Allows earlier approval of drugs to treat serious diseases and those that fill an unmet medical need based on a surrogate endpoint.

Accredited Persons Program
FDA program that accredits third parties to conduct the primary review of 510(k)s for eligible devices.

ACE
Adverse Clinical Event

ACRP
Association for Clinical Research Professionals

Glossary

Action Letter
Official communication from FDA informing an NDA or BLA sponsor of an agency decision; includes approvable, not approvable and clinical hold.

Active Ingredient
Any drug component intended to furnish pharmacological activity or other direct effect in the diagnosis, cure, mitigation, treatment or prevention of disease, or to affect the structure or any function of the body of man or other animals.

ADE
Adverse Drug Event or Adverse Drug Experience

ADME
Absorption, Distribution, Metabolism and Excretion

ADR
Adverse Drug Reaction

ADUFA
Animal Drug User Fee Act of 2003

ADUFA II
Animal Drug User Fee Amendments of 2008

Adulterated
Product containing any filthy, putrid or decomposed substance; or prepared under unsanitary conditions; or not made according to GMPs; or containing an unsafe color additive; or does not meet the requirements of an official compendium. (*FD&C Act*, SEC. 501 [351])

AdvaMed
Advanced Medical Technology Association

Advisory Committee
Committees and panels used by FDA to obtain independent expert advice on scientific, technical and policy matters.

AE
Adverse Event

AERS
See FAERS.

AFDO
Association of Food and Drug Officials

AGDUFA
Animal Generic Drug User Fee Act of 2008

AHRQ
Agency for Healthcare Research and Quality

AIA
America Invents Act of 2011

AIP
Application Integrity Policy. FDA's approach to reviewing applications that may be affected by wrongful acts that raise significant questions regarding data reliability.

AMDUCA
Animal Medicinal Drug Use Clarification Act of 1994

Amendment
Additions or changes to an ANDA, NDA, BLA, PMA or PMA supplement still under review. Includes safety updates. Any updates to an IND or an IDE prior to approval are also called amendments.

AMS
Agricultural Marketing Service (USDA)

ANADA
Abbreviated New Animal Drug Application

ANDA
Abbreviated New Drug Application. Used for generic drugs.

Animal Drugs@FDA
Database that allows users to search for approved animal drug products, suitability petitions, sponsors, the *Green Book*, CFR, *FR*, patents and exclusivity.

Animal Rule
Provides for approval of certain new drug and biological products based on animal data when adequate and well-controlled efficacy studies in humans cannot be ethically conducted because the studies would involve administering a potentially lethal or permanently disabling toxic substance or organism to healthy human
volunteers and field trials are not feasible prior to approval.

Anti-Kickback Statute
Prohibits offering, paying, soliciting or receiving anything of value to induce or reward referrals or generate federal healthcare program business.

Annual Report
An annual periodic report or progress report that must be submitted to FDA. Depending on the type of application for which the report is submitted, it may include new safety, efficacy and labeling information; preclinical and clinical investigation summaries; CMC updates;

nonclinical laboratory studies; and completed unpublished clinical trials.

ANPR
Advance Notice of Proposed Rulemaking

APhA
American Pharmacists Association

APHIS
Animal and Plant Health Inspection Service

API
Active Pharmaceutical Ingredient

APLB
Advertising and Promotional Labeling Branch (CBER)

Approved
FDA designation given to drugs, biologics and medical devices that have been granted marketing approval.

AQL
Acceptable Quality Level

ASTM
American Society of Testing and Materials

ASQ
American Society for Quality (formerly ASQC)

ASR
Analyte Specific Reagents

ATF
Bureau of Alcohol, Tobacco, Firearms and Explosives

AUT
Actual Use Trials

B

BA/BE Studies
Bioavailability and bioequivalence studies.

Bad Ad Program
Truthful Prescription Drug Advertising and Promotion. Education program for healthcare providers to ensure that prescription drug advertising and promotion is truthful and not misleading. Administered by CDER's Office of Prescription Drug Promotion (OPDP).

BACPAC
Bulk Actives Chemical Postapproval Changes

Banned Device
Device presenting a substantial deception, unreasonable risk of injury or illness, or unreasonable direct and substantial danger to public health.

BIMO
Bioresearch Monitoring Program

BIO
Biotechnology Industry Organization

Bioequivalence
The absence of a significant difference in the rate and extent to which the active ingredient or active moiety in pharmaceutical equivalents or pharmaceutical alternatives becomes available at the site of drug action when administered at the same molar dose under similar conditions in an appropriately designed study.

Biologic
A virus, therapeutic serum, toxin, antitoxin, vaccine, blood, blood component or derivative, allergenic product, protein (except any chemically synthesized polypeptide), or analogous product, or arsphenamine or derivative of arsphenamine (or any other trivalent organic arsenic compound) applicable to the prevention, treatment or cure of a disease or condition of human beings.

Biosimilar
Under the *BPCI Act*, a biological product may be demonstrated to be "biosimilar" if data show that, among other things, the product is "highly similar" to an already-approved biological product.

Bioterrorism Act
Public Health Security and Bioterrorism Preparedness and Response Act of 2002

BLA
Biologics License Application

Blinded Study
Clinical trial in which the patient (single-blind) or patient and investigator (double-blind) are unaware of which treatment the patient receives. Involves use of multiple treatment groups such as other active, placebo or alternate dose groups. Sometimes referred to as "masked."

BPCA
Best Pharmaceuticals for Children Act of 2002

Glossary

BPCI Act
Biologics Price Competition and Innovation Act of 2009

BPDR
Biological Product Deviation Report

C

CAPA
Corrective and Preventive Actions

CBE-30
Changes Being Effected in 30 days. A submission to an approved application reporting changes that FDA has identified as having moderate potential to adversely affect drug product identity, strength, quality, purity and potency. The supplement must be received by FDA at least 30 days before product distribution.

CBER
Center for Biologics Evaluation and Research

CBP
US Customs and Border Protection

CDC
Centers for Disease Control and Prevention

CDER
Center for Drug Evaluation and Research

CDRH
Center for Devices and Radiological Health

CECATS
CDRH Export Certification Application and Tracking System

CF
Consent Form. Document used to inform a potential subject of the risks and benefits of a clinical trial per the Declaration of Helsinki. Sometimes referred to as ICF (Informed Consent Form) or ICD (Informed Consent Document).

CFG
Certificate to Foreign Government. Required by certain countries to prove that an exported product can be legally marketed in the US.

CFR
Code of Federal Regulations

CFSAN
Center for Food Safety and Applied Nutrition

CGMP
Current Good Manufacturing Practice

CGTP
Current Good Tissue Practice

CH
Clinical Hold

CIOMS
Council for International Organizations of Medical Sciences

CIR
Cosmetic Ingredient Review

Class I Device
Low-risk device requiring general controls to ensure safety and effectiveness.

Class II Device
Requires general and special controls to ensure safety and effectiveness. Special controls may include mandatory performance standards, patient registries for implantable devices and postmarket surveillance. Requires 510(k), unless exempted; may require clinical trials.

Class III Device
Requires general controls, special controls and premarket approval (PMA); includes devices that are life-sustaining, life-supporting or pose significant potential for risk to patient, or are not substantially equivalent to Class I or Class II devices. PMAs almost always require clinical trials.

Clearance
Devices that receive marketing permission through the 510(k) process based on demonstrating substantial equivalence to a pre-amendment device or another device reviewed under section 510(k) of the *FD&C Act*.

CLIA
Clinical Laboratory Improvement Amendments of 1988

Clinical Hold
FDA order to delay proposed clinical investigation or suspend an ongoing investigation.

Clinical Investigator
A medical researcher in charge of carrying out a clinical trial's protocol.

ClinicalTrials.gov
A registry and results database of federally and privately supported clinical trials conducted in the US and around the world. Operated by NIH.

CLSI
Clinical and Laboratory Standards Institute (formerly National Committee for Clinical Laboratory Standards)

CMC
Chemistry, Manufacturing and Controls

CME
Continuing Medical Education

CMS
Centers for Medicare & Medicaid Services

COA
Clinical outcomes assessment. Directly or indirectly measures how patients feel or function and can be used to determine whether a drug has been demonstrated to provide a treatment benefit.

Codex Alimentarius Commission
Develops harmonized international food standards, guidelines and codes of practice to protect the health of consumers and ensure fair practices in the food trade.

CoDx
Companion Diagnostics

COE
Certificate of Exportability. Required by certain countries for the export of unapproved devices not sold or offered for sale in the US; issued by FDA to the exporter.

Combination Product
Defined in 21 CFR 3.2(e) as a combination of two or more different types of regulated products, i.e.:
- a drug and a device
- a device and a biological product
- a drug and a biological product
- a drug, a device and a biological product

Commercial Distribution
Any distribution of a device intended for human use, which is offered for sale but does not include: internal or interplant transfer within the same parent, subsidiary or affiliate company any device with an approved exemption for investigational use.

Common Rule
Requires the research institution's IRB to ensure that each research protocol contains adequate provisions to protect a subject during the course of the study.

Complaint
Any written, electronic or oral communication alleging deficiencies related to a product's identity, quality, durability, reliability, safety, effectiveness or performance after release for distribution.

Component
Any ingredient or part intended for use in the manufacture of a drug, device, cosmetic, biologic or IVD product, including those that may not appear in the finished product.

COOL
Country of Origin Labeling. Requirements for source labeling for food products (USDA)

Cosmetic
Articles intended to be rubbed, poured, sprinkled or sprayed on, introduced into or otherwise applied to the human body or any part thereof for cleansing, beautifying, promoting attractiveness or altering appearance; and, articles intended for use as a component of any such article; except that such term shall not include soap.

CPG
Compliance Policy Guide

CPGM
Compliance Program Guidance Manual

CPI
Critical Path Initiative

CPMP
Committee for Proprietary Medicinal Products (EU)

CPSC
Consumer Product Safety Commission

CRA
Clinical Research Associate

CRADA
Cooperative Research and Development Agreement (with a government agency such as NIH and FDA)

CRC
Clinical Research Coordinator

Glossary

CRF
Case Report Form. Paper or electronic document used to record data collected in a clinical trial.

Critical Path Initiative
FDA's effort to stimulate and facilitate a national effort to modernize the scientific process through which a potential human drug, biological product or medical device is transformed from a discovery or "proof of concept" into a medical product.

CR Letter
Complete response letter. Communicates FDA's decision to a drug company that its new drug application (NDA) or abbreviated new drug application (ANDA) to market a new or generic drug will not be approved in its present form.

CRO
Contract Research Organization

CSO
Consumer Safety Officer. Often the FDA contact person for sponsors. Also known as the regulatory project manager.

CTD
Common Technical Document

CTFA
Cosmetic, Toiletry and Fragrance Association

CTP
Center for Tobacco Products

Custom Device
A device that:
- deviates from devices generally available
- deviates from an applicable performance standard or PMA requirement in order to comply with the order of a physician or dentist
- is not generally available in finished form for purchase or dispensing by prescription
- is not offered for commercial distribution through labeling or advertising, is intended for use by an individual patient named in the order of a physician or dentist, and is to be made in a specific form for that patient
- is intended to meet the special needs of the physician or dentist

CVB
Center for Veterinary Biologics (USDA)

CVM
Center for Veterinary Medicine (FDA)

D

DARRTS
Document Archiving, Reporting, and Regulatory Tracking System (CDER)

D&D
Design and Development Plan

DDT
Drug Development Tools

DEA
Drug Enforcement Administration

Dear Health Care Professional (DHCP) letter
Correspondence mailed by a manufacturer and/or distributor to physicians and/or other health care professionals to convey important information about drugs. DHCP letters are considered promotional labeling. These letters can be requested by FDA or initiated by the applicant.

Debarment
An official action in accordance with 21 CFR 1404 to exclude a person from directly or indirectly providing services in any capacity to a firm with an approved or pending drug or device product application. A debarred corporation is prohibited from submitting or assisting in the submission of any NDA or ANDA. Equivalent to disqualification for devices requiring a PMA submission.

Declaration of Helsinki
Ethical principles for medical research involving human subjects. Trials conducted under Good Clinical Practice generally follow the Declaration of Helsinki.

***De Novo* Process**
Provides a route to market for medical devices that are low to moderate risk, but that have been classified in Class III because FDA has found them to be "not substantially equivalent" (NSE) to legally marketed predicate devices.

DESI
Drug Efficacy Study Implementation

DFUF
Device Facility User Fee

DHF
Design History File. Describes a finished device's design.

DHHS
Department of Health and Human Services

DHR
Device History Record. Contains a device's production history.

DIA
Drug Information Association

Discipline Review Letter
Used by FDA to convey early thoughts on possible deficiencies found by a discipline review team for its portion of the pending application at the conclusion of the discipline review.

DMC
Data Monitoring Committee

DMEPA
Division of Medication Error Prevention and Analysis (CBER)

DMETS
Division of Medication Errors and Technical Support (CDER)

DMF
Drug Master File. Submission to FDA that may be used to provide confidential detailed information about facilities, processes or articles used in the manufacturing, processing, packaging and storing of one or more human drugs.

DMPQ
Division of Manufacturing and Product Quality (CBER)

DMR
Device Master Record. Compilation of records containing a finished device's procedures and specifications.

DNCE
Division of Nonprescription Clinical Evaluation

DRC
Direct Recall Classification

DRLS
Drug Registration and Listing System

Drug
Any article intended for use in the diagnosis, cure, mitigation, treatment or prevention of disease in man.

Drugs@FDA
A searchable database of brand-name and generic prescription and OTC human drugs and biological therapeutic products approved since 1939.

"Drug Facts" Label
Labeling requirement for all nonprescription, over-the-counter (OTC) medicine labels with detailed usage and warning information so consumers can properly choose and use the products.

Drug Product
A finished dosage form (e.g., tablet, capsule, solution, etc.) that contains an active drug ingredient. It is generally, but not necessarily, also associated with inactive ingredients. This includes a finished dosage form that does not contain an active ingredient but is intended to be used as a placebo.

DSHEA
Dietary Supplement Health and Education Act of 1994

DSMICA
Division of Small Manufacturers, International, and Consumer Assistance (CDRH)

DSNDCA
Dietary Supplement and Nonprescription Drug Consumer Protection Act

DTC
Direct-to-Consumer (advertising)

D-U-N-S
Data Universal Numbering System. A unique nine-digit sequence provided by Dun & Bradstreet, which is specific to each physical location of an entity (e.g., branch, division and headquarter).

E

EA
Environmental Assessment

eBPDR
Electronic Biological Product Deviation Reports

EC
European Commission, European Community or Ethics Committee

ECO
Emergency Change Order

eCTD
Electronic Common Technical Document

eDRLS
Electronic Drug Registration and Listing System

Glossary

EFTA
European Free Trade Association

EIR
Establishment Inspection Report

EMA
European Medicines Agency (formerly European Medicines Evaluation Agency)

Emergency Use IND
FDA authorization for shipping a drug for a specific emergency use for a life-threatening or serious disease for which there is no alternative treatment.

EPA
Environmental Protection Agency

ERS
Expedited Review Status. Program for veterinary products.

Establishment Listing and Registration
In accordance with 21 CFR 807, manufacturers (both domestic and foreign) and initial distributors (importers) of medical devices must electronically register their establishments with FDA. Manufacturers must also list their devices with FDA.

ETASU
Elements to Ensure Safe Use

EU
European Union has 27 Member States: Belgium, Germany, France, Italy, Luxembourg, The Netherlands, Denmark, Ireland, the United Kingdom, Greece, Spain, Portugal, Austria, Finland, Sweden, Cyprus, the Czech Republic, Estonia, Hungary, Latvia, Lithuania, Malta, Poland, Slovakia, Slovenia, Bulgaria and Romania. EU policies also apply to members of the European Free Trade Association: Iceland, Norway, Switzerland and Liechtenstein.

EUnetHTA
European network for Health Technology Assessment

Excipient
An ingredient contained in a drug formulation that is not a medicinally active constituent.

Expected Life
Time a device is expected to remain functional after being placed into service.

Expiration Date
Date printed on product label indicating the end of the product's useful life. Expiration period length is determined by stability studies and negotiated with FDA.

F

FAERS
FDA Adverse Event Reporting System. A database that contains information on adverse event and medication error reports submitted to FDA (CDER).

FALCPA
Food Allergen Labeling and Consumer Protection Act of 2004

FAR
Field Alert Report

Fast Track
FDA program to facilitate the development and expedite the review of new drugs intended to treat serious or life-threatening conditions that demonstrate the potential to address unmet medical needs. Accelerated NDA review.

FCA
False Claims Act

FCC
Federal Communications Commission

FD&C Act
Federal Food, Drug, and Cosmetic Act of 1938

FDA
Food and Drug Administration

FDAAA
Food and Drug Administration Amendments Act of 2007

FDA ESG
FDA Electronic Submissions Gateway. Enables the secure submission of regulatory information for review.

FDAMA
FDA Modernization Act of 1997

FDASIA
Food and Drug Administration Safety and Innovation Act of 2012

FDERA
Food and Drug Export Reform and Enhancement Act of 1996

FDLI
Food and Drug Law Institute

FIFRA
Federal Insecticide, Fungicide, and Rodenticide Act

FMECA
Failure Mode, Effects and Critical Analysis

FOIA
Freedom of Information Act

FPI
Full prescribing information

FPLA
Fair Packaging and Labeling Act

FPS
Fraud Prevention Systems

FR
Federal Register

FSIS
Food Safety and Inspection Service

FSMA
Food Safety Modernization Act of 2011

FTC
Federal Trade Commission

FURLS
FDA Unified Registration and Listing System for establishment registration of medical device operators and distributors.

G

GADPTRA
Generic Animal Drug and Patent Term Restoration Act of 1988

GAIN Act
Generating Antibiotic Incentives Now Act of 2011

GAO
Government Accountability Office

GCP
Good Clinical Practice. Regulations and requirements with which clinical studies must comply. These regulations apply to manufacturers, sponsors, clinical investigators and institutional review boards.

GDEA
Generic Drug Enforcement Act of 1992

GDUFA
Generic Drug User Fee Amendments

GE
Genetically engineered

GeMCRIS
Genetic Modification Clinical Research Information System. Allows public users to access basic reports about human gene transfer trials registered with NIH and to develop specific queries based on their own information needs.

Generic Drug
Drugs manufactured and approved after the original brand-name drug has lost patent protection. Sponsor files Abbreviated New Drug Application (ANDA) for marketing approval.

GGP
Good Guidance Practice

GLP
Good Laboratory Practice. Regulations governing the conduct of nonclinical laboratory studies that support or are intended to support applications for research or marketing applications.

GMP
Good Manufacturing Practice (for devices, see Quality System Regulation).

GPO
Government Printing Office

GPR
General Purpose Reagents

Grandfathered
Tacit approval of drugs marketed before 1938 and devices marketed before May 1976.

GRADE
Grading of Recommendations Assessment, Development and Evaluation

GRAS(E)
Generally Recognized as Safe (and Effective)

Glossary

Green Book
FDA-published listing of all animal drug products approved for safety and effectiveness. Updated monthly.

GRP
Good Review Practice

GTP
Good Tissue Practice

Guidance
Documents published by FDA to provide current interpretation of regulations.

H

HAACP
Hazard Analysis and Critical Control Point (inspection technique)

Hatch-Waxman Act
Drug Price Competition and Patent Restoration Act of 1984

HCT/P
Human Cells, Tissues and Cellular and Tissue-Based Products

HDE
Humanitarian Device Exemption

HeartNet
A subnetwork of MedSun (CDRH's adverse event reporting program) that focuses on identifying, understanding, and solving problems with medical devices used in electrophysiology laboratories.

HIPAA
Health Insurance Portability and Accountability Act of 1996, also known as the Privacy Rule, established the minimum federal requirements for protecting the privacy of individually identifiable health information.

HMO
Health Maintenance Organization

Homeopathic Drug
Any drug labeled as being homeopathic listed in the Homeopathic Pharmacopeia of the United States (HPUS), an addendum to it or its supplements. The practice of homeopathy is based on the belief that disease symptoms can be cured by small doses of substances which produce similar symptoms in healthy people.

HPC-C
Hematopoietic progenitor cells derived from cord blood

HPCUS
Homeopathic Pharmacopoeia Convention of the United States

HPUS
Homoeopathic Pharmacopoeia of the United States

HTA
Health Technology Assessment

HUD
Humanitarian Use Device

I

IB
Investigator's Brochure

IC (ICF) (ICD)
Informed Consent (Form) (Document)

ICA
Intercenter Agreement

ICCR
International Cooperation on Cosmetic Regulations

ICH
International Conference on Harmonisation of Technical Requirements for Registration of Pharmaceuticals for Human Use (participants include Europe, Japan and US; observers include Australia and Canada).

IDE
Investigational Device Exemption

IDMC
Independent Data Monitoring Committee

IMDRF
International Medical Device Regulators Forum. A voluntary group of medical device regulators from around the world who have come together to build on the strong foundational work of the Global Harmonization Task Force on Medical Devices (GHTF) and aims to accelerate international medical device regulatory harmonization and convergence.

Inactive Ingredient
Any drug product component other than the active ingredient, such as excipients, vehicles and binders.

INAD
Investigational New Animal Drug (application)

INCI
International Nomenclature of Cosmetic Ingredients

IND
Investigational New Drug (application)

Information Amendment
Includes most submissions under an active IND, such as new protocols, final study reports, safety reports, CMC information, etc. The initial IND ends with 000; each serial amendment receives the next consecutive number.

INHATA
International Network of Agencies for Health Technology Assessment

INN
International Nonproprietary Names

Intended Use
Objective labeled use of a device.

Investigator IND
Protocol and IND submitted by an individual investigator instead of a manufacturer. A letter of authorization allows FDA to review the sponsor's DMF or cross-reference CMC information. The investigator, not the manufacturer, is responsible for maintaining the IND.

IOM
Investigations Operations Manual and Institute of Medicine

IRB
Institutional Review Board or Independent Review Board

IR Letter
A communication sent by FDA to an applicant during an application or supplement review to request further information or clarification that is needed or would be helpful to complete the discipline review.

ISO
International Organization for Standardization

IUO
Investigational Use Only

IVD
In Vitro Diagnostic

K

KidNet
A subnetwork of MedSun (CDRH's adverse event reporting program) that focuses on identifying, understanding and solving problems with medical devices used in neonatal and pediatric intensive care units.

L

Label
Any display of written, printed or graphic matter on the immediate container or package of, or affixed to, any article.

Labeling
All written, printed or graphic matter accompanying an article at any time while such article is in interstate commerce or held for sale after shipment in interstate commerce; includes user manuals, brochures, advertising, etc.

LDT
Laboratory developed test

LOA
Letter of Authorization. A letter from the holder of a Drug Master File to FDA, authorizing another party to reference the DMF (also Letter of Agreement).

LoD
Limit of Detection

M

Market Withdrawal
Firm-initiated removal or correction of a device, drug or biologic product involving a minor violation of the *FD&C Act*, not subject to legal action by FDA, or which involves no violation, e.g., normal stock rotation practices, routine equipment adjustments and repairs, etc.

MAF
Device Master File. Analogous to a drug master file; submission to FDA that may be used to provide confidential detailed information about a medical device or a component used in the manufacture of a medical device to FDA in support of another party's obligation.

Glossary

MAPP
Manual of Policy and Procedures. Approved instructions for internal practices and procedures followed by CDER staff to help standardize the new drug review process and other activities.

MAUDE
Manufacturer and User Facility Device Experience database. Contains reports of adverse events involving medical devices.

MCB
Master Cell Bank. A collection of cells of uniform composition derived from a single source prepared under defined culture conditions.

MCSR
Minor changes and stability report (for animal drugs). An annual report that is submitted to the application once each year within 60 days before or after the anniversary date of the application's original approval or on a mutually agreed upon date.

MDR
Medical Device Reporting

MDUFA III
Medical Device User Fee Amendments of 2012

MDUFMA
Medical Device User Fee and Modernization Act of 2002

MedDRA
Medical Dictionary for Regulatory Activities. Global standard international medical terminology designed to supersede or replace all other terminologies used within the medical product development process including COSTART and WHO-ART.

Medical Device
An instrument, apparatus, implement, machine, contrivance, implant, in vitro reagent or other similar or related article, including any component, part or accessory that is:
- recognized in the official *National Formulary* or *US Pharmacopeia*, or any supplement to them
- intended for use in diagnosis of disease or other conditions, or in cure, mitigation, treatment or prevention of disease in man or other animals intended to affect the structure or any function of the body of man or other animals, and which does not achieve its primary intended purposes through chemical action within or on the body of man or other animals, and which is not dependent upon being metabolized for the achievement of its primary intended purposes. (*FD&C Act* Section 201(h))

Medical Food
A food that is formulated to be consumed or administered enterally under the supervision of a physician and is intended for the specific dietary management of a disease or condition for which distinctive nutritional requirements, based on recognized scientific principles, are established by medical evaluation.

Medication Guide
Paper handouts that come with many prescription medicines that address issues specific to particular drugs and drug classes, which contain FDA-approved information that can help patients avoid serious adverse events.

MedSun
Medical Product Safety Network. An adverse event reporting program for healthcare professionals launched in 2002 by CDRH.

MedWatch
FDA program for voluntary and mandatory reporting of AEs and product problems. (Form FDA 3500 or 3500A)

Misbranded
Designation given to a product that is incorrectly labeled (i.e., false or misleading or fails to include information required by law). Other violations may also render a product misbranded (e.g., failure to obtain a 510(k) for a device).

MMA
Medicare Prescription Drug, Improvement and Modernization Act of 2003

Modular PMA
Allows a company to file the completed portions or modules of a PMA for an ongoing review by FDA.

MOU
Memorandum of Understanding. An agreement between FDA and another country's regulatory authority that allows mutual recognition of inspections.

MSDS
Material Safety Data Sheet

MTD
Maximum Tolerated Dose

MUMS
Minor Use and Minor Species Animal Health Act of 2004

N

NADA
New Animal Drug Application

NAF
Notice of Adverse Findings

NAFTA
North American Free Trade Agreement

NAI
No Action Indicated. Most favorable FDA post-inspection classification.

NCE
New Chemical Entity

NCTR
National Center for Toxicological Research

NDA
New Drug Application

NDA Field Alert
Report filed with FDA within three working days of obtaining information on any distributed drug product that has contamination, significant chemical or physical change, deterioration, batch failure or labeling causing mistaken identity.

NDC
National Drug Code. The first five digits identify establishment and last five digits identify drug name, package size and drug type.

NDF
New Dosage Form

NF
National Formulary (incorporated into the *USP-NF*)

NICE
National Institute for Health and Care Excellence (UK)

NIDPOE
Notice of Initiation of Disqualification Proceedings and Opportunity to Explain Letter

NIH
National Institutes of Health

NLEA
Nutrition Labeling and Education Act of 1990

NLM
National Library of Medicine

NME
New Molecular Entity

NORD
National Organization for Rare Disorders

NOV
Notice of Violation letter

NRC
National Research Council or Nuclear Regulatory Commission

NSE
Not Substantially Equivalent. Designation for device that does not qualify for 510(k) clearance; generally requires a PMA.

NSR
Nonsignificant Risk

Nuremberg Code of 1947
A set of research ethics principles for human experimentation that was created as a result of atrocities involving medical experimentation on humans during World War II.

O

OAI
Official Action Indicated. Serious FDA post-inspection classification.

OBRR
Office of Blood Research and Review (CBER)

OC
Office of the Commissioner (FDA)

OCBQ
Office of Compliance and Biologics Quality (CBER)

OCC
Office of the Chief Counsel (FDA)

OCET
Office of Counterterrorism and Emerging Threats (FDA)

OCI
Office of Criminal Investigation (FDA)

Glossary

OCP
Office of Combination Products (FDA)

OCTGT
Office of Cellular, Tissue and Gene Therapies (CBER)

ODA
Orphan Drug Act of 1983

ODE
Office of Device Evaluation (FDA)

OPDP
Office of Prescription Drug Promotion (CDER, formerly Division of Drug Marketing, Advertising, and Communications (DDMAC))

OECD
The Organization for Economic Cooperation and Development

Off-Label Drug Use
When a drug is used in a way that is different from that described in the FDA-approved drug label.

Office of the Chief Scientist
Includes the following offices:
- Office of Counterterrorism and Emerging Threats
- Office of Regulatory Science and Innovation
- Office of Scientific Integrity
- Office of Scientific Professional Development

OGD
Office of Generic Drug Products (CDER)

OIG
Office of the Inspector General (FDA)

OIP
Office of International Programs (FDA)

OIRA
Office of Information and Regulatory Affairs (OMB)

OIVD
Office of In Vitro Diagnostic Device Evaluation and Safety (FDA)

OMUMS
Office of Minor Use & Minor Species Animal Drug Development (CVM)

ONADE
Office of New Animal Drug Evaluation (CVM)

OND
Office of New Drugs (CDER)

ONPLDS
Office of Nutritional Products, Labeling and Dietary Supplements (CFSAN)

OOPD
Office of Orphan Products Development (FDA)

OPA
Office of Public Affairs (FDA)

Open Label Study
A clinical trial in which subjects and investigators are aware of the treatment received.

ORA
Office of Regulatory Affairs (FDA); oversees FDA's field organization.

Orange Book
FDA-published listing of Approved Drug Products with Therapeutic Equivalence Evaluations generally known as generics (original print version had an orange cover).

Orphan Drug
Drugs for a disease or condition that affects fewer than 200,000 persons in the US or occurs in more than 200,000 and for which there is no reasonable expectation that drug development and manufacturing costs will be recovered from US sales.

OSB
Office of Surveillance and Biometrics (CDRH)

OSHA
Occupational Safety Health Administration

OSI
Office of Scientific Integrity (FDA)

OTC
Over-the-Counter. Nonprescription drugs receive this designation.

OTC Monograph
Rules for a number of OTC drug categories.

OVRR
Office of Vaccine Research and Review (CBER)

P

PADER
Periodic Adverse Drug Experiences Report

PAI
Preapproval Inspection

PAS
Prior Approval Supplement or Postapproval Study

PAT
Process Analytical Technology

PBRER
Periodic benefit:risk evaluation reports

PCPC
Personal Care Products Council (formerly Cosmetic, Toiletry and Fragrance Association)

PD
Pharmacodynamics. Study of the reactions between drugs and living structures.

PDA
Parenteral Drug Association

PDMA
Prescription Drug Marketing Act of 1987

PDP
Product Development Protocol (for medical devices) or Principal Display Panel (for product labels)

PDUFA
Prescription Drug User Fee Act of 1992

PDUFA II
Prescription Drug User Fee Act of 1997

PDUFA III
Prescription Drug User Fee Act of 2002

PDUFA IV
Prescription Drug User Fee Act of 2007

PDUFA V
Prescription Drug User Fee Act of 2012

Pediatric Rule
Requires manufacturers to assess the safety and effectiveness of certain drug and biological products in pediatric patients.

PEPFAR
President's Emergency Plan for AIDS Relief

PGx
Pharmacogenomics. The study of variations of DNA and RNA characteristics as related to drug response.

Pharmaceutical equivalents
Drug products that contain the same active ingredient(s), are of the same dosage form and route of administration and are identical in strength or concentration.

Pharmacovigilance
Adverse event monitoring and reporting

PhRMA
Pharmaceutical Research and Manufacturers of America

Phase I
Initial clinical safety studies in humans. May be as few as 10 subjects, often healthy volunteers, includes PK, ADME and dose escalation studies. Usually open label.

Phase II
Well-controlled clinical trials of approximately 100–300 subjects who have the condition of interest, includes PK, dose ranging, safety and efficacy.

Phase III
Larger, well-controlled clinical trials of hundreds to thousands of subjects, including both safety and efficacy data. Generally, two well-controlled studies are needed to establish efficacy for drug products.

Phase IV
Postmarket clinical trials performed to support labeling and advertising or fulfill FDA safety requirements noted at the time of NDA approval.

PHI
Protected Health Information

PHS
Public Health Service

PI
Package Insert (approved product labeling) or Principal Investigator

PK
Pharmacokinetics. The study of the processes of ADME of chemicals and medicines.

Glossary

Placebo
A drug product fashioned to look like an active drug but containing no active ingredient. Used in clinical trials to blind or mask the patient, investigator or both as to the treatment received.

PLR
Physician Labeling Rule

PMA
Premarket Approval. Marketing application required for Class III devices.
- Traditional PMA: The complete PMA application is submitted to FDA at once. This method is generally used if the device has already undergone clinical testing and has been approved in a country with established medical device regulations.
- Modular: The complete contents of a PMA are broken down into well-delineated components (or module) and each component is submitted to FDA as soon as the applicant has completed the module, compiling a complete PMA over time.
- Streamlined: A pilot program in the Division of Clinical Laboratory Devices. A complete PMA is submitted as in a traditional PMA; however, the Streamlined PMA is for a device in which the technology and use are well known to FDA.
- Product Development Process (PDP): The clinical evaluation of a device and the development of necessary information for marketing approval are merged into one regulatory mechanism. Ideal candidates for the PDP process are those devices in which the technology is well established in industry.

PMC
Postmarketing commitment. Studies or clinical trials that a sponsor has agreed to conduct, but that are not required by a statute or regulation.

PMN
Premarket Notification. A premarket notification is also called a 510(k).

PMOA
Primary Mode of Action. The single mode of action of a combination product that provides the most important therapeutic action of the combination product; used to assign a combination product to a lead FDA center.

PMR
Postmarketing Requirements. Studies and clinical trials that sponsors are required to conduct under one or more statutes or regulations

PMS
Postmarketing Surveillance. Ongoing monitoring of the safety of approved medical products; may include Phase IV studies and AE reporting.

PNSI
Prior Notice System Interface. Used to provide prior notice for food products entering the US.

POCs
Physician-owned companies

PPA
Poison Prevention Act

PPACA
Patient Protection and Affordable Care Act of 2010

PPI
Patient Package Insert

PPIA
Poultry Products Inspection Act

PREA
Pediatric Research Equity Act of 2003

Preclinical Studies
Animal studies of PK and toxicity generally performed prior to clinical studies. These studies must comply with GLP.

Pre-Sub Meeting
Provides the opportunity for an applicant to obtain FDA feedback prior to intended submission of an IDE or marketing application.

Priority Review
FDA review category for drugs that appear to represent an advance over available therapy. NDA or BLA receives a faster review than standard applications.

PRO
Patient-reported outcome

Protocol
Document describing a clinical trial's objectives, design and methods. All GLP and GCP studies must follow a protocol.

PSUR
Periodic Safety Update Report

PTC
Points to Consider. Type of guidance published by FDA, usually by CBER.

PTCC
Pharmacology/Toxicology Coordinating Committee (CDER)

PTO
Patent and Trademark Office

***Public Health Security and Bioterrorism Preparedness and Response Act* of 2002**
Also known as *Bioterrorism Act*

PWR
Pediatric Written Request. *BPCA* authorizes FDA (in consultation with NIH) to issue a written request for the conduct of pediatric studies to holders of approved NDAs and ANDAs for drugs on the NIH list.

Q

QA
Quality Assurance

QALY
Quality Adjusted Life Year

QAU
Quality Assurance Unit

QC
Quality Control

QbR
Question-based review (CDER). Chemistry, Manufacturing, and Controls (CMC) evaluation of ANDAs that incorporates the most important scientific and regulatory review questions focused on critical pharmaceutical attributes essential for ensuring generic drug product quality.

QdB
Quality by Design. The focus of this concept is that quality should be built into a product with a thorough understanding of the product and process by which it is developed and manufactured along with a knowledge of the risks involved in manufacturing the product and how best to mitigate those risks.

QIDP
Qualified Infectious Disease Product

QoL
Quality of Life

QSIT
Quality System Inspection Technique

QSR
Quality System Regulation (21 CFR 820). Identifies GMPs for medical devices.

R

R&D
Research and Development

RAC
Reviewer Affairs Committee (CDER) or Regulatory Affairs Certification

RAPS
Regulatory Affairs Professionals Society

RCT
Randomized Clinical Trial or Randomized Controlled Trial

Real Time PMA Supplement
A supplement to an approved premarket application or premarket report under section 515 that requests a minor change to the device, such as a minor change to the design of the device, software, sterilization or labeling, and for which the applicant has requested and the agency has granted a meeting or similar forum to jointly review and determine the status of the supplement.

Recall
A firm's removal or correction of a marketed product that FDA considers to be in violation of the laws it administers and against which the agency would initiate legal action, e.g., seizure. Recall does not include a market withdrawal or a stock recovery.

Recall Classification
Assigned by FDA and applicable to firm-initiated device recalls based upon reasonable probability and relative degree of health hazard.
- Class I: violative device would cause serious adverse health consequences.
- Class II: violative device may cause temporary or medically reversible adverse health consequences or such consequences are remote.
- Class III: violative device is not likely to cause adverse health consequences.

Regulation
Refers to Code of Federal Regulations

Glossary

REMS
Risk Evaluation and Mitigation Strategy

Restricted Device
A device restricted, by regulation, to sale, distribution and/or use only upon the written or oral authorization of a licensed practitioner or other conditions prescribed by the commissioner.

RFA
Request for Application

RFD
Request for Designation. A written submission to OCP requesting designation of the center with primary jurisdiction for a combination or non-combination product.

RFR
Request for Reconsideration. A request that OCP reconsider an RFD determination.

RFR
Reportable Food Registry. An electronic portal used to report foods suspected of causing serious adverse health consequences.

RiskMAP
Risk Minimization Action Plan. A strategic safety program designed to meet specific goals and objectives in minimizing known risks of a product while preserving its benefits.

RLD
Reference Listed Drug. Drug product listed in the Approved Drug Products with Therapeutic Equivalence Evaluations book (also known as the *Orange Book*).

Rolling NDA Submission
Allows a company to file the completed portions of an NDA for an ongoing review by FDA. Only permitted for drugs and biologics that have received Fast Track designation from FDA.

RPM
Regulatory Procedures Manual. A reference manual for FDA personnel containing information on internal procedures to be used in processing domestic and import regulatory and enforcement matters.

RTA Policy
Refuse to accept. FDA staff will conduct an acceptance review of all traditional, special or abbreviated 510(k)s based on objective criteria using the applicable Acceptance Checklist to ensure that the 510(k) is administratively complete.

RTF
Refusal to File. Letter sent by FDA when incomplete NDA or ANDA is filed. FDA will not review the application until complete. Letter is sent within 60 days of submission.

RUO
Research Use Only

Rx
Prescription Use Only

Rx to OTC Switch
The process of transferring FDA-approved prescription medications to nonprescription, over-the-counter (OTC) for the same dosage form, population and route of administration.

S

SAE
Serious Adverse Event

SBA
Summary Basis of Approval

SC
Study Coordinator

SD
Standard Deviation

SDWA
Safe Drinking Water Act

SE
Substantially Equivalent

S&E
Safety and Efficacy

SECG
Small entity compliance guide

Sentinel Initiative
FDA program aimed at developing and implementing a proactive system that will complement existing systems the agency has in place to track reports of adverse events linked to the use of its regulated products.

Shelf Life
Maximum time a device will remain functional from the date of manufacture until it is used in patient care (See Expiration Date).

Significant Risk Device
An investigational device that:
- is intended as an implant
- is represented to be for use in supporting or sustaining human life
- is for a use of substantial importance in diagnosing, curing, mitigating or treating disease or otherwise preventing impairment of human health and presents a potential for serious risk to the subject's health, safety or welfare

SMDA
Safe Medical Devices Act of 1990

SME
Significant Medical Event

SMP
Senior medical protocol

SNDA
Supplemental New Drug Application

SoCRA
Society of Clinical Research Associates

SOP
Standard Operating Procedure

Source Documents
Original documents and records containing information captured in a clinical study. Case Report Forms are monitored against source documents. Includes office charts, laboratory results, x-rays, etc.

SPA
Special Protocol Assessment

SPL
Structured Product Label. Content of package insert in XML format.

SR
Significant Risk (device)

Sponsor
Company, person, organization or institution taking responsibility for initiating, managing or financing a clinical trial.

SSED
Summary of Safety and Effectiveness Data. An FDA document intended to present a reasoned, objective, and balanced summary of the scientific evidence, both positive and negative, that served as the basis of the decision to approve or deny the PMA.

SST
System Suitability Testing. Required by USP and FDA to check and ensure on-going performance of analytical systems and methods.

Standard Review (S)
FDA review category for drugs with therapeutic qualities similar to those already approved for marketing.

Subject
Clinical trial participant; may be a healthy volunteer or a patient.

Subpart E
21 CFR 312. Accelerated review for life-threatening and severely debilitating illness.

Subpart H
21 CFR 314.500. Approval based upon a surrogate endpoint or a product approved with restrictions and/or requirements for Phase IV trials.

Substantial Equivalence
Comparison of a new device to a legally marketed predicate device; substantial equivalence establishes a device is as safe and as effective as another 510(k) cleared device.

Suitability Petition
A request to FDA to submit an ANDA for a product that varies from a Reference Listed Drug in indication, strength, dosage form, route of administration, etc.

SUPAC
Scale Up and Post Approval Changes

Supplement (sNDA)
NDA submission for changes to an approved NDA, including SUPAC.

Supplement (sPMA)
PMA submission for changes to an approved PMA that affect the device's safety or effectiveness.

Surrogate Endpoint
A laboratory or physical sign that is used in trials as a substitute for a clinically meaningful endpoint that is a direct measure of how a patient feels, functions or survives and is expected to predict the effect of the therapy.

Glossary

T

Target Product Profile (TPP)
A format for a summary of a drug development program described in terms of labeling concepts. A TPP can be prepared by a sponsor and then shared with the appropriate FDA review staff to facilitate communication regarding a particular drug development program.

TEA
Time and extent application. Demonstrates that a drug product can meet the statutory standard of marketing to a material extent and for a material time

Team Biologics
A group of specialized investigators who conduct routine and CGMP follow-up inspections of manufacturers of biological products regulated by CBER. Partnership program between ORA and CBER.

TFM
Tentative Final Monograph

Third-party Review
Under *FDAMA*, FDA has accredited third parties that are authorized to conduct the primary review of 510(k)s for eligible devices.

THOMAS
Public federal legislation database (Library of Congress)

TK
Toxicokinetics

Tobacco Control Act
The Family Smoking Prevention and Tobacco Control Act of 2009

TOPRA
The Organisation for Professionals in Regulatory Affairs

TPLC
Total product lifecycle

TPP
Target Product Profile

Transitional Device
Devices that were regulated as drugs prior to the 28 May 1976, the date the *Medical Device Amendments* were signed into law. Any device that was approved by the New Drug Application process is now governed by the PMA regulations.

Treatment IND (tIND)
Allows limited use of an unapproved drug for patients with a serious or life-threatening disease.

Truthful Prescription Drug Advertising and Promotion (Bad Ad Program)
Educational outreach program to help healthcare providers recognize misleading prescription drug promotion and provide them with an easy way to report this activity to the agency.

TTB
Tax and Trade Bureau

U

UADE
Unexpected Adverse Device Effect. Any serious adverse effect on health or safety or any life-threatening problem or death caused by, or associated with, a device, if that effect, problem or death was not previously identified in nature, severity or degree of incidence in the investigational plan or application, or any other unanticipated serious problem associated with a device that relates to the rights, safety or welfare of subjects.

UDI
Unique Device Identification. Would require the label of a device to bear a unique identifier, unless an alternative location is specified by FDA or unless an exception is made for a particular device or group of devices.

Unexpected AE
An AE whose nature or severity is not described in the Investigator's Brochure (for an unapproved product) or in the package insert (for an approved product).

USAN
US Adopted Name

USANC
US Adopted Names Council

USC
US Code

USCA
US Code Annotated

USDA
US Department of Agriculture

User Fees
Fees authorized by Congress to fund various FDA activities. The fee schedule for different application types is published annually in the *Federal Register*. Initially established by the *Prescription Drug User Fee Act* and later extended to medical devices, generic drugs and animal drugs.

USP
United States Pharmacopeia

V

VA
Department of Veterans Affairs

VAERS
Vaccine Adverse Event Reporting System

VAI
Voluntary Action Indicated. Moderately serious FDA post-inspection classification.

VCRP
Voluntary Cosmetic Registration Program. An FDA post-market reporting system for use by manufacturers, packers and distributors of cosmetic products that are in commercial distribution in the US.

VICH
Veterinary International Conference on Harmonization

W

Warning Letter (WL)
Serious enforcement letter issued by FDA notifying a regulated entity of violative activity; requires immediate action within 15 days.

Warning Letter Database
Contains Warning Letters issued from November 1996 to the present. Searchable by company, subject, issuing office or date.

WCB
Working Cell Bank. Cells derived from one or more vials of cells from the master cell bank, which are expanded by serial subculture.

Well-Characterized Biologic
A biological product whose identity, purity, impurities, potency and quantity can be determined and controlled.

WHO
World Health Organization

Glossary

Index

15-Day Alert Reports, 145–146, 296
180-day exclusivity, 25, 180, 184–185
351(a), 132
351(k), 132
505(b)(1), 27, 132
505(b)(2), 39, 132, 181, 192
505(j), 132, 192, 195
510(k)
    abbreviated submissions, 228–229
    approval pathways, 227–228
    modifications, 228
    overview and exemptions, 41–42, 223
    PMA reclassification requirements, 222–223
    refuse-to-accept policy, 230
    special, 229–230
513(g), 44, 46, 223

A

Abbreviated New Animal Drug Application (ANADA), 392–394
Abbreviated new drug application (ANDA)
    180-day marketing exclusivity, 180, 184–185
    approval process, 156–164
    certification requirements, 181
    CMC requirements, 24–25
    Hatch-Waxman Act authorized generic submission requirements, 15, 24–26, 132
    inactivation/withdrawal, 152
    non-patent market exclusivity, 181–182
    OTC drug approval, 195
    paragraph IV litigation, 183–184
    postapproval change reporting requirements, 143–145
    transfer of ownership/sponsor, 152–153
    user fee requirements, 163–164
Accelerated approval, 126, 303–304
Active moiety, 136–137, 180
Active pharmaceutical ingredient (API)
    GMP/CGMP requirements, 142
Administrative License Action Letters, 297
Administrative meetings, 48, 51. *See also* Food and Drug Administration (FDA) -- communications/meetings types and requirements
Administrative Procedure Act (1946), 12, 16
Adulteration, 384–385, 395–396, 402, 410–411, 439
AdvaMed Code, 448
Adverse drug reaction (ADR)/Adverse drug experience (ADE), 123, 145–146, 149, 212–217
Adverse event reporting
    biologics, 291–292, 296
    combination products, 316–317
    devices, 252–253
    dietary supplements, 38, 373–375
    drugs, 123, 212–217
    medical foods, 432
Advertising
    biologic requirements, 303–307
    cosmetic product requirements, 386–387
    device/IVD requirements, 263–264
    dietary supplement requirements, 367–371
    food product requirements, 406–410
    help-seeking, 308
    homeopathic drug requirements, 378–379
    OTC drug requirements, 196–197
    prescription drug requirements, 148–149, 205–208
Advisory committees
    CBER, 286, 328

Index

legislative history, 36, 135
meeting overview and preparation requirements, 52–53, 57–63
pediatric, 360
Advisory opinion, 48. *See also* Regulatory communications
Agency for Healthcare Research and Quality (AHRQ), 76–77
Alcohol and Tobacco Tax and Trade Bureau. *See* Tax and Trade Bureau (TTB)
Analyte-specific reagents (ASRs). *See* Reagents
Animal Drug Availability Act (ADAA) (1996), 394
Animal Drug User Fee Act (ADUFA) (2003), 394
Animal Drug User Fee Amendments (ADUFA II) (2008), 394
Animal drugs. *See* Veterinary products
Animal feeds, 396
Animal Generic Drug User Fee Act (AGDUFA) (2008), 394–495
Animal grooming aids, 397
Animal Rule, 281
Animal Medicinal Drug Use Clarification Act (AMDUCA) (1994), 397
Annual Reports
  biologic requirements, 285–286, 293–295, 303
  combination product requirements, 321, 323
  drug requirements, 147–148
  veterinary product requirements, 397
Anti-Kickback Statute (1987), 209, 446–448
Antibiotic drugs, 136, 185, 188

B

Bad Ad program, 205
Belmont Report (1979), 93
Best Pharmaceuticals for Children Act (2002), 182–183, 355, 357–358
Bioequivalence, 24–25, 108, 157, 161–163
Biological marker. *See* Biomarker
Biological Product Deviation Reporting (BPDR), 297, 329–330
Biologics
  advertising and promotional labeling requirements, 284, 303–307
  CMC requirements, 279–280
  compared with drugs, 27
  definition, development and approval pathway, 22–23, 26–27, 44, 121, 123–124, 274
  GMP/CGMP requirements, 107, 287–288
  IND requirements, 275–276
  inspection requirements, 294
  labeling requirements, 131, 300–307
  licensing compliance standards, 290–293
  lot release requirements, 287

  market exclusivity, 286
  postapproval application requirements, 284–286, 294–295
  postmarket surveillance requirements, 293–294, 296
  preclinical/clinical safety issues, 276–279
  product application meetings, 48–50
  product naming requirements, 292
  safety reporting requirements, 213–214
  therapeutic products, 125
  veterinary products, 398–399
Biologics Control Act (1902). *See Virus Serum and Toxin Act (VSTA)* (1902)
Biologics License Application (BLA)
  application format/content & CTD/eCTD requirements, 131–132, 281
  application types, 132
  briefing book requirements for AC meeting, 60
  CMC requirements, 279–280
  companion diagnostic product requirements, 424–425
  cord blood product requirements, 332
  HPC-C requirements, 350
  licensing compliance requirements, 290–291
  package insert/labeling requirements, 202–203, 300–303
  postapproval change reporting requirements, 143–145, 302–303
  presubmission requirements, 130–131
  submission, review and approval requirements, 27–29, 123–124, 133–136, 274, 281, 283–284
Biologics Price Competition and Innovation Act (BPCI Act) (2009), 26, 274, 286–287, 323
Biomarker, 125
Bioresearch Monitoring Program (BIMO), 88, 135, 291, 293
Biosimilars, 26–27, 132, 286–287
Biotechnology products, 405–406
Bioterrorism Act (2002), 14, 371, 375, 413
Blood Action Plan, 328–239
Blood establishments, 330–331
Blood/blood products
  donor eligibility, 328–330
  establishment registration, 330–331
  GMP/CGMP requirements, 330
  legislative history, 327–328
Board of inquiry, 51–52
Breakthrough therapy designation, 30, 127–128

C

Cellular and tissue-based products, 336–337, 350
Center for Biologics Evaluation and Research (CBER)
  Advertising and Promotional Labeling Staff (APLS), 263, 284, 303–306

advisory committees, 286
blood/blood products oversight, 327–332
cell and tissue product oversight, 331–332, 336
companion diagnostic product oversight, 423–424
enforcement authority, 297–298
manuals of standard operating procedures and policies (SOPPs), 23
mission and scope of regulatory authority, 5, 222, 274–275
pre-license inspection requirements, 292–293
proprietary name oversight, 292
role in BLA review, 27, 281, 283–284
role in reviewing blood collection, cellular therapies and vaccine submissions, 40–41
role in therapeutic biologic product review, 124–125

Center for Devices and Radiological Health (CDRH)
companion diagnostic product oversight, 424
Export Certification and Tracking System (CECATS), 249
MedSun, 252–253
mission and scope of regulatory authority, 6, 221–223
postapproval studies program, 255–256
Postmarket Transformation Leadership Team, 252
risk communication activities, 254–255
role in reviewing/approving CLIA laboratory tests, 7

Center for Drug Evaluation and Research (CDER)
Antibacterial Drug Development Task Force, 136
companion diagnostic product oversight, 423–424
Drug Safety and Risk Management Advisory Committee, 215
manuals of policies and procedures (MAPPs), 23
role in drug/biologic review and oversight, 124–125, 127, 274
scope of regulatory authority, 5

Center for Food Safety and Applied Nutrition (CFSAN), 6, 384, 389

Center for Medicare and Medicaid Services (CMS)
health technology assessment activities, 77
scope of regulatory authority, 7, 448

Center for Tobacco Products (CTP), 6
Center for Veterinary Medicine (CVM), 6, 392–397
Centers for Disease Control and Prevention (CDC), 335
Certificate for Foreign Government (CFG), 248, 294
Certificate of Exportability (COE), 250, 294
Changes Being Effected supplement(CBE)/Changes Being Effected in 30 days supplement (CBE-30), 144–145, 285, 294–295, 303, 396–397

Chemistry, manufacturing and controls (CMC)
ANDA application requirements, 24–25
ANDA/NDA/BLA postapproval change reporting requirements, 143–145
biologic product requirements, 279–280, 291, 293–295

Citizen petitions, 39, 48, 193. *See also* Regulatory communications

Claims
biologic products, 305
cosmetics, 386–387
dietary supplements, 367–371
food products, 409–410
prescription drug products, 206–207

Classification
IVDs, 268–271
medical devices, 40, 45, 222–223

Clinical Laboratory Improvement Amendments (*CLIA*), 7, 80, 269–270

Clinical outcomes assessment (COA), 125

Clinical trials
AE/ADR reporting requirements, 212–217
biologic requirements, 277–279
pediatric medical device requirements, 359–360
purpose and history, 92–93, 101–102
study site/investigator requirements, 100–103

Clinical Trials Data Bank, 16, 34
Code of Federal Regulations (CFR), 12, 22–23, 94
Code of Medical Ethics (AMA), 92
College of American Pathologists (CAP), 81
Color Additive Amendments (1960), 14–15
Color additives, 405
Color Certification Program, 14

Combination products
definition and regulatory scope, 223–224, 311–312
development and approval program review, 43–44, 46, 312–315
GMP/CGMP requirements, 108, 315–316
postmarket safety reporting requirements, 316–317
premarket review requirements, 315
user fees, 317–318

Common Technical Document (CTD)
biologic IND submission requirements, 275–276
DMF submission requirements, 150
eCTD submission requirements, 35, 131–132
initial IND submission requirements, 34
modules overview, 31–32, 45

Companion diagnostics (CoDx)
approval pathways, 424–425
CDER/CBER meetings, 423–424
legislative history and definition, 421–422
postapproval requirements, 425
regulatory roles of drug/diagnostic companies, 423

Consumer Healthcare Product Association (CHPA), 197
Consumer Product Safety Act (*CPSA*), 7

Consumer Product Safety Commission (CPSC)
child-resistant packaging requirements, 196, 443
scope of regulatory authority, 7, 470

Cord blood products, 331–332, 350
Corrective and preventive action (CAPA), 109–110

Cosmeceuticals, 388
Cosmetic Ingredient Review (CIR), 385, 388
Cosmetic, Toiletry and Fragrance Association (CTFA), 386
Cosmetics
    adulteration, 384–385
    advertising, labeling and misbranding, 385–387, 389
    establishment registration requirements, 388
    GMP/CGMP requirements, 384, 387
    import/export requirements, 388
    legislative history and definition, 15, 383–384
    with drug/device components, 387–388
Council of Better Business Bureaus, 197
Country of Origin Labeling (COOL), 408
Creutzfeldt-Jacob Disease (CJD), 330
Crisis management
    definition, 65
    external, 67
    internal, 66–67
    overview, 65–66
    post-resolution assessment, 68
Critical Path Initiative (CPI), 4
current Good Manufacturing Practices (CGMPs). *See* Good maufacturing practices (GMPs)/current good manufacturing practices (CGMPs)
Customs and Border Protection (CBP), 403, 408

D

De Novo process, 223, 270
Debarment, 440
Declaration of Conformity, 229
Declaration of Geneva (1948), 92–93
Declaration of Helsinki (1964), 93
Delaney clause, 14, 404–405
Device History Record (DHR), 245
Device Master Record (DMR), 245
Device Registration Listing Module (DRLM), 242–243
Dietary Supplement and Nonprescription Drug Consumer Protection Act (2006), 38, 373–375
Dietary Supplement Health and Education Act (DSHEA) (1994), 14, 38, 45, 365–366, 369–372
Dietary supplements
    adverse event reporting requirements, 373–375
    definition, 366
    GMP/CGMP requirements, 365, 371–373
    import/export requirements, 375–376
    labeling/advertising requirements, 367–371
    legislative history, 38, 45, 365–366
    NDI notifications, 366–367
Direct-to-consumer (DTC), 16, 194, 207–208, 284, 304
Division of Drug Marketing, Advertising and Communications (DDMAC). *See* Office of Prescription Drug Promotion (OPDP)

Division of Small Manufacturers, International, and Consumer Assistance (DSMICA), 10
Donor eligibility, 328–331
Drug Amendments. See Kefauver-Harris Amendments (1962)
Drug Efficacy Amendments (1962), 156
Drug Efficacy Study Implementation (DESI) program, 24, 156
Drug Enforcement Administration (DEA), 9
Drug Facts Label Regulation (1999), 39, 195–196
Drug History File (DHF), 229
Drug Master File (DMF), 150, 164, 229, 280, 315
Drug Price Competition and Patent Term Restoration Act (1984). *See Hatch-Waxman Act*
Drug Registration Listing System (DRLS), 130
Drugs
    505(b)(2) submission requirements, 37–38
    application and approval pathways, 132
    breakthrough therapy designation, 31
    compared with biologics, 26–27
    compared with OTC drugs, 123
    crisis management, 65
    definition and development, 22–23, 27–28, 44, 122–126
    electronic submission requirements, 35
    establishment registration/listing requirements, 129–130, 151–152
    exclusivity, 136–137
    expedited drug review pathways, 126–127
    fast track designation, 30–31, 44–45, 126–127
    generic/ANDA application requirements, 23, 25–27
    GMP/CGMP and quality system requirements, 107–111, 141–143
    import/export requirements, 150–151
    IND submission requirements, 32–34
    labeling requirements, 131, 201–203, 206
    legislative history, 12–16
    NDA/BLA submission and review process requirements, 35, 133–135
    orphan, 28–30
    presubmission meetings, 130–131
    product application meetings, 48–50
    proprietary name requirements, 128–129
    risk assessment/REMS, 35–36
    safety reporting requirements, 213–214
    user fees, 15
Durham Humphrey Amendment (1951), 13, 39, 191–192
Dykstra Report, 366

E

eBPDR. *See* Biological Product Deviation Reporting (BPDR)

eCTD. *See* Common Technical Document (CTD)
Elements to Assure Safe Use (ETASU), 128, 296
Emergency use, 98
Enantiomers, 188
Enforcement
  biologic, 297–298, 308–309
  cosmetics, 388–389
  device, 265–266
  food product, 412–413
  overview of FDA activities, 439–443
Environmental Protection Agency (EPA)
  GLP requirements, 80
  memorandum of agreement with FDA, 9
  pesticide requirements, 399
  scope of regulatory authority, 9
Establishment Inspection Report (EIR), 439
Establishment registration
  biologic, 287–288
  blood/blood products, 329–331
  cosmetics, 388
  device, 43, 46, 240–243
  drug, 36–37, 129–130, 151–152
EUnetHTA, 71–72
European Medicines Agency (EMA)
  common orphan drug application with OOPD, 30, 323
  health technology assessment activities, 71
  pediatric product oversight, 360
Evidentiary hearing, 51
Excipients, 160–161
Expedited review, 234–235, 394–395
Extended Machine Language. *See* XML

F

Fair balance, 206–207, 305–306
Fair Packaging and Labeling Act (*FPLA*) (1967), 14, 385, 429
False Claims Act (*FCA*) (1863), 209, 446
Family Smoking Prevention and Tobacco Control Act, 6
Fast track designation, 30–31, 44, 126–127
FDA Adverse Event Reporting System (FAERS), 146, 218
FDA Electronic Submissions Gateway (FDA ESG), 133
FDA Unified Registration and Listing System (FURLS), 241–243
Federal Advisory Committee Act (*FACA*) (1972), 36, 286
Federal Alcohol Administration Act (*FAAA*), 8
Federal Food, Drug, and Cosmetic Act (*FD&C Act*) (1938)
  505(b)(1) provision, 27
  animal drug/feed provisions, 392–396
  biologic provisions, 274
  combination product provisions, 312–315
  cosmetic product provisions, 383–384
  device provisions, 13–14
  drug product exclusivity provisions, 181–182, 184–185
  FDA inspectional authority and enforcement provisions, 435–436, 439–443
  FDA prescription drug labeling authority provisions, 201
  food-related products/food additive provisions, 402–403, 406–407, 410–411
  generic drug/ANDA provisions, 157–162
  GMP/CGMP regulatory provisions, 107–109
  import/export provisions, 150–151
  labeling provisions, 300–301
  legislative history, 2, 13–16, 22–23
  medical device regulatory provisions, 221–223, 239
  medical food provisions, 428
  prescription drug/NDA regulatory provisions, 122–123
Federal Insecticide, Fungicide, and Rodenticide Act (*FIFRA*) (1947), 399
Federal Register (*FR*), 16–17, 22, 94
Federal Trade Commission (FTC)
  advertising and labeling jurisdiction, 13, 196–197, 263–264, 371–372, 385–386, 388, 443
  memorandum of understanding with FDA, 7, 263
  scope of regulatory authority, 6, 470
Federal Trade Commission Act (*FTC Act*) (1914), 7, 263
Financial disclosure, 99–100
Food additives, 403–405
Food Additives Amendment (1958), 14
Food Allergen Labeling and Consumer Protection Act (*FALCPA*) (2004), 367, 408, 430
Food and Drug Administration (FDA)
  advertising, labeling and promotion authority, 24, 201–203, 206–209
  advisory committee activities, 52–53, 57–59, 286
  AE/ADE reporting oversight, 145–146, 212–218
  ANDA approval process oversight, 156–164
  ANDA/NDA/BLA postapproval change reporting requirements, 143–145
  blood/blood product oversight, 327–332
  cell and tissue product oversight, 335–337, 350–351
  combination product oversight, 223–224, 312–318
  communications/meetings types and requirements, 47–53, 55–57
  companion diagnostic oversight, 421–425
  consumer/industry resources, 9–10
  cosmetic product oversight, 383–389
  device establishment registration/listing requirements, 240–243

device/IVD advertising, promotion and labeling authority, 260–265
device/IVD classification and submission requirements, 268–271
dietary supplement oversight, 365–375
DMF requirements, 150
drug advertising, labeling and promotional authority, 201–203, 205–209
drug establishment registration/listing requirements, 151–152
enforcement activities
    biologics, 297–298, 308–309
    cosmetics, 388–389
    devices, 265–266
    food product, 412–413
    overview, 439–443
food-related products/food additives oversight, 402–405
GCP/clinical trial requirements, 93–96, 213–214
GLP authority and inspection requirements, 79–88
GMP/CGMP compliance and quality system inspection requirements, 107–112, 141–143
Good Guidance Practice (GGP) regulations, 12
homeopathic drug oversight, 376–379
import/export oversight, 248–251
IND sponsor requirements, 28–29
inspectional authority, 135, 245–246, 435–439
interagency cooperation, 4–5, 7–9
investigational product approval requirements, 97–98
IVD review, 270–272
legislative history and mission, 1–2, 12–15
medical device reporting requirements, 247
medical device tracking requirements, 251–252
medical food oversight, 428–432
mission, 1–2
NDA/BLA review and approval, 133–135, 152–153
off-label promotion authority, 446–447
organizational structure, 2–6, 23 (*See also* specific Centers & Offices)
orphan drug joint application with EMA, 323
OTC drug oversight, 192–197
patent exclusivity approval, 180–185, 188
pediatric regulatory oversight, 354–360
PMA review, 230–235
postmarket device authority, 252
pre-IDE meetings and submission program, 226–227, 270–271
prescription drug market approval, 122–125
proprietary name review, 128–129
recall authority, 149–150, 247–248
REMS review, 128, 147
role in 510(k)/PMA submission review, 228–235

role in expedited drug review/fast track designation, 30–31, 44, 126–127
role in harmonizing medical device standards, 244
role in presubmission meetings, 130–131
Sentinel Initiative, 123, 220
sponsor meetings, 27–28, 280–281
veterinary product oversight, 392–397
Food and Drug Administration Amendments Act (FDAAA) (2007)
    180-day exclusivity provision, 185
    advisory committee provisions, 52, 57, 135
    Clinical Trials Data Bank registry certification requirement, 34
    drug/biologic postmarketing surveillance provision, 293–294
    establishment registration/drug listing provisions, 129, 242–243
    legislative history, 16
    medical device provisions, 240
    NDA safety labeling change provisions, 202
    pediatric research provisions/*BPCA* and *PREA*, 355–358
    REMS provision, 123, 128, 147, 218–219, 296, 302
    Sentinel Initiative provision, 123, 220
Food and Drug Administration Modernization Act (FDAMA) (1997), 15–16
    Accredited Persons Program, 230
    antibiotic drug application exemptions, 185
    biological license provision, 330–331
    de novo provision, 270
    dietary supplement claim provisions, 368–371
    establishment registration provisions, 242
    fast track drug program provisions, 30
    medical device classification provision, 223, 240
    medical device reporting provision, 247
    medical device tracking provision, 251
    nutrition content/health claim provisions, 409–410
    orphan drug provisions, 29
    PMA provisions, 230
    reprint provisions, 209
    scientific dissemination, off-label provision, 265
Food and Drug Administration Safety and Innovation Act (FDASIA) (2012), 15
    180-day exclusivity provision, 185
    antibiotic incentive provision, 136
    breakthrough therapy provisions, 31, 127–128
    de novo classification provision, 223
    establishment registration provisions, 129–130, 242
    esubmission requirements provision, 131
    FDA extraterritorial jurisdiction provision, 436
    orphan drug accelerated approval provisions, 29
    PDUFA V provisions, 123–124, 284
    pediatric research provisions/*BPCA* and *PREA*, 355–358

risk-based inspection schedule provision, 437
Food and Drug Export Reform and Enhancement Act (FDERA) (1996), 249, 294
Food and Drugs Act (1906), 2, 12–13, 239
Food products
 adulteration, 410–411
 GMP/CGMP requirements, 411–412
 import/export requirements, 413
 labeling and advertising requirements, 406–410
 legislative history, 12–14, 402–403
Food Safety Modernization Act (FSMA) (2011), 14–15, 371, 412–413, 430–431, 436
Food-contact substance (FCS), 403–405
Forms
 FDA 1571, 32
 FDA 1932, 397
 FDA 2253, 148, 284, 303
 FDA 2567, 302
 FDA 2656, 36, 151
 FDA 2657, 37, 151
 FDA 2658, 151
 FDA 3500, 432
 FDA 3500A, 216–217, 296, 374
 FDA 3537, 376, 430
 FDA 356h, 281
 FDA 483, 438

G

General purpose reagents (GPRs). *See* Reagents
Generally recognized as safe and effective (GRASE) substances, 14, 192, 366, 403, 405
Generating Antibiotic Incentives Now (GAIN), 136, 188
Generic Animal Drug and Patent Term Restoration Act (GADPTRA) (1988), 395
Generic Drug Enforcement Act (GDEA) (1992), 440
Generic Drug User Fee Amendments (GDUFA) (2012), 163–164
Generic drugs
 branded and authorized, 26
 development and approval pathways, 23, 25–27, 158–164
 GMP/CGMP requirements, 108
 Hatch-Waxman Act authorization, 15
 regulatory history and scope, 156–157
 two-way crossover studies, 25
 user fees, 163–164
Genetically engineered products, 405–406
Global Harmonization Task Force (GHTF). *See* International Medical Device Regulator Forum (IMDRF)
Good Clinical Practices (GCPs)
 clinical trial requirements overview, 92–93, 103

federal/state requirements, 94–96
Good Laboratory Practices (GLPs), 79–87
Good manufacturing practices (GMPs)/current good manufacturing practices (CGMPs)
 ANDA certification requirements, 181
 biologics requirements, 287–288
 blood/blood products requirements, 331
 cell and tissue product requirements, 337
 combination product requirements, 315–316
 cosmetic product requirements, 384, 386
 device quality system requirements, 43, 239–240, 243–245
 dietary supplement requirements, 38, 45, 365, 371–373
 drug quality system requirements, 110–111, 141–143
 drug/device legislative overview, 106–109
 facilities and equipment system and microorganisms management, 111–116
 food product requirements, 411–412
 homeopathic drug requirements, 379
 inspection requirements, 135
 Kefauver-Harris Amendments, 13, 24
 laboratory control system requirements, 117
 materials system requirements, 116
 medical food requirements, 430–431
 packaging and labeling system requirements, 117
 process validation, 119–120
 product complaint filing requirements, 149
 production system requirements, 116–117
 records management, 118–119
 standard operating procedures and training, 117–118
 veterinary product requirements, 393–394
Government in the Sunshine Act (1976), 16
Guaranty clause, 443
Guidance documents, 12, 32, 48

H

Hatch-Waxman Act
 505(b)(2) provision, 132
 antibiotic drug exclusivity provision, 185, 188
 generic drug/ANDA provisions, 24
 legislative history, 15, 44
 new drug product exclusivity provision, 136–137, 181–182
 patent term extension provision, 36, 157, 180–181
Hazard Analysis and Critical Control Points (HACCP), 9, 411–412
Health Canada, 360
Health Care Financing Administration (HCFA). *See* Center for Medicare and Medicaid Services (CMS)

Index

Health Care Fraud Prevention and Enforcement Act Team (HEAT), 452
Health Insurance Portability and Accountability Act (HIPAA), 7, 95, 129
Health Research and Health Services Amendments (HRSA) (1976), 428
Health technology assessment (HTA)
    agency activities, 76–77
    overview and definition, 71–72
    process, 72–76
Healthcare fraud and abuse
    compliance programs, 452–453
    legislative overview, 445–446
    state laws, 451–452
    types of, 447–450
Hematopoietic progenitor cells (HPC-C), 350
Herceptest (HER2), 421–422
Homeopathic drugs
    approval process, 377–378
    GMP/CGMP requirements, 379
    labeling and advertising, 378–379
    legislative history and definition, 376–377
Homeopathic Pharmacopeia Convention of the United States (HPCUS), 376–378
Homeopathic Pharmacopeia of the United States (HPUS), 376–378
Human cells, tissues and cellular/tissue-based products (HCT/Ps), 335–337, 350
Human immunodeficiency virus (HIV), 328, 330, 335–336
Human subject protection, 92–96
Humanitarian device exemption (HDE), 41, 234, 239, 320, 324–325, 360
Humanitarian use devices (HUDs), 14–15, 41, 234, 320, 324–325

I

Imports/Exports
    biologic product requirements, 294
    cosmetic product requirements, 388
    device product requirements, 248–251
    dietary supplement requirements, 375–376
    drug product requirements, 150–151
    food product requirements, 413
In vitro diagnostic (IVD) devices
    classification requirements, 268–269
    companion products, 421–422
    labeling requirements, 260–264
    regulatory scope and definition, 268–269
    software classification requirements, 271
    submission and approval pathways, 270–271
Inactive ingredients. *See* Excipients
Individual case safety report (ICSR), 215—216

Informed consent, 24, 93, 96
Informed consent form, 103
Initial filing review, 133
Inspections
    blood establishments, 331
    FDA authority, 435–439
    food product manufacturing facilities, 412–413
    GMP/CGMP, 142
    HCT/Ps, 350
    preapproval (PAI), 135, 437
Institute of Medicine (IOM)
    FDA inspection procedures, 437–438
    report on 510(k) progress, 235
Institutional Review Board (IRB)
    GCP compliance responsibilities, 93, 96–97
    role in HUD approval, 324–325
    role in IDE approval, 226
    role in reviewing ANDA bioequivalence studies, 25
Interagency cooperation
    FDA and CMS, 7
    FDA and CPSC, 7
    FDA and DEA, 9
    FDA and DOC, 9
    FDA and EMA, 30, 323
    FDA and EPA, 9
    FDA and FTC, 7, 263
    FDA and NCTR, 4
    FDA and NIH/NLM, 16
    FDA and OSHA, 8
    FDA and SEC, 7–8
    FDA and TTB, 9
    FDA and USDA, 9
    FDA Office of International Programs, 5
International Conference on Harmonisation (ICH), 470
    and FDA role, 5
    biologic preclinical/clinical guidelines, 276–279
    clinical trial safety reporting requirements, 212
    CTD requirements, 31–32, 45, 131
    GCP/clinical trial guidelines, 93–94, 96
    GMP/CGMP and quality system guidelines, 110, 142–143
    PSUR requirements, 146
International Cooperation on Harmonisation of Technical Requirements for Registration of Veterinary Products (VICH), 393–394
International Medical Device Regulator Forum (IMDRF), 244, 470
International Network of Agencies for Health Technology Assessment (INHATA), 71
International Nomenclature Cosmetic Ingredient (INCI), 386
Investigational device exemption (IDE)
    clinical study requirements, 97
    companion diagnostic product requirements, 424

product application meeting requirements, 50, 226–227
submission and approval process, 42–43, 224–226, 270–271
supplemental submission requirements, 226
Investigational New Animal Drug (INAD) exemption, 392–395
Investigational new drug (IND)
biologic submission requirements, 275–276, 279–280, 290–291
companion diagnostic product requirements, 424
fast track designations, 126
FDA-sponsor meetings, 28–29
GMP/CGMP requirements, 108
HPC-C requirements, 350
proprietary name review requirements, 35
safety reporting requirements, 34, 213–214, 291–292
submission requirements and review process, 32–34, 44–45
Investigational products
FDA approval requirements, 97–98

K

Kefauver-Harris Amendments (1962), 13, 23, 25, 37, 203
Kickbacks, 447–448

L

Labeling
ANDA/NDA/BLA postapproval change reporting requirements, 143–145
biologics, 300–308
companion diagnostic products, 425
cosmetic products, 385–387, 389
devices and IVDs, 260–264
dietary supplements, 38, 367–371
FD&C Act provisions, 12–13
food product requirements, 14, 406–409
GMP/CGMP, 429–430
investigational products, 97–98
medical foods, 429–430
OTC drugs, 39
prescription drugs, 148–149, 201–203, 206–207
reagents, 261
veterinary biologic products, 398–399
Laboratory developed tests (LDTs), 271–272, 422–423
Lanham Act (1946), 210, 266
Laws and regulations
compared, 22
development and definition, 12, 22
Leahy-Smith America Invents Act (2011), 188

Licensing, biologics, 290–291
Lookback procedures, 330
Lot release, 287

M

MedDRA, 31, 44
Medical Device Amendments (*MDA*) (1976), 13, 40, 108, 233, 239, 249, 263–264
Medical Device Amendments (MDA) (1992), 13–14, 239–240, 247
Medical Device Reporting Regulation (MDR) (1996), 246–247
Medical Device User Fee Amendments (*MDUFA III*) (2012), 14, 42
Medical Device User Fee and Modernization Act (*MDUFMA*) (2002), 14, 240
modular PMA provision, 233
OCP established, 43, 46, 312
third party review provision, 245–246
Medical Device User Fee and Modernization Act III (*MDUFMA III*) (2012), 240
Medical devices
510(k) submission requirements, 227–229
class III PMA submission requirements, 42–43, 45, 230–234
classification, 40, 45
clinical labeling requirements, 98
crisis management, 65
definition and development, 14, 22–23, 39–41, 45
establishment registration requirements, 43, 46, 240–243
exemptions, 223
expedited review, 234–235
export requirements, 248–250
GMP/CGMP and quality system requirements, 107–110
HUD requirements, 41
IDE approval requirements, 224–226
import requirements, 250–251
labeling requirements, 260–264
legislative history and scope, 13–14, 39–41, 221–222, 239–240
pediatric approvals, 358–360
postmarket surveillance requirements and activities, 219, 246, 252
product application meetings, 50–51
QSR history, 243–245
recalls, corrections and removals, 247–248
reclassification, 222–223
reporting requirements, 246–247
tracking, 16, 251–252
UDI requirements, 253
veterinary product requirements, 397

with cosmetic components, 387–388
Medical foods
   adverse event reporting requirements, 432
   GMP/CGMP requirements, 430–431
   labeling, 429–430
   legislative history and definition, 410, 428–429
Medical Product Safety Network. *See* MedSun
Medicare and Medicaid Patient Protection Act of 1987. *See Anti-Kickback Statute* (1987)
Medicare Prescription Drug, Improvement, and Modernization Act (*MMA*) (2003), 159, 184–185
Medicated feeds, 396
Medication Guide, 128, 201, 203, 296, 302
Medicines and Healthcare Products Regulatory Agency (UK), 71
MedSun, 219, 252–253
MedWatch, 146, 374–375, 432
Meetings
   advisory committee, 52–53, 57–63
   agreement, 50, 226 (*See also* Medical devices -- product application meetings)
   companion diagnostic products, 423–424
   determination, 50–51, 226 (*See also* Medical devices -- product application meetings)
   drug/biologics product applications, 48–50
   FDA-sponsor requirements, 27, 55–57, 280–281
   medical device product applications, 50–51
   PMA Day-100, 51
   pre-IDE, 51, 226, 270–271
   pre-IND, 33
   pre-NDA, 34
   pre-PMA, 51
Microorganisms, 112–116
Minor Use or Minor Species Act (MUMS), 394–395
Misbranding, 439–440
   cosmetics, 385–387
   devices, 264
   foods, 402, 406
   HUDs, 325
   veterinary products, 395–396
Monogram HIV Tropism test, 422

N

National Center for Toxicological Research (NCTR), 4
National Childhood Vaccine Injury Act (1986), 298
National Drug Code (NDC), 36, 129–130, 152
National Formulary (*NF*), 12, 395–396
National Institutes of Health
   National Library of Medicine, 16, 34
   pediatric regulatory oversight, 354–355
   role in biologic products regulatory history, 27, 274

National Oceanic and Atmospheric Administration (NOAA), 9
National Research Council (NRC), 24
New Animal Drug Application (NADA), 392–395
New chemical entities. *See* New drugs
New dietary ingredient (NDI) notifications, 366–367
New drug application (NDA)
   505(b)(2) submission requirements, 39
   amendments, 37
   application format/content & CTD/eCTD requirements, 131–132
   application types, 132
   briefing book requirements for AC meetings, 60
   companion diagnostic product requirements, 424–425
   direct-to-OTC drugs, 194
   eCTD submission requirements, 35
   inactivation/withdrawal, 152
   Orange Book patent listing, 181
   OTC drug approval pathways, 192–195
   package insert/labeling requirements, 35, 202–203
   paragraph IV litigation, 183–184
   patent term extensions, 180–181
   postapproval change reporting requirements, 143–145
   preapproval inspections, 36
   presubmission requirements, 130–131
   proprietary name review requirements, 35
   submission, review and approval requirements, 29, 34–35, 45, 123–124, 133–136
   transfer of ownership/sponsor, 152–153
New drugs, 27–28, 122
Non-significant risk device, 224
Notice of Change (NOC), 15
Notice of Violation (NOV) letters, 203, 265, 297, 308
Notifications, 254–255
Nuremberg Code (1947), 92–93
Nutrition Labeling and Education Act (1990), 14, 366–368, 407, 429–430

O

Occupational Safety and Health Administration (OSHA), 8
Off-label, 98, 123, 206, 264, 446–447
Office for Human Research Protections (OHRP), 94–95
Office of Blood Research and Review (OBRR), 269
Office of Combination Products (OCP), 43–44, 46, 312–315
Office of Compliance (OC), 263
Office of Compliance and Biologics Quality (OCBQ), 263, 290–292, 303, 329–330
Office of Counterterrorism and Emerging Threats (OCET), 3

Office of Critical Path Programs (OCPP), 4
Office of Drug Evaluation (ODE), 196, 226
Office of Foods and Veterinary Medicine (OFVM), 6
Office of Generic Drugs (OGD), 24–25, 163–164
Office of In Vitro Diagnostic Device Evaluation and Safety (OIVD), 269–271
Office of Inspector General (OIG), 452
Office of International Programs (OIP), 5
Office of Medical Products and Tobacco (OMPT), 5, 23
Office of New Drug Quality Assessment (ONDQA), 33
Office of New Drugs (OND), 124, 274
Office of Nutritional Products, Labeling and Dietary Supplements (ONPLDS), 366, 371
Office of Orphan Products Development (OOPD), 30, 234, 319–324
Office of Postmarketing Drug Risk Assessment (OPDRA), 36
Office of Prescription Drug Promotion (OPDP), 148, 205–206, 208, 263, 308
Office of Regulatory Affairs (ORA), 80
Office of Regulatory Science and Innovation (ORSI), 3–4
Office of Scientific Integrity (OSI), 4
Office of Scientific Professional Development (OSPD), 4
Office of Special Medical Programs (OSMP), 5
Office of Surveillance and Epidemiology (OSE), 215
Office of the Chief Counsel (OCC), 2–3
Office of the Chief Scientist (OCS), 3
Office of the Commissioner (OC), 2
Office of the Ombudsman, 6, 10
On-label, 206
Orange Book, 149, 157–158, 162–163, 181
Oregon Drug Effectiveness Review Project (DERP), 77
Organisation for Economic Cooperation and Development (OECD), 80
Orphan devices. *See* Humanitarian use devices (HUDs)
Orphan Drug Act (1983), 15, 29–30, 44, 183, 319–320, 322, 354, 428–430
Orphan Drug Amendments (*ODA*) (1988), 428
Orphan drugs
    annual report requirements, 321, 323
    designation/application process requirements, 29–30, 320–322
    incentives, 321
    legislative history and definition, 319–320
    patent exclusivity, 183, 322–323
    postmarket approval requirements, 323
OTC drug monographs, 192–193
Over-the-counter (OTC) drugs
    advertising requirements, 196–197
    approval pathways, 192–195
    compared with prescription drugs, 122
    labeling requirements, 195–196
    legislative history and scope, 39, 45, 191–192
    packaging requirements, 196
    with cosmetic components, 387–388

P

Package insert (PI), 35, 201–202, 300–301
Packaging, 117
Pan American Health Organization (PAHO), 5
Paragraph IV certification, 181, 183–184
Patent and Trademark Office (PTO), 37
Patent Protection and Affordable Care Act (*PPACA*) (2010), 26, 358, 449, 451
Patents
    Hatch-Waxman Act term extension provisions, 15, 37, 180–181
    marketing exclusivity for pediatric drug products, 357
    Orange Book submissions for exclusivity, 149
    orphan drugs exclusivity, 322–323
Patient reported outcome (PRO), 125–126
Pediatric
    device approval tracking, 358
    device clinical trial study requirements, 359–360
    exclusivity, 182–183, 357
    legislative history, 354–358
Pediatric Medical Device Safety and Improvement Act (*PMDSIA*) (2007), 358–359
Pediatric Pharmacology Research Unit (PPRU) Network, 354
Pediatric Research Equity Act (*PREA*) (2003, 2007), 16, 158, 355–358
Pediatric Rule (1998), 355
Penalties (sanctions/seizures/injunctions), 441–442
Periodic Benefit-Risk Evaluation Report (PBRER), 146
Periodic Safety Update Report (PSUR), 146
Periodic Adverse Drug Experience Reports (PADER), 145–146
Pesticide regulation, 9, 399
Petitions, 17
Pharmaceutical and Medical Devices Agency (Japan), 360
Pharmaceutical Research and Manufacturers of America (PhRMA) Code. *See* PhRMA Code
Pharmacogenomics, 322
Pharmacovigilance, 212–218
PhRMA Code, 207, 448
Physican self-referrals, 448
Physician Labeling Rule (PLR) (2006), 35, 201–202
Physician Payment Sunshine Act (2010), 451–452
Postapproval
    changes to approved ANDAs/NDAs/BLAs, 143–145, 284–286, 294–295, 302–303
    companion diagnostic product requirements, 425

device studies, 255–256
orphan drug product requirements, 323
veterinary products, 396–397
Postmarket surveillance
combination product requirements, 316–317, 323
device requirements, 219, 240, 246, 252, 256
drug and biologic requirements, 135–136, 145–146, 212–218, 293–294, 296
medical food requirements, 432
pediatric device requirements, 360
Preapproval inspection (PAI), 36, 135
Preclinical development, 276–277
Predicate device, 41–42, 227, 270
Premarket approval (PMA) application
amendments, 232
briefing book requirements for AC meetings, 60
combination product review, 315
companion diagnostic product requirements, 424–425
determination meeting requirements, 50–51
IDE requirements, 42–43, 270–271
IVD requirements, 270
modular, 233–234
reclassifying device to 510(k), 222–223
submission and approval process, 40, 45, 230–232
supplements, 232–233
Premarket notification (PMN). *See* 510(k)
Prescription Drug User Fee Act (*PDUFA*) (1992), 15, 36, 127
Prescription Drug User Fee Act II (*PDUFA II*) (1997), 28
Prescription Drug User Fee Act IV (*PDUFA IV*) (2007), 147
Prescription Drug User Fee Act V (*PDUFA V*) (2012), 123–124, 133–134, 284
President's Emergency Plan for AIDS Relief (PEPFAR), 136, 158
Price reporting fraud, 448–449
Primary mode of action (PMOA), 223–224, 312–315
Prior approval supplement (PAS), 144–145, 285, 294–295, 303, 396–397
Priority review, 127, 136
Process validation, 119–120
Product application meetings, 48–51. *See also* Food and Drug Administration (FDA) -- communications/meetings types and requirements
Product development protocol (PDP), 50–51, 233
Professional labeling. *See* Packaging insert
Promotion
biologic labeling and advertising requirements, 303–307
drug labeling and advertising requirements, 201–203, 205–209
Proprietary names

BLA submission requirements, 292
IND/NDA submission and review requirements, 36, 128–129, 218
Protected Health Information (PHI), 7
Protocols, 29
Public administrative meetings, 48, 51–53. *See also* Food and Drug Administration (FDA) -- communications/meetings types and requirements
Public comments, 17
Public Health Service (PHS), 23, 26–27
Public Health Service Act (*PHS Act*) (1944)
biologic product provisions, 26–27, 121, 294
blood/blood product provisions, 327, 331
device provisions, 256
tissue and cell product provisions, 336–337
Public hearing, 52
Pure Food and Drug Act (1906). *See Food and Drugs Act* of 1906

Q

QI Program Supplemental Funding Act (2008), 185, 188
Quality System Regulation (QSR) (1996), 43, 108–110, 246, 325
Quality systems
device quality system requirements, 239–240
drug quality system requirements, 110–112, 142–143
drug/device legislative overview and GMP/CGMP requirements, 43, 107–109, 243–245
HUD requirements, 325
Quality Systems Inspection Technique (QSIT), 246
Question-based review (QbR), 24–25

R

Rare diseases, 15, 29–30, 41, 319–322, 395
Reagents, 261–262, 268
Recalls
biologic, 298
device, 247–248
drug, 149–150, 203
food product, 413
Reclassification, 222–223
Records management, 118–119
Reference Listed Drug (RLD), 25–26, 38, 157–163
Refuse-to-Accept, 230
Refuse-to-File (RTF), 133, 281, 283
Regulatory communications, 48, 471. *See also* Food and Drug Administration (FDA) -- communications/meetings types and requirements

Regulatory resources
    book publishers, 455–457
    commercial databases
        business intelligence, 463–464
        regulatory intelligence, 462–463
    electronic newsletters, 457–459
    fee-based association, 461–462
    fee-based industry, 459–461
    global organizations, 470
    government databases
        federal agencies, 465, 467–469
        legislative and regulatory tracking, 464–465
    industry associations, 470
    US government agencies, 469–470
    web 2.0 tools, 471
Reimbursement, 448
Reminder labeling, 207, 307
Reportable Food Registry (RFR), 413, 431
Reprints, 209
Request for Designation (RFD), 44, 46, 223, 312–315
Risk communication, 254–255, 305–306
Risk Evaluation and Mitigation Strategy (REMS), 35–36, 123, 128, 147, 218–219, 296–297, 302
Rolling review, 126–127
Rulemaking process, 16–17
Rx-to-OTC switch, 39, 194–195

S

Safe Drinking Water Act (*SDWA*), 9
Safe Medical Devices Act (*SMDA*) (1990), 13–16, 40, 239
    combination product provision, 43–44, 223–224, 312
    medical device tracking provision, 251
    orphan drug provision, 324
Scale-Up and Postapproval Changes (SUPAC), 144–145
Scientific dissemination
    off-label, 265, 307–308
Searle (GD) and Company, 81
Securities and Exchange Commission (SEC), 7–8
Senior Medical Patrols (SMP) (AoA), 453
Sentinel Initiative, 123, 220
Serious adverse event (SAE), 34
Significant risk device, 224
Sinclair, Upton, 2, 12
Social networking, 471
Special dietary uses, 428–429
Special protocol assessment (SPA), 28–29, 44
Sponsors
    510(k) submission requirements, 227–230
    advertising/labeling requirements, 148–149, 303–304

AE/ADE reporting requirements, 145–148, 215–217
GCP/clinical trial compliance responsibilities, 98–99, 213–214
PMA submission requirements, 230–235
role in advisory committee meeting preparation, 57–63
role in ANDA/NDA/BLA postapproval change reportng requirements, 143–145
role in pre-IDE meetings, 226
role in presubmission meetings, 130–131
role in requesting/executing FDA meetings, 48–53, 280–281
Stark Law, 446, 448
Structured product label (SPL), 35, 131, 151, 203, 287, 302
Substantial equivalence, 41–42, 123, 206, 227, 270, 305–306
Suitability petitions, 26, 48, 158–159. *See also* Regulatory communications
Suspected adverse reaction, 213
Sweden, 71

T

Target Product Profile, 35, 125
Tax and Trade Bureau (TTB), 8–9
Therapeutic equivalence, 157–158, 161–163
Third-party review, 230, 240, 245–246
Time and Extent Application (TEA), 193
Title 18 (USC), 440
Traceability, 251–252
Transfusions, 330
Trilateral Cooperation, 5
Tropical diseases, 136
Truthful Prescription Drug Advertising and Promotion. *See* Bad Ad program

U

Unique device identification (UDI), 253
United States Adopted Names Council (USANC), 292
United States Code (USC), 12, 22, 440
United States Pharmacopeia (USP), 12, 395–396
Untitled letters. *See* Notice of Violation (NOV) letters
US Department of Agriculture (USDA)
    Bureau of Chemistry, 2, 12–13
    Center for Veterinary Biologics (CVB), 398–399
    Food Safety and Inspection Service (FSIS), 9, 399, 406, 408
US Department of Commerce (DOC), 9
US Department of Health and Human Services (DHHS)
    blood/blood products oversight, 328
    drug advertising enforcement, 209
    FDA jurisdiction, 1–2, 23

human subject protection regulations, 93–94
human tissue products oversight, 336
Orphan Products Board, 320
Physician Payment Sunshine Act responsibilities, 451–452
US Department of Justice (DOJ)
drug advertising oversight and enforcement, 209–210
off-label promotion, 446–447
seizures, injunctions, and criminal prosecution, 441–443
US Department of Veterans Affairs (VA), 77
US Patent and Trademark Office (PTO), 180–181
US Statutes-at-Large, 12
US Trademark Act. *See Lanham Act* (1946)
User fees
combination products, 317–18
generic drug, 163–164
PDUFA requirements, 36

V

Vaccine Act of 1813, 2
Vaccine Adverse Event Reporting System (VAERS), 296

Veterinary products
biologic requirements, 398–399
device requirements, 397
legislative overview, 392
postapproval reporting requirements, 396–397
product approval pathways, 392–396
Virus Serum and Toxin Act (*VSTA*)(1902), 27, 398

W

Warning letters
biologic, 297, 308–309
cosmetics, 388–389
device, 265–266
prescription drug, 203, 205
Wiley Act, 2
Wiley, Harvey W., 2, 12
World Health Organization (WHO), 5, 96, 470
World Medical Association (WMA), 92–93
Written Request, 357–358

X

XML, 35, 131, 203